COMPLETE
DIABETIC
COOKBOOK

Healthy, Delicious Recipes the Whole Family Can Enjoy

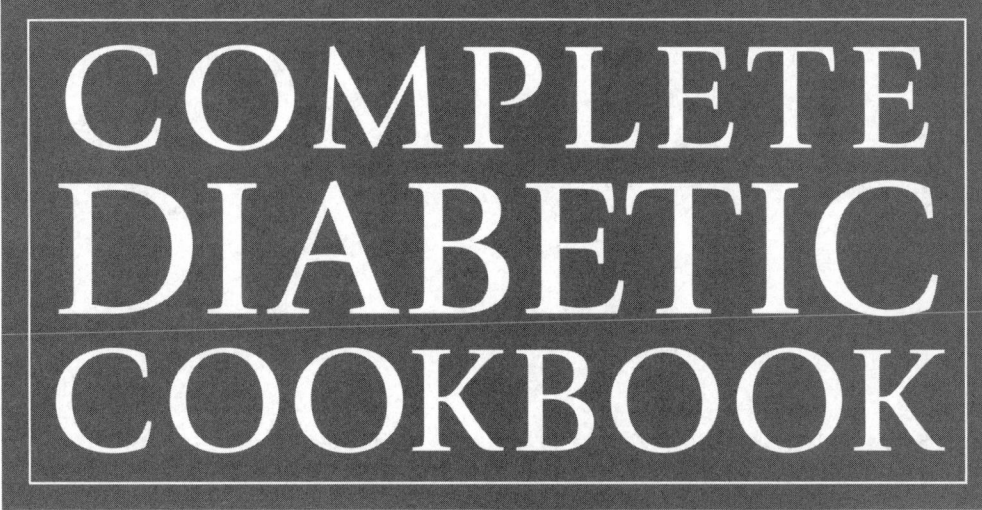

COMPLETE DIABETIC COOKBOOK

by **Mary Jane Finsand, Karin Cadwell, Ph.D., R.N.**
and **Edith White, M.Ed.**

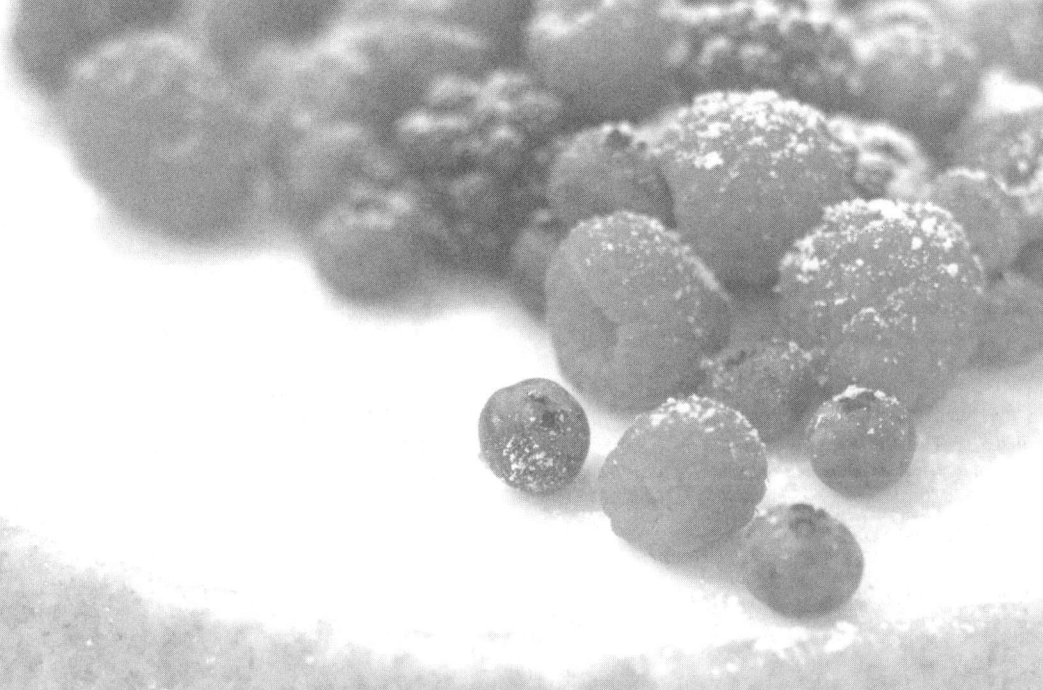

Library of Congress Cataloguing in Publication Data
Available on file

Published by
Black Dog & Leventhal Publishers
151 West 19th Street
New York, NY 10011

Distributed by
Workman Publishing Company
225 Varick Street
New York, NY 10014

*The material in this book is provided for information only and should not be construed as medical
advice or instruction. Always consult with your physician or other appropriate health professionals
before making any changes in diet, physical activity, and/or drug therapy.*

Manufactured in the United States of America
Jacket and interior design by Christina Gaugler
Composition by Compset Inc.

ISBN: 978-1-57912-926-2

g f e d c b a

CONTENTS

Fruits and Vegetables

Breakfast Banana Split

1	banana	1
½ t.	lemon juice	2 mL
4	lettuce leaves	4
¼ c.	fresh grapefruit sections	60 mL
¼ c.	seedless purple grapes	60 mL
4	fresh orange sections	4

Peel and cut banana in half crosswise. Cut each half banana into 4 lengthwise sections. Sprinkle with lemon juice. Place 2 sections of banana on a leaf of lettuce. Evenly distribute the grapefruit inside of the banana slices among the 4 plates. Distribute the purple grapes evenly among the plates. Top each plate with an orange slice. Serve immediately or cover with plastic wrap and keep refrigerated until serving time.

Yield: 4 servings

Exchange, 1 serving: 1 fruit
Each serving contains: Calories: 41, Carbohydrates: 10 g

Broiled Grapefruit

A simple, but often forgotten breakfast starter.

1	grapefruit	1
½ t.	butter	2 mL
1 t.	granulated sugar replacement	5 mL
dash	ground cinnamon	dash
dash	ground or grated nutmeg	dash

Cut grapefruit in half crosswise. Loosen sections with a sharp knife or grapefruit spoon. Place ¼ t. (1 mL) butter in middle of each half. Sprinkle each half with ½ t. (2 mL) granulated sugar replacement, cinnamon and nutmeg. Broil 4 in. (10 cm) from heat for 6 to 8 minutes. Serve hot.

Yield: 2 servings

Exchange, 1 serving: 1 fruit, ½ fat
Each serving contains: Calories: 60, Carbohydrates: 12 g

Citrus Cup

4	oranges	4	
½ c.	fresh shredded coconut, chopped	125 mL	
8 oz. can	Featherweight grapefruit segments, drained	227 g can	
8 oz. can	Featherweight pineapple, drained and cut into eighths	227 g can	

Cut off top third of oranges. Scoop out pulp, slice into pieces and put into a bowl. Set orange shells in custard cups. Reserve 1 T. (15 mL) coconut. Add remaining coconut, grapefruit and pineapple to orange pieces; toss gently. Spoon fruit into orange shells. Top with reserved coconut.

Yield: 4 servings

Exchange, 1 serving: 4 fruit, ½ fat
Each serving contains: Calories: 192, Carbohydrates: 29 g

Based on a recipe from Featherweight Brand Foods.

Fried Fruit Turnovers

2 T.	cold butter	30 mL
1 c.	sifted all-purpose flour	250 mL
1	egg yolk	1
3 T.	hot skim milk	45 mL
9 T.	puréed baby food fruit	135 mL

Cut butter into flour. Blend egg yolk and milk together; then add to flour mixture. Knead well to make a smooth dough. Roll out to ⅛ in. (4 mm) thickness. Cut into six pastry rounds. Place 1½ T. (21 mL) of puréed fruit in center of each round. Fold over turnover-style and seal or pinch edges securely. Fry in hot fat at 365°F (180°C) until brown.

Yield: 6 servings

Exchange, 1 serving: 1¼ starch/bread, 1 fat
Each serving contains: Calories: 132, Carbohydrates: 16 g

Mixed Fruit Cocktail

8 oz. can	Featherweight sliced peaches, drained, reserve 1 T. (15 mL) liquid	227 g can
8 oz. can	Featherweight pear halves, drained and cut in quarters	227 g can
8 oz. can	Featherweight sliced pineapple, drained and cut in quarters	227 g can
8 oz. can	Featherweight purple plums, drained, pitted and cut in halves	227 g can
½ c.	Featherweight apricot preserves	125 mL

Combine drained fruit in a bowl. Mix preserves and reserved peach liquid in a small saucepan; heat thoroughly. Pour over fruit and stir.

Yield: 4 servings

Exchange, 1 serving: 3 fruit
Each serving contains: Calories: 117, Carbohydrates: 37 g

All-American Hash Browns

2 lbs.	potatoes	1 kg
2	large onions	2
¼ c.	low-calorie margarine	60 mL
1 t.	salt	5 mL
	pepper to taste	

The day before: Peel and dice the potatoes. Place in a heavy saucepan and cover with water. Heat to the boiling point; reduce heat and simmer until potatoes are barely tender. Drain and cool to room temperature. Refrigerate in a covered container. Dice onions and place in tightly sealed bag and refrigerate in a covered container.

Day of brunch: Melt margarine in a large nonstick skillet and allow margarine to brown slightly. Add onions and sauté until limp. Add potato cubes and sauté, turning occasionally, until browned on all sides. Sprinkle with salt and pepper. Turn into heated serving dish.

Yield: 8 servings

Exchange, 1 serving: 1 bread, ½ fat
Each serving contains: Calories: 94, Carbohydrates: 15 g

New Potato Roast

2 lbs.	small new potatoes	1 kg
2 T.	olive oil	30 mL
⅓ c.	low-calorie margarine	90 mL
	salt and pepper to taste	
2 T.	fresh parsley, finely snipped	30 mL

Peel and trim potatoes into smooth ovals. Heat olive oil in a heavy skillet. Add potatoes and sauté over high heat, rotating potatoes until they are golden on all sides. (You may need to do these in several batches.) With a slotted spoon, place potatoes in a baking dish or casserole. Drain any excess oil from skillet. Melt margarine in same skillet and brown slightly. Add salt and pepper to the margarine and pour over potatoes. Bake at 350°F (175°C) for 15 to 20 minutes until potatoes are tender, stirring occasionally. Transfer to a heated serving dish. Sprinkle with fresh parsley.

Yield: 8 servings

Exchange, 1 serving: 1 bread, 1½ fat
Each serving contains: Calories: 137, Carbohydrates: 15 g

Cauliflower au Gratin

10 oz. pkg.	cauliflower, thawed	280 g

Sauce

1 T.	butter	15 mL
1 T.	Stone-Buhr all purpose flour	15 mL
¼ t.	salt	1 mL
dash	pepper	dash
1 t.	dry mustard	5 mL
¾ c.	skim milk	190 mL
½ c.	cheddar cheese, grated	125 mL

Topping

¼ c.	Stone-Buhr wheat germ	60 mL
¼ c.	Stone-Buhr branflakes	60 mL
2 t.	butter, melted	10 mL
¼ t.	dried sage	1 mL
dash	dry mustard	dash
dash	salt	dash

Spread cauliflower in bottom of ungreased 1 qt. (1 L) casserole. To prepare cheese sauce, melt butter in a saucepan and blend in flour and seasonings; stir until smooth. Remove from heat and stir in milk. Heat to boiling, stirring constantly. Add grated cheese and stir until melted and mixture is thickened. Pour sauce over cauliflower.

Combine the topping ingredients and sprinkle over the sauce. Bake uncovered at 325°F (165°C) for 15 minutes or until vegetable is heated through and crispy-tender.

Microwave: Combine ingredients as above. Cook at Medium for 3 minutes; turn and cook 2 minutes longer.

Yield: 5 servings

Exchange, 1 serving: 2 vegetable, 1 fat
Each serving contains: Calories: 88, Carbohydrates: 10 g

Cauliflower Crunch

½ c.	Kretschmer regular wheat germ	125 mL
¼ c.	Parmesan cheese, grated	60 mL
1 t.	paprika	5 mL
½ t.	dried tarragon, crushed	2 mL
½ t.	salt	2 mL
dash	pepper	dash
¼ c.	margarine. melted	60 mL
1 head	cauliflower, cut into florets	1 head

Combine wheat germ, cheese, paprika, tarragon, salt and pepper in a plastic bag. Toss together the melted margarine and cauliflower in a bowl until coated. Shake cauliflower, a third at a time, with crumb mixture in plastic bag until coated. Place on 15½ × 10½ × 1 in. (39 × 25 × 3 cm) jelly roll pan. Bake at 375°F (190°C) for 10 to 12 minutes until crisp-tender.

Yield: 6 servings

Exchange, 1 serving: 1 vegetable, ½ bread, 1½ fat
Each serving contains: Calories: 123, Carbohydrates: 7 g

With the courtesy of Kretschmer Wheat Germ/International Multifoods.

Baked Red Onions

So easy to prepare, this vegetable dish features red onions—try it!

2 large	red onions	2 large
1 T.	red wine vinegar	15 mL
3 T.	water	45 mL
2 t.	granulated sugar replacement	10 mL
½ t.	salt	2 mL
¼ t.	ground sage	1 mL
¼ t.	dry mustard	1 mL
2 T.	margarine	30 mL

Peel and cut onions in half crosswise. Place side by side, cut side up, in a shallow 8 in. (20 cm) baking pan. In a small bowl, blend together the vinegar, water, sugar replacement, salt, sage and mustard. Pour over onion halves. Cover tightly. Bake at 350°F (175°C) for 50 to 60 minutes or until onions are tender.

Microwave: Reduce water to 2 T. (30 mL). Cook on High for 5 to 10 minutes, turning dish every 3 minutes.

Yield: 4 servings

Exchange, 1 serving: 1 vegetable
Each serving contains: Calories: 30, Carbohydrates: 9 g

Sautéed Oriental Beans

2 T.	low calorie margarine	10 mL
¼ c.	white onion, chopped	60 mL
2 c.	bean sprouts	500 mL
1 T.	soy sauce	15 mL

Melt margarine in a nonstick saucepan. Over medium treat, lightly sauté onions until translucent. Add bean sprouts. Reduce heat. Cover and cook 3 minutes. Toss with soy sauce. Serve immediately.

Yield: 4 servings

Exchange, 1 serving: 1 vegetable
Each serving contains: Calories: 28, Carbohydrates: 4 g

Stir-Fried Broccoli

2 T.	Mazola corn oil	30 mL
1 lb.	broccoli, cut in florets, and stems sliced	500 g
1¼ c.	mushrooms	310 mL
1 clove	garlic, minced	1 clove
¼ t.	dried thyme	1 mL
¼ t.	black pepper	1 mL

In a large skillet, heat oil over medium high heat. Add remaining ingredients. Stir-fry 5 to 8 minutes or until tender.

Yield: 4 servings

Exchange, 1 serving: 2 vegetable, 1 fat
Each serving contains: Calories: 110, Carbohydrates: 10 g

"A Diet for the Young at Heart" by Mazola.

Brussels Sprouts in Yogurt Sauce

2 lbs.	brussels sprouts	1 kg	
8 oz.	Dannon plain low-fat yogurt	227 g	
2 T.	cream of wheat cereal	30 mL	
	freshly ground pepper		
	salt to taste		

Trim any wilted leaves or woody stem sections from the brussels sprouts. Put brussels sprouts in a steamer over boiling water and cook until just tender (be careful not to overcook). Combine yogurt and cereal in a small saucepan. Cook and stir over low heat until mixture thickens. Pour sauce over hot brussels sprouts. Sprinkle with pepper and salt.

Yield: 8 servings

Exchange, 1 serving: 1 vegetable, ½ nonfat milk
Each serving contains: Calories: 61, Carbohydrates: 87 g

Brussels Sprouts with Cream Sauce

3 c.	fresh brussels sprouts	750 mL	
2 T.	margarine	30 mL	
2 T.	Stone-Buhr dark rye flour	30 mL	
¼ t.	salt	1 mL	
1 c.	skim milk	250 mL	

Trim off the stem and discolored leaves from the brussels sprouts; cook in salted water for 15 minutes. Drain and cover with boiling salted water. Cook, uncovered, just until tender, about 15 minutes. Meanwhile, to make the sauce, melt the margarine in a pan. Add the flour and salt and mix thoroughly. Stir in the milk and bring to a boil, stirring occasionally. Set aside over low heat until brussels sprouts are cooked. Drain brussels sprouts and place in a heated serving bowl. Pour sauce over vegetables and serve.

Yield: 6 servings

Exchange, 1 serving: 1 vegetable, 1 fat
Each serving contains: Calories: 62, Carbohydrates: 11 g

With the compliments of Arnold Foods Company, Inc.

Broccoli and Pasta with Cheese

A side dish that includes a bread, vegetable and fat exchange.

1¼ lbs.	fresh broccoli	625 g
2 T.	salt	30 mL
½ lb.	small shell pasta	250 g
16	cherry tomatoes halved	16
1 clove	garlic, minced	1 clove
4 c.	Parmesan cheese, grated	60 mL

Cut florets from broccoli head and slice stems crosswise into ½ in. (13mm) pieces. In a large saucepan, heat 2 qts. (2 L) water to the boiling point. Add broccoli and 1 T. (15 mL) of the salt. Cook 4 to 5 minutes or until crisp-tender. Drain in strainer or colander. In the same pan, bring 3 qts. (3 L) water to the boiling point. Add pasta and 1 T. (15 mL) salt to water; cook until pasta is *al dente* ("firm to the teeth"). Remove from heat but do not drain. Add tomato halves and garlic to hot pasta and water. Cover and allow to rest for 5 minutes. Add broccoli and reheat slightly. Drain in strainer or colander. While in strainer, sprinkle mixture with half the cheese, toss lightly and repeat with remaining cheese. Pour into hot serving bowl.

Yield: 8 servings

Exchange, 1 serving: 1 bread, 1 vegetable, 1 fat
Each serving contains: Calories: 146, Carbohydrates: 14 g

Crumb-Topped Zucchini and Tomatoes

¾ c.	Kellogg's branflakes cereal	190 mL
2 t.	margarine	10 mL
½ t.	lemon peel, grated	2 mL
3 c.	zucchini, cut in ¼ in. (6-mm) slices	750 mL
2 T.	margarine	30 mL
¼ t.	salt	1 mL
dash	pepper	dash
1 T.	lemon juice	15 mL
3	tomatoes, cut in wedges	3

Crush cereal to make crumbs. Melt the 2 t. (10 mL) margarine in small skillet. Stir in cereal crumbs. Cook over low heat, stirring constantly, until lightly browned. Remove from heat. Stir in lemon peel. Set aside for topping.

In large skillet, cook zucchini in the 2 T. (30 mL) margarine until almost tender, stirring frequently. Sprinkle with salt and pepper. Stir in lemon juice and tomato wedges. Continue cooking until tomatoes are heated. Spoon vegetable mixture into serving bowl. Top with cereal mixture. Serve immediately.

Yield: 6 servings

Exchange, 1 serving: 2 vegetables, 1 fat
Each serving contains: Calories: 85, Carbohydrates: 11 g

From Kellogg's Test Kitchens.

Peppers and Tomatoes

1 med.	onion, chopped	1 med.
2 cloves	garlic, minced	2 cloves
1 T.	vegetable oil	15 mL
1 c.	green pepper, sliced into sticks	250 mL
½ c.	sweet red pepper, cut into chunks	125 mL
5	tomatoes, cored and quartered	5
1	bay leaf	1
2 T.	fresh parsley, chopped	30 mL

In a heavy pan, sauté onion and garlic in the oil until golden brown. Add peppers. Reduce heat, cover and cook 5 minutes. Add tomatoes and bay leaf. Cover and cook for 5 minutes longer. Pour into serving dish. Season with salt and pepper. Garnish with parsley and serve warm.

Yield: 6 servings

Exchange, 1 serving: 1 vegetable, ½ fat
Each serving contains: Calories: 42, Carbohydrates: 8 g

Zucchini Patties

⅓ c.	Kretschmer regular wheat germ	90 mL
⅓ c.	all-purpose flour	90 mL
¼ c.	Parmesan cheese, grated	60 mL
¼ t.	baking powder	1 mL
¼ t.	oregano, crushed	1 mL
dash	salt	dash
2 c.	zucchini (about 2 med), shredded	500 mL
2	eggs, slightly beaten	2

Combine wheat germ, flour, cheese, baking powder, oregano and salt in a bowl. Stir well to blend. Add zucchini and eggs. Stir just to blend. Preheat griddle to 350°F (175°C). It is ready when drops of water skitter on the surface. Grease hot griddle for the first patties. Drop batter by spoonfuls onto griddle, spreading to flatten slightly. Bake until golden brown, about 3 to 4 minutes. Turn and bake other side about 3 to 4 minutes. Continue making patties. Serve with favorite main dish, if desired.

Yield: 12 small patties

Exchange, 2 patties: 2 vegetables, ½ fat
Each serving contains: Calories: 80, Carbohydrates: 6 g

With the courtesy of Kretschmer Wheat Germ/International Multifoods.

Creamed Beets

The lovely color invites you to any table.

2 T.	butter	30 mL
3 T.	all-purpose flour	45 mL
1 c.	water	250 mL
2 T.	lemon juice	30 mL
1 small	bay leaf	1 small
2 c.	small beets, cooked and diced	500 mL
1 env.	aspartame sweetener	1 env.
	salt to taste	

Melt butter in a heavy or nonstick fry pan. Add flour and stir over low heat for 1 minute. Mix water with lemon juice; slowly add to pan, stirring constantly, to blend into a smooth mixture. Add bay leaf. Cook until thickened. Add beets and cook until hot. Remove from heat and discard bay leaf. Add aspartame sweetener and salt.

Yield: 6 servings

Exchange, 1 serving: 1 vegetable, 1 fat
Each serving contains: Calories: 76, Carbohydrates: 7 g

Spicy Cabbage

3 c.	cabbage, shredded	750 mL
1 t.	mixed pickling spices	5 mL
2 cloves	garlic, minced	2 cloves
¼ c.	wine vinegar	60 mL
1 t.	salt	5 mL
¼ t.	red pepper	1 mL

Combine all ingredients in large saucepan. Cover, cook until cabbage is tender. Drain.

Yield: 4 servings

Exchange, 1 serving: ½ vegetable
Each serving contains: Calories: 11, Carbohydrates: 4 g

Sweet Cabbage

Don't snub this dish until you try it. It's delicious!

¼ c.	water	60 mL
6 c.	cabbage, finely shredded	½ L
2 T.	cider vinegar	30 mL
½ t.	salt	2 mL
2 med.	apples, unpeeled and finely sliced	2 med.
½ t.	granulated sugar replacement	2 mL

In a large saucepan, bring water to boil, add cabbage, vinegar and salt. Stir to mix. Cover and cook over medium heat for 20 to 25 minutes or until cabbage is tender. Add apple slices and sugar replacement to cabbage. Cook for 5 minutes longer. Serve hot.

Microwave: Place cabbage in 2 qt. (2-L) casserole. Add 2 T. (30 mL) water, vinegar and salt. Stir to mix. Cover tightly. Cook on High for 8 to 10 minutes, turning dish once. Add apples and sugar replacement. Cover and cook for 3 minutes.

Yield: 5 c. (1¼ L)

Exchange, 1 c. (250 mL): 1 fruit or 1½ vegetable
Each serving contains: Calories: 40, Carbohydrates: 11 g

Sweet and Sour Sauerkraut

This is a delicious way to serve sauerkraut.

3 c.	homemade or canned sauerkraut, drained	750 mL
1 c.	crushed pineapple in its juice	250 mL
1 large	white onion	1 large
1 t.	pepper	5 mL

Combine ingredients in saucepan. Cover and cook over medium heat until onion is tender and most of the liquid has evaporated. Serve hot.

Yield: 6 servings

Exchange, 1 serving: 1 fruit
Each serving contains: Calories: 43, Carbohydrates: 9 g

Light and Lively Cabbage Dish

This is microwave-fast to prepare and looks so pretty at the table.

1 c.	cabbage, finely shredded	250 mL
1 c.	cauliflower, chopped	250 mL
1 med.	carrot, thinly sliced	1 med.
2 T.	water	30 mL
2 t.	butter	10 mL
1 t.	salt	5 mL
½ t.	white pepper	2 mL

Combine cabbage, cauliflower, carrot and water in a serving bowl. Cover tightly with plastic wrap. Microwave on High for 8 minutes, turning dish once. Drain any excess water. Add butter, salt and white pepper. Stir to mix.

Yield: 2 c. (500 mL)

Exchange, ½ c. (125 mL): ½ vegetable, ½ fat
Each serving contains: Calories: 37, Carbohydrates: 3 g

Corn on the Grill

I have grilled corn on the cob many times, but this is my favorite version. This recipe is suggested for just one ear of corn. Repeat this procedure for each cob you plan to serve.

5 in. long ear	corn, unhusked	12 cm long ear
1 t.	butter, melted	5 mL
½ t.	soy sauce	2 mL
	salt and pepper to taste	

Carefully, turn back husk from corn. Remove and discard corn silk. Wash corn, allowing husk to get wet. Add butter to soy sauce and brush corn with the mixture, then rewrap husk around corn. Wrap cob in aluminum foil. Grill 6 in. (15 cm) over heated coals for 10 to 12 minutes. Remove foil and husk. Season with salt and pepper.

Yield: 1 serving

Exchange, 1 serving: 3 vegetable, 1 fat
Each serving contains: Calories: 115, Carbohydrates: 14 g

Corn Custard

Fresh or frozen corn can be substituted for canned corn in this no-fuss corn casserole.

2 T.	all-purpose flour	30 mL
½ t.	salt	2 mL
dash	pepper	dash
16 oz. can	whole kernel corn, drained	456 g
1	egg	1
¾ c.	nonfat milk	190 mL
1 T.	margarine, melted	15 mL
⅓ c.	All-Bran cereal	90 mL

Stir together the flour, salt and pepper. Toss with corn. In another bowl, beat egg slightly. Combine with milk and margarine and stir into corn mixture. Pour into round 1 qt. (1 L) casserole. Sprinkle with cereal. Bake at 325°F (165°C) for about 50 minutes or until knife inserted near middle comes out clean.

Yield: 4 servings

Exchange, 1 serving: 1 bread, 2 vegetable, 1 fat
Each serving contains: Calories: 170, Carbohydrates: 20 g

From Kellogg's Test Kitchens.

Colorful Carrot and Green Bean Ring

A pretty vegetable dish—like this one—pleases both the eye and the appetite.

2 large	carrots, peeled	2 large
1 c.	green beans, canned	250 mL
1 large	snow-white mushroom, chopped	1 large
	salt and black pepper to taste	

Cut carrots into large pieces and finely grate them. Ring a plate or flat soup bowl with the grated carrots. Add a few drops of water. Cover tightly with plastic wrap. Microwave on High for 4 minutes. Meanwhile, chop the green beans and mushroom but keep them separated. Uncover carrots and place green beans in the central section of the ring. Top the very middle with the chopped mushroom. Cover tightly with plastic. Microwave on Medium for 4 minutes. Season with salt and pepper.

Yield: 4 servings

Exchange, 1 serving: 1 vegetable
Each serving contains: Calories: 25, Carbohydrates: 6 g

Asparagus to Perfection

1 lb.	fresh asparagus	500 g
½ lb.	fresh mushrooms	250 g
1 T.	butter	15 mL
½ t.	salt	2 mL
1 t.	La Choy soy sauce	5 mL
½ c.	water	125 mL
½ t.	cornstarch	2 mL

Wash asparagus and break off and discard the woody parts. Place spears on cutting board and slice diagonally into thin slices. Clean and slice mushrooms. Melt butter in a skillet; add asparagus and mushrooms. Stir to coat. Add salt and soy sauce; cook, stirring, for 4 minutes. Combine water and cornstarch in bowl or shaker jar. Blend completely. Add to asparagus. Cook until cornstarch mixture clears and slightly thickens.

Yield: 4 servings

Exchange, 1 serving: 1 vegetable, 1 fat
Each serving contains: Calories: 65, Carbohydrates: 3 g

Baked Spinach

This is a perfect dish for dinner parties. It can be made up in advance and popped into the oven at the last minute.

2 lbs.	fresh spinach	1 kg
2 T.	salad oil	30 mL
2 c.	onion, chopped	500 mL
1 clove	garlic, minced	1 clove
2	eggs, beaten	2
½ c.	Parmesan cheese, grated	125 mL

Thoroughly wash and clean spinach. Drain. In a large frying pan, heat oil. Add onion and garlic, cook and stir until onion is transparent but not browned. Add spinach; cover tightly. Reduce heat and cook until spinach wilts. Pour spinach mixture into a greased casserole. In a bowl, combine the eggs with the cheese. Pour over top of spinach. (You may now refrigerate spinach until ready to bake.) Bake, uncovered, at 375°F (190°C) for about 15 minutes.

Yield: 8 servings

Exchange, 1 serving: 1 vegetable, ½ lean meat, 1 fat
Each serving contains: Calories: 102, Carbohydrates: 8 g

Creamed Spinach

An Italian touch for spinach.

1 T.	butter	15 mL
1 c.	onion, finely chopped	250 mL
2 cloves	garlic, minced	2 cloves
2 T.	all-purpose flour	30 mL
¾ c.	skim milk	190 mL
¼ t.	ground oregano	1 mL
	salt and pepper to taste	
2 lbs.	fresh spinach, cleaned and cooked	1 kg

Melt butter in a skillet. Add onion and garlic; cook over medium heat until onion is soft. Stir in flour; blend well. Remove pan from heat, slowly stir in milk, oregano, salt and pepper. Return to heat and cook 1 minute. Remove skillet from heat; add spinach and fold to mix. Turn into a well-greased baking dish. Bake uncovered at 375°F (190°C) for 12 to 15 minutes.

Yield: 6 servings

Exchange, 1 serving: 2 vegetable, ½ fat
Each serving contains: Calories: 72, Carbohydrates: 9 g

Heavenly Eggplant Slices

A bouquet of spicy flavors for eggplant.

1 large	eggplant	1 large
2 T.	vegetable oil	30 mL
3	tomatoes, cored and cubed	3
1 med.	yellow onion, finely chopped	1 med.
1 t.	granulated sugar replacement	5 mL
1 t.	ginger root, finely chopped	5 mL
¼ t.	ground ginger	1 mL
¼ t.	salt	1 mL
dash	pepper	dash
3 T.	fresh parsley, chopped	45 mL

Slice unpeeled eggplant in 1 in. (2.5 cm) slices. Brush oil on both sides. Arrange in single layer in a baking dish. Place tomatoes in blender; blend to a purée. In a large saucepan, combine tomato purée, onion, sugar replacement, ginger root, ground ginger, salt and pepper. Cook and stir over medium heat until onions are translucent. Pour sauce over eggplant slices. Bake at 400°F (200°C) for 20 to 30 minutes or until eggplant is tender. Garnish with parsley.

Yield: 6 servings

Exchange, 1 serving: ½ vegetable, 1 fat
Each serving contains: Calories: 55, Carbohydrates: 12 g

Celery with Pearl Onions

1 qt.	celery, thickly sliced	1 L
1 c.	pearl onions, peeled	250 mL
3 T.	dry sherry	45 mL
2 T.	water	30 mL
¼ t.	ground or grated nutmeg	1 mL
½ t.	salt	2 mL
¼ t.	black pepper	1 mL
1 T.	butter	15 mL

Combine celery and onions in large microwave bowl. Mix together the sherry, water and nutmeg. Pour over vegetables. Microwave on High for 7 minutes, turning bowl once. Drain any excess liquid. Mix in salt, pepper and butter. Serve hot.

Yield: 6 servings

Exchange, 1 serving: 1 vegetable, ½ fat
Each serving contains: Calories: 40, Carbohydrates: 5 g

A Side Dish of Mushrooms

Here is a very quick way to prepare an impressive dish of mushrooms.

1 lb.	fresh mushrooms	500 g
2 T.	water	30 mL
1 T.	soy sauce	15 mL
	black pepper to taste (optional)	

Clean and slice mushrooms. Heat a nonstick skillet. Add water and soy sauce. Heat slightly and add mushrooms. Cook and stir until mushrooms are tender. Season with pepper, if desired. Serve hot.

Yield: 4 servings

Exchange, 1 serving: 1 vegetable
Each serving contains: Calories: 25, Carbohydrates: 5 g

Butternut Squash

2 lbs.	butternut squash	1 kg
1 clove	garlic, minced	1 clove
	water	
2 T.	sesame seeds, toasted	30 mL
2 T.	wheat germ, toasted	30 mL
	salt and pepper to taste	

Wash and cut off stern of butternut squash. Cut squash into thin slices and arrange in large skillet. Sprinkle with minced garlic. Add just enough water to steam the squash; cover and cook over medium heat. When squash is tender, drain off any excess water. Place on heated serving platter. Sprinkle with sesame seeds. wheat germ, salt and pepper.

Yield: 9 servings

Exchange, 1 serving: 2 vegetables
Each serving contains: Calories: 42, Carbohydrates: 18 g

Stewed Tomatoes and Green Beans

2 cloves	garlic, minced	2 cloves
1 med.	onion, sliced into rings	1 med.
½ c.	green pepper, chopped	125 mL
½ c.	celery, sliced	125 mL
2 T.	low-calorie margarine	30 mL
2 c.	fresh tomatoes, chopped	500 mL
2 c.	fresh green beans, snapped	500 mL
	salt and pepper to taste	

In a nonstick skillet, sauté garlic, onion rings, green pepper and celery in margarine for 4 minutes. Add tomatoes, green beans, salt and pepper. Stir to mix. Reduce heat, cover and cook for about 15 minutes or until green beans are *al dente*.

Yield: 4 servings

Exchange, 1 serving: 2 vegetable
Each serving contains: Calories: 50

Orange Slices in Amaretto

1	orange	1
¼ c.	amaretto (liqueur)	60 mL
¼ c.	orange juice	60 mL

Peel and remove membrane from the orange. Slice the orange crosswise into very thin circles. Combine amaretto and orange juice in a glass bowl or wide-mouthed jar. Gently place the orange slices into the mixture; cover tightly. Refrigerate overnight or longer. (You may add other orange slices to any remaining liquid.)

Yield: 4 servings

Exchange, 1 serving: ½ fruit
Each serving contains: Calories: 22, Carbohydrates: 7 g

Green Grapes in Jamaican Rum

½ c.	seedless green grapes	125 mL
¼ c.	Jamaican rum	60 mL

Remove stems from grapes and wash. Place grapes in a small glass jar cover with the rum. Cover tightly and refrigerate at least overnight. (You may add more grapes to the remaining liquid.)

Yield: 2 servings

Exchange, 1 serving: 1 fruit
Each serving contains: Calories: 38, Carbohydrates: 13 g

Banana Sauté

Arrange these bananas in a fan shape on a glass plate. Add a sprig of mint for garnish.

4 T.	unsalted butter	60 mL
6	bananas, firm but ripe	6
4 T.	granulated fructose	60 mL
⅓ c.	dark rum	90 mL

Melt butter in a large nonstick skillet. Peel and cut bananas in half lengthwise and crosswise. Add the bananas and sauté until coated with the butter. Remove from heat and sprinkle fructose over the bananas. Slowly add the rum. Return to heat and cook and stir until bananas are coated. Fan bananas on a serving plate. Pour any remaining sauce over bananas.

Yield: 12 servings

Exchange, 1 serving: 1½ fruit, 1 fat
Each serving contains: Calories: 105, Carbohydrates: 17 g

Golden Apricot Mold

2 16 oz. cans	apricot halves in their own juice	2 454 g cans	
¼ c.	vinegar	60 mL	
1 t.	whole cloves	5 mL	
4 in.	cinnamon stick	10 cm	
1 pkg.	dietetic orange gelatin	1 pkg.	

Drain juice from apricots into a saucepan and reserve the apricots. Add vinegar, cloves, and cinnamon to the juice; bring to the boil. Add the apricots, reduce heat, and simmer for 5 minutes. With a slotted spoon, remove apricots to 10 individual molds. Strain liquid and measure; add enough boiling water to make 2 c. (500 mL). Add the gelatin and stir to completely dissolve. Pour gelatin mixture over apricots in molds. Chill until firm. Turn out onto plates.

Yield: 10 servings

Exchange, 1 serving: 1 fruit
Each serving contains: Calories: 43, Carbohydrates: 11 g

Fresh Fruit Plate

1	fresh pineapple	1	
6	fresh peaches	6	
1 pt.	fresh strawberries	500 mL	
¼ c.	orange juice	60 mL	

Clean the pineapple and cut into 12 ring slices. Cut peaches in half and discard the pits. Clean the strawberries. On a chilled plate, place peach halves in the middle. Encircle the peaches with the pineapple rings. Place strawberries around edge of plate. Sprinkle with orange juice. Cover with plastic wrap and refrigerate until ready to serve.

Yield: 12 servings

Exchange, 1 serving: 2 fruit
Each serving contains: Calories: 76, Carbohydrates: 19 g

Cranberry Salad

Red and green for a cool and crisp look.

2 c.	cranberries	500 mL	
3 env.	Equal low-calorie sweetener	3 env.	
1 c.	seedless green grapes	250 mL	
2 T.	walnuts, broken	30 mL	
½ c.	nondairy whipped topping, prepared	125 mL	

Place cranberries in a food processor. Using a steel blade, process until coarsely chopped. Place in a glass refrigerator bowl. Stir in the sweetener; cover and refrigerate overnight. Drain thoroughly to remove any excess liquid. Cut grapes in half. Add grape halves and walnuts to the well-drained cranberries. Just before serving, fold in the topping. Serve immediately.

Yield: 8 servings

Exchange, 1 serving: 1 fruit
Each serving contains: Calories: 42, Carbohydrates: 6 g

Melon with Prosciutto

1	large honeydew melon	1	
¼ lb.	prosciutto ham, sliced paper-thin	125 g	
1	lemon, sliced paper-thin	1	

Cut melon in half; remove seeds and peel off the rind. Cut each melon half into 10 thin slices. Arrange on a chilled platter. (If prosciutto slices are large, cut in half or thirds to make sure you have at least 20 slices.) Fold prosciutto slices in half. Place alternately between melon slices. Garnish with lemon slices. Cover with plastic wrap and refrigerate until ready to serve. Optional: Sprinkle with freshly ground black pepper.

Yield: 20 servings

Exchange, 1 serving: 1 fruit, ⅓ high-fat meat
Each serving contains: Calories: 82, Carbohydrates: 11 g

Red Fruit

1 qt.	strawberries	1 L	
10 oz. pkg.	frozen raspberries, partially thawed	280 g	
1 c.	nondairy whipped topping, prepared	250 mL	

Clean and arrange strawberries in a pyramid on a chilled serving dish. Drain excess liquid from the raspberries. Break raspberries into large chunks and place in a blender. Process at high speed into a thick purée. Pour over the strawberries. Serve with nondairy whipped topping.

Yield: 10 servings

Exchange, 1 serving: 1⅓ fruit
Each serving contains: Calories: 56, Carbohydrates: 12 g

Pears with Cinnamon

1 lb. can	pear halves in their own juice	454 g can	
3 in.	cinnamon stick	7.5 cm	
1 t.	Tone's imitation vanilla extract	5 mL	

Carefully spoon pear halves into a glass jar or bowl and save the juice. Break cinnamon stick in half; add to pears. Add the vanilla. Pour in the juice from can and cover tightly. Store in refrigerator for at least 1 week. Remove pear halves to 4 chilled serving dishes.

Yield: 4 servings

Exchange, 1 serving: 1 fruit
Each serving contains: Calories: 42, Carbohydrates: 9 g

Peaches with Clove

1 lb. can	peaches in their own juice	454 g can
10	whole cloves	10

Pour peaches with juice in a glass jar or bowl. Add the cloves; cover tightly and refrigerate for at least 1 week. Carefully remove peaches to plate that has been lined with paper towels. Drain slightly. Place peach halves on 4 chilled serving dishes. Reserve juice to make Peach and Clove Jelly.

Yield: 4 servings

Exchange, 1 serving: 1 fruit
Each serving contains: Calories: 39, Carbohydrates: 9 g

Dried Fruit Medley

Make this dish at least a day before you plan to serve this medley so the flavors have some time to mingle.

½ c.	dried apples	125 mL
½ c.	dried apricots	125 mL
⅓ c.	dried peaches	90 mL
⅓ c.	dried pears	90 mL
¼ c.	lemon juice	60 mL
3 env.	Equal low-calorie sweetener	3 env.

Combine all dried fruits in a saucepan. Cover with water; cover pan and simmer until fruits are almost tender. Add the lemon juice. Continue cooking until fruits are tender, adding extra water, if needed. Cool to room temperature. Stir in the sweetener. Chill thoroughly. This will stay fresh in a tightly covered refrigerator bowl for your morning breakfast for at least 2 weeks.

Yield: 12 servings

Exchange, 1 serving: 1 fruit
Each serving contains: Calories: 45, Carbohydrates: 11 g

Alabama Apricots

16 oz. can	whole apricots in their own juice	454 g can
½ c.	rum	125 mL
¼ c.	raisins	60 mL
1 t.	nutmeg	5 mL
	mint leaves (optional)	

Pour contents of apricots and juice into glass refrigerator container with cover. Add remaining ingredients. Stir slightly to mix. Cover and refrigerate for at least 4 days. With a slotted spoon, remove apricots to chilled serving dishes. Garnish with raisins. Pour the chilled liquid into small glasses and serve on the side. Optional: Decorate with mint leaves.

Yield: 5 servings

Exchange, 1 serving: 1 fruit
Each serving contains: Calories: 42, Carbohydrates: 15 g

Winter Fruit Sauce

10	prunes, pitted	10
8	figs, stems removed	8
½ c.	dates, pitted	125 mL
½ c.	raisins	125 mL
6	dried apricots	6
2 c.	water	500 mL
1 T.	cornstarch	15 mL
⅓ c.	white grape juice	90 mL

Combine fruits in a food processor. With a steel blade, process into small chunks. Combine water and cornstarch in a saucepan. Cook and stir until just starting to thicken. Add fruit chunks and grape juice. Continue cooking until clear and thickened. Serve hot or cold.

Yield: 15 servings

Exchange, 1 serving: 1 fruit
Each serving contains: Calories: 48, Carbohydrates: 12 g

Summertime Compote

1	lemon, sliced	1
¾ c.	water	190 mL
¾ c.	granulated sugar replacement	190 mL
4	pears, halved and cored	4
8	purple plums, halved and pitted	8
4	peaches, halved and pitted	4
4	apricots, halved and pitted	4

Combine the lemon slices, water, and granulated sugar replacement in a saucepan. Bring to the boiling point and fold in the fruits. Reduce heat, cover, and simmer until tender. Pour into a serving dish and refrigerate. Compote will keep for several days.

Yield: 20 servings

Exchange, 1 serving: 1 fruit
Each serving contains: Calories: 39, Carbohydrates: 10 g

Easy Fruit Compote

This recipe is delicious all year long.

16 oz. can	pear halves in their own juice	454 g can
16 oz. can	peach halves in their own juice	454 g can
16 oz. can	whole apricots in their own juice	454 g can
16 oz. can	plums in their own juice	454 g can
	peel from 1 orange	
1 t.	ground cinnamon	5 mL

Drain juice from all canned fruits into a saucepan, add orange peel and cinnamon to the juice. Bring to the boil, reduce heat and simmer to reduce liquid to half. Place fruits in a large bowl. Gently fold to mix, while pouring hot fruit liquid over fruit. Remove the orange peel. Chill thoroughly before serving.

Yield: 16 servings

Exchange, 1 serving: 1½ fruit
Each serving contains: Calories: 60, Carbohydrates: 15 g

Potato Puffs

½ c.	potatoes. cooked and mashed or whipped	125 mL
1 c.	flour	250 mL
1½ t.	baking powder	8 mL
½ t.	salt	3 mL
1	egg, well beaten	1
½ c.	milk	125 mL
	oil for deep-fat frying	

With a fork, break up and mash enough potatoes to fill a small cup. Combine with remaining ingredients, except oil. Beat well. Heat oil to 375°F (190°C). From tablespoon, drop a walnut-size piece of dough into hot fat. Remove when puff rises to the surface (about 2–3 minutes) and is golden brown. Repeat with remaining dough. Drain.

Yield: 24 puffs

Exchange, 2 puffs: 1 bread, 1½ fat
Each serving contains: Calories: 160, Carbohydrates: 58 g

Potato Dumplings

1 small	cooked potato	1 small
1	egg, beaten	1
2 T.	flour	30 mL
	salt and pepper to taste	

With a fork, break up and mash the potato. Combine with the remaining ingredients. Beat until light and fluffy. Drop by tablespoonfuls on top of boiling salted water or beef broth. Boil for 5 minutes, or until dumplings rise to surface. Good with Sauerbraten.

Yield: 3 or 4 dumplings

Exchange, 1 serving: 1 bread, 1 meat
Each serving contains: Calories: 140, Carbohydrates: 13 g

Baked Sweet Potato

¼ c.	sweet potato or yam, mashed	60 mL
dash each	salt, pepper, nutmeg	dash each
1 T.	milk	15 mL

Combine all ingredients. Beat until smooth and creamy. Bake at 350° F (175°C) for 20 minutes.

Yield: 1 serving

Exchange, 1 serving: 1 bread
Each serving contains: Calories: 75, Carbohydrates: 20 g

Corn Pudding

16 oz. can	corn	500 g can
1	egg, beaten	1
1 t.	pimiento, chopped	5 mL
1 t.	green pepper	5 mL
1 t.	margarine, melted	5 mL
1 t.	sugar replacement	5 mL
¾ c.	milk	180 mL
	salt and pepper to taste	
	vegetable cooking spray	

Combine all ingredients, except vegetable cooking spray. Pour into baking dish coated with vegetable cooking spray. Bake at 325°F (165°C) for 35 to 40 minutes, or until firm.

Yield: 6 servings

Exchange, 1 serving: 1 bread, 1 fat
Each serving contains: Calories: 55

Creamed Potatoes au Gratin

2 lbs.	small potatoes, scrubbed	1 kg
1¼ c.	skim milk	310 mL
2 t.	cornstarch	10 mL
½ t.	lemon juice	2 mL
	salt and pepper to taste	
2 T.	Parmesan cheese, grated	30 mL

Place potatoes in a saucepan and cover with water. Heat to the boiling point; cover and reduce heat. Simmer until potatoes are barely fork-tender. Drain and rinse potatoes under cold water. Meanwhile, pour the milk into a heavy saucepan. Cook until milk is reduced by a third; cool. Blend in the cornstarch; return to heat and cook until slightly thickened. Peel and slice the potatoes. Add potatoes, lemon juice, salt, and pepper to milk. Fold until potatoes are coated. Spoon potatoes and creamed mixture into a greased baking dish. Sprinkle with the cheese. Place under broiler, 2 in. (5 cm) from heat until top is golden brown.

Yield: 8 servings

Exchange, 1 serving: 1 bread, ¼ nonfat milk
Each serving contains: Calories: 87, Carbohydrates: 28 g

Potato Béarnaise

3 c.	frozen hash brown potatoes	750 mL
½ c.	celery, sliced	125 mL
1 pkg.	béarnaise sauce dry mix	1 pkg.
1 env.	Butter Buds natural butter-flavored mix	1 env.
1 c.	water	250 mL

Place frozen potatoes and celery in a lightly oiled casserole. Combine sauce mix, butter-flavored mix, and water in a saucepan. Cook and stir for 1 minute or until well blended. Pour sauce over potatoes; fold to mix. Bake at 350°F (175°C) for 1 hour.

Yield: 6 servings

Exchange, 1 serving: 2 bread, ½ fat
Each serving contains: Calories: 163, Carbohydrates: 31 g

Stuffed Baked Potato

A perfect accompaniment with sausages.

3	baking potatoes	3
¼ c.	low-calorie margarine	60 mL
1 t.	salt	5 mL
¼ t.	black pepper	1 mL
¼ t.	ground nutmeg	1 mL
4	egg yolks	4
¼ c.	nondairy whipped topping	60 mL

Scrub the potatoes; pierce several times with a fork. Bake or microwave until tender. Halve the potatoes lengthwise. Scoop potato from skins; reserve skins. Rice the potatoes directly into a bowl. Stir in the margarine, salt, pepper, and nutmeg. Add egg yolks, one at a time, beating well after each addition. Fold in the topping. Spoon mixture into the reserved potato shells; place on cookie sheet. Bake at 450°F (230°C) for about 10 minutes until tops are golden brown.

Yield: 6 servings

Exchange, 1 serving: 1 bread, 2½ fat
Each serving contains: Calories: 186, Carbohydrates: 17 g

Southern-Style Corn Pudding

3 c.	frozen corn, thawed	750 mL
3	eggs, well beaten	3
1 c.	skim milk, warmed	250 mL
2 T.	low-calorie margarine, melted	30 mL
1 T.	granulated sugar replacement	15 mL
1 t.	salt	5 mL
¼ t.	black pepper	1 mL

Combine all ingredients in a bowl; stir to thoroughly blend. Pour into well-greased baking dish. Bake at 325°F (165°C) for 35 to 40 minutes or until set.

Yield: 6 servings

Exchange, 1 serving: 1 bread, 1½ medium-fat meat
Each serving contains: Calories: 104, Carbohydrates: 15 g

Baked Lima Beans

These will stay hot for a long time on a serving table.

3 T.	low-calorie margarine	45 mL
3 T.	all-purpose flour	45 mL
1¼ c.	skim milk	310 mL
3½ c.	lima beans, cooked	875 mL
½ c.	onion, very finely chopped	125 mL
2	eggs, well beaten	2
½ t.	salt	2 mL
¼ t.	black pepper	1 mL
½ c.	dry bread crumbs	125 mL

Melt margarine in a skillet; stir in the flour and gradually add the milk. Over low heat, cook and stir until thickened. Combine milk sauce and lima beans in food processor or bowl; whip until puréed. Add onion, eggs, salt, and pepper; stir to blend. Transfer to a well-greased baking dish. Sprinkle with bread crumbs. Bake at 375°F (175°C) for 20 to 25 minutes.

Yield: 8 servings

Exchange, 1 serving: 2 bread, 1 medium-fat meat
Each serving contains: Calories: 216, Carbohydrates: 30 g

Boston Baked Beans

Because of the long baking time, I start these several days in advance and bake them about 4 hours at a time. Then I reheat the beans for 1 or 2 hours before serving them. Any leftover beans can be frozen.

1 lb.	pea beans	500 g
¼ lb.	salt pork	125 g
2 t.	salt	10 mL
1½ T.	granulated brown sugar replacement	22 mL
¼ c.	dietetic maple syrup	60 mL
½ t.	Tone's dry mustard	2 mL
1 c.	boiling water	250 mL

Wash and sort beans. Soak beans overnight in cold water. Drain and cover with fresh water. Simmer until skins split; drain. Pour beans into a bean pot. Cut salt pork into small pieces; press into the beans. Combine remaining ingredients in a bowl. Stir to blend and pour over beans. Cover and bake at 300°F (150°C) for about 8 hours. Add extra water when needed. Uncover to brown during last half hour of baking.

Yield: 20 servings

Exchange, 1 serving: 1 bread, 3¼ fat
Each serving contains: Calories: 114, Carbohydrates: 14 g

Carrot Ring

1 lb. can	carrots, diced and drained	485 g can
3	eggs, well beaten	3
1 c.	skim milk	250 mL
1 t.	onion, minced	5 mL
1 t.	salt	5 mL
⅛ t.	Tone's black pepper	½ mL

Combine all ingredients in a bowl; stir well to mix. Pour into a well-greased ring mold. Bake at 350°F (175°C) for 40 minutes or until set. Unmold onto a heated serving plate.

Yield: 6 servings

Exchange, 1 serving: ½ bread, ½ medium-fat meat
Each serving contains: Calories: 74, Carbohydrates: 7 g

Ratatouille

2 T.	olive oil	30 mL
2	yellow onions	2
3	garlic cloves	3
2	eggplants, cubed	2
4	small zucchini, cubed	4
2	green bell peppers, sliced	2
2 t.	fennel seed	10 mL
1 lb.	plum tomatoes, chopped	500 g
1 t.	basil	5 mL
1 t.	salt	5 mL
½ t.	parsley	2 mL
2 t.	cornstarch	10 mL
¼ c.	cold water	60 mL

Heat the olive oil in a large nonstick skillet or wok. Add the onions and garlic; sauté for 2 minutes, tossing lightly. Add the eggplant, zucchini, green pepper, and fennel seed; stir to mix well. Add the tomatoes and seasonings. Cover and cook over medium heat for 3 minutes, stirring occasionally. Combine cornstarch and water in a cup or shaker; blend thoroughly. Pour over the vegetables. Cook and stir until mixture is clear and thickened. Serve hot.

Yield: 10 servings

Exchange, 1 serving: 1 vegetable
Each serving contains: Calories: 24, Carbohydrates: 6 g

Sautéed Cauliflower

This is easy to prepare and can be served hot or cold.

1	cauliflower head	1
	salt	
2 T.	peanut oil	30 mL
	pepper to taste	
2 T.	lemon juice	30 mL

Clean and wash the cauliflower under cool running water. Dissolve 1 t. (5 mL) salt in 2 c. (500 mL) cold water in a large bowl. Add the cauliflower and enough extra water to completely cover the cauliflower. Cover and refrigerate for at least 1 hour. Drain and wash cauliflower again under cool water; cut into florets. Place florets in a saucepan with enough water to cover bottom of pan. Cook until florets are barely tender; drain thoroughly. Heat the oil in large skillet. Sauté florets quickly over high heat until browned on all sides. Season with salt and pepper to taste. Add the lemon juice and quickly toss. Serve hot or cold.

Yield: 6 servings

Exchange, 1 serving: 1 vegetable, 1 fat
Each serving contains: Calories: 70, Carbohydrates: 6 g

Italian-Style Cold Vegetables

Make this dish a day or two before serving.

2 T.	olive oil	30 mL
2	small yellow onions, sliced in rings	2
2	celery stalks, thinly sliced	2
3	small unpeeled eggplants, cut in strips	3
¾ lb.	plum tomatoes, chopped	350 g
2	garlic cloves, sliced	2
1 t.	salt	5 mL
½ t.	freshly ground black pepper	2 mL
1 t.	basil	5 mL
⅓ c.	capers	90 mL
10	pitted black olives	10
1	lemon, thinly sliced	1
¼ c.	fresh parsley, finely snipped	60 mL

Heat the olive oil in a nonstick skillet or wok. Sauté onions and celery just until limp. Add eggplant and toss to coat with oil. Add the tomatoes and garlic; cook for 2 minutes, stirring occasionally. Season with salt, pepper, and basil. Stir in the capers, olives, and lemon slices. Cook, uncovered, for 1 minute; stir occasionally. Spoon into a serving dish or bowl. Cover and refrigerate for a day or two. Just before serving, sprinkle with parsley.

Yield: 6 servings

Exchange, 1 serving: 1 vegetable, ¼ fat
Each serving contains: Calories: 33, Carbohydrates: 5 g

Autumn Vegetable Medley

1 T.	unsalted butter	15 mL
1	white onion, chopped	1
1 c.	green beans, snapped	250 mL
½ c.	water	125 mL
1	green bell pepper, chopped	1
6	small yellow squash, sliced	6
2	plum tomatoes, cut into eighths	2
1 c.	corn kernels	250 mL
	salt and pepper to taste	

Melt butter in a nonstick skillet. Add the onion and sauté until lightly browned. Add beans and water. Cover and cook until beans are tender. Add the remaining ingredients; cover and cook until vegetables are tender.

Yield: 10 servings

Exchange, 1 serving: 1 vegetable
Each serving contains: Calories: 26, Carbohydrates: 6 g

Sautéed Asparagus

1 lb.	asparagus with firm tips	500 g
⅓ c.	water	90 mL
½ t.	salt	2 mL
2 T.	low-calorie margarine	30 mL
1 T.	unsalted butter	15 mL
2 t.	cornstarch	10 mL
2 T.	water	30 mL
⅛ t.	Tone's black pepper	½ mL

Peel the asparagus and cut into 2 in. (5 cm) pieces. Combine the water and salt in a nonstick skillet. Bring to the boiling point and add asparagus. Cover and cook for about 2 minutes. Add the margarine and butter; stir until melted. Combine cornstarch and water in a cup or shaker. Mix and pour over asparagus. Add the pepper. Gently stir over medium heat until mixture is clear and thickened. Add a small amount of extra water, if mixture becomes too thick.

Yield: 4 servings

Exchange, 1 serving: 3¼ vegetable, 1 fat
Each serving contains: Calories: 66, Carbohydrates: 3 g

Mixed Summer Vegetables

A delightful dish using many fresh summer vegetables and herbs.

1 lb.	tomatoes, sliced	500 g
1 lb.	tiny new potatoes, sliced	500 g
1 lb.	small red onions, quartered	500 g
1 lb.	small zucchini, thickly sliced	500 g
3	celery stalks, cut in 2 in. (5 cm) lengths	3
⅓ c.	fresh parsley, snipped	90 mL
1 T.	fresh dill seed	15 mL
1 t.	fresh marjoram	5 mL
	salt and pepper to taste	
3 T.	low-calorie Italian dressing	45 mL

In an oiled casserole, layer the vegetables in order given above. Sprinkle with the herbs and dressing. Cover and bake at 400°F (200°C) for 30 minutes. Remove cover and bake another 20 minutes.

Yield: 10 servings

Exchange, 1 serving: 1⅓ vegetables, ½ bread
Each serving contains: Calories: 61, Carbohydrates: 9 g

Globe Artichokes

Something a little special for just the two of you. You can make more for larger groups.

2	fresh globe artichokes	2
½ t.	salt	2 mL

To cook: Wash artichokes in salted water and drain, bottoms up. Remove the thick, loose leaves around the base and clip off any sharp tips. Place artichokes in a saucepan or an artichoke holder. Cover with boiling water. Add the salt and simmer for 30 minutes. Drain with bottoms up. Serve hot.

To eat: Pull off a leaf; hold by the tip. Remove the fleshy part of the base of the leaf with the teeth and discard the remainder of the leaf. When all the leaves are removed, discard the choke (hairy part) and eat the artichoke heart with a fork.

Yield: 2 servings

Exchange, 1 serving: ½ vegetable
Each serving contains: Calories: 13, Carbohydrates: 3 g

Steamed Fresh Spinach

1 lb.	fresh spinach	500 g
1 t.	fresh lemon juice	5 mL
	salt	
¼ t.	black pepper, freshly ground	1 mL

Discard stems from spinach and rinse the leaves thoroughly to remove any sand particles; drain. Place spinach in a steamer over boiling water. Cover and steam until leaves are tender. Remove from steamer and turn spinach into a heated serving dish. Sprinkle with lemon juice, salt, and pepper; toss to completely coat.

Yield: 4 servings

Exchange, 1 serving: 1 vegetable
Each serving contains: Calories: 21, Carbohydrates: 4 g

Added Touch: Crush a couple of whole garlic cloves and put them in the water before you bring it to a boil. The spinach will have a delicious hint of garlic.

Jerusalem Artichokes

Several people have asked how to cook these roots that taste a little like a potato.

2 lbs.	fresh Jerusalem artichokes	1 kg	
1 t.	salt	5 mL	

Wash, scrape, and rinse the Jerusalem artichokes in cold water. Place in a large saucepan or kettle; cover with boiling water. Add the salt and simmer for about 20 to 30 minutes until tender. Drain thoroughly. Season as desired, with salt and pepper.

Yield: 4 servings

Exchange, 1 serving: ½ vegetable
Each serving contains: Calories: 11, Carbohydrates: 3 g

Vegetable ABC's

1 c.	asparagus pieces	250 mL
1 c.	broccoli florets	250 mL
1 c.	carrot slices	250 mL
1 c.	spinach, chopped	250 mL
	vegetable cooking spray	
11 oz. can	condensed cream of mushroom soup	300 g can
2 T.	onions, finely chopped	30 mL
1 t.	thyme	5 mL
½ c.	water	125 mL
	salt and pepper to taste	

Layer asparagus, broccoli, carrots, and spinach in a baking dish coated with vegetable cooking spray. Blend remaining ingredients. Pour over vegetables. Cover. Bake at 350°F (175°C) for 30 to 40 minutes, or until vegetables are tender.

Yield: 8 servings

Exchange, 1 serving: 1 vegetable, ½ bread, ½ fat
Each serving contains: Calories: 42, Carbohydrates: 6 g

Baked Eggplant

1 slice	eggplant	1 slice
1 slice	onion	1 slice
1 oz.	sharp cheddar cheese, shredded	30 g
2 T.	condensed tomato soup	30 mL
1 t.	dry bread crumbs	5 mL
¼ t.	thyme	1 mL
¼ t.	salt	1 mL
dash	pepper	dash

Cook eggplant and onion in small amount of water until, tender. Drain; reserve liquid. Place eggplant and onion in small baking dish. Top with cheese. Blend condensed soup, 1 T. (15 mL) of the eggplant liquid, bread crumbs, thyme, salt, and pepper. Pour over eggplant; cover. Bake at 350°F (175°C) for 30 minutes.

Microwave: Uncover. Cook on High for 5 minutes. Turn after 2 minutes.

Yield: 1 serving

Exchange, 1 serving: 1 high-fat meat, 1 vegetable
Each serving contains: Calories: 161, Carbohydrates: 28 g

Okra and Tomatoes

2 c.	okra	500 mL
¼ c.	vinegar	60 mL
2 c.	tomatoes, cut into eighths	500 mL
1 c.	onions, coarsely chopped	250 mL
½ c.	green pepper, coarsely chopped	125 mL
sprig	parsley, chopped	sprig
1 T.	mint, chopped	15 mL
1 t.	garlic powder	5 mL
	salt and pepper to taste	
	vegetable cooking spray	

Soak okra in vinegar for 5 minutes. Drain. Pat okra slightly dry. Combine all ingredients (except vinegar) in baking dish coated with vegetable cooking spray. Cover. Bake at 350°F (175 °C) for 45 minutes.

Yield: 5 servings

Exchange, 1 serving: 1 vegetable
Each serving contains: Calories: 31, Carbohydrates: 8 g

Kohlrabi

2 c.	kohlrabi, cut into strips	500 mL
2 t.	butter	10 mL
2 T.	fresh parsley, chopped	30 mL
	salt and pepper to taste	

Cook kohlrabi in boiling salted water until soft; drain. Melt butter or margarine in saucepan. Add parsley; sauté over low heat for 2 minutes. Add kohlrabi. Toss to coat. Add salt and pepper.

Yield: 4 servings

Exchange, 1 serving: 1 vegetable, ½ fat
Each serving contains: Calories: 36, Carbohydrates: 4 g

Italian Asparagus

½ lb.	asparagus spears (cooked or canned) vegetable cooking spray	250 g
¼ c.	Tomato Sauce	60 mL
¼ c.	water	60 mL
½ t.	oregano	3 mL
¼ t.	garlic powder	1 mL
	salt and pepper to taste	
¼ c.	Swiss cheese, grated	60 mL

Lay asparagus spears in shallow baking dish coated with vegetable cooking spray. Blend Tomato Sauce, water, oregano, garlic powder, salt, and pepper. Spread evenly over spears. Top with grated cheese. Bake at 350°F (175°C) for 20–25 minutes.

Microwave: Cook on High for 5–6 minutes.

Yield: 4 servings

Exchange, 1 serving: ½ vegetable, ½ medium-fat meat
Each serving contains: Calories: 58, Carbohydrates: 4 g

Brussels Sprouts and Mushrooms au Gratin

1 T.	butter	15 mL
2 c.	brussels sprouts	500 mL
1 c.	mushroom pieces	250 mL
	salt and pepper to taste	
2 oz.	Swiss cheese, grated	60 g

Melt butter in skillet. Lightly sauté brussels sprouts and mushrooms. Add salt and pepper. Remove from heat and pour into baking dish. Cover with cheese. Bake at 350°F (175°C) for 20 to 25 minutes.

Microwave: Cook on Medium for 10 minutes. Turn once.

Yield: 4 servings

Exchange, 1 serving: 1 high-fat meat, ½ vegetable
Each serving contains: Calories: 65, Carbohydrates: 5 g

Baked Vegetable Medley

1 c.	2 in. (5 cm) cubes eggplant	250 mL
1 c.	2 in. (5 cm) slices okra	250 mL
1 c.	bean sprouts	250 mL
½ c.	small mushrooms	125 mL
1	onion, cut into eighths	1
	vegetable cooking spray	
11 oz. can	condensed cream of celery soup	300 g can
¼ c.	water	60 mL
	salt and pepper to taste	
1 slice	bread, finely crumbled	1 slice

Combine all vegetables in baking dish coated with vegetable cooking spray. Blend condensed soup and water; add salt and pepper. Pour over vegetables. Top with bread crumbs. Cook at 325°F (165°C) for 25 to 30 minutes, or until hot, and crumbs are golden brown.

Yield: 8 servings

Exchange, 1 serving: 1 vegetable, ½ bread
Each serving contains: Calories: 49, Carbohydrates: 8 g

Shredded Cabbage

1 head	cabbage, shredded	1 head
2 t.	butter	10 mL
½ t.	nutmeg	2 mL
	salt and pepper to taste	

Cook cabbage in a small amount of boiling salted water until tender; drain. Press out excess moisture or pat dry. Melt butter in skillet. Add nutmeg; stir to blend. Add cabbage; toss to coat. Add salt and pepper.

Yield: 4 servings

Exchange, 1 serving: ½ vegetable, ½ fat
Each serving contains: Calories: 32, Carbohydrates: 17 g

Irish Vegetables

1	bay leaf	1
1 c.	water	250 mL
2 T.	wine vinegar	30 mL
½ c.	corn	125 mL
½ c.	celery, sliced	125 mL
½ c.	broccoli florets	125 mL
½ c.	carrot, sliced	125 mL
½ c.	cauliflower florets	125 mL
¼ c.	pimiento, chopped	60 mL
	salt and pepper to taste	

Combine bay leaf, water, and wine vinegar in medium saucepan. Bring to a boil; add vegetables. Simmer until vegetables are tender. Drain; remove bay leaf. Add salt and pepper.

Yield: 5 servings

Exchange, 1 serving: 1 bread
Each serving contains: Calories: 51, Carbohydrates: 6 g

Spiced Bean Sprouts

2 c.	bean sprouts	500 mL
½ t.	caraway seeds	2 mL
½ t.	basil	2 mL
2 t.	butter	10 mL
	salt and pepper to taste	

Combine bean sprouts, caraway seeds, and basil in saucepan with small amount of water. Cook until hot and tender; drain. Place in serving dish; top with butter, salt, and pepper. Toss to coat.

Yield: 4 servings

Exchange, 1 serving: ¼ vegetable, ½ fat
Each serving contains: Calories: 25, Carbohydrates: 3 g

German Green Beans

2 c.	green beans	500 mL
1 slice	bacon	1 slice
¼ c.	onion, chopped	60 mL
1 t.	flour	5 mL
¼ c.	vinegar	60 mL
½ c.	water	125 mL
2 T.	sugar replacement	30 mL

Cook green beans in boiling salted water until tender; drain. Cut bacon into ½ in. (12 mm) pieces. Place in skillet; add onion. Sauté until bacon is crisp and onion is tender; drain. Blend flour, vinegar, water, and sugar replacement in screwtop jar. Pour over bacon and onion. Cook over low heat to thicken slightly. Add green beans.

Yield: 4 servings

Exchange, 1 serving: ½ vegetable, ¼ bread, ½ fat
Each serving contains: Calories: 52, Carbohydrates: 9 g

Pizza Beans

2 c.	green beans	500 mL
1 T.	lemon juice	15 mL
¼ t.	oregano	1 mL
1 t.	pimiento, chopped	5 mL
dash each	garlic powder, salt	dash each

Cook green beans in boiling salted water until tender; drain. Combine lemon juice, oregano, pimiento, garlic powder, and salt. Pour over beans; toss.

Yield: 5 servings

Exchange, 1 serving: 1 vegetable
Each serving contains: Calories: 32, Carbohydrates: 1 g

Whipped Summer Squash

3 c.	summer squash	750 mL
¼ c.	evaporated milk	60 mL
2 t.	butter	10 mL
	salt and pepper to taste	

Peel and cut squash into small pieces. Place in saucepan with small amount of water. Bring to a boil; reduce heat and simmer until squash is crisp-tender. Drain. Beat squash with rotary beater; add evaporated milk and butter. Beat until light and fluffy. Add salt and pepper.

Yield: 4 servings

Exchange, 1 serving: 1 vegetable, 1 fat
Each serving contains: Calories: 68, Carbohydrates: 7 g

Spiced Beets

½ c.	wine vinegar	125 mL
¼ c.	water	60 mL
1	bay leaf	1
1	whole clove	1
1 t.	black pepper	5 mL
3 T.	sugar replacement	45 mL
2 c.	beets, sliced	500 mL

Combine all ingredients except beets. Bring to a boil. Add beets; simmer for 10 minutes, or until tender.

Microwave: Combine all ingredients, except beets. Cook on High for 2 minutes. Add beets. Cook on Medium for 2 minutes.

Yield: 4 servings

Exchange, 1 serving: 1 bread
Each serving contains: Calories: 36, Carbohydrates: 9 g

Indian Squash

2 c.	acorn squash, cubed	500 mL
2 t.	margarine	10 mL
1 t.	orange rind	5 mL
¼ c.	orange juice	60 mL
2 T.	sugar replacement	30 mL

Cook squash in small amount of boiling water until crisp-tender; drain. Melt margarine in saucepan. Add orange rind, juice, and sugar replacement, Cook over low heat until sugar is dissolved. Add squash; cover. Continue cooking until squash is tender.

Yield: 4 servings

Exchange, 1 serving: 1 bread, ½ fat
Each serving contains: Calories: 60, Carbohydrates: 1 g

Asian Green Beans

1½ c.	French-cut green beans, cooked	375 mL
2 T.	almonds, blanched and slivered	30 mL
½ c.	mushroom pieces	125 mL
2 t.	butter	10 mL
	salt and pepper to taste	

Heat green beans; drain. Sauté almonds and mush-rooms in butter. Add green beans. Add salt and pepper.

Microwave: Melt butter in bowl. Add almonds and mushrooms. Cover. Cook on High for 30 seconds. Add green beans. Cook on Medium for 2 to 3 minutes.

Yield: 4 servings

Exchange, 1 serving: ½ vegetable, ½ fat
Each serving contains: Calories: 45, Carbohydrates: 5 g

Vegetable Casserole

1 c.	peas	250 mL
1 c.	green beans	250 mL
1 c.	carrots, sliced	250 mL
1 c.	mushrooms	250 mL
1	egg	1
1 t.	margarine, melted	5 mL
½ c.	milk	125 mL
	salt and pepper to taste	
	vegetable cooking spray	

Cook vegetables in small amount of boiling salted water until crisp-tender; drain. Chop vegetables fine. Whip egg until lemon colored; add margarine and milk. Blend well. Add chopped vegetables, salt, and pepper. Pour into baking dish coated with vegetable cooking spray. Cover. Bake at 350°F (175°C) for 45 minutes, or until set.

Yield: 8 servings

Exchange, 1 serving: 1 vegetable
Each serving contains: Calories: 36, Carbohydrates: 4 g

Pea Pod–Carrot Sauté

1 c.	pea pods	250 mL
1 c.	carrots, sliced	250 mL
1 t.	salt	5 mL
2 t.	margarine	10 mL
1 T.	Worcestershire sauce	15 mL

Combine pea pods and carrots in saucepan. Cover with water; add salt. Cook until tender; drain. Melt margarine in saucepan. Add Worcestershire sauce; stir to blend. Add pea pods and carrots. Toss to coat.

Yield: 4 servings

Exchange, 1 serving: ½ bread, ½ fat
Each serving contains: Calories: 50, Carbohydrates: 4 g

Circus Carrots

2 c.	carrots, finger- or julienne-cut	500 mL
2 t.	butter	10 mL
2 T.	lemon juice	30 mL
2 t.	parsley flakes	10 mL

Cook carrots in boiling salted water until tender; keep warm. Melt butter; add lemon juice and parsley flakes. Add warm carrots; toss to coat.

Microwave: Cook carrots in small amount of water on High for 2 minutes. Drain. Add remaining ingredients. Cover. Cook on High for 2 minutes. Toss to mix.

Yield: 4 servings

Exchange, 1 serving: ¼ fat, 1 bread
Each serving contains: Calories: 59, Carbohydrates: 4 g

Candied Carrot Squares

4	carrots	4
1 t.	salt	5 mL
2 T.	brown sugar replacement	30 mL
2 t.	butter	10 mL
½ c.	low-calorie cream soda	125 mL

Cut carrots into lengths to make squares. Place carrots in saucepan and cover with water; add salt. Cook until crisp-tender; drain. Place in baking dish. Sprinkle carrots with brown sugar replacement; dot with butter; add cream soda. Bake at 350°F (175°C) for 30 minutes. Turn carrots gently two or three times during baking.

Yield: 4 servings

Exchange, 1 serving: 1 bread, ½ fat
Each serving contains: Calories: 47, Carbohydrates: 14 g

Spinach with Onion

2 lb.	fresh spinach	1 kg
2 t.	margarine	10 mL
½ c.	onion, sliced	125 mL
dash each	nutmeg, thyme, salt, pepper	dash each

Rinse spinach thoroughly; place in top of double boiler and heat until wilted. Drain and chop coarsely. Melt margarine in skillet; add onion. Sauté over high heat until onion is brown on the edges. Add seasonings. Stir to blend. Add spinach and toss to blend.

Yield: 4 servings

Exchange, 1 serving: ½ vegetable, ½ fat
Each serving contains: Calories: 37, Carbohydrates: 36 g

Zucchini Florentine

4 small	zucchini	4 small
2 t.	margarine	10 mL
1 c.	fresh spinach, chopped	250 mL
1 c.	skim milk	250 mL
3	eggs, slightly beaten	3
1 t.	salt	5 ml
¼ t.	pepper	1 mL
¼ t.	thyme	1 mL
¼ t.	paprika	1 mL

Cut zucchini into thin slices. Melt margarine in baking dish; add zucchini. Bake at 400°F (200°C) for 15 minutes. Add spinach. Blend skim milk, eggs, salt, pepper, and thyme. Pour over vegetables. Sprinkle with paprika. Bake at 350°F (175°C) for 40 minutes, or until set.

Yield: 6 servings

Exchange, 1 serving: 1 vegetable, ½ high-fat meat
Each serving contains: Calories: 82, Carbohydrates: 6 g

Zucchini Wedges

4 small	zucchini	4 small
2 t.	margarine	10 mL
2 t.	onion, grated	10 mL
1 cube	beef bouillon	1 cube
2 T.	boiling water	30 mL

Cut zucchini in half lengthwise. Melt margarine in skillet. Add onion and bouillon cube. Press bouillon cube against bottom of skillet to crush. Stir to blend. Place zucchini cut side down in skillet. Sauté until golden brown; turn. Add boiling water; cover. Cook over low heat for 10 minutes, or until tender.

Yield: 4 servings

Exchange, 1 serving: ½ vegetable, ½ fat
Each serving contains: Calories: 37

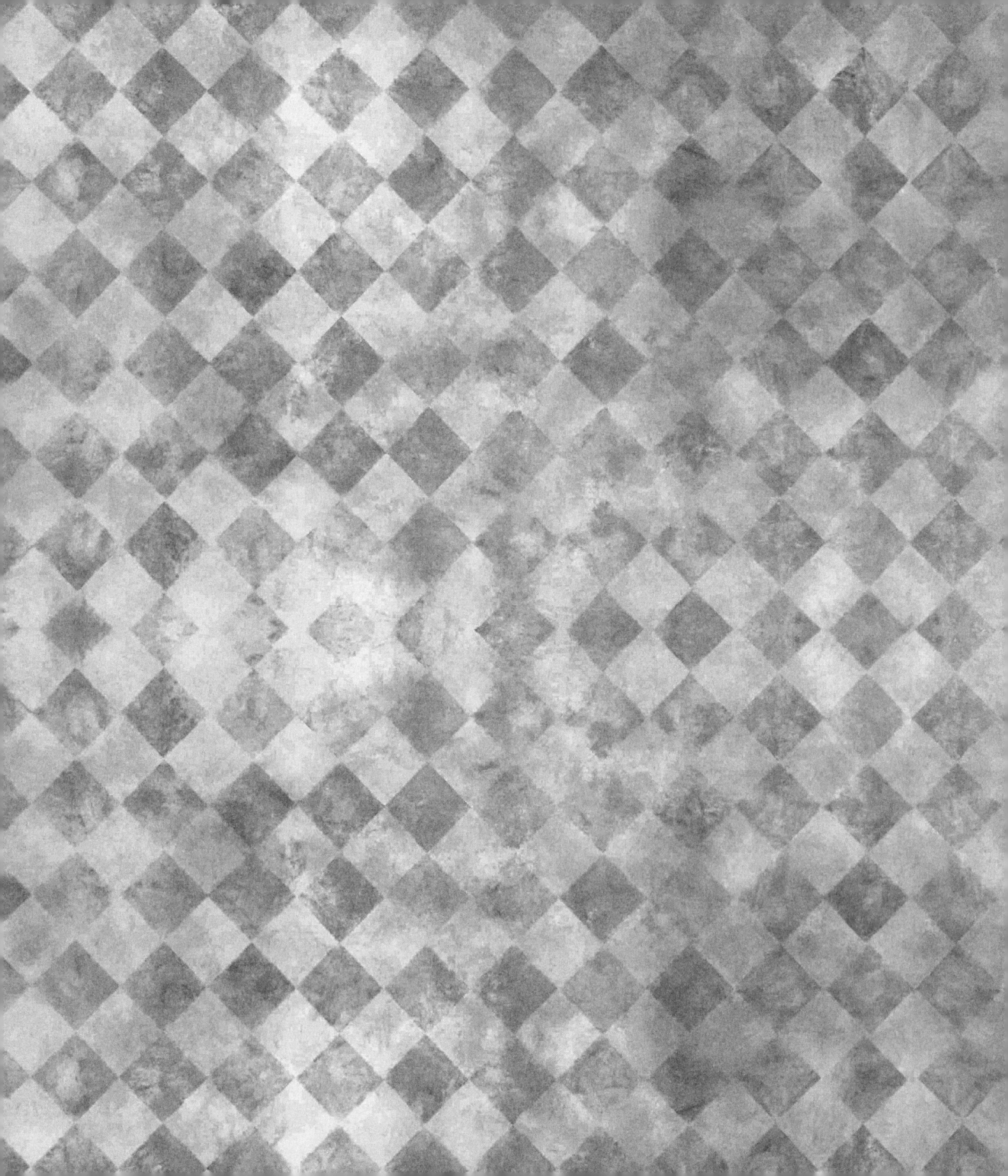

Poultry

Turkey Breast

A real calorie and exchange saver.

2 lbs.	turkey breast	1 kg
2 T.	low-calorie margarine, melted	30 mL
	salt and pepper to taste	
	paprika	

Place turkey breast, skin side up, in a baking dish. Add small amount of water to pan. Season with salt and pepper to taste; cover tightly. Bake at 325°F (165°C) for 45 to 60 minutes or until meat is tender. Remove from oven. Discard the skin. Brush with melted margarine and sprinkle lightly with paprika. Place under broiler until just slightly browned. Serve hot or cold in slices.

Yield: 18 servings

Exchange, 1 serving: 1 lean meat
Each serving contains: Calories: 56, Carbohydrates: negligible

Turkey Legs

Turkey is low in calories and tasty, and turkey legs and thighs are usually inexpensive.

4 lbs.	turkey legs and thighs	2 kg
¼ c.	low-calorie margarine	60 mL
2	garlic cloves, minced	2
1	onion, sliced and separated into rings	1
2 c.	celery, sliced	500 mL
1½ c.	carrots, sliced	375 mL
2 c.	water	500 mL
1 t.	salt	5 mL
¼ t.	black pepper	1 mL
1 T.	all-purpose flour	15 mL

Cut turkey legs from the thighs. Brown turkey in margarine in a large skillet; remove turkey from pan. Add the garlic, onion, celery, and carrots to skillet and sauté until onions are soft. Stir in the water, salt, and pepper. Place turkey back in skillet. Bring to the boil, reduce heat, and cover. Simmer for 3 hours or until turkey is very tender. Remove turkey from pan; strain the juice. Cool turkey and remove meat from bones; discard turkey skin and bones and vegetables. Refrigerate the juice. (This much can be done the day before.) Skim and discard any fat from the turkey juice. Spoon into skillet. Heat until just melted. Blend in flour. Add turkey pieces to skillet. Cook and stir until mixture is hot and thick. Spoon into heated serving dish.

Yield: 10 servings

Exchange, 1 serving: 1½ lean meat
Each serving contains: Calories: 92, Carbohydrates: 2 g

Baked Turkey and Eggplant

1	eggplant, large	1
	salt	
1½ c.	onion, chopped	375 mL
1 T.	low-calorie margarine	15 mL
1 lb.	ground turkey	500 g
2 c.	tomatoes, chopped	500 mL
1 t.	paprika	1 mL
1 t.	ground nutmeg	5 mL
½ t.	black pepper	2 mL

Topping

1 c.	fresh bread crumbs, soft	250 mL
1 T.	low-calorie margarine	15 mL
¼ c.	cheddar cheese, grated	60 mL

Wash and slice the eggplant; sprinkle with salt and set aside. Sauté the onion in margarine; add the tomatoes and sauté for 3 minutes. Add the turkey, paprika, nutmeg, and black pepper. Cook and stir until turkey is browned. Drain eggplant and rinse in cold water. In a flat baking dish, alternate layers of turkey mixture and eggplant. Cover and bake at 350°F (175°C) for 30 minutes. Combine the bread crumbs, margarine and cheese; sprinkle on top of turkey and eggplant. Bake, uncovered, for 10 minutes more.

Yield: 10 servings

Exchange, 1 serving: 1 medium-fat meat, ¼ bread
Each serving contains: Calories: 95, Carbohydrates: 3 g

Scalloped Turkey and Cauliflower

2 c.	fresh cauliflower, broken into florets	500 mL
1½ c.	turkey stock	375 mL
2 T.	whole wheat flour	30 mL
1 t.	parsley flakes	5 mL
2 t.	onion flakes	10 mL
1 t.	salt	5 mL
¼ t.	black pepper	1 mL
½ lb.	turkey breast, cooked	250 g

Cook cauliflower in boiling, salted water for 6 minutes or until almost tender. Drain. Combine stock, flour and seasonings in a small saucepan. Cook and stir until mixture is slightly thickened. Place turkey breast in a greased baking pan. Arrange cauliflower around turkey breast. Pour sauce over turkey and cauliflower. Bake in a 350°F (175°C) oven for 20 to 25 minutes or until heated through.

Yield: 4 servings

Exchange, 1 serving: 1 medium-fat meat, 1 vegetable
Each serving contains: Calories: 112, Carbohydrates: 8 g

Turkey Divan

10 oz. pkg.	frozen broccoli spears	285 g pkg.
½ lb.	unsalted, cooked turkey breast, thickly sliced	250 g
2 pkg.	Estee low-sodium mushroom soup mix	2 pkg.
½ c.	skim milk	125 mL
⅓ c.	cheddar cheese, shredded	90 mL

Cook broccoli until just tender as directed on package; drain. With stems towards the middle, arrange broccoli in a 1½ qt. (1½ L) casserole or round 9 in. (23 cm) baking dish. Place turkey slices in an even layer on top. Combine soup mix with ½ c. (125 mL) boiling water. Blend in milk and cheese. Pour sauce over turkey. Bake at 375°F (190°C) for 25 minutes or until sauce begins to bubble.

Yield: 4 servings

Exchange, 1 serving: 2½ lean meat, 1 vegetable
Each serving contains: Calories: 140, Carbohydrates: 12 g

For you from The Estee Corporation.

Country Style Chicken Loaf

2 c.	chicken, cooked	500 mL
1 c.	bread crumbs	50 mL
½ c.	skim milk, warmed	125 mL
1	egg	1
½ c.	carrot, grated	125 mL
½ c.	celery, finely chopped	125 mL
2 T.	onion, minced	30 mL
2 T.	green pepper, finely chopped	30 mL
1 t.	salt	5 mL
¼ t.	black pepper	1 mL
10 oz. can	cream of mushroom soup	304 g can
¼ can	water	¼ can
5	mushrooms, sliced	5

Combine chicken, bread crumbs, milk, and egg in a food processor. With the steel blade, mix until blended. Pour into a bowl. Add carrot, celery, onion, green pepper, salt, and pepper. Stir to mix thoroughly. Place in well-greased loaf pan. Bake at 350°F (175°C) for 40 minutes or until firm. About 10 minutes before serving, combine soup, water, and sliced mushrooms in a saucepan. Heat over low heat until fresh mushrooms are limp. Serve in a separate dish with chicken loaf.

Yield: 8 servings

Exchange, 1 serving: 1 lean meat, 1 bread
Each serving contains: Calories: 137, Carbohydrates: 13 g

Cold Chicken Ring

This is a particularly nice recipe for a group because it can be made at least a day ahead.

3 c.	chicken, cooked	750 mL
2 c.	skim milk, hot	500 mL
1 c.	bread crumbs, dry	250 mL
2	eggs, slightly beaten	2
½ c.	celery, chopped	125 mL
1	green pepper, chopped	1
1 T.	lemon juice	15 mL
1 t.	Worcestershire sauce	5 mL
½ t.	salt	2 mL
¼ t.	paprika	1 mL

In a bowl, combine ingredients in the order listed. Stir until bread is moist. Place a damp cloth over bowl and allow to sit for 1 hour. Spoon mixture into well-greased ring mold. Bake at 300°F (150°C) for 45 to 60 minutes or until knife inserted in middle comes out clean. Allow to rest 10 to 15 minutes before unmolding. Cool completely. Place chicken ring on a serving plate. Wrap tightly with plastic wrap. Refrigerate until ready to use.

Yield: 12 servings

Exchange, 1 serving: 1 lean meat, ⅔ bread
Each serving contains: Calories: 109, Carbohydrates: 8 g

Sweet and Sour Chicken

It's a good idea to brown the chicken and make the sauce the day before and store them in the refrigerator until ready to bake. You can double this recipe for a group. Add only 45 minutes more cooking time when doubling, or chicken will be too well done.

2	bacon slices	2
2 lbs.	chicken	1 kg
½ c.	water	125 mL
1 c.	Fruit-Full Pineapple Preserves	250 mL
1	onion	1
1 T.	vinegar	15 mL
½	sweet red pepper	½

In a skillet, fry the bacon until crisp; set bacon aside and discard the fat. Cut chicken in serving-sized pieces. In the same skillet over low heat, thoroughly brown each chicken piece; do not crowd pan. Discard fat as it accumulates. Place chicken in a flat casserole that has been coated with vegetable spray. Add the water to the skillet. With a wooden spoon, scrape up any browned residue on the bottom. Place skillet over low heat; add the pineapple preserves and stir until dissolved. Cut onion across into eighths and separate the ring slices. Add to skillet and stir in the vinegar. Cover and simmer for 5 minutes. Cut red pepper into chunks; add to sauce. Cover and simmer until onion is translucent. Cut bacon slices into large squares; add to the sauce. Pour sauce over chicken; cover tightly. Bake at 325°F (165°C) for 1 hour.

Yield: 10 servings

Exchange, 1 serving: 1 medium-fat meat, ½ fruit
Each serving contains: Calories: 99, Carbohydrates: 7 g

Savory Chicken Breasts

2 (4 oz. each)	boneless chicken breasts	2 (120 g each)
6	pressed ham slices	6
½ oz.	Port du Salut cheese	15 g
4	saltine crackers	4
¼ t.	basil	1 mL
⅛ t.	fennel, finely crushed	½ mL
1	egg	1
1 T.	water	15 mL
1½ t.	cider vinegar	2 mL
	vegetable oil for frying	

Remove skins from the chicken breasts. With a flat plate or platter, press the chicken as flat as possible. Place 3 slices of ham on each breast. Lay cheese on top, in the middle of ham. Enfold the cheese: fold one side of chicken and ham over the cheese; fold in the ends; fold over other side. Wrap tightly in plastic wrap; place in freezer until slightly frozen. Meanwhile, crush saltines in a blender until very fine; pour into bottom of a flat dish. Stir in the basil and fennel. Combine egg, water, and vinegar in another flat bowl; beat to blend. Remove chicken from plastic wrap and roll in egg mixture. With your hand, remove any excess egg. Roll chicken in cracker crumbs. Wrap in plastic wrap and place in freezer until slightly frozen. Heat oil to 365°F (184°C). Remove plastic and fry chicken in deep oil until deep brown.

Yield: 2 servings

Exchange, 1 serving: 1¾ lean meat
Each serving contains: Calories: 98, Carbohydrates: 2 g

Festive Party Chicken

12 6 oz.	chicken breasts	12 180 g
1½ qts.	long-grain rice, cooked	1½ L
1½ c.	golden raisins	375 mL
2¼ c.	salt	11 mL
4 5 oz. cans	La Choy chow mein noodles	4 150 g cans
6 T.	butter, melted	90 mL
7½ c.	pineapple chunks in their juice	1875 mL
4 c.	mandarin oranges	1 L
1½ T.	lemon juice	22 mL
6 T.	cornstarch	90 mL
6 T.	La Choy soy sauce	90 mL
6 T.	butter, cut into bits	90 mL
2 8 oz. cans	La Choy water chestnuts, drained and sliced	2 240 g cans

Cut chicken breasts in half, remove bones and cut through thickest part of each piece to form a pocket. In a bowl, mix rice, raisins, salt and 3 c. (750 mL) of the chow mein noodles. Stuff ½ c. (125 mL) of the mixture into each breast; fasten with toothpicks and tie with string. Place chicken in buttered shallow baking pans and brush with melted butter; bake at 350°F (175°C) for 30 minutes. In a heavy pan, drain juice from pineapple and oranges and blend with lemon juice, cornstarch and soy sauce. Cook over medium heat, stirring constantly until sauce is thick and transparent. Remove from heat and add butter, pineapple, oranges and water chestnuts; mix well. Spoon over chicken and cover with aluminum foil. Bake at 325°F (165°C) for 30 minutes longer or until chicken is tender. Remove toothpicks and string. Serve sauce over chicken with remaining noodles on the side.

Yield: 24 servings

Exchange, 1 serving: 1 bread, 3 lean meat
Each serving contains: Calories: 220, Carbohydrates: 58 g

Sweet Chicken

The sweet touches of pineapple and cherries add flavor and fiber to this colorful entrée.

2 T.	margarine	30 mL
4 4 oz.	chicken breasts, boned	4 120 g
16 oz. can	tart cherries	454 g can
8 oz. can	crushed pineapple in its own juice	227 g can
¼ c.	dry sherry	60 mL
2 T.	soy sauce	30 mL
1 clove	garlic, minced	1 clove
1 T.	ginger, chopped	15 mL
1 c.	celery, sliced	250 mL
½ c.	sweet red pepper, cut into chunks	125 mL
1 T.	cornstarch	15 mL
¼ c.	water	60 mL

Melt margarine in a skillet and brown chicken breasts. Drain juices from cherries and pineapple into a mixing bowl. Reserve the fruit and add sherry, soy sauce, garlic and ginger to the juices. Stir to blend. Pour juice mixture over chicken. Cover and simmer 30 minutes. Remove chicken to warm serving dish and keep hot. Combine cherries, pineapple, celery, and red pepper in the pan. Dissolve cornstarch in the water and stir into pan. Cook and stir until mixture thickens. Pour over chicken.

Yield: 4 servings

Exchange, 1 serving: 2 fruit, 1 high-fat meat
Each serving contains: Calories: 188, Carbohydrates: 3 g

Crowned Chicken Breasts

3 T.	margarine	45 mL
4 4 oz.	chicken breasts, boned	4 120 g
2 T.	celery, very finely chopped	30 mL
1 T.	onion, very finely chopped	15 mL
1 lb.	mushrooms	500 g
2 t.	flour	10 mL

Melt 1 T. (15 mL) of the margarine in a nonstick skillet. Curl or roll breasts and fasten with toothpicks or poultry pins. Over low heat, brown chicken breasts on all sides. Lift and place breasts, skin side up in a 10 in. (25 cm) pie pan. Remove toothpicks or pins. In the same skillet, melt 1 T. (15 mL) of the margarine. Add celery and onion; cook and stir until onion is tender. Slice mushrooms in half (if mushrooms are large, slice into thirds). Add mushrooms to pan and continue cooking: occasionally flip with a spatula until mushrooms are partially tender. Remove celery, onion and mushrooms from pan and set aside. Melt remaining 1 T. (15 mL) margarine in the skillet and stir in the flour. Cook and stir until flour is brown. Add enough water to make a thin sauce. Return mushrooms to skillet and stir to mix. Pour mushroom sauce over chicken breasts. Cover with aluminum foil. Bake at 300°F (150°C) for 40 to 45 minutes.

Yield: 4 servings

Exchange, 1 serving: 2 high-fat meat
Each serving contains: Calories: 205, Carbohydrates: 13 g

Bran Parmesan Chicken

1½ c.	Kellogg's branflakes cereal	375 mL
1	egg	1
¼ c.	milk	60 mL
¼ c.	all-purpose flour	60 mL
dash	salt	dash
dash	pepper	dash
¼ t.	ground sage	1 mL
3 T.	Parmesan cheese, grated	45 mL
1 lb.	chicken, cut in pieces	500 g
1 T.	margarine, melted	15 mL

Crush enough cereal to measure ¾ c. (190 mL) in a shallow dish. Lightly beat together the egg and milk. Add flour, salt, pepper, sage, and cheese. stirring until smooth. Dip chicken pieces in the egg mixture. Coat with crushed cereal. Place in a single layer, skin side up, in greased or foil-lined, shallow baking pan. Drizzle with margarine. Bake, uncovered, at 350°F (175°C) for about 45 minutes or until tender, without turning chicken while baking.

Yield: 4 servings

Exchange, 1 serving: 1 bread, 3 lean meat, 1 fat
Each serving contains: Calories: 272, Carbohydrates: 13 g

From Kellogg's Test Kitchens.

Crispy Wheat Germ Chicken

1 c.	Kretschmer regular wheat germ	250 mL
1 t.	dried tarragon, crushed*	5 mL
1 t.	lemon rind, grated*	5 mL
¼ c.	milk	60 mL
3 lb.	broiler-fryer chicken, cut up and skinned	1 ½ kg

Combine wheat germ, tarragon and lemon rind in a shallow container. Stir well to blend. Pour milk into another shallow container. Dip chicken pieces in milk, then in wheat germ mixture, coating evenly. Place on foil-lined 15½ × 10½ × 1 in. (39 × 25 × 3 cm) jelly roll pan. Bake, uncovered, at 375°F (190°C) for 40 to 50 minutes until tender.

Yield: 4 servings

Exchange, 1 serving: 1 bread, 5 lean meat
Each serving contains: Calories: 357, Carbohydrates: 15 g

* One teaspoon crushed oregano and a dash of garlic powder may be used instead of the tarragon and lemon rind.

With the courtesy of Kretschmer Wheat Germ/International Multifoods.

Chicken El Dorado

½ c.	chicken broth	125 mL
½ oz.	fresh oysters	15 g
1 t.	margarine	5 mL
1 T.	carrot, grated	15 mL
2 T.	celery, chopped	30 mL
1 t.	parsley, chopped	5 mL
1 oz.	cooked chicken, diced	30 g
	salt and pepper to taste	

Heat chicken broth to a boil; add oysters. Cook until edges roll; drain. Heat margarine in heavy skillet. Add carrot, celery, and parsley. Sauté until crisp-tender. Add chicken, oysters, and 1 T. (15 mL) of the chicken broth. Cook until thoroughly heated. Drain, if necessary. Add salt and pepper.

Yield: 1 serving

Exchange, 1 serving: 1½ lean meat, 2 fat
Each serving contains: Calories: 80, Carbohydrates: 3 g

Chicken Livers

3 oz.	chicken livers	90 g
½ c.	skim milk	125 mL
2 T.	flour	30 mL
	salt and pepper to taste	
2 t.	margarine	10 mL

Soak chicken livers in skim milk overnight. Drain. Combine flour, salt, and pepper in shaker bag. Add livers, one at a time; shake to coat. Remove livers from bag and shake off excess flour. Melt margarine in small skillet; add livers. Cook until lightly browned and tender.

Yield: 1 serving

Exchange, 1 serving: 3 lean meat, 2 fat
Each serving contains: Calories: 190, Carbohydrates: 3 g

Duck with Pineapple

3 lbs.	duck	1½ kg
2 c.	boiling water	500 mL
2 T.	soy sauce	30 mL
1 lb. can	pineapple chunks with the juice	454 g can
	salt and pepper to taste	

Cut duck into serving pieces; wash thoroughly. Place in a saucepan and cover with boiling water. Simmer for about 45 minutes or until almost tender. Add soy sauce, juice from pineapple chunks (reserve the chunks), salt, and pepper. Simmer 30 minutes longer; drain. Place on heated serving dish. Top with pineapple chunks.

Yield: 12 servings

Exchange, 1 serving: 2½ high-fat meat, ½ fruit
Each serving contains: Calories: 268, Carbohydrates: 6 g

Roast Duck à l'Orange

4 to 5 lb.	duck	2 to 3 kg	
2 med.	oranges	2 med.	
	salt to taste		
	Orange Sauce		

Wash inside and outside of duck thoroughly. Remove any fat from tail or neck opening. Salt interior of bird. Cut each orange (with peel) into 8 sections. Place inside of duck. Secure tail and neck skin, legs and wings with poultry pins. Salt exterior of duck. Place breast side up on a rack in roasting pan. Bake at 350°F (175°C) for 4 hours. During the final hour, baste with Orange Sauce every 15 minutes.

Exchange, 1 oz. (30 g): 1 high-fat meat
Each serving contains: Calories: 96, Carbohydrates: 11 g

Roast Goose

5 to 6 lb.	goose	2½ to 3 kg	
	salt to taste		

Wash and dry goose thoroughly. Salt cavity and exterior. Fill cavity loosely with stuffing. Close cavity and secure tightly. Place breast side up in roasting pan. Roast at 350°F (175°C) for 30 to 40 minutes per pound, or about 3 to 4 hours. Cover with a loose tent of aluminum foil for the last hour to prevent excess browning.

Yield: 8 to 10 servings

Exchange, 1 oz. (30 g): 1 high-fat meat (without skin)
Each serving contains: Calories: 120 (without skin), Carbohydrates: 0 g

Pork, Beef, and Sausages

Pork Tenderloin with Apricots

1½ lbs.	pork tenderloin	750 g
¼ 1b.	dried apricots	140 g

With a sharp knife, cut tenderloin in half lengthwise and flatten. Cut tenderloin in half across the grain. In a saucepan, cook apricots in a small amount of water until very soft. Drain and process to a purée in a blender. Spread apricot purée on one half of the tenderloin. Cover with remaining half of tenderloin. Secure sides together with poultry pins along the edges. Bake at 350°F (175°C) for 1 hour or until done.

Yield: 10 servings

Exchange, 1 serving: 2⅓ medium-fat meat, ¼ fruit
Each serving contains: Calories: 204, Carbohydrates: 8 g

Mushroom-Stuffed Pork Chops

2 T.	mushroom pieces	30 mL
1 t.	onion, chopped	5 mL
½ t.	parsley, chopped	2 mL
1 t.	raisins, soaked	5 mL
¼ t.	nutmeg	1 mL
1	double pork chop	1

Combine ingredients for stuffing; stir to blend. Split meaty part of chop down to bone; do not split through bone. Fill with stuffing; secure with poultry pins. Place on baking sheet. Bake uncovered at 350°F (175°C) for 35 to 40 minutes, or until tender. Turn once.

Yield: 1 chop

Exchange, 1 oz. (30 g): 1 high-fat meat
Each serving contains: Calories: 109, Carbohydrates: 12 g

Teriyaki Pork Steak

1	pork steak, thinly sliced	1
½ c.	soy sauce	125 mL
1 T.	wine vinegar	15 mL
2 T.	lemon juice	30 mL
¼ c.	water	60 mL
2 T.	sugar replacement	30 mL
1½ t.	ginger	7 mL
½ t.	garlic powder	2 mL

Place slices of pork steak in shallow dish. Combine remaining ingredients; pour over pork. Marinate 1 to 2 hours; turn once. Broil pork 5 to 6 inches (12 to 15 cm) from heat, for 2–3 minutes per side. Turn and broil second side.

Exchange, 1 oz. (30 g): 1 medium-fat meat
Each serving contains: Calories: 89, Carbohydrates: 21 g

Sesame Pork

8	lean side pork slices	8
1	egg, slightly beaten	1
2 T.	skim milk	30 mL
3 T.	all-purpose flour	45 mL
2 T.	sesame seeds	30 mL
½ t.	salt	2 mL
⅛ t.	black pepper	1/2 mL

Cut each slice of side pork in half. In a bowl, combine the egg and milk; stir to blend. Combine the flour, sesame seeds, salt, and pepper in another bowl. Dip the side pork pieces in the egg mixture. Then roll in the flour mixture. Place in a flat baking dish. Bake uncovered at 350°F (175°C) for 30 to 40 minutes or until brown and crispy.

Yield: 16 servings

Exchange, 1 serving: ½ high-fat meat
Each serving contains: Calories: 55, Carbohydrates: 1 g

Smoked Loin of Pork and Kielbasa

These two meats cooked together make a classic combination.

2 lbs.	boneless smoked pork loin	1
1	onion, chopped	1
2	garlic cloves, chopped	2
1 c.	sauerkraut juice	250 mL
1 c.	dry red wine	250 mL
1 recipe	Kielbasa, prepared in links in casings	1 recipe

Place smoked pork loin in a large saucepan. Cover with water and bring to the boil; reduce heat and simmer for 30 minutes. Drain. Add remaining ingredients to saucepan. Bring to the boil; reduce heat and simmer for 20 minutes. Remove meats to a heated serving platter. Cut the loin and kielbasa into very thin slices.

Yield: 20 servings

Exchange, 1 serving: 2 medium-fat meat
Each serving contains: Calories: 152, Carbohydrates: 2 g

Sweet and Sour Smoked Pork Chops

8 (2 lbs.)	smoked pork chops	8 (1 kg.)
2 T.	olive oil	30 mL
1 c.	chicken broth	250 mL
3 T.	cornstarch	45 mL
2 T.	soy sauce	30 mL
2 T.	granulated brown sugar replacement	30 mL
2 T.	cider vinegar	30 mL
1	green pepper, sliced	1
1	white onion, chopped	1
1 c.	fresh pineapple chunks	250 mL

In a skillet, brown chops on both sides in the olive oil. Add the broth and cover; simmer for 20 minutes. Combine cornstarch, soy sauce, brown sugar replacement, and vinegar in a bowl; stir to blend. Add to pan, stirring until thickened. Add the green pepper, onion, and pineapple. Cover and simmer for 5 to 10 minutes or until heated.

Yield: 8 servings

Exchange, 1 serving: 2 high-fat meat, ⅓ fruit
Each serving contains: Calories: 227, Carbohydrates: 4 g

Pork Cube Sauté

Easy to make for a quick meal.

⅓ c.	all-purpose flour	90 mL
1 t.	salt	5 mL
¼ t.	black pepper	1 mL
1 lb.	pork, cut in bite-sized cubes	500 g
2 T.	olive oil	30 mL
1	garlic clove, finely chopped	1
½ t.	rosemary	2 mL

Combine the flour, salt, and pepper in a shaker bag. Add the pork cubes and shake to coat with flour mixture. Shake off any excess. Heat olive oil in nonstick skillet. Add the garlic and rosemary. Add pork cubes and sauté until golden brown on all sides. Pour entire contents of skillet into a baking dish. Bake uncovered at 350°F (175°C) for 20 to 25 minutes.

Yield: 6 servings

Exchange, 1 serving: 1½ high-fat meat, ⅓ bread
Each serving contains: Calories: 168, Carbohydrates: 5 g

Sweet Ham Steak

1 lb.	lean ham steak	500 g
1 t.	white wine vinegar	5 mL
1 T.	granulated brown sugar replacement	15 mL
1 c.	water, boiling	250 mL
¼ c.	cream sherry	60 mL

Rub both sides of the ham steak with vinegar and sprinkle with brown sugar replacement. Allow to stand for 15 minutes at room temperature. Spray a nonstick skillet with vegetable cooking spray. Brown ham on both sides. Add the boiling water and sherry. Cook slowly, uncovered, until liquid has almost evaporated and ham is tender.

Yield: 4 servings

Exchange, 1 serving: 2 ¼ medium-fat meat
Each serving contains: Calories: 180, Carbohydrates: 2 g

Ham Corncake

1 T.	margarine	15 mL
¼ c.	onion, chopped	60 mL
¼ c.	green pepper, chopped	60 mL
1¼ c.	Featherweight corn flour	310 mL
½ c.	Featherweight oat flour	125 mL
5 t.	Featherweight baking powder	25 mL
1	salt	5 mL
1	egg, beaten	1
1 c.	milk	250 mL
3 T.	margarine, melted	45 mL
8 oz. can	Featherweight golden corn, drained	227 g can
16 oz. can	Featherweight ham, drained and chopped	454 g can
	Cheese Sauce (recipe follows)	

Melt 1 T. (15 mL) margarine in a saucepan. Add onion and green pepper: cook until tender. Set aside to cool. In a bowl, combine dry ingredients—corn flour, oat flour, baking powder and salt. In another bowl, beat together the egg, milk and 3 T. (45 mL) melted margarine; add to dry ingredients and mix well. Add cooked onion and green pepper, corn and ham: stir to mix. Turn into a greased 9 × 9 × 2 in. (23 × 23 × 5 cm) pan. Bake at 400°F (200°C) about 30 minutes or until lightly browned. Serve hot with Cheese Sauce.

Yield: 6 servings

Exchange, 1 serving with Cheese Sauce: 2 bread, 3 medium-fat meat
Each serving contains: Calories: 374, Carbohydrates: 40 g

Cheese Sauce

2 T.	margarine	30 mL
1 T.	cornstarch	15 mL
½ t	Featherweight mustard	1 mL
1 c.	milk	250 mL
½ c.	Featherweight cheddar cheese, shredded	125 mL

Melt margarine in a saucepan. Blend in cornstarch. Remove from heat. Mix in mustard. Add milk gradually, stirring until smooth. Cook and stir over medium heat until mixture boils; boil 1 minute. Add cheese and stir until cheese melts. Serve hot.

Yield: 6 2⅔ T. or 40 mL servings

Exchange, 1 serving: 1 high-fat meat
Each serving contains: Calories: 101, Carbohydrates: 5 g

Based on recipes from Featherweight Brand Foods.

Steak Roberto

¼ c.	margarine	60 mL
1 t.	garlic powder	5 mL
1 lb.	beef tenderloin (8 slices)	500 g
½ t.	steak sauce	3 mL
¼ t.	bay leaf, crushed	1 mL
1 T.	lemon juice	15 mL
½ t.	salt	2 mL
dash	pepper	dash

Melt margarine and combine with garlic powder. Set aside for 20 minutes to allow flavor to develop. Heat 1 T. (15 mL) of the garlic margarine in heavy skillet until very hot. Place as many beef tenderloin slices as possible in skillet; brown on both sides. Remove to warm steak platter. Repeat with remaining beef, if necessary. Reduce heat. Add remaining garlic margarine to pan. Add steak sauce, bay leaf, lemon juice, salt, and pepper; blend thoroughly. Pour over beef tenderloin on platter.

Yield: 8 servings

Exchange, 1 serving: 2 medium-fat meat, ½ fat
Each serving contains: Calories: 155, Carbohydrates: 0 g

Swiss Steak

1 t.	margarine	5 mL
3 oz.	beef minute steak	90 g
	salt and pepper to taste	
¼ c.	celery, sliced	60 mL
1 T.	onion, chopped	15 mL
¼ c.	tomato, crushed	60 mL
¼ c.	water	60 mL

Heat margarine until very hot. Salt and pepper the steak. Brown both sides; drain. Place in individual baking dish. Add salt, pepper, and remaining ingredients. Cover. Bake at 375°F (175°C) for 1 hour, or until steak is tender.

Microwave: Cook on High 8 to 10 minutes. Uncover at last minute.

Yield: 1 serving

Exchange, 1 serving: 3 medium-fat meat, 1 fat
Each serving contains: Calories: 220, Carbohydrates: 14 g

Steak Hawaiian

3 oz.	beef top round steak, sliced	90 g
½ t.	mace	2 mL
2 T.	unsweetened pineapple juice	30 mL
1	pineapple slice, unsweetened	1

Pound slices of round steak with mallet or edge of plate until thin. Sprinkle both sides with mace. Place in aluminum foil. Sprinkle with pineapple juice; top with pineapple slice. Secure foil tightly. Place in baking dish. Bake at 350°F (175°C) for 40 to 45 minutes.

Microwave: Place in plastic wrap. Cook on High for 10 to 12 minutes.

Yield: 1 serving

Exchange, 1 serving: 3 lean meat, 1 fruit
Each serving contains: Calories: 200, Carbohydrates: 10 g

Breakfast Steak Roll-Ups

4 oz. (4 slices)	breakfast steaks (from beef sirloin tip)	120 g (4 slices)	
½ lb.	spinach	250 g	
1	garlic clove, chopped	1	
3 T.	onion, chopped	45 mL	
dash	lemon juice	dash	
dash	salt and pepper	dash	
10 oz. can	cream of mushroom soup	304 g can	
½ c.	water	125 mL	

Place steaks between wax paper. With a rolling pin, roll steaks as flat as possible. Combine spinach, garlic, onion, and lemon juice in a saucepan with a small amount of water. Cook until spinach is limp. Drain and cool. Wring spinach with your hands to remove any excess water. Chop in a food processor or with a knife until fine. Divide evenly among the 4 beef slices; roll up. Place in a lightly greased pan. Combine the soup and ½ c. (125 mL) water in a bowl; stir to blend. Pour over steaks. Bake at 350°F (175°C) for 30 to 40 minutes.

Yield: 4 servings

Exchange, 1 serving: 1 lean meat, 1 vegetable, ½ fat
Each serving contains: Calories: 98, Carbohydrates: 5 g

Brisket of Beef with Horseradish

3 to 4 lb.	beef brisket	1½ to 2 kg	
	salt and pepper to taste		
1 med.	onion, sliced	1 med.	
1	bay leaf	1	
1 T.	lemon juice	15 mL	
½ c.	horseradish, grated	125 mL	
	salt and pepper to taste		

Place brisket in large kettle; add salt and pepper. Add onion, bay leaf, and enough water to cover brisket. Bring to a boil. Reduce heat and simmer for 2 hours. Remove brisket from water. Combine lemon juice and horseradish. Rub surface of brisket with horseradish mixture. Return brisket to kettle; cover. Cook 1 hour longer.

Exchange, 1 oz. (30 g): 1 medium-fat meat
Each serving contains: Calories: 84, Carbohydrates: 2 g

Beef with Vegetables

½ lb.	round steak (13 mm) thick	250 g	
2	yellow onions	2	
4	tomatoes	4	
1	green pepper	1	
¼ c.	water	60 mL	
1 T.	soy sauce	15 mL	
2 t.	cornstarch	10 mL	
½ t.	salt	2 mL	
3 T.	vegetable oil	45 mL	
1 slice	ginger root	1 slice	

Cut steak across the grain into ⅛ in. (3 mm) thick and 2 in. (5 cm) long strips. Slice onions, tomatoes and green pepper into ½ in. (1.3 cm) wedges. Combine water, soy sauce, cornstarch, salt and 1 t. (5 mL) of the oil. Stir to blend and set aside. Heat remaining oil in wok or skillet; add beef strips and the ginger root. Stir and cook until well-browned. Add onions and stir-fry 1 minute. Add pepper and stir-fry 1 minute longer. Stir in cornstarch mixture and cook until sauce is clear. Add tomatoes and heat slightly.

Yield: 4 servings

Exchange, 1 serving: 1 vegetable, 2 medium-fat meat, ½ fat
Each serving contains: Calories: 202, Carbohydrates: 11 g

Beef with Cauliflower

½ lb.	flank steak	250 g
1 t.	salt	5 mL
1 T.	cornstarch	15 mL
3 T.	soy sauce	45 mL
1 large	yellow onion	1 large
2	carrots, peeled	2
½ head	cauliflower, cleaned	½ head
4 T.	vegetable oil	60 mL
2 cloves	garlic, crushed	2 cloves
½ t.	sesame seeds	2 mL
½ c.	water	125 mL

Trim off any fat from the steak. Cut across grain into ⅛ in. (3 mm) strips. Put meat in a mixing bowl, add salt, 1 t. (5 mL) of the cornstarch and 2 t. (10 mL) of the soy sauce. Stir to marinate meat; set aside for 30 minutes, stirring occasionally. Meanwhile, cut onion in half lengthwise; lay cut side down and slice crosswise ¼ in. (6 mm) slices. Place onions in a separate bowl. Cut carrots in half on a long diagonal; slice on the diagonal into ¼ in. (6 mm) slices. Put carrots in a separate bowl. Cut cauliflower on the diagonal into ¼ in. (6 mm) slices. Add to the carrots. Heat a wok or heavy pan on high heat with 2 T. (30 mL) of the oil. Add garlic and sesame seeds; cook 20 seconds. Add remaining oil, heat; add meat and stir-fry quickly until brown. Remove meat from wok; keep warm. Add ¼ c. (60 mL) of the water to the wok. Add onions, cook and stir 2 minutes. Add carrots and cauliflower. Stir to mix. Cover and cook just until cauliflower is crisp-tender, stirring occasionally. Combine remaining cornstarch, soy sauce and water in a bowl or jar. Shake or stir to completely blend. Add meat to wok, stir to mix. Push meat and vegetables to side of wok. Add cornstarch mixture, cook and stir until thickened. Mix with the meat and vegetables. Pour onto hot serving platter.

Yield: 4 servings

Exchange, 1 serving: ⅔ bread, 1 vegetable, 3 medium-fat meat
Each serving contains: Calories: 328, Carbohydrates: 11 g

Sauerbraten

4 oz.	lean beef roast	120 g
½ c.	beef broth	125 mL
¼ c.	water	60 mL
¼ c.	cider vinegar	60 mL
¼ t.	salt	1 mL
dash	garlic powder	dash
1 t.	margarine	5 mL

Place beef in glass pan or bowl. Combine remaining ingredients, except margarine; pour over beef. Marinate 4 to 5 days in refrigerator. Turn beef at least once a day. Melt margarine in small skillet; add beef and brown. Reduce heat. Add half of the marinade to the skillet. Simmer until beef is tender.

Yield: 1 serving

Exchange, 1 serving: 4 medium-fat meat
Each serving contains: Calories: 300, Carbohydrates: 4 g

Klip Klops

4 slices	bread, crust removed	4 slices
½ c.	skim milk	125 mL
½ t.	garlic powder	2 mL
1 t.	onion salt	5 mL
1 lb.	lean ground beef	500 g
1	egg, beaten	1
1 qt.	water	1 L
1 small	bay leaf	1 small
1 t.	salt	5 mL
1	clove	1

Soak bread in skim milk. Add garlic powder, onion salt, ground beef, and egg; mix thoroughly. Form into 8 balls. Combine water, bay leaf, salt, and clove. Bring to boil. Drop balls into boiling water. Cook until beef is done (about 15 minutes). Drain before placing on hot platter.

Yield: 8 servings

Exchange, 1 serving: 2 high-fat meat, 1 bread
Each serving contains: Calories: 190, Carbohydrates: 1 g

Calf's Liver

1 T.	flour	15 mL
½ t.	bay leaf, finely crushed	2 mL
¼ t.	nutmeg	1 mL
	salt and pepper to taste	
½ c.	beef broth	125 mL
3 oz.	calf's liver	90 g
	vegetable cooking spray	

Combine flour, bay leaf, nutmeg, salt, and pepper in shaker bag. Add liver; shake to coat. Remove liver from bag and shake off excess flour. Brown liver in heavy skillet coated with vegetable cooking spray. Reduce heat. Add beef broth; cover. Simmer for 25 to 30 minutes, or until tender.

Yield: 1 serving

Exchange, 1 serving: 3 lean meat
Each serving contains: Calories: 132, Carbohydrates: 1.5 g

Curried Veal with Rice

4 T.	Mazola corn oil	60 mL
1 lb.	boneless veal, cut into ½ in. (13 mm) cubes	500 g
2 c.	green apple, coarsely chopped	500 mL
1 c.	onion, finely chopped	250 mL
½ c.	sweet red pepper, cut into thin strips	125 mL
1 clove	garlic, minced	1 clove
2 T.	curry powder	30 mL
1 t.	ginger	5 mL
1 c.	apple juice	250 mL
¾ c.	chicken broth	190 mL
2 t.	cornstarch	10 mL
¼ c.	cold water	60 mL
⅔ c.	regular rice, cooked without salt	165 mL
½ c.	unsalted peanuts	125 mL
½ c.	raisins	125 mL
½ c.	green onion, sliced	125 mL

In a Dutch oven, heat 2 T. (30 mL) of the oil over medium-high heat. Add veal, half at a time and cook, turning occasionally, about 5 minutes or until brown. Remove. Heat remaining oil and add next 6 ingredients. Cook, stirring, 2 minutes or until onion is tender. Return veal to Dutch oven. Stir in juice and broth. Bring to a boil, reduce heat and simmer 20 minutes or until veal is tender. Mix the cornstarch and water. Add to veal mixture. Stirring constantly, bring to a boil and boil 1 minute. Serve over rice with peanuts, raisins and onion.

Yield: 4 servings

Exchange, 1 serving: 2 bread, 3 fruit, 1 vegetable, 3½ high-fat meat
Each serving contains: Calories: 660, Carbohydrates: 53 g

"A Diet for the Young at Heart" by Mazola.

Veal Roast

2 to 3 lb.	veal roast	1 to 1½ kg
2 c.	beef broth	500 mL
1 med.	onion, sliced	1 med.
1	bay leaf	1
¼ t.	thyme	1 mL
	salt and pepper to taste	

Place roast in heavy kettle or roasting pan. Combine remaining ingredients. Pour over roast. Bake at 375°F (190°C) for 2 to 2½ hours, or until meat is very tender. While baking, baste with pan juices.

Exchange, 1 oz. (30 g): 1 lean meat
Each serving contains: Calories: 55, Carbohydrates: 2 g

Veal Scalopine

2 oz.	veal steak, boned	60 g	
¼ c.	tomato, sieved	60 mL	
2 T.	green pepper, chopped	30 mL	
1 T.	mushroom pieces	15 mL	
1 T.	onions, chopped	15 mL	
¼ t.	parsley	1 mL	
dash each	garlic powder, oregano	dash each	
	salt and pepper to taste		

Place veal on bottom of individual baking dish. Add remaining ingredients; cover. Bake at 350°F (175°C) for 45 minutes, or until meat is tender.

Microwave: Cook on High for 10 to 12 minutes. Turn and uncover last 2 minutes.

Yield: 1 serving

Exchange, 1 serving: 2 lean meat, 1 vegetable
Each serving contains: Calories: 164, Carbohydrates: 14 g

Veal Roll

1 oz.	veal, thin slice	30 g	
	salt and pepper to taste		
½ oz.	prosciutto, thin slice	15 g	
½ oz.	Swiss cheese, thin slice	15 g	
	vegetable cooking spray		

Pound veal slice with mallet or edge of plate until very thin. Add salt and pepper. Place prosciutto on top and roll up. Secure with poultry pin. Brown in heavy skillet coated with vegetable cooking spray. Top with cheese slice. Cover. Cook over low heat just until cheese melts slightly. Serve on hot plate.

Yield: 1 serving

Exchange, 1 serving: 2 medium-fat meat
Each serving contains: Calories: 156, Carbohydrates: 1 g

Roast Leg of Lamb

5 to 6 lb.	leg of lamb	2½ to 3 kg	
½ c.	low calorie Italian dressing	125 mL	
½ c.	water	125 mL	
3 T.	lemon juice	45 mL	
1 t.	garlic powder	5 mL	
½ t.	rosemary, ground	2 mL	
½ t.	thyme	2 mL	
½ t.	mace	2 mL	
1 t.	salt	5 mL	
¼ t.	pepper	1 mL	

Wipe lamb with damp cloth. Puncture lamb with long sharp spear or poultry pin. Place on a rack in roasting pan, fat side up. Blend remaining ingredients; pour over lamb. Roast uncovered at 325°F (165°C) for 3 to 3½ hours. Baste with pan juices every ½ hour. Add more Italian dressing and water, if necessary.

Exchange, 1 oz. (30 g): 1 medium-fat meat
Each serving contains: Calories: 75, Carbohydrates: 6 g

Lamb Shish Kebab

4 lb.	lean lamb	2 kg
3	garlic cloves, crushed	3
1½ t.	salt	7 mL
1	bay leaf	1
½ t.	pepper	3 mL
½ t.	ground allspice	3 mL
½ t.	ground clove	3 mL
1 t.	white vinegar	5 mL
1 c.	skim milk	250 mL

Cut lamb into 2 in. (5 cm) cubes. Combine remaining ingredients; blend thoroughly. Pour over lamb in bowl; cover. Refrigerate overnight. Place lamb on skewers. Barbecue or broil 10 to 15 minutes. Turn once.

Exchange, 1 oz. (30 g): 1 medium-fat meat
Each serving contains: Calories: 89, Carbohydrates: 4 g

Meat Ring

2 lbs.	lean ground beef	1kg
1 lb.	lean ground pork	500 g
1 c.	salted cracker crumbs	250 mL
¾ c.	skim milk	190 mL
⅓ c.	onion, minced	90 mL
1 t.	yellow prepared mustard	5 mL
¼ t.	black pepper	1 mL

Combine all ingredients in a large bowl. Stir or work with your hands to blend. Press into well-greased ring mold. Bake at 350°F (175°C) for 1½ hours. Allow to rest for 10 minutes before unmolding.

Yield: 20 servings

Exchange, 1 serving: 1¼ high-fat meat, ½ bread
Each serving contains: Calories: 151, Carbohydrates: 5 g

Meatloaf

2 lb.	lean ground beef	1 kg
¼ c.	onion, grated	60 mL
1 c.	soft bread crumbs	250 mL
1	egg	1
¼ c.	parsley, finely snipped	60 mL
1¼ t.	salt	6 mL
dash each	pepper, thyme, marjoram	dash each
1 t.	evaporated milk	5 mL

Combine all ingredients. Add just enough water to form firm ball. Press into baking dish. Bake at 350°F (175°C) for 1½ hours.

Microwave: Cook on High for 15 minutes. Turn dish halfway through cooking time. Allow to rest for 5 minutes before serving.

Yield: 12 servings

Exchange, 1 serving: 2½ high-fat meat, ¼ bread
Each serving contains: Calories: 237, Carbohydrates: 3 g

Soy Flour Meatloaf

1 lb.	ground meat	500 g
2	eggs	2
1 c.	milk	250 mL
2½ t.	salt	12 mL
½ c.	Stone-Buhr soy flour	125 mL
¼ c.	Stone-Buhr quick-cooking rolled oats	60 mL
½ c.	onion, minced	125 mL
¼ t.	black pepper	1 mL

Combine all ingredients and mix well. Shape the loaf and place in a 9 × 5 in. (23 × 13 cm) loaf pan. Bake at 350°F (175°C) for 50 minutes or until done.

Yield: 6 servings

Exchange, 1 serving: ¾ bread, 2 medium-fat meat
Each serving contains: Calories: 217, Carbohydrates: 8 g

With the compliments of Arnold Foods Company. Inc.

Swedish Meatballs

1 c.	dry bread crumbs	250 mL
1 c.	skim milk	250 mL
¾ 1b.	lean ground beef	375 g
¼ 1b.	lean ground pork	125 g
1	egg	1
¼ c.	onion, minced	60 mL
½ t.	salt	2 mL
dash	black pepper and nutmeg	dash

In a large bowl, soak the bread crumbs in the milk until soft. Add remaining ingredients. Stir or work with your hands until blended. Shape into 36 small meatballs. Bring a large pan of salted water to the boiling point. Drop each meatball into the boiling water. When meatball is brown and firm, remove with a slotted spoon to a baking sheet. Bake at 350°F (175°C) for 20 to 25 minutes or until meatballs are browned, turning occasionally.

Yield: 36 servings

Exchange, 1 serving: ⅓ medium-fat meat, ⅓ bread
Each serving contains: Calories: 38, Carbohydrates: 3 g

Sweet Meat Roll

The raisins in this onion-sage filling give it a unique flavor.

1½ lbs.	lean ground beef	750 g
½ lb.	ground ham	250 g
2 t.	salt	10 mL
¼ t.	black pepper	1 mL
1	egg	1
⅓ c.	raisins	90 mL
4 c.	dry bread crumbs	1 L
½ c.	onion, finely chopped	125 mL
1 t.	ground sage	5 mL
⅔ c.	water	180 mL

Combine the meats, salt, pepper, and egg in a bowl. Stir or work with your hands until well blended. Spread on wax paper into a ½ in. (1.3 cm) thick square. Mix the remaining ingredients. Spread filling evenly over meat. Roll up jelly-roll fashion. Place in oiled pan, seam side down. Bake at 350°F (175°C) for 1½ hours. Occasionally baste with meat juices.

Yield: 12 servings

Exchange, 1 serving: 2 medium-fat meat, 2 bread, ¼ fruit
Each serving contains: Calories: 289, Carbohydrates: 28 g

DIRECTIONS FOR ALL SAUSAGES

Mix sausage the old-fashioned way with clean hands until thoroughly blended. Wrap sausage in plastic and refrigerate for several hours or overnight to allow herbs, spices and seasonings to permeate the meat. Sausage can be formed into patties or stuffed into natural casings, using standard stuffing procedures. Make 16 patties or links per recipe unless recipe specifies 8 patties or links. Fresh pork sausage should be refrigerated and used within a day or two. Pan-fry or bake sausage until brown and juicy. Pork must be cooked thoroughly. Cooked or uncooked sausage can be individually wrapped with waxed paper, placed in a freezer bag and frozen for future use.

Kielbasa

3 T.	water	90 mL
¼ t.	celery seed	1 mL
⅛ t.	ground allspice	½ mL
½ t.	garlic powder	2 mL
¼ t.	ground marjoram	1 mL
¼ t.	ground nutmeg	1 mL
½ t.	ground paprika	2 mL
¾ t.	black pepper, freshly ground	4 mL
1 t.	salt	5 mL
¼ t.	ground thyme	1 mL
½ lb.	pork, coarsely ground	125 g
½ lb.	beef, coarsely ground	125 g
2–3 ft.	natural hog casings	1 m

Pour water into a large bowl. Grind celery seed with mortar and pestle. Add remaining seasonings and stir. Add the meats and mix the old-fashioned way.

Yield: 16 servings

Exchange, 1 serving: 1 high-fat meat
Each serving contains: Calories: 96, Carbohydrates: 2 g

Quick Sausage Dish

1 recipe	Hot Pork Breakfast Sausage	1 recipe
1	white onion, chopped	1
2 c.	chow mein noodles	500 mL
10 oz. can	vegetable beef soup	304 g can
10 oz. can	tomato soup	304 g can
10 oz. can	cream of mushroom soup	304 g can

Brown the sausage and onion in a nonstick skillet; drain thoroughly. Combine the soups in a bowl and stir to blend. Add the browned sausage and onion, and the noodles; stir and mix thoroughly. Cover bowl and refrigerate overnight. Pour into a well-greased casserole. Bake at 350°F (175°C) for 40 to 45 minutes or until set.

Yield: 12 servings

Exchange, 1 serving. 1½ high-fat meat, ¾ bread
Each serving contains: Calories: 269, Carbohydrates: 9 g

Sausage Brunch Dish

Serve as a main dish for brunch.

6	bread slices	6
1 recipe	Hot Pork Breakfast Sausage	1 recipe
1 c.	Swiss cheese, grated	250 mL
1 T.	Dijon-style mustard	15 mL
3	eggs, slightly beaten	3
1¼ c.	skim milk	310 mL
¾ c.	skim evaporated milk	190 mL
1 T.	Worcestershire sauce	15 mL
½ t.	salt	2 mL
⅛ t.	black pepper	½ mL
⅛ t.	mace	½ mL

Trim crusts from bread slices and reserve separately. Coat the bottom of a 9 × 13 in. (23 × 33 cm) cake pan with vegetable spray. Place the bread slices in the pan. Crumb the bread crusts; brown in a nonstick skillet; reserve. Fry and crumble the sausage over low heat until browned; drain thoroughly. Sprinkle the cheese over the bread slices in the pan. Top with the browned sausage. Combine remaining ingredients in a bowl and stir to blend completely. Pour over the sausage mixture. Bake at 350°F (175°C) for 30 to 35 minutes or until set. Serve hot.

Yield: 12 servings

Exchange, 1 serving: 2 high-fat meat, ⅓ nonfat milk
Each serving contains: Calories: 230, Carbohydrates: 4 g

Upside-Down Sausage Bake

1 recipe	Hot Pork Breakfast Sausage	1 recipe
½ c.	onion, chopped	125 mL
½ t.	salt	2 mL
¼ t.	black pepper	1 mL
1 c.	all-purpose flour	250 mL
1 c.	yellow cornmeal	250 mL
2	eggs	2
1 c.	skim milk	250 mL
1 T.	baking powder	15 mL
2 t.	granulated sugar replacement	10 mL

Combine the sausage, onions, salt, and pepper in a skillet. Cook and stir until sausage is browned and onion is tender; drain thoroughly. Spoon into a 9 in. (23 cm) square pan. Combine the remaining ingredients in a bowl; beat to blend. Pour over the sausage mixture. Bake at 375°F (190°C) for 20 to 30 minutes or until done. Remove by inverting on a heated serving plate.

Yield: 12 servings

Exchange, 1 serving: 1 bread, 1⅛ high-fat meat
Each serving contains: Calories: 278, Carbohydrates: 16 g

Sweet Pork and Raisin Bran Breakfast Sausage

½ c.	ice-cold orange juice	125 mL
½ t.	celery flakes	2 mL
¼ t.	ground nutmeg	1 mL
¾ t.	ground black pepper	4 mL
½ t.	ground sage	2 mL
¾ t.	salt	4 mL
¼ t.	ground thyme	1 mL
1 lb.	freshly ground pork	500 g
1½ c.	raisin bran flakes	375 mL

Pour orange juice into a large bowl. Add seasonings and stir. Add ground pork and raisin bran flakes. Mix sausage the old-fashioned way.

Yield: 16 servings

Exchange, 1 serving: 1 medium-fat meat
Each serving contains: Calories: 80, Carbohydrates: 5 g

Sweet Beef with Apples Breakfast Sausage

½ c.	ice-cold apple juice	125 mL
½ t.	ground cinnamon	2 mL
½ t.	parsley flakes	2 mL
¼ t.	ground marjoram	1 mL
¾ t.	ground black pepper	4 mL
½ t.	ground sage	2 mL
¾ t.	salt	4 mL
1 lb.	freshly ground beef	500 g
1 c.	uncooked oatmeal	250 mL
3 T.	dried apple, diced	45 mL

Pour apple juice into large bowl. Add seasonings and stir. Add ground beef, oatmeal and dried apple. Mix sausage the old-fashioned way.

Yield: 16 servings

Exchange, 1 serving: 1 lean meat
Each serving contains: Calories: 46, Carbohydrates: 6 g

Hot Pork Breakfast Sausage

1	egg	1
¼ c.	ice-cold tomato juice	60 mL
¼ t.	ground allspice	1 mL
¼ t.	ground basil	1 mL
½ t.	parsley flakes	2 mL
¼ t.	ground ginger	1 mL
1 t.	ground paprika	5 mL
¾ t.	cayenne pepper	4 mL
¼ t.	cayenne pepper flakes	1 mL
½ t.	ground sage	2 mL
½ t.	salt	4 mL
1 lb.	freshly ground pork	500 g
1 c.	wheat germ	250 mL

In a large bowl, combine egg and tomato juice. Blend seasonings into the liquid. Add pork and wheat germ. Mix sausage the old-fashioned way.

Yield: 16 servings

Exchange, 1 serving: 1 high-fat meat
Each serving contains: Calories: 93, Carbohydrates: 4 g

Added touch: Although this is an excellent breakfast sausage, it's great at a picnic when grilled on an outdoor charcoal barbecue and served on a bun.

Yield: 8 servings

Exchange, 1 serving: 2 high-fat meat
Each serving contains: Calories: 187, Carbohydrates: 7 g

Note: Add exchanges and calories for bun and condiments.

GERMAN BRATWURST

Bratwurst is a plump traditional sausage that originated in Nuremberg, Germany. In the German language, brat means "to fry" and wurst means "sausage." Bratwurst, well-known throughout the world, is a common cookout favorite in the United States Midwest, especially in the Sheboygan/Milwaukee, Wisconsin area.

Bratwurst can be made of pork, beef and/or veal. There are countless ways to make bratwurst. Each sausage maker (wurstmacher) blends his or her own bratwurst variation, according to personal, regional and ethnic preferences. Bratwurst tastes best when charcoal-grilled and served with your favorite condiments on a German-style bun. The following bratwurst recipes are only a sampling of the hundreds of delightful variations that bratwurst fans have created. Although bratwurst is usually an all-meat sausage, these high-fiber variations retain the authentic style and flavor of the original recipes.

Smoky Pork Bratwurst

1	egg	1
¼ c.	ice water	60 mL
1 t.	liquid smoke	5 mL
1 t.	caraway seeds	5 mL
½ t	celery flakes	2 mL
¼ t.	parsley flakes	1 mL
¼ t.	ground ginger	1 mL
½ t.	ground dry orange peel	2 mL
¼ t.	ground nutmeg	1 mL
1 t.	onion powder	5 mL
½ t.	ground white pepper	2 mL
¾ t.	salt	4 mL
¼ t.	brown sugar	1 mL
1 lb.	freshly ground pork	500 g
1¼ c.	40% bran flakes	310 mL

In a large bowl, combine the egg, water and liquid smoke. Crush caraway seasonings into the liquid. Add pork and bran flakes. Mix sausage the old-fashioned way. Make eight patties or links per recipe.

Added touch: Bake fresh or frozen bratwurst with sauerkraut for a delectable main dish.

Yield: 8 servings

Exchange, 1 serving: 2 medium-fat meat
Each serving contains: Calories: 151, Carbohydrates: 6 g

Smoky Beef and Pork Bratwurst

1	egg	1
1 t.	liquid smoke	5 mL
¼ c.	ice water	60 mL
¼ t.	allspice	1 mL
½ t.	caraway seeds	2 mL
1½ L	celery flakes	7 mL
¼ t.	ground ginger	1 mL
1 t.	ground dry lemon peel	5 mL
¼ t.	ground mace	1 mL
1 t.	onion flakes	5 mL
¾ t.	ground black pepper	4 mL
4 t.	salt	4 mL
dash	brown sugar	dash
½ lb.	freshly ground beef	250 g
½ lb.	freshly ground pork	250 g
1 c.	wheat germ	250 mL

Add egg, liquid smoke and water to large bowl. Crush caraway seeds and celery flakes in a mortar with pestle. Blend seasonings into the liquid. Add beef, pork, and wheat germ. Mix sausage the old-fashioned way. Make 8 patties or links per recipe.

Added touch: Use diced, sliced or crumbled bratwurst as a pizza topping.

Yield: 8 servings

Exchange, 1 serving: 2 medium-fat meat
Each serving contains: Calories: 169, Carbohydrates: 7 g

Note: Add exchanges and calories of pizza dough and other toppings.

Spicy Beef Bratwurst

1	egg	1
¼ c.	cold milk	60 mL
¼ t.	caraway seeds	1 mL
1 t.	parsley flakes	5 mL
¼ t.	ground coriander	1 mL
1 t.	ground dry lemon peel	5 mL
¼ t.	ground mace	1 mL
¼ t.	ground mustard	1 mL
1 T.	onion or leek, diced	15 mL
1 T.	onion powder	15 mL
¼ t.	paprika	1 mL
¾ t.	ground white pepper	4 mL
1 t.	salt	5 mL
¼ t.	brown sugar	1 mL
1 lb.	freshly ground beef	500 g
1 c.	uncooked oatmeal	250 mL

Combine egg and milk in a large bowl. Crush caraway seeds and parsley flakes in mortar with pestle. Blend all seasonings into the liquid. Add beef and oatmeal. Mix sausage the old-fashioned way. Make 8 patties or links per recipe.

Yield: 8 servings

Exchange, 1 serving: 1 high-fat meat
Each serving contains: Calories: 119, Carbohydrates: 3 g

Viennese Sausage

Viennese Sausage is delightful when smothered in hot tomato sauce and served as an appetizer or as the meat in your favorite casserole.

½ c.	ice-cold milk	125 mL
1 T.	all-purpose flour	15 mL
½ t.	ground coriander	2 mL
¼ t.	ground mace	1 mL
1 T.	onion, diced	15 mL
½ t.	ground paprika	2 mL
¼ t.	cayenne pepper	1 mL
1 t.	salt	5 mL
¼ t.	sugar	1 mL
½ lb.	freshly ground beef	250 g
½ lb.	freshly ground pork	250 g
1 c.	white cornmeal	250 mL

Pour milk into a q. (L) jar. Sprinkle flour into the jar, cover shake to blend. Pour milk and flour solution into a large bowl. BIend seasonings into the liquid. Add beef, pork, and cornmeal. Mix sausage the old-fashioned way.

Yield: 16 servings

Exchange, 1 serving: 1⅔ high-fat meat
Each serving contains: Calories: 173, Carbohydrates: 1 g

Note: Add exchanges and calories for all other foods used with Viennese Sausage.

Parisienne Sausage

½ c.	Burgundy wine, chilled	125 mL
1 T.	white flour	15 mL
¼ t.	ground bay leaf	1 mL
¼ t.	ground clove	1 mL
¼ t.	ground coriander	1 mL
¼ t.	ground ginger	1 mL
¼ t.	ground mace	1 mL
½ t.	ground nutmeg	2 mL
1 t.	ground black pepper	5 mL
1¼ t.	salt	6 mL
½ t.	ground savory	2 mL
¼ t.	sugar	1 mL
¼ t.	ground tarragon	1 mL
¼ t.	ground thyme	1 mL
½ lb.	fresh ground pork	250 g
½ lb.	fresh ground beef	250 g
1 c.	yellow cornmeal	250 mL

Pour chilled wine into a large bowl. Blend flour and seasonings into the wine. Add pork, beef and cornmeal. Mix sausage the old-fashioned way.

Yield: 16 servings

Exchange, 1 serving: 1 medium-fat meat
Each serving contains: Calories: 66, Carbohydrates: 7 g

Loukanika

Loukanika can be served as a main dish for dinner or on Greek-style bread as a luncheon meal.

½ c.	rose wine, chilled	125 mL
2 T.	orange juice, chilled	30 mL
¼ t.	ground allspice	1 mL
¼ t.	ground cinnamon	1 mL
¼ t.	ground cumin	1 mL
1 clove	garlic, minced	1 clove
¼ t.	ground nutmeg	1 mL
2 T.	orange peel, grated	30 mL
¼ t.	ground black pepper	1 mL
½ t.	peppercorns, cracked	2 mL
1 t.	salt	5 mL
1 t.	dried savory	5 mL
¼ t.	brown sugar	1 mL
½ lb.	freshly ground veal	250 g
½ lb.	freshly ground pork	250 g
1 c.	bulgur	250 mL

Mix wine and orange juice in a large bowl. Blend all seasonings into the liquid. Add veal, pork, and bulgur. Mix sausage the old-fashioned way. Make 8 patties or links per recipe.

Yield: 8 servings

Exchange, 1 serving: 2 medium-fat meat
Each serving contains: Calories: 139, Carbohydrates: 14 g

Note: Add exchanges and calories for all other foods used with loukanika.

ITALIAN SAUSAGE

Italian sausage is a worldwide favorite. Sweet or hot Italian sausage can be served as a main dish, on a slice of hot Italian bread, as the meat sauce on spaghetti or as a pizza topping. Use your imagination to create delightful menus using the following delicious sausages.

Sweet Italian Sausage

½ c.	ice water	125 mL
¾ t.	aniseed	4 mL
½ t.	ground coriander	2 mL
½ t.	ground paprika	2 mL
¼ t.	ground black pepper	1 mL
¼ t.	ground cayenne pepper	1 mL
¼ t.	cayenne pepper flakes	1 mL
¾ t.	salt	4 mL
¼ t.	brown sugar	1 mL
1 lb.	freshly ground pork	500 g
1 c.	bulgur	250 mL

Pour ice water into a large bowl. Crush aniseed with mortar and pestle. Blend seasonings into the liquid. Add pork and bulgur. Mix sausage the old-fashioned way. Make 8 patties or links per recipe.

Yield: 8 servings

Exchange, 1 serving: 1½ high-fat meat
Each serving contains: Calories: 156, Carbohydrates: 13 g

Hot Italian Sausage

½ c.	dry Italian red wine	125 mL
½ t.	fennel seed	2 mL
1 t.	liquid smoke	5 mL
1 t.	paprika	5 mL
1 t.	cayenne pepper	5 mL
¾ t.	cayenne pepper flakes	4 mL
1 t.	salt	5 mL
1 lb.	freshly ground pork	500 g
1 c.	40% bran flakes	250 mL

Chill the wine. Pour into a large bowl. Crush fennel seed with mortar and pestle. Blend all seasonings into the liquid. Add pork and bran flakes. Mix sausage the old-fashioned way. Make 8 patties or links per recipe.

Yield: 8 servings

Exchange, 1 serving: 2 medium-fat meat
Each serving contains: Calories: 151, Carbohydrates: 4 g

Luganega: Northern Italian Sausage

½ c.	Italian white vermouth	125 mL
2 T.	orange juice	30 mL
4 T.	Parmesan cheese, grated	45 mL
¼ t.	ground coriander	1 mL
1 clove	garlic, minced	1 clove
¼ t.	ground dry lemon peel	1 mL
¼ t.	ground nutmeg	1 mL
¼ t.	ground dry orange peel	1 mL
¼ t.	ground black pepper	1 mL
¾ t.	salt	4 mL
1 lb.	fresh ground pork	500 g
1 c.	wheat germ	250 mL

Chill vermouth and pour into a large bowl. Blend seasonings into the liquid. Add pork and wheat germ. Mix sausage the old-fashioned way. Make 8 patties or links per recipe.

Yield: 8 servings

Exchange, 1 serving: 2 high-fat meat
Each serving contains: Calories: 188, Carbohydrates: 7 g

Near Eastern Sausage

Serve as a main meat dish, baked with your favorite casserole or on pita bread with condiments.

½ c.	ice water	125 mL
dash	ground allspice	dash
¼ t.	ground cloves	1 mL
2 cloves	garlic, minced	2 cloves
¼ t.	ground oregano	1 mL
½ t.	ground black pepper	2 mL
½ t.	ground rosemary	2 mL
1 t.	salt	5 mL
¼ t.	sugar	1 mL
1 lb.	freshly ground lamb	500 g
1 c.	bran flakes	250 mL

Pour ice water into a large bowl. Blend seasonings into the liquid. Add lamb and bran flakes. Mix sausage the old-fashioned way. Make 8 patties or links per recipe.

Yield: 8 servings

Exchange, 1 serving: 1 high-fat meat or 2 lean meat
Each serving contains: Calories: 118, Carbohydrates: negligible

Note: Add calories and exchanges for condiments or other foods served with Near Eastern Sausage.

POLISH SAUSAGE

Polish style sausage, a favorite throughout the Western World, can be served on a whole wheat or rye bun with your favorite condiments. This sausage is great as a main dish all by itself or cooked with sauerkraut. You can be creative and develop your own favorite menus featuring Polish sausage.

Mild Polish Sausage

½ c.	ice water	125 mL
¼ t.	celery seed	1 mL
½ t.	garlic powder	2 mL
¼ t.	ground marjoram	1 mL
dash	ground or grated nutmeg	dash
½ t.	ground black pepper	2 mL
1 t.	salt	5 mL
¼ t.	brown sugar	1 mL
¼ t.	ground thyme	1 mL
½ lb.	freshly ground beef	250 g
½ lb.	freshly ground pork	250 g
1 c.	40% bran flakes	250 mL

Pour water into a large bowl. Blend seasonings into the liquid. Add beef, pork, and bran flakes. Mix sausage the old-fashioned way. Make 8 patties or links per recipe.

Yield: 8 servings

Exchange, 1 serving: 2 medium-fat meat
Each serving contains: Calories: 122, Carbohydrates: 4 g

Spicy Polish Sausage

½ c.	ice-cold beer	125 mL
1 t.	liquid smoke	5 mL
¼ t.	ground allspice	1 mL
½ t.	celery seed	2 mL
¼ t.	ground coriander	1 mL
2 cloves	garlic, minced	2 cloves
½ t.	ground marjoram	2 mL
¼ t.	ground mace	1 mL
1 t.	ground paprika	5 mL
1 t.	ground white pepper	5 mL
¾ t.	salt	4 mL
½ t.	ground thyme	2 mL
¼ lb.	freshly ground beef	125 g
¾ lb.	freshly ground pork	375 g
1 c.	bulgur	250 mL

Pour beer into a large bowl. Blend seasonings into the beer. Add beef, pork, and bulgur. Mix sausage the old-fashioned way. Make 8 patties or links per recipe.

Yield: 8 servings

Exchange, 1 serving: 1½ high-fat meat
Each serving contains: Calories: 147, Carbohydrates: 13 g

Russian Kielbasa

½ c.	ice water	125 mL
1 t.	vinegar	5 mL
¼ t.	dillseed	1 mL
¼ t.	ground allspice	1 mL
¼ t.	celery flakes	1 mL
¼ t.	cinnamon	1 mL
2 cloves	garlic, minced	2 cloves
½ t.	ground marjoram	2 mL
¼ t.	paprika	1 mL
1	ground black pepper	5 mL
¾ t.	salt	4 mL
1 lb.	freshly ground beef	500 g
½ c.	oatmeal	125 mL
½ c.	wheat germ	125 mL

Combine water and vinegar in a large bowl. Crack dillseed in a mortar and pestle. Blend seasonings into the liquid. Add beef, oatmeal and wheat germ. Mix sausage the old-fashioned way. Make 8 patties or links per recipe.

Yield: 8 servings

Exchange, 1 serving: 1¼ high-fat meat
Each serving contains: Calories: 126, Carbohydrates: 4 g

Note: Add calories and exchanges for condiments or other foods served with Russian Kielbasa.

Scandinavian Potato Sausage

Scandinavian Potato Sausage can be served on a bun with condiments, as a meat entree, or as the meat in a delicious stew.

¼ c.	ice-cold milk	60 mL
1	egg	1
¼ t.	allspice	1 mL
dash	ground mace	dash
¼ t.	ground nutmeg	1 mL
4 T.	onion, minced	60 mL
1 t.	ground black pepper	5 mL
1 t.	suet	5 mL
¼ t.	brown sugar	1 mL
½ lb.	freshly ground beef	250 g
½ lb.	freshly ground pork	250 g
½ c.	bran flakes	125 mL
½ c.	dried instant potatoes	125 mL

Combine egg and milk in a large bowl. Blend seasonings into the liquid. Add beef, pork, bran flakes and potatoes. Mix sausage the old-fashioned way. Make 8 patties or links per recipe.

Yield: 8 servings

Exchange, 1 serving: 1½ high-fat meat or 2 medium-fat meat
Each serving contains: Calories: 143, Carbohydrates: 13 g

Chorizo

½ c.	red wine, chilled	125 mL
1 T.	cider vinegar	15 mL
1 T.	dark corn syrup	5 mL
½ t.	fennel seed	2 mL
1 t.	chili powder	5 mL
½ t.	ground cumin	2 mL
2 cloves	garlic, minced	2 cloves
1 T.	onion powder	15 mL
1 t.	ground oregano	5 mL
2 t.	ground paprika	10 mL
1 t.	cayenne pepper	5 mL
1 t.	cayenne pepper flakes	5 mL
¾ t.	salt	4 mL
1 lb.	freshly ground pork	500 g
1 c.	wheat germ	250 mL

Mix wine, vinegar and corn syrup in a large mixing bowl. Crush fennel seed in mortar with pestle. Blend seasonings into the liquid. Add pork and wheat germ. Mix sausage the old-fashioned way. Make 8 patties or links per recipe.

Yield: 8 servings

Exchange, 1 serving: 2 high-fat meat
Each serving contains: Calories: 196, Carbohydrates: 3 g

Seafood

Breaded Slipper Lobster

1 pkg.	Island Queen slipper lobster tails	1 pkg.
2	white bread slices	2
	salt and pepper to taste	
1	egg white, slightly beaten	1
	vegetable oil for frying	

Cook the lobster as suggested on the package; cool. Discard shells and set the lobster aside. Toast bread until almost burnt. While hot, break into pieces; whip into crumbs at high speed in a blender. Pour crumbs into a shaker bag; add salt and pepper. Dip lobsters (if large, cut in half) into egg white; then shake in bread crumbs. Fry in deep oil at 365°F (180°C) until golden brown. Drain on paper towels. Serve warm or chilled.

Yield: 12 servings

Exchange, 1 serving: ½ lean meat
Each serving contains: Calories: 23, Carbohydrates: 3 g

Breakfast Salt Cod

¾ 1b	salt cod, boneless and skinless	375 g
¼ c.	all-purpose flour	60 mL
1 t.	oregano	5 mL
½ t.	black pepper	2 mL
¼ c.	onion, finely chopped	60 mL
¼ c.	vegetable oil	60 mL
3 T.	low-calorie margarine	45 mL
12	eggs, beaten	12

Rinse cod thoroughly under cold running water. Place in a large glass baking dish and cover with cold water. Cover and refrigerate for 36 hours; change water 2 to 3 times during that period. Drain thoroughly and rinse under cold running water. Place on absorbent towel and squeeze excess water from cod; cut into bite-sized cubes. Combine flour, oregano, and pepper in a flat bowl; stir to blend. Coat cod cubes with flour mixture and shake off excess. Heat oil in a nonstick skillet. When hot, add cod in small batches. Fry until golden on all sides. Push cod to side of pan and add onion. Sauté until onion is transparent. Remove cod and onion. Drain skillet and wipe clean. Heat margarine in the same skillet. Add the cod; reduce heat to medium. Add eggs and cook and stir slightly to scramble the eggs. Transfer to heated platter or plates.

Yield: 12 servings

Exchange, 1 serving: 1½ medium-fat meat, ½ fat
Each serving contains: Calories: 127, Carbohydrates: 3 g

Poached Salmon

Poaching water

1½ qts.	water	1½ L
1 c.	white wine	250 mL
¼ c.	white wine vinegar	60 mL
1	onion, sliced	1
8	peppercorns	8
2	whole allspice	2
2	bay leaves	2
1 t.	salt	5 mL

Fish

2 lbs.	fresh whole salmon with skin, cleaned	1 kg
	lemon wedges	
	dill	

In a large saucepan, combine all ingredients for poaching water (do not add salmon). Bring to the boil, reduce heat, and simmer for 30 minutes; cool to room temperature. Wrap salmon in cheesecloth and secure. Place salmon in poaching water and add extra water to completely cover salmon. Place over medium heat and heat until simmering. Cover and cook for about 10 minutes until salmon is opaque. Lift salmon from water and unwrap; remove skin and bones. Chill or serve hot with lemon wedges and a dill garnish.

Yield: 12 servings

Exchange, 1 serving: 1 high-fat meat
Each serving contains: Calories: 106, Carbohydrates: negligible

Glorified Salmon

1 lb. can	salmon, drained, boned, and flaked	500 g can
2 c.	fresh bread crumbs	500 mL
1	small onion, finely chopped	1
½ c.	cheddar cheese, shredded	125 mL
½ c.	fresh parsley, finely snipped	125 mL
2 T.	pimiento	30 mL
3	eggs	3
1 c.	skim milk	250 mL
¼ c.	lemon juice	60 mL
	salt and pepper to taste	

Combine salmon, bread crumbs, onion, cheese, parsley, and pimiento in a large bowl; work with your hands or a spoon to mix. Beat together the eggs, milk, lemon juice, salt, and pepper. Pour and stir into the salmon mixture. Turn into a greased 1½ qt. (1½L) casserole. Place salmon casserole in a baking dish that contains 1 in. (2.5 cm) of hot water. Bake at 350°F (175°C) for 1 hour or until knife inserted in middle comes out clean.

Yield: 10 servings

Exchange, 1 serving: 1¾ medium-fat meat, ⅓ bread
Each serving contains: Calories: 148, Carbohydrates: 5 g

Slipper Lobster Casserole

1 pkg.	Island Queen slipper lobster tails	1 pkg.
2 T.	butter	30 mL
1 T.	onion, minced	15 mL
2 t.	salt	10 mL
1½ t.	paprika	7 mL
½ t.	black pepper	2 mL
1 qt.	skim milk	1 L
3 T.	all-purpose flour	45 mL
½ c.	dry sherry	125 mL
12 oz. pkg.	wide noodles, cooked	338 g pkg.

Cook lobster as directed on the package; cool. Discard shells and cut lobster into bite-sized pieces. Melt butter in a skillet. Add the onion, salt, paprika, and pepper. Combine milk and flour in a bowl; mix to completely blend and pour into the skillet. Cook and stir sauce over low heat until thickened; stir in the sherry. Combine noodles, sauce, and half of the lobster pieces in a 3 qt. (3 L) casserole. Bake, uncovered, at 375°F (190°C) for 25 minutes or until hot and bubbly. Place remaining lobster pieces on top of noodle casserole. Return to oven for 10 more minutes.

Yield: 6 servings

Exchange, 1 serving: 1 lean meat, 1 nonfat milk, ½ bread
Each serving contains: Calories: 157, Carbohydrates: 20 g

Sautéed Shrimp

6 oz. bag	Brilliant cooked frozen shrimp	170 g bag
1 T.	low-calorie margarine	15 mL
2 T.	onion, minced	30 mL

Thaw and drain shrimp thoroughly. Melt margarine in small skillet. When margarine bubbles, add the onion; stir and sauté until onion is translucent but not browned. Add the drained shrimp. Stir-fry until completely heated. Turn out onto 3 heated plates.

Yield: 3 servings

Exchange, 1 serving: ¾ lean meat
Each serving contains: Calories: 46, Carbohydrates: negligible

Shrimp Special

1 T.	low-calorie margarine	15 mL
3 T.	onion, chopped	45 mL
2 T.	parsley, finely snipped	30mL
6 oz. bag	Brilliant cooked frozen shrimp, thawed	170 g bag
2	eggs, slightly beaten	2

Melt margarine in a nonstick skillet. Add the onion and parsley. Cook and stir for 1 minute; remove from heat. Drain the liquid from the shrimp package into the beaten eggs. Pour shrimp into skillet. Place skillet over medium heat and cook until most of the moisture has evaporated. Beat the shrimp liquid into the eggs; pour eggs over the onion, parsley, and shrimp in the skillet. Reduce heat, cover, and cook until eggs are firm. Turn over onto a heated serving plate.

Yield: 3 servings

Exchange, 1 serving: 1¾ lean meat
Each serving contains: Calories: 99, Carbohydrates: negligible

Whitefish Florentine

Terrific with hot rolls.

2 10 oz. pkg.	frozen spinach	2 280 g pkg.
1 lb.	whitefish	500 g
10 oz. can	cream of mushroom soup	304 g can
10	mushrooms, sliced	10
¼ c.	skim milk	60 mL

Thaw and drain spinach thoroughly; spread evenly on the bottom of a well-greased baking dish. Place whitefish in a nonstick skillet. Cover with water and simmer for 10 minutes. Drain thoroughly and lay fish on the spinach in the baking dish. Combine mushroom soup, mushrooms, and milk in a bowl; stir to blend and pour over the fish. Bake, uncovered, at 400°F (200°C) for 20 minutes.

Yield: 6 servings

Exchange, 1 serving: 1 high-fat meat, 1½ vegetable
Each serving contains: Calories: 134, Carbohydrates: 7 g

Crisp Oven Trout

4	pan trout, dressed	4
	salt and pepper	
3 T.	low-calorie margarine	45 mL
½ c.	fresh parsley, finely snipped	125 mL
1	egg	1
3 T.	skim milk	45 mL
½ c.	fresh bread crumbs, toasted	125 mL

Wash and pat trout with a towel to dry. Season both the cavity and the outside with salt and pepper. With a fork, blend together the margarine and parsley. Spread mixture inside the cavity of the trout. In a flat pan, beat together the egg and milk. Dip each fish in the egg mixture. Roll trout in the bread crumbs and shake off any excess. Place in well-greased flat baking dish. Bake at 500°F (290°C) for 15 to 20 minutes or until trout is brown and tender.

Yield: 4 servings

Exchange, 1 serving: 2 medium-fat meat, ¼ bread
Each serving contains: Calories: 180, Carbohydrates: 4 g

Sole and Mushroom Bake

1 lb.	sole fillets	500 g
2 T.	low-calorie margarine	30 mL
½ lb.	mushrooms, sliced	250 g
1	onion, chopped	1
¼ c.	parsley, snipped	60 mL
½	sweet red bell pepper, sliced	½
¼ c.	dry white wine	60 mL

Melt margarine in a skillet. Sauté mushrooms, onion, parsley, and red pepper until soft. Place sole fillets in a well-greased casserole. Cover with the vegetables. Pour on the wine. Bake, uncovered, at 350°F (175°C) for 15 minutes, Drain off any excess liquid from the food. Cover casserole and return to oven. Bake 5 to 10 minutes longer or until sole flakes easily with a fork.

Yield: 6 servings

Exchange, 1 serving: 1 medium-fat meat, ¾ vegetable
Each serving contains: Calories: 96, Carbohydrates: 5 g

Chinese-Style Shrimp and Broccoli

Make sure you do not overcook this dish—this dish is best when the shrimp is tender and the broccoli is still a little crunchy.

10 oz.	shrimp, cleaned	300 g
¼ c.	vegetable oil	60 mL
1 clove	garlic	1 clove
2 c.	broccoli florets	500 mL
⅔ c.	water	180 mL
1 t.	salt	5 mL
2 c.	fresh or frozen peas	500 mL
1 T.	cornstarch	15 mL

Cut shrimp into ½ in. (13 mm) lengths. Heat oil in wok or skillet, add garlic and cook until transparent. Stir in the shrimp and cook just until their color changes. Remove shrimp from wok and keep hot. Add broccoli to wok and cook 1 minute. Carefully, add water and salt. Cover and bring water to the boiling point. Add peas, cook 5 minutes. Return shrimp to wok. Blend cornstarch with 2 T. (30 mL) cold water: add to pan. Simmer and stir until mixture thickens and is clear.

Yield: 4 servings

Exchange, 1 serving: ½ bread, 1 vegetable, 2 medium-fat meat
Each serving contains: Calories: 217, Carbohydrates: 12 g

Crab à la Lourna

This dish makes for an easy and elegant dinner.

2 T.	unsalted butter	30 mL
½ lb.	small snow-white mushrooms	250 g
½ lb.	snow peas	250 g
½ lb.	crab meat, cut into bite-size pieces	250 g
1 T.	all-purpose flour	15 mL
1 T.	cornstarch	15 mL
1 c.	cold water	250 mL
½ c.	2% milk	125 mL
	salt and pepper to taste	
1 c.	wild rice, cooked	250 mL
2 c.	brown rice, cooked	500 mL

Heat a large skillet and melt 1 T. (15 mL) of the butter. Add mushrooms and sauté until tender; remove from heat. Meanwhile, clean snow peas and cut into 1 in. (2.5 cm) pieces. With a slotted spoon, remove mushrooms from skillet and return pan to medium heat. Add snow peas and cook until peas are tender; remove peas from pan. Melt remaining 1 T. (15 mL) butter. Add crab meat and sauté until lightly browned. Remove from pan. Dissolve flour and cornstarch in the water. Pour into skillet, add milk and simmer over low heat until mixture thickens. Season with salt and pepper. Return mushrooms, peas and crab, heat and fold mixture gently until hot. Combine hot wild and brown rice. Serve over the hot rice.

Yield: 6 servings

Exchange, 1 serving: 1 bread, 1 vegetable, 1 medium-fat meat
Each serving contains: Calories: 178, Carbohydrates: 20 g

Crab Fried Rice

2 T.	margarine	30 mL
2	eggs, lightly beaten	2
1 c.	mushrooms, sliced	250 mL
1 c.	celery, sliced	50 mL
½ c.	onion, chopped	125 mL
¼ c.	bamboo shoots	60 mL
¼ c.	water chestnuts, sliced	60 mL
3 c.	brown rice, cooked	750 mL
3 T.	soy sauce	45 mL
½ lb.	crab meat, cut in chunks	500 g
	salt and pepper, if needed	

Melt 1 T. (15 mL) of the margarine in a large nonstick skillet. Add eggs and cook over low heat until set; remove to cutting board. Chop or cut eggs into large strips. Melt remaining 1 T. (15 mL) margarine in the same pan. Add vegetables, cook and stir until celery is tender. Remove vegetables from pan. Stir the rice into pan and add soy sauce. Mix until completely blended. Add vegetables, crab and egg. Cover and cook over low heat until mixture is hot.

Yield: 6 servings

Exchange, 1 serving: 1 bread, 1 vegetable, 1 medium-fat meat
Each serving contains: Calories: 176, Carbohydrates: 15 g

Tuna Patties

2	eggs	2
2 6½ oz. cans	chunk light tuna in water	2 185 g cans
⅓ c.	milk	90 mL
dash	pepper	dash
1 t.	lemon juice	5 mL
2 T.	pickle relish	30 mL
1 c.	Kellogg's branflakes cereal	250 mL
	fresh parsley, snipped	

Beat eggs lightly. Add remaining ingredients except parsley. Mix well. Shape into 6 patties. Place on lightly greased baking sheet. Bake at 350°F (175°C) about 25 minutes, turning patties after 15 minutes. Sprinkle with parsley.

Yield: 6 servings

Exchange, 1 serving: 2 lean meat, ⅓ bread
Each serving contains: Calories: 125, Carbohydrates: 8 g

Based on a recipe from Kellogg's Test Kitchens.

Casseroles, Pilafs, and Pastas

Yam-Pecan Casserole

4 lbs.	yams, scrubbed	2 kg
½ c.	skim milk	125 mL
⅓ c.	low-calorie margarine	90 mL
2	eggs, slightly beaten	2
½ c.	granulated brown sugar replacement	125 mL
½ c.	skim evaporated milk	125 mL
½ c.	pecans, coarsely chopped	125 mL
1 t.	vanilla extract	5 mL
¼ t. each	ground cinnamon, nutmeg, and salt	1 mL each

Place yams in baking dish; bake at 350°F (175°C) until tender. Remove and cool until able to handle. Peel or remove soft pulp from yams. Whip pulp until smooth. Scald the milk in a small heavy saucepan. Remove from heat and add the margarine; stir to melt margarine. Cool slightly; then beat in eggs and ¼ c. (60 mL) brown sugar replacement. Beat into yams. Spread yam mixture on bottom of 13 × 9 in. (33 × 23 cm) baking dish. Combine evaporated milk, remaining brown sugar replacement, pecans, vanilla, and spices in a small heavy saucepan. Simmer and stir for 5 minutes. Pour mixture over yams, spreading evenly. Bake at 350°F (175°C) for about 30 minutes until top is set.

Yield: 12 servings

Exchange, 1 serving: ½ bread, ⅓ nonfat milk, 1 fat
Each serving contains: Calories: 114, Carbohydrates: 10 g

Beef Stroganoff

3 oz.	lean beef, cubed	90 g
1 t.	margarine	5 mL
½	onion, cut into large pieces	½
¼ t.	garlic, minced	1 mL
2 T.	mushroom pieces	30 mL
½ c.	condensed cream of mushroom soup	125 mL
1 T.	low-calorie sour cream	15 mL
1 t.	ketchup	5 mL
dash each	Worcestershire sauce, ground bay leaf, salt, pepper	dash each
1 c.	noodles	250 mL

Brown beef cubes in margarine. Add onion, garlic, and mushrooms. Cook over low heat until onion is partially cooked; remove from beat. Combine condensed soup, sour cream, ketchup, and seasonings; blend well. Pour over beef mixture; beat thoroughly. *Do not boil.* Serve over noodles.

Yield: 1 serving

Exchange, 1 serving: 3 high-fat meat, 2 ½ bread
Each serving contains: Calories: 470, Carbohydrates: 58 g

Quick Kabobs

2 oz.	cooked beef roast, cut in 1 in. (2.5 cm) cubes	60 g
6	green peppers, cut in 1 in. (2.5 cm) squares	6
6	cherry tomatoes	6
6	zucchini, cut in 1 in. (2.5 cm) cubes	6
6	unsweetened pineapple chunks	6
2 T.	low-calorie French dressing	30 mL

Alternate beef, vegetables, and fruit on 2 skewers. Brush with 1 T. (15 mL) of the French dressing. Broil 5 to 6 in. (12 to 15 cm) from heat for 8 minutes. Brush with remaining French dressing. Broil 4 minutes longer.

Yield: 1 serving (2 kabobs)

Exchange, 1 serving: 2 medium-fat meat, 1 vegetable, 1 fruit
Each serving contains: Calories: 150, Carbohydrates: 107 g

Beef and Rice Casserole

3 oz.	ground beef	90 g
1 T.	onion, chopped	15 mL
1 T.	celery, chopped	15 mL
¾ c.	condensed chicken gumbo soup	180 mL
¼ c.	water	60 mL
½ c.	rice, uncooked	125 mL
¼ c.	condensed cream of mushroom soup	60 mL
	salt and pepper to taste	

Combine ground beef, onion, and celery with a small amount of water in a saucepan. Boil until onion is tender; drain. Combine condensed chicken gumbo soup, water, and rice. Simmer until all moisture is absorbed. Mix beef mixture, rice, and mushroom soup; pour into a small greased casserole dish. Add salt and pepper. Bake at 350°F (175°C) for 25 minutes.

Microwave: Cook on Medium for 8 to 10 minutes.

Yield: 1 serving

Exchange, 1 serving: 3 high-fat meat, 2 bread
Each serving contains: Calories: 380, Carbohydrates: 103 g

German Goulash

3 oz.	lean ground beef	90 g
1 t.	onion, chopped	5 mL
1 T.	green pepper, chopped	15 mL
1 T.	celery, chopped	15 mL
¼	bay leaf, crushed	¼
½ c.	kidney beans, cooked	125 mL
½ c.	elbow macaroni, cooked	125 mL
¼ c.	carrot (sliced)	60 mL
	salt and pepper to taste	

Brown ground beef, onion, green pepper, and celery over low heat; drain. Add crushed bay leaf, kidney beans, macaroni, and carrots; mix gently. Add salt and pepper. Pour into casserole dish; cover. Bake at 350°F (175°C) for 40 minutes.

Microwave: Cook on Medium for 7 minutes.

Yield: 1 serving

Exchange, 1 serving: 3 medium-fat meat, 2½ bread
Each serving contains: Calories: 413, Carbohydrates: 46 g

Stuffed Peppers

1	green pepper	1
2 T.	rice	30 mL
2 oz.	lean ground beef	60 g
1	egg	1
1 t.	onion flakes	5 mL
1 T.	mushrooms, finely chopped	5 mL
	salt and pepper to taste	
1 t.	Tomato Sauce	5 mL

Cut green pepper in half, lengthwise. Remove membrane and seeds; rinse, drain and reserve shells. Boil rice with ½ c. (125 mL) of water for 5 minutes; drain. Combine ground beef, rice, egg, onion flakes, and mushrooms; blend thoroughly. Add salt and pepper. Fill green pepper cavities with beef mixture; top with Tomato Sauce. Place in baking dish; cover. Bake at 350°F (175°C) for 20 to 25 minutes.

Microwave: Cook on High for 10 minutes.

Yield: 1 serving

Exchange, 1 serving: 3 medium-fat meat, 1 bread, 1 vegetable
Each serving contains: Calories: 255, Carbohydrates: 40 g

Lasagne

2 oz.	ground beef	60 g
1 T.	onion, chopped	15 mL
½ c.	Tomato Sauce	125 mL
3 T.	water	45 mL
¼ t.	garlic powder	1 mL
½ t.	oregano	3 mL
	salt and pepper to taste	
1½ c.	lasagne noodles, cooked	375 mL
1 oz.	mozzarella cheese, grated	30 g
1 oz.	provolone cheese, grated	30 g

Crumble beef in small amount of water; add onion. Boil until meat is cooked; drain. Blend Tomato Sauce, 3 T. (45 mL) water, garlic powder, oregano, salt, and pepper. Add beef-onion mixture; stir to blend. Spread small amount of sauce into bottom of individual baking dish. Layer noodles, sauce, mozzarella and provolone cheese. Bake at 375°F (190°C) for 30 minutes.

Microwave: Cook on High for 10 minutes.

Yield: 1 serving

Exchange, 1 serving: 4 high-fat meat, 3 bread
Each serving contains: Calories: 485, Carbohydrates: 90 g

Hamburger Pie

2 lb.	lean ground beef	1 kg
½ c.	cornflakes, crushed	125 mL
¼ t.	garlic powder	1 mL
½ t.	onion, finely chopped	3 mL
1	egg	1
	salt and pepper to taste	
2¼ c.	water	560 mL
1 c.	skim milk	250 mL
1 t.	salt	5 mL
2 c.	instant mashed potatoes	500 mL
1 t.	margarine	5 mL

Combine ground beef, cornflakes, garlic powder, onion, and egg; mix well. Add salt and pepper. Place beef mixture in 9 in. (23 cm) pie pan. Pat to cover bottom and sides evenly. Bake at 425°F (220°C) for 30 minutes; drain off excess fat. Heat water, skim milk, and salt just to a boil; remove from heat. Add potato granules; mix thoroughly. Add margarine; blend well. Cover and allow to stand 5 minutes, or until potatoes thicken. Spread evenly over meat mixture. Return to oven and bake until potatoes are golden brown. Allow to rest 10 minutes before cutting pie into wedges.

Microwave: Cover beef mixture. Cook on Medium for 10 to 12 minutes; drain. Cover with potatoes. Cook on Medium for 2 minutes. Hold 5 minutes.

Yield: 8 servings

Exchange, 1 serving: 4 high-fat meat, 1 bread, ½ fat
Each serving contains: Calories: 372, Carbohydrates: 46 g

Cheese Lasagne

½ c.	Tomato Sauce	125 mL
3 T.	water	45 mL
1 T.	onion	15 mL
¼ t.	garlic powder	1 mL
½ t.	oregano	3 mL
	salt and pepper to taste	
¼ c.	large curd cottage cheese	60 mL
1	egg	1
1½ c.	lasagne noodles, cooked	375 mL
2 oz.	mozzarella cheese	60 g
1 T.	Parmesan cheese	15 mL

Combine Tomato Sauce, water, onion, garlic powder, oregano, salt, and pepper. Thoroughly blend together cottage cheese and egg. Spread small amount of sauce into bottom of individual baking dish. Alternate layers of noodles, sauce, cottage cheese mixture, and mozzarella cheese. Top with Parmesan cheese. Bake at 375°F (190°C) for 30 minutes.

Microwave: Cook on High for 10 minutes.

Yield: 1 serving

Exchange, 1 serving: 3 high-fat meat, 3 bread
Each serving contains: Calories: 350, Carbohydrates: 104 g

Clam Pilaf

2 oz.	clams, minced	60 g
½ c.	rice, cooked	125 mL
2 T.	onion, chopped	30 mL
1 med.	fresh tomato, peeled and cubed	1 med.
dash each	ground bay leaf, thyme, salt, pepper	dash each
2 T.	grated Cheddar cheese	30 mL

Combine clams, rice, onion, tomato, and seasonings in baking dish; top with cheese. Bake at 350°F (175°C) for 25 minutes.

Microwave: Combine clams, rice, onion, tomato, and seasonings. Cook on High for 5 minutes; top with cheese. Reheat on High for 1 minute.

Yield: 1 serving

Exchange, 1 serving: 2 lean meat, 1 bread
Each serving contains: Calories: 170, Carbohydrates: 76 g

Macaroni and Cheese Supreme

1 c.	elbow macaroni	250 mL
11 oz. can	condensed cream of mushroom soup	300 g can
6 oz.	cheese, shredded	180 mL
1 t.	yellow mustard	5 mL
1 t.	salt	5 mL
dash	pepper	dash
2 c.	cooked spinach, drained	500 mL
12 oz.	lean meat, diced	360 g

Cook macaroni as directed on package; drain. Combine mushroom soup, cheese, mustard, salt, and pepper. Add macaroni; stir well. Spread cooked spinach on bottom of lightly greased 13 × 9 in. (33 × 23 cm) baking dish. Top with meat. Spoon macaroni mixture evenly over entire surface. Bake at 375°F (190°C) for 40 minutes. Allow to cool 15 minutes before serving.

Microwave: Cook on Medium for 12 to 15 minutes. Turn dish halfway through cooking time. Allow to rest 15 minutes before serving.

Yield: 6 servings

Exchange, 1 serving: 2 bread, 3 high-fat meat, 1 vegetable
Each serving contains: Calories: 287, Carbohydrates: 11 g

Turkey à la King

¼ c.	White Sauce	60 mL
1 oz.	cooked turkey, diced	30 g
¼ c.	mushroom pieces	60 mL
2 T.	green pepper, chopped	30 mL
1 T.	stuffed green olives, chopped	15 mL
	salt and pepper to taste	
	dough for 1 baking powder biscuit	

Heat White Sauce. Combine sauce, turkey, mushrooms, green pepper, and olives; add salt and pepper. Pour into lightly greased individual baking dish. Top with biscuit dough. Bake at 375°F (190°C) for 15 to 20 minutes, or until biscuit is golden brown.

Yield: 1 serving

Exchange, 1 serving: 1 medium-fat meat, 1 vegetable, 1 bread
Each serving contains: Calories: 168, Carbohydrates: 31 g

Chicken Gambeano

¼ c.	condensed cream of chicken soup	60 mL
3 T.	skim milk	45 mL
¼ c.	zucchini, cubed	60 mL
¼ c.	green beans	60 mL
2 oz.	cooked chicken, cubed	60 g
¼ t.	poultry seasoning	2 mL
	salt and pepper to taste	
1¼ c.	linguine, cooked	310 mL

Blend condensed soup and skim milk; place in saucepan. Add zucchini and green beans. Cook over Medium heat until vegetables are partially tender. Add chicken and seasonings; reheat. Serve over linguine.

Microwave: Blend condensed soup and skim milk in bowl. Add zucchini and green beans; cover. Cook on High for 5 to 7 minutes, or until vegetables are partially tender. Add chicken and seasonings; reheat on Medium for 4 minutes. Serve over linguine.

Yield: 1 serving

Exchange, 1 serving: 3 bread, 2 medium-fat meat, ½ vegetable
Each serving contains: Calories: 300, Carbohydrates: 169 g

Mostaccioli with Oysters

8 oz. can	oysters with liquid, minced	225 g
4 oz.	mushroom pieces	120 g
½ c.	green pepper, sliced	125 mL
1 T.	parsley	15 mL
1 t.	garlic powder	5 mL
	salt and pepper to taste	
3 c.	mostaccioli noodles, cooked	750 mL

Combine minced oysters with liquid, mushrooms, green pepper, and parsley in saucepan. Add garlic powder. Cook until green pepper is crispy tender. Add salt and pepper. Serve over mostaccioli noodles.

Microwave: Combine minced oysters with liquid, mushrooms, green pepper, parsley, and garlic powder in bowl. Cook on High for 4 minutes or until green pepper is crispy tender. Add salt and pepper. Serve over mostaccioli noodles.

Yield: 2 servings

Exchange, 1 serving: 4 lean meat, 1½ bread
Each serving contains: Calories: 195, Carbohydrates: 92 g

Veal Steak Parmesan

1 T.	flour	15 mL
1 t.	salt	5 mL
dash each	poultry seasoning, salt, pepper, paprika	dash each
4 oz.	veal steak, cut in half	120 g
1 t.	shortening	5 mL
½ c.	wide noodles, cooked	125 mL
½ c.	sour cream sauce	125 mL
3 T.	hot water	45 mL
1 t.	Parmesan cheese	5 mL

Combine flour, salt, and seasonings in shaker bag. Add veal steak; shake to coat. Remove veal from bag and shake off excess flour. Heat shortening in small skillet. Brown veal on both sides; place in small baking dish. Cover with noodles. Blend sour cream sauce and hot water. Pour over noodles. Top with Parmesan cheese. Bake at 350°F (175°C) for 45 minutes, or until veal is tender.

Microwave: Cover. Cook on Medium to High for 15 minutes, or until meat is tender.

Yield: 1 serving

Exchange, 1 serving: 4¼ medium-fat meat, 2 bread
Each serving contains: Calories: 390, Carbohydrates: 39 g

Ham and Scalloped Potatoes

2 oz.	lean ham, diced	60 g
1 med.	potato, peeled and sliced	1 med.
2 T.	onion	30 mL
2 t.	parsley	10 mL
	vegetable cooking spray	
¼ c.	condensed cream of celery soup	60 mL
¼ c.	milk	60 mL
	salt and pepper to taste	

Combine ham, potato, onion, and parsley in baking dish coated with vegetable cooking spray. Blend condensed soup and milk; pour over potato mixture; cover. Bake at 350°F (175°C) for 1 hour, or until potatoes are tender. Add salt and pepper.

Microwave: Cook on high for 10 minutes, or until potatoes are tender. Add salt and pepper.

Yield: 1 serving

Exchange, 1 serving: 2 high-fat meat, 1½ bread, ½ milk
Each serving contains: Calories: 365, Carbohydrates: 41 g

Tuna Soufflé

11 oz. can	condensed cream of celery soup	300 g can
2 t.	parsley, finely chopped	10 mL
1 t.	salt	5 mL
dash	pepper	dash
½ t.	marjoram	3 mL
7 oz. can	tuna, in water	200 g can
6	eggs, separated	6
1 c.	mixed vegetables, cooked	250 mL

Combine condensed soup, parsley, salt, pepper, marjoram, and tuna in saucepan. Heat, stirring constantly, until mixture is hot. Remove from beat and cool slightly. Add egg yolks, one at a time, beating well after each addition. Stir in vegetables. Beat egg whites until soft peaks form. Fold small amount of beaten egg whites into egg yolk mixture, then fold egg yolk mixture into remaining egg whites. Pour into lightly greased 10 in. (25 cm) soufflé dish. Bake at 325°F (165°C) for 50 minutes, or until firm and golden brown. Serve immediately.

Yield: 8 servings

Exchange, 1 serving: 1½ lean meat, 1 bread
Each serving contains: Calories: 134, Carbohydrates: 6 g

Carrot Soufflé

3 T.	low-calorie margarine	45 mL
3 T.	all-purpose flour	45 mL
1 c.	skim milk	250 mL
¼ t.	salt	1 mL
1 c.	baby food carrots	250 mL
4	eggs, separated	4

Melt margarine in a skillet. Stir in the flour and blend thoroughly. Slowly add the milk; cook, stirring over low heat until sauce is smooth and thickened. Add salt and remove from heat. Beat egg yolks in a bowl until light and lemon-colored. Add to cooled sauce. Blend in the carrots. In a bowl, beat the egg whites until stiff. Fold half of the beaten whites into sauce-carrot mixture; gently fold in the remaining whites. Carefully pour into a greased 2 qt. (2-L) baking dish. Bake at 375°F (190°C) for 35 to 40 minutes or until lightly browned and puffy. Serve immediately.

Yield: 4 servings

Exchange, 1 serving: 1 medium-fat meat, 1 bread
Each serving contains: Calories: 149, Carbohydrates: 15 g

Apricot Soufflé

3 T.	low-calorie margarine	45 mL
3 T.	all-purpose flour	45 mL
1 c.	baby food apricots	250 mL
1 T.	lemon juice	15 mL
4	eggs, separated	4

Melt margarine in a skillet over low heat. Stir in the flour and cook until blended. Add the apricots and cook until thickened; remove from heat. Add the lemon juice. In a bowl, beat egg yolks until thick and lemon-colored. Stir apricot mixture into the yolks. In another bowl, beat egg whites until stiff. Fold apricot-yolk mixture into the whites. Pour mixture into a greased 1½ qt. (1½ L) baking dish. Bake at 375°F (190°C) for 25 to 30 minutes or until lightly browned and puffed.

Yield: 4 servings

Exchange, 1 serving: 1 medium-fat meat, ½ fruit, ¼ bread
Each serving contains: Calories: 118, Carbohydrates: 9 g

Butter Soufflé

A light puff of buttery egg.

1 T.	low-calorie margarine	15 mL
1 T.	all-purpose flour	15 mL
⅓ c.	skim milk	90 mL
1 env.	Butter Buds natural butter-flavored mix	1 env.
	salt and pepper to taste	
2	eggs, separated	2

Melt margarine in a small saucepan; blend in the flour and stir to mix thoroughly. Slowly add the milk; cook and stir until thickened. Stir in Butter Buds; remove from heat and allow to cool. In a bowl, beat egg yolks until thick and lemon-colored; add yolks to butter mixture. In another bowl, beat egg whites until stiff. Fold egg whites into butter-yolk mixture. Pour in an oiled baking dish. Bake at 375°F (190°C) for 17 to 20 minutes or until knife inserted in middle comes out clean.

Yield: 2 servings

Exchange, 1 serving: 1 high-fat meat, ⅓ bread
Each serving contains: Calories: 120, Carbohydrates: 5 g

Cheese Soufflé

3 T.	low-calorie margarine	45 mL
3 T.	all-purpose flour	45 mL
¼ t.	dry mustard	1 mL
1 c.	skim milk	250 mL
½ c.	sharp cheddar cheese	125 mL
½ t.	salt	2 mL
¼ t.	black pepper	1 mL
6	eggs, separated	6

Melt margarine in a skillet. Stir in the flour and dry mustard until well blended. Slowly add the milk; cook, stirring over low heat until smooth and thickened. Add the cheese, salt, and pepper. Cook until cheese melts. Remove cheese sauce from heat and allow to cool. In a bowl, beat egg yolks until thick and lemon-colored, Fold beaten yolks into the cheese sauce. In another bowl, beat egg whites until stiff. Gently fold cheese sauce into beaten whites. Turn into an oiled 3 qt. (3 L) baking dish. Set baking dish into a pan of hot water. Bake at 350°F (175°C) for 35 to 40 minutes or until a knife inserted in middle comes out clean. Serve immediately.

Yield: 6 servings

Exchange, 1 serving: 1½ medium-fat meat, ¾ bread
Each serving contains: Calories: 170, Carbohydrates: 11 g

Tuna Casserole

½ c.	condensed cream of chicken soup	125 mL
2 oz.	chunk tuna, in water	60 g
2 T.	celery, diced	30 mL
1 T.	onion, chopped	15 mL
1	egg, hard cooked	1
4 T.	potato chips, crushed	60 mL

Combine condensed soup, tuna, celery, and onion; mix thoroughly. Pour into small casserole. Slice egg; layer egg, then crushed potato chips. Bake at 350°F (175°C) for 20 minutes.

Microwave: Cook on Medium for 7 to 10 minutes.

Yield: 1 serving

Exchange, 1 serving: 1⅓ bread, 3 medium-fat meat
Each serving contains: Calories: 297, Carbohydrates: 130 g

Casserole of Shrimp

2 t.	margarine	30 mL
1 T.	parsley, chopped	15 mL
1 T.	sherry	15 mL
dash each	garlic powder, paprika, cayenne	dash each
½ c.	soft bread crumbs	125 mL
3 oz.	large shrimp, cooked	90 g

Melt margarine over low heat. Add parsley, sherry, and seasonings; cook slightly. Add bread crumbs; toss to mix. Place shrimp in small baking dish. Top with bread crumb mixture. Bake at 325°F (165°C) for 20 minutes.

Microwave: Melt margarine; add parsley, sherry, and seasonings. Cook on High for 2 minutes. Add bread crumbs; toss to mix. Place shrimp in small baking dish. Top with bread crumb mixture. Cook on Medium for 5 to 7 minutes.

Yield: 1 serving

Exchange, 1 serving: 3 high-fat meat, 1 bread
Each serving contains: Calories: 204, Carbohydrates: 11 g

Stuffed Cabbage Rolls

2 large	cabbage leaves	2 large
2 oz.	ground veal	60 g
2 oz.	ground lean beef	60 g
3 T.	skim milk	45 mL
1 slice	dry bread, crumbled	1 slice
1 t.	onion, grated	5 mL
dash each	salt, pepper, nutmeg	dash each
½ c.	beef broth	125 mL
1 T.	flour	15 mL

Cook cabbage leaves in boiling salted water until tender; drain. Combine ground veal, beef, skim milk, bread crumbs, onion, salt, pepper, and nutmeg; mix thoroughly. Place half of meat mixture in a cabbage leaf and roll up, tucking ends in. Secure with toothpicks. Place in small baking dish. Repeat with remaining meat mixture and cabbage leaf. Blend beef broth and flour; pour over cabbage rolls. Bake at 350°F (175°C) for 45 to 50 minutes.

Microwave: Cook on Medium for 10 to 12 minutes.

Yield: 1 serving

Exchange, 1 serving: 4 medium-fat meat, 1 vegetable, 1 bread
Each serving contains: Calories: 396, Carbohydrates: 28 g

Fresh Potato-Carrot Casserole

2 t.	margarine	10 mL
1 c.	Kellogg's bran flakes cereal	250 mL
dash	ground thyme	dash
1½ c.	potatoes, sliced	375 mL
1½ c.	carrots, sliced	375 mL
2 T.	margarine	30 mL
5 t.	all-purpose flour	25 mL
½ t.	salt	2 mL
dash	pepper	dash
dash	dried rosemary	dash
1 c.	milk	250 mL

Melt 2 t. (10 mL) margarine. Stir in ¾ c. (190 mL) of the cereal and the thyme. Set aside for the topping.

Place potatoes and carrots in medium saucepan with salted water to cover. Bring to boil. Boil, uncovered, for 5 minutes. Remove from heat. Drain. In a large saucepan, melt the margarine over low heat. Stir in flour, salt, pepper and rosemary. Add milk gradually, stirring until smooth. Increase heat to medium and cook, stirring constantly. until mixture boils and thickens. Remove from heat. Gently stir in potatoes, carrots and remaining ¼ c. (60 mL) of the cereal. Pour into a round 1½ qt. (1½ L) casserole. Sprinkle with the topping. Bake at 350°F (175°C) about 25 minutes or until vegetables are tender.

Yield: 6 servings

Exchange, 1 serving: 2 vegetable, 1 fat
Each serving contains: Calories: 105, Carbohydrates: 28 g

From Kellogg's Test Kitchens.

Soybean Casserole

1 c.	Stone-Buhr soybeans, soaked in water overnight	250 mL
2 T.	salt pork, diced	30 mL
1 c.	celery, sliced	250 mL
2 T.	onion, chopped	30 mL
1 T.	green pepper, sliced	15 mL
3 T.	Stone-Buhr all-purpose flour	45 mL
1 c.	2% milk	250 mL
¼ t.	salt	5 mL
¼ c.	Stone-Buhr wheat germ	60 mL

Cook soybeans in pressure cooker at 15 pounds pressure until tender, about 30 minutes; drain. Brown the salt pork in a skillet. Add the celery, onion and green pepper and cook for about 5 minutes or until vegetables are tender. Add the flour and mix well. Gradually add the milk and salt, stirring until it reaches the boiling point. Stir in the soybeans and pour the mixture into a baking dish. Cover with wheat germ. Bake at 350°F (175°C) for 30 minutes or until the wheat germ is golden brown.

Yield: 6 servings

Exchange, 1 serving: 1 bread
Each serving contains: Calories: 78, Carbohydrates: 15 g

With the compliments of Arnold Foods Company, Inc.

Herbed Spinach Pasta

¼ c.	Kellogg's All-Bran cereal	60 mL
¼ c.	Parmesan cheese, grated	60 mL
dash	black pepper	dash
¼ t.	dried basil	1 mL
½ t.	oregano leaves	2 mL
1 t.	fresh parsley, snipped	5 mL
3½ c.	spinach pasta ribbons	875 mL
2 T.	margarine	30 mL

Crush cereal into crumbs. Stir in the cheese, pepper, basil, oregano and parsley. Set aside. Cook pasta ribbons according to package directions just until tender. Drain. Gently toss hot pasta with margarine. Add cereal mixture, tossing until well combined. Serve immediately.

Yield: 5 servings

Exchange, 1 serving: 2 bread, ½ lean meat, 1 fat
Each serving contains: Calories: 210, Carbohydrates: 78 g

From Kellogg's Test Kitchens.

Soybeans and Millet Casserole

1 c.	Stone-Buhr soybeans	250 mL
1 c.	Stone-Buhr millet	250 mL
½ c.	onions, chopped	125 mL
½ c.	green pepper, chopped	125 mL
¾ c.	mushrooms, chopped	190 mL
1 t.	vegetable oil	5 mL
2	eggs, beaten	2
2 T.	margarine	30 mL
¼ c.	tomato juice	190 mL
1 t.	fresh marjoram, chopped	5 mL
¼ c.	brown sugar replacement	60 mL
	salt to taste	

Cook soybeans and millet according to package directions. Set aside. Sauté onions, green peppers and mushrooms in the oil for 10 minutes. Mix in remaining ingredients. Bake in well-greased casserole at 325°F (165°C) for about 45 to 60 minutes.

Yield: 6 servings

Exchange, 1 serving: 1 bread, 1 medium-fat meat
Each serving contains: Calories: 142, Carbohydrates: 30 g

With the compliments of Arnold Foods Company. Inc.

Golden Barley

You don't always have to serve potatoes. Try barley for a new side dish.

½ c.	cheddar cheese soup	125 mL
2 T.	hot water	30 mL
1 T.	catsup	15 mL
1½ c.	barley, cooked	375 mL
¼ c.	fresh parsley, chopped	60 mL

Combine cheese soup, hot water and catsup in a mixing bowl. Stir to blend. Add barley and thoroughly mix. Spoon into a greased microwave baking dish. Cover tightly. Microwave on medium for 7 minutes. Turn dish and stir slightly. Return to microwave, cook 3 minutes more. Remove cover, garnish with parsley.

Oven method: Increase water to ¼ c. (60 mL). Combine as above. Spoon into a greased baking dish or casserole. Cover tightly. Bake at 350°F (175°C) for 25 to 30 minutes or until mixture is bubbly. Garnish with parsley.

Yield: 4 servings

Exchange, 1 serving: 1 bread
Each serving contains: Calories: 69, Carbohydrates: 21 g

Savory Bran-Rice Pilaf

½ c.	long-grain brown rice	125 mL
1	chicken bouillon cube	1
¼ c.	margarine	60 mL
¼ c.	onion, chopped	60 mL
½ c.	celery, chopped	125 mL
½ c.	mushrooms, sliced and drained	125 mL
¼ c.	water chestnuts, sliced	60 mL
1 c.	Kellogg's All-Bran cereal	250 mL
¼ t.	ground sage	1 mL
½ t.	dried basil	2 mL
dash	pepper	dash
½ c.	water	125 mL

Cook rice according to package directions, adding bouillon cube instead of the salt and butter called for in the directions. While rice is cooking, melt margarine in a large skillet. Stir in onion, celery, mushrooms, and water chestnuts. Cook over medium heat, stirring occasionally, until celery is almost tender. Gently stir in the cooked rice, cereal, sage, basil, pepper and water. Cover and cook over very low heat about 15 minutes. Serve immediately.

Yield: 6 servings

Exchange, 1 serving: 1 bread, 1 vegetable, 2 fat
Each serving contains: Calories: 185, Carbohydrates: 8 g

From Kellogg's Test Kitchens.

Easy Lentils

I like this side dish with hamburgers instead of french fries.

1 slice	bacon	1 slice
⅓ c.	green onions, chopped	90 mL
¼ c.	celery, chopped	60 mL
1¼ c.	vegetable juice	310 mL
½ c.	lentils	125 mL

In a small saucepan, brown the bacon. Remove and set aside; crumble when cool. Add onions and celery to pan, cook slightly. Add vegetable juice. Bring to a boil and stir in the lentils. Cover and reduce heat. Cook until lentils are tender, but not mushy, and liquid has been absorbed, stirring occasionally. Add crumbled bacon.

Yield: 4 servings

Exchange, 1 serving: 1 bread
Each serving contains: Calories: 68, Carbohydrates: 158 g

Eggplant Casserole

1 c.	Stone-Buhr brown rice	250 mL
3 c.	water, salted and boiling	750 mL
4 c.	eggplant, cubed	1 L
½ c.	onion, chopped	125 mL
1 lb.	lean ground beef	500 g
1¾ c.	canned tomatoes, drained	440 mL
½ c.	white wine	125 mL
1 c.	Parmesan cheese, grated	250 mL
1½ t.	salt	7 mL
¼ t.	pepper	1 mL
½ t.	granulated sugar replacement	2 mL

Stir brown rice into 3 c. (750 mL) of the boiling water. Cover and cook about 35 minutes. Rice should be almost tender, but still slightly firm: drain rice well. Pour boiling salted water over eggplant; soak eggplant for 5 minutes. Drain eggplant. Brown onion and ground beef. Add tomatoes and wine; bring to boil and simmer 5 minutes. Add drained eggplant, rice and all remaining ingredients. Transfer to a 3 qt. (3 L) casserole. Cover and bake at 350°F (175°C) for 30 minutes. Remove cover; increase heat to 400°F (200°C) and bake 15 minutes or until golden brown on top.

Yield: 8 servings

Exchange, 1 serving: 1 bread, 2 medium-fat meat, 1 vegetable
Each serving contains: Calories: 258, Carbohydrates: 11 g

With the compliments of Arnold Foods Company, Inc.

Barley Hash

This is wonderful for a quick lunch or supper. It is also a good recipe to help you use leftover beef.

1½ c.	water	375 mL
¾ c.	quick-cooking barley	190 mL
2 t.	salt	10 mL
¼ lb.	beef roast, cooked and cut into small pieces	120 g
¼ c.	onion, finely chopped	60 mL
¼ c.	green pepper, finely chopped	60 mL
2 T.	water	30 mL
	salt and pepper	

Bring water to a boil: stir in the barley and salt. Reduce heat, cover and simmer for 10 to 12 minutes or until barley is tender; drain thoroughly. Meanwhile, combine beef, onion and green pepper in nonstick skillet over medium heat. Add the 2 T. (30 mL) water, cover and heat until vegetables are tender. Drain off any excess water. Add barley and heat thoroughly. Season with salt and pepper to taste.

Yield: 4 servings

Exchange, 1 serving: 2 bread, 1 lean meat
Each serving contains: Calories: 194, Carbohydrates: 31 g

Bulgur Pilaf

1 T.	margarine	15 mL
1 c.	bulgur wheat	250 mL
2 c.	beef broth, hot	500 mL
¼ c.	chive, chopped	60 mL
3 T.	sweet red pepper	45 mL
3 T.	fresh parsley, chopped	45 mL
	salt and pepper to taste	

Melt margarine in a medium saucepan. Add bulgur and sauté for 1 minute, stirring constantly. Add broth, chive and red pepper. Stir to mix. Simmer, covered, over low heat for 15 minutes or until broth is absorbed, Stir in parsley. Season with salt and pepper. Spoon into serving dish.

Yield: 4 servings

Exchange, 1 serving: 2 bread
Each serving contains: Calories: 132, Carbohydrates: 27 g

Baked Rice

1 cube	beef bouillon	1 cube
1 c.	hot water	250 mL
¼ c.	rice	60 mL
1	green onion, chopped	1
2 T.	celery, chopped	30 mL
3 T.	dry bread crumbs	45 mL

Dissolve bouillon in hot water. Add rice, green onion, and celery; cover. Cook for 5 minutes. Add bread crumbs. Pour into small baking dish. Bake at 350°F (175°C) for 25 to 30 minutes, or until top is lightly crusted.

Yield: 1 serving

Exchange, 1 serving: 1½ bread
Each serving contains: Calories: 115, Carbohydrates: 62 g

Rice Pilaf

½ c.	rice	125 mL
1 t.	butter	5 mL
½ t.	salt	3 mL
1 T.	lemon juice	15 mL
1 c.	boiling water	250 mL

Sauté rice in butter over low heat in large saucepan. Add remaining ingredients. Bring to a boil. Reduce heat; cover. Simmer until water is absorbed. Fluff with fork before serving.

Yield: 1 c. (250 mL)

Exchange, 1 serving: 2 bread, 1 fat
Each serving contains: Calories: 150, Carbohydrates: 38 g

Spanish Rice

3	bacon slices	3
1	white onion, chopped	1
1 t.	salt	5 mL
1 c.	long-grain rice	250 mL
2 c.	tomato juice, heated	500 mL
1 t.	Tone's paprika	5 mL

Fry bacon until crisp; drain and crumble. Combine bacon and remaining ingredients in a well-greased casserole; stir to blend. Cover and bake at 350°F (175°C) for 30 minutes or until rice is tender and liquid is absorbed; add extra water, if needed.

Yield: 10 servings

Exchange, 1 serving: 1 bread, ¼ fat
Each serving contains: Calories: 89, Carbohydrates: 16 g

Tamale Casserole

1½ lbs.	lean ground beef	750 g
1 med.	green pepper, chopped	1 med.
1 large	onion, chopped	1 large
1 lb. can	whole tomatoes, undrained	500 g can
8 oz. can	tomato sauce	240 g can
¼ c.	Kretschmer regular wheat germ	60 mL
2 t.	chili powder	10 mL
1½ t.	salt	7 mL
dash	hot pepper sauce	dash
1 recipe	wheat germ cornbread	1 recipe
1 c.	sharp cheddar cheese, grated	250 mL

Cook beef, green pepper and onion over medium heat until beef is lightly browned. Drain. Stir in tomatoes, tomato sauce, wheat germ, chili powder, salt and hot pepper sauce. Simmer while preparing the batter for wheat germ cornbread. Pour hot meat mixture into greased 3 qt. (3 L) casserole. Spread evenly with the batter. Bake at 400°F (200°C) for 25 to 30 minutes until corn bread is golden brown. Sprinkle with cheese. Bake for 2 to 3 minutes longer until cheese melts.

Yield: 8 servings

Exchange with 1 serving corn bread: 1 bread, 2 ½ medium-fat meat
Each serving contains: Calories: 224, Carbohydrates: 24 g

With the courtesy of Kretschmer Wheat Germ/International Multifoods.

Great Bean Casserole

A quick Saturday lunch to make ahead and have extra time while it's baking.

2 c.	Great Northern beans, cooked	500 mL
1 cube	chicken bouillon	1 cube
1 c.	boiling water	250 mL
1 t.	cornstarch	5 mL
3 T.	cold water	45 mL
1 c.	broccoli stems, chopped	250 mL
3 T.	onion, chopped	45 mL
½ lb.	freshly ground pork, cooked	250 g
1 t.	salt	5 mL

Place beans in 1½ qt. (1½ L) casserole. Dissolve bouillon cube in boiling water; pour over beans. Dissolve cornstarch in cold water; add to beans. Add broccoli, onion. pork and salt. Stir to completely mix. Cover tightly. Bake at 350°F (175°C) for 2 hours or until beans are completely tender, adding more water, if needed.

Yield: 4 servings

Exchange, 1 serving: 1 bread, 1 vegetable, 2 lean meat
Each serving contains: Calories: 220, Carbohydrates: 33 g

Vegetable Linguine

12 oz. pkg.	enriched linguine	360 g pkg.
4 small	stalks broccoli, thinly sliced lengthwise	4 small
1 med	butternut squash, thinly sliced	1 med
1 large	carrot, shredded	1 large
1 T.	onion, chopped	15 mL
32 oz. jar	meatless spaghetti sauce	900 g jar
½ c.	Parmesan cheese, grated	125 mL
½ c.	bean sprouts	125 mL

Cook linguine as package directs for 7 minutes. Add vegetables; cook 5 minutes and drain. In a medium saucepan, simmer spaghetti sauce 5 minutes or until thoroughly heated. Place pasta and vegetables in a large bowl. Add sauce and cheese; toss well. Serve 6 equal portions topped with the bean sprouts.

Yield: 6 servings

Exchange, 1 serving: 3½ bread, 2 vegetable, 1 medium-fat meat
Each serving contains: Calories: 382, Carbohydrates: 54 g

Vegetarian Supper Pie

1 c.	soda cracker crumbs (about 26 crackers)	250 mL
¾ c.	Kretschmer regular wheat germ	190 mL
½ c.	margarine, melted	125 mL
1 lb.	zucchini, sliced	500 g
1 med.	onion, sliced	1 med.
1 t.	dried marjoram, crushed	5 mL
½ t.	salt	2 mL
¼ t.	pepper	1 mL
¼ t.	dried tarragon, crushed	1 mL
1 c.	Monterey Jack cheese, grated	250 mL
½ c.	Parmesan cheese, grated	125 mL
2	eggs	2
⅓ c.	nonfat milk	90 mL
1 med	tomato, thinly sliced	1 med

Combine cracker crumbs, ¼ c. (60 mL) of the wheat germ and 6 T. (90 mL) margarine in small bowl. Stir well. Press evenly on bottom and about 1 in. (2.5 cm) up sides of 9 in. (23 cm) springform pan or on bottom and sides of 9 in. (23 cm) pie pan. Bake at 400°F (200°C) for 7 to 9 minutes until very lightly browned. Remove from oven.

Sauté zucchini and onion in remaining 2 T. (30 mL) margarine until crisp-tender. Add seasonings to vegetable mixture; stir well. Place half the vegetables in the crumb crust. Sprinkle with 3 T. (45 mL) of the wheat germ. Top with ½ c. (125 mL) Monterey Jack, ½ c. (125 mL) Parmesan cheese, remaining vegetables, and 3 T. (45 mL) wheat germ. Beat together the eggs and milk; pour over vegetable mixture. Arrange tomato slices on top. Sprinkle with remaining cheese and wheat germ. Bake at 325°F (165°C) for 40 to 45 minutes until hot and bubbly. Let stand 5 minutes before cutting and serving.

Yield: 6 servings

Exchange, 1 serving: 1 bread, 1 low-fat milk, ½ medium-fat meat, 4 fat
Each serving contains: Calories: 420, Carbohydrates: 9 g

With the courtesy of Kretschmer Wheat Germ/International Multifoods.

Light Eggplant Parmigiana

8 slices	eggplant, ¼ in. (6-mm) thick	8 slices
1 T.	Mazola corn oil	15 mL
8 t.	Corn Oil Herb Blend (recipe follows)	40 mL
4 oz.	skim-milk mozzarella cheese, thinly sliced	120 g
8 slices	tomato	8 slices
4 t.	Parmesan cheese, grated	20 mL

Lightly brush 1 side of eggplant slices with oil. On a cookie sheet, place eggplant slices with the oil side down. Spread top of each eggplant slice with 1 T. (15 mL) of the herb mixture. Top with mozzarella, tomato, and cheese. Bake at 375°F (190°C) for 15 minutes or until eggplant is tender.

Corn Oil Herb Blend

¼ c.	Mazola corn oil	60 mL
1 c.	fresh parsley	250 mL
1 t.	dried basil	5 mL
1 t.	dried marjoram	5 mL
dash	black pepper	dash

In blender container, place the corn oil, parsley, basil, marjoram and pepper; cover. Blend on medium speed until smooth.

Yield: 4 servings

Exchange, 1 serving: 1 vegetable, 1½ high-fat meat
Each serving contains: Calories: 210, Carbohydrates: 15 g

Stuffed Eggplant Italiano

1 lb.	eggplant	500 g
⅓ c.	All-Bran cereal	90 mL
1 c.	fresh mushrooms, sliced	250 mL
1 c.	Parmesan cheese, grated	60 mL
¼ c.	onion, chopped	60 mL
¼ c.	green pepper, finely chopped	60 mL
2 T.	margarine, melted	30 mL
1 small clove	garlic, finely chopped	1 small clove
½ t.	salt	2 mL
½ t.	dried basil	2 mL
dash	black pepper	dash
⅓ c.	mozzarella cheese, shredded	90 mL

Cut eggplant in half lengthwise. Place halves, cut side down, in shallow baking pan. Bake at 350°F (175°C) for 15 minutes. Remove from oven. Cool slightly. Scoop out pulp, leaving ⅜ in. (1 cm) shell. Place shells, cut side up, in baking pan. Coarsely chop eggplant pulp. Combine with remaining ingredients except mozzarella cheese. Fill eggplant shells, pressing firmly. Cover with foil. Pierce foil in several places to allow steam to escape. Bake at 350°F (175°C) about 40 minutes or until vegetables are tender. Remove foil and sprinkle with the mozzarella. Bake, uncovered, about 2 minutes longer or until cheese melts. Cut each half into 2 pieces to serve.

Yield: 4 servings

Exchange, 1 serving: 2 medium-fat meat
Each serving contains: Calories: 150, Carbohydrates: 13 g

From Kellogg's Test Kitchens.

Stuffed Green Peppers

½ c.	Stone–Buhr long-grain brown rice	125 mL
¼ c.	salt	1 mL
8 med.	green peppers	8 med.
1 lb.	ground beef chuck	500 g
⅓ c.	onion, minced	90 mL
8 oz. can	tomato sauce	227 g can
1 t.	salt	5 mL

Place rice in saucepan with 1½ c. (375 mL) water. Add salt and bring to a boil. Cover and simmer until rice is tender and until all the water has been absorbed, about 40 minutes. Cut off and reserve tops of green peppers: scoop out and discard seeds. Place peppers upright in a baking dish. Mix together beef, onion, tomato sauce, salt, and cooked rice. Stuff green peppers and replace tops. Pour ½ c. (125 mL) water in bottom of baking dish and bake in a 350° (175°C) oven for about 1 hour.

Yield: 8 servings

Exchange, 1 serving: 1 bread, 1 lean meat
Each serving contains: Calories: 166, Carbohydrates: 14 g

With the compliments of Arnold Foods Company. Inc.

Simple Sunday Brunch

1 qt.	bread cubes	1 L
2 c.	ham, cooked and cubed	500 mL
1 c.	cheddar cheese, shredded	250 mL
2 c.	skim milk	500 mL
3	eggs	3

Place bread cubes on a cookie sheet; toast and dry in oven. Spray a 9 × 13 in. (23 × 33 cm) pan with vegetable spray. Layer bread cubes, ham cubes, and cheese. Combine milk and eggs in a bowl; beat to blend. Pour over ham mixture. Cover and refrigerate over night. Bake at 350°F (175°C) for 40 to 45 minutes or until set. Serve hot.

Yield: 12 servings

Exchange, 1 serving: 2 medium-fat meat, 1⅓ bread
Each serving contains: Calories: 177, Carbohydrates: 5 g

Sausage and Hominy Brunch

29 oz. can	white hominy, drained	850 g can
¼ t.	ground nutmeg	1 mL
¼ t.	ground cinnamon	1 mL
1 lb.	pork link sausages	500 g

Combine the hominy, nutmeg, and cinnamon in a bowl; stir to blend. Place in 9 in. (23 cm) square baking pan. Set a wire cake rack over the same baking pan and lay the sausages on the rack. Bake at 350°F (175°C) for 1 hour or until sausages are browned. Drain the hominy. Mound hominy in middle of heated platter. Surround with sausages.

Yield: 12 servings

Exchange, 1 serving: 2 high-fat meat, ¾ bread
Each serving contains: Calories: 235, Carbohydrates: 11 g

Eggs

Simple Baked Egg

1	egg	1	
½ t.	low-calorie margarine	2 mL	
	salt and pepper to taste		

Melt margarine in a custard cup. Break egg into the cup. Sprinkle with salt and pepper. Bake at 350°F (175°C) for about 15 minutes or until the egg is firm but not hard. Serve hot.

Yield: 1 serving

Exchange: 1 medium-fat meat, ½ fat
Each serving contains: Calories: 100, Carbohydrates: negligible

Baked Egg and Cheese

An easy alternative to an omelette.

1	egg	1	
½ t.	low-calorie margarine	2 mL	
1 t.	sharp cheddar cheese, shredded	5 mL	

Melt margarine in a custard cup. Break egg into the cup and top with cheddar cheese. Bake at 350°F (175°C) for 15 minutes or until egg is firm and cheese is melted. Serve hot.

Yield: 1 serving

Exchange: 1 medium-fat meat, 1 fat
Each serving contains: Calories: 122, Carbohydrates: negligible

Eggs in Tomato Nests

4	tomatoes	4	
4	eggs	4	
4 t.	butter	20 mL	
	salt and pepper to taste		

Cut tops from the tomatoes. Scoop out a hollow in the middle of each tomato large enough to hold the egg. Place 1 t. (5 mL) of butter in each tomato hollow. Break an egg into each hollow. Place tomatoes on a baking sheet or 8 or 9 in. (20 or 23 cm) pie pan. Bake at 350°F (175°C) for 15 to 18 minutes or until eggs are firm and tomato is cooked.

Yield: 4 servings

Exchange, 1 serving: 1 medium-fat meat, 1 vegetable, 1 fat
Each serving contains: Calories: 150, Carbohydrates: 6 g

Eggs à la King

This is such a pretty dish, I like to serve it on a foggy or rainy day to brighten things up.

2 T.	butter	30 mL
3 T.	all-purpose flour	45 mL
2 c.	skim milk	500 mL
	salt and pepper to taste	
6	eggs, hard-cooked	6
3	small carrots, sliced and cooked	3
⅓ c.	peas, cooked	90 mL
⅓ c.	snow-capped mushrooms, sliced and cooked	90 mL
1	medium pimiento, sliced and cooked	1
	fresh parsley for garnish (optional)	
6	bread slices, toasted	6

Melt butter in top of a double boiler. Blend in the flour; add the milk and stir until sauce thickens. Season with salt and pepper and cook 3 minutes longer. Slice or chop the eggs. Gently fold eggs, carrots, peas, and mushrooms into the sauce. Place toast on heated serving plates. Evenly divide egg mixture among the 6 pieces of toast. Arrange pimiento slices in crisscross fashion over the top of egg mixture. If desired, garnish plate with fresh parsley.

Yield: 6 servings

Exchange, 1 serving: 1 medium-fat meat, 1½ bread
Each serving contains: Calories: 186, Carbohydrates: 22 g

French-Style Eggs

1 T.	butter	15 mL
3 T.	all-purpose flour	45 mL
¾ c.	2% milk	190 mL
½ t.	paprika	2 mL
¼ t.	salt	1 mL
dash	black pepper, freshly ground	dash
6	hard-cooked eggs	6
¼ c.	dry bread crumbs, finely ground	60 mL
	vegetable oil for deep-fat frying	
½ c.	Quick Tomato Sauce	125 mL

Melt butter in a saucepan; blend in the flour. Add milk and seasonings. Cook over low heat until sauce thickens, stirring constantly. Dip eggs in the sauce; cool eggs and roll in bread crumbs. Heat oil to 375°F (190°C). Fry eggs until brown. Serve hot with the tomato sauce.

Yield: 6 servings

Exchange, 1 serving: 1 bread, 1 medium-fat meat, 1 vegetable
Each serving contains: Calories: 172, Carbohydrates: 19 g

Egg Croquettes

2 T.	low-calorie margarine	30 mL
3 T.	all-purpose flour	45 mL
¾ c.	2% milk	190 mL
½ t.	salt	2 mL
⅛ t.	paprika	½ mL
4	eggs, hard-cooked	4
1	raw egg	1
2 T.	water	30 mL
⅓ c.	salted cracker crumbs	90 mL

Melt margarine in top of a double boiler; add the flour and stir constantly until blended. Add the milk, salt, and paprika. Cook and stir until mixture thickens. Chop the hard-cooked eggs; add to creamed mixture. Remove from heat and allow to cool. Combine the raw egg and water in small narrow bowl; beat until well blended. When egg/cream mixture is cold, shape into 6 large or 12 small croquettes. Roll in the cracker crumbs; then dip in egg-water and again in the crumbs. Refrigerate until completely chilled. Fry in deep fat, heated to 375°F (190°C), for about 3 to 5 minutes until golden brown. Serve hot.

Yield: 6 servings

Exchange, 1 serving: 1 bread, 1 medium-fat meat
Each serving contains: Calories: 98, Carbohydrates: 16 g

Mushroom-Capped Eggs

These eggs have a pixie look that children love.

6	eggs, hard-cooked	6
12	mushroom caps	12
1 c.	mushroom soup	250 mL
1 t.	paprika	5 mL
½ t.	salt	2 mL
	black pepper, freshly ground	

Cut eggs in half. Place a mushroom cap on top of the yolk. Arrange mushroom-capped eggs in a single layer in a baking pan. Top with the soup. Sprinkle with paprika, salt, and pepper. Bake at 350°F (175°C) for 12 to 15 minutes or until thoroughly heated. Serve hot.

Yield: 12 servings

Exchange, 1 serving: ½ medium-fat meat, ½ bread
Each serving contains: Calories: 63, Carbohydrates: 5 g

Bacon-Ringed Eggs

A nice Sunday brunch dish for the family or just for a single serving.

1	bacon slice	1
1	egg	1
½ c.	mashed potatoes	125 mL
	salt and pepper to taste	
	fresh parsley for garnish	

Lightly oil the bottom of a custard cup. Curl the bacon slice around the inside of the cup. (If you prefer the bacon crisp, fry slightly before lining the cup.) Break the egg inside the bacon ring. Season with salt and pepper to taste. Bake at 350°F (175°C) for about 15 to 20 minutes or until egg is firm but not hard. (Cooking time will vary with the number of bacon and egg dishes you are baking.) Carefully remove egg and bacon together from the cup. Place in the middle of the mashed potatoes. Garnish with parsley. Serve hot.

Yield: 1 serving

Exchange: 1 bread, 1½ medium-fat meat
Each serving contains: Calories: 188, Carbohydrates: 15

New Orleans Eggs

5	tomatoes, peeled and chopped	5
½	green pepper, chopped	½
½ c.	celery, chopped	125 mL
¼ c.	white onion, chopped	60 mL
1	bay leaf	1
½ t.	salt	2 mL
¼ t.	black pepper, freshly ground	1 mL
¾ c.	fine bread crumbs	190 mL
6	eggs	6
½ c.	American cheese, grated	125 mL

In a saucepan, combine the tomatoes, green pepper, celery, onion, bay leaf, salt, and pepper. Cook and stir over medium heat for 10 minutes. Remove bay leaf. Stir in the bread crumbs. Spread the mixture into a lightly oiled casserole. With the back of a spoon, make 6 small hollows in the mixture and break the eggs into the hollows. Sprinkle with cheese. Bake at 350°F (175°C) for 15 to 20 minutes until eggs are firm and cheese has melted. Serve hot.

Yield: 6 servings

Exchange, 1 serving: 1½ medium-fat meat, ¾ bread, 1 vegetable
Each serving contains: Calories: 190, Carbohydrates: 16 g

Eggs Baked in Shells

This is a lovely dish to serve.

¼ c.	low-calorie margarine, melted	60 mL
¼ c.	all-purpose flour	60 mL
½ t.	salt	5 mL
⅛ t.	black pepper	½ mL
2 c.	skim milk	500 mL
½ c.	sharp cheddar cheese	125 mL
6	eggs	6

Combine the margarine, flour, salt, pepper, and milk in a saucepan; stir to thoroughly blend. Cook and stir until mixture just starts to thicken. Stir in the cheese; cook until cheese melts. Divide evenly among 6 shell baking dishes; allow to cool slightly to thicken. With the back of the spoon, make a hollow or indentation in the cheese sauce and break 1 egg in each. Season with salt and pepper. Place filled shells on a baking sheet. Cover lightly with aluminum foil. Bake at 350°F (175°C) for 15 to 20 minutes or until eggs are firm but not hard.

Yield: 6 servings

*Exchange, 1 serving: 1½ medium-fat meat, ¾ bread,
    ½ low-fat milk*
Each serving contains: Calories: 235, Carbohydrates: 16 g

Eggs with Mornay Sauce

2 T.	low-calorie margarine	30 mL
2 T.	all-purpose flour	30 mL
½ t.	salt	2 mL
	pepper to taste	
1	small bay leaf	1
1½ t.	fresh parsley, minced	7 mL
2 t.	onion, minced	10 mL
1 c.	skim milk	250 mL
2 T.	Gruyère cheese	30 mL
6	eggs	6

Melt margarine in a saucepan. Add flour, salt, pepper, bay leaf, parsley, and onion; stir to blend. Slowly add the milk. Cook and stir until thickened; remove the bay leaf. Stir in the cheese; remove pan from heat. Arrange 6 custard cups on a baking pan. Pour 1 T. (15 mL) of the sauce into each cup; break an egg over the sauce. Cover egg with an additional 2 T. (30 mL) of the sauce. Bake at 350°F (175°C) for 15 to 20 minutes or until eggs are firm but not hard. Serve immediately.

Yield: 6 servings

Exchange, 1 serving: ⅓ bread, 1 high-fat meat
Each serving contains: Calories: 114, Carbohydrates: 4 g

Baked Potato with Egg

3	medium potatoes	3	
3 T.	skim milk	45 mL	
	salt and pepper to taste		
6	eggs	6	
	paprika		

Wash and scrub the potatoes. Bake at 425°F (220°C) about 40 minutes or until tender. Reduce oven heat to 350°F (175°C). Cut potatoes lengthwise in half. Carefully scoop out potatoes in a small bowl without breaking the skin. Mash potatoes with the milk. (If potatoes seem dry, add a small amount of hot water.) Beat until light and fluffy. Fill potato skins, leaving a hollow in the middle. Break an egg in each hollow. Season with salt and pepper and sprinkle with paprika. Place back in oven and bake for about 7 minutes until egg is firm but not hard.

Yield: 6 servings

Exchange, 1 serving: 1 medium-fat meat, ½ bread
Each serving contains: Calories: 115, Carbohydrates: 8 g

Eggs on Spanish Rice

2 c.	long-grain rice, cooked	500 mL
6 oz. can	tomato paste	180 g can
1½ c.	water	375 mL
½ c.	onion, chopped	125 mL
½ t.	salt	2 mL
1	bay leaf	1
2	whole cloves	2
2 T.	butter, melted	30 mL
2 T.	all-purpose flour	30 mL
6	eggs	6

Arrange rice in layer on bottom of well-greased baking dish. To make the Spanish sauce, combine tomato paste, water, onion, salt, bay leaf, and cloves in a saucepan. Cook and stir over medium heat for 10 minutes or until well blended and hot; remove bay leaf and cloves. Blend in the butter and flour; cook and stir until mixture is smooth and thickened. Make 6 hollows or indentations in the rice and break an egg into each indentation. Pour the sauce over eggs and rice. Bake at 350°F (175°C) for 15 to 20 minutes or until eggs are firm but not hard. Serve hot.

Yield: 6 servings

Exchange, 1 serving: 1 bread, 1 medium-fat meat
Each serving contains: Calories: 148, Carbohydrates: 16 g

Herbed Eggs in Ramekins

4	eggs, hard-cooked	4
1 t. each	basil, thyme, sweet marjoram, and parsley	5 mL each
2 T.	low-calorie margarine	30 mL
2	eggs, slightly beaten	2
¼ c.	skim evaporated milk	60 mL
¼ c.	skim milk	60 mL
	salt and pepper to taste	

Melt margarine in a saucepan. Add the herbs and sauté for several minutes. Mince the hard-cooked eggs. Remove saucepan from heat and add remaining ingredients; stir to blend. Divide mixture evenly among 4 well-greased ramekins or custard cups. Place ramekins in a pan of hot water. Bake at 350°F (175°C) for 20 minutes or until firm.

Yield: 4 servings

Exchange, 1 serving: 2 medium-fat meat
Each serving contains: Calories: 160, Carbohydrates: 2 g

Old-Fashioned Poached Egg

2 c.	water	500 mL
1 t.	white vinegar	5 mL
½ t.	salt	2 mL
¼ t.	black pepper	1 mL
1	egg	1
1	bread slice, toasted	1

Heat water to the boiling point in a small skillet. Add the vinegar, salt, and pepper. Break egg into a cup and gently slip into the boiling water. With a spoon or fork, make a whirlpool effect in the water. Reduce heat to allow water to simmer. Cook until egg is firm. Remove egg with a skimmer; drain and serve on toast.

Yield: 1 serving

Exchange: 1 medium-fat meat, 1 bread
Each serving contains: Calories: 148, Carbohydrates: 14 g

Eggs Florentine

A must recipe for any breakfast or brunch cookbook. This is a favorite dish for many people.

3 c.	spinach, cooked	750 mL
6	eggs	6
	salt and pepper to taste	
½ c.	sharp cheddar cheese	125 mL
½ c.	skim evaporated milk	125 mL
½ c.	skim milk	125 mL
2 c.	bread crumbs, toasted	500 mL

Place cooked spinach in bottom of shallow baking dish; make 6 hollows in the spinach. Drop an egg into each hollow and season with salt and pepper. To prepare the cheese sauce, mix the cheese, evaporated milk, and skim milk in the top of a double boiler over boiling water; heat until the cheese melts and the sauce thickens. Pour the hot sauce over the eggs and spinach. Sprinkle with bread crumbs. Bake at 350°F (175°C) for about 25 minutes until brown. Serve hot.

Yield: 6 servings

Exchange, 1 serving: 1 medium-fat meat, 1 vegetable, 2 bread
Each serving contains: Calories: 235, Carbohydrates: 36 g

Poached Eggs with Wine

1 t.	butter	5 mL
½ c.	Rhine wine	125 mL
4	eggs	4
	salt and pepper to taste	
2 T.	blue cheese, crumbled	30 mL

Melt butter in a skillet. Add the wine. Carefully slip eggs into skillet. Season with salt and pepper. Cover and cook over medium heat until egg whites are set but egg is still loose. Sprinkle with the cheese. Cover and continue cooking until eggs are done as you like them and cheese is melted.

Yield: 4 servings

Exchange, 1 serving: 1 medium-fat meat, ½ bread
Each serving contains: Calories: 114, Carbohydrates: 7 g

Egg-Mushroom Cream Sauce on Muffins

4	eggs, hard-cooked	4
½ c.	skim milk	125 mL
¼ c.	evaporated skim milk	60 mL
2 t.	all-purpose flour	10 mL
½ c.	snow-capped mushrooms, sliced	125 mL
¼ lb.	cheddar cheese, grated	250 g
	salt and pepper to taste	
3	English muffins	3
	fresh parsley for garnish (optional)	

Slice or chop the eggs. Scald ¼ c. (60 mL) milk and the evaporated milk in top of a double boiler. In a bowl, blend remaining milk and flour into a smooth paste. Stir flour mixture into the scalded milk. Add eggs, mushrooms, and cheese. Season with salt and pepper. Cook and stir over simmering water until cheese melts. Break muffins in half and toast. Place each half muffin on a heated plate. Evenly divide cream sauce among the 6 muffins. If desired, garnish with fresh parsley. Serve immediately.

Yield: 6 servings

Exchange, 1 serving: 1 bread, 1 high-fat meat, ½ fat
Each serving contains: Calories: 198, Carbohydrates: 17 g

Delightful Eggs

An easy way to deliver eggs and meat to the table and still have time for your guests.

1 c.	corned beef, chopped finely	250 mL
1 c.	dry bread crumbs, finely crushed	250 mL
⅓ c.	skim milk	90 mL
4 c.	mashed potatoes	1 L
8	eggs, poached	8
2	tomatoes, sliced	2
8	green pepper rings	8

Mix the corned beef, bread crumbs, and milk in a bowl to make a paste. (If more moisture is needed, add small amounts of water to get the desired paste consistency.) Spread the meat-bread mixture on the bottom of a lightly greased tart pan; do not let mixture touch sides of pan. Place mashed potatoes in a pastry tube fitted with a large decorative opening. Pipe an edging around the meat-bread mixture. Divide the central circle of meat-bread mixture into 8 even triangles by piping the remaining mashed potatoes into a spoke design. Slip a poached egg into each triangle. Bake at 425°F (220°C) until potato is browned. Garnish with tomato slices and pepper slices. Serve immediately.

Yield: 8 servings

Exchange, 1 serving: 1½ medium-fat meat, 1½ bread
Each serving contains: Calories: 251, Carbohydrates: 21 g

Creamed Bacon and Eggs

3	bacon slices	3
⅓ c.	celery, sliced	90 mL
¼ c.	onion, chopped	60 mL
1 c.	skim milk	250 mL
1 T.	all-purpose flour	15 mL
2	eggs, hard-cooked	2
	salt and pepper to taste	
4	bread slices, toasted	4

Fry bacon until crisp in a skillet. Remove bacon from pan and discard all but 1 T. (15 mL) of bacon grease. Sauté celery and onion in the skillet until onion is slightly browned and celery is tender; set aside. Combine milk and flour in top of a double boiler. Cook and stir over simmering water until mixture thickens. Crumble the bacon. Chop the eggs. Add celery, onion, bacon, and eggs to the creamed mixture. Season with salt and pepper. Place toast slices on 4 warm plates. Spoon mixture evenly over toast. Serve immediately.

Yield: 4 servings

Exchange, 1 serving: 1 bread, 1 high-fat meat
Each serving contains: Calories: 159, Carbohydrates: 17 g

Poached Eggs, Chinese Style

1 T.	low-calorie margarine	15 mL
¼ c.	celery, thinly sliced	60 mL
2 T.	broccoli, chopped	30 mL
2 T.	red bell pepper, chopped	30 mL
1 T.	white onion, chopped	15 mL
3	snow mushrooms, sliced	3
½ c.	rice, cooked	25 mL
2	eggs, poached	2

Melt the margarine in a small nonstick skillet. Add vegetables and sauté until crisp-tender. Divide rice on 2 very warm serving dishes. Place poached egg in middle of each rice bed. Top with sautéed vegetables.

Yield: 2 servings

Exchange, 1 serving: 1 medium-fat meat, ½ bread, ½ vegetable
Each serving contains: Calories: 125, Carbohydrates: 9 g

Poached Eggs in Nests of Rice

1 c.	2% milk	250 mL
2 T.	low-calorie margarine	30 mL
2 T.	all-purpose flour	30 mL
½ c.	cheddar cheese, shredded	125 mL
1 c.	rice, cooked	250 mL
4	eggs, poached	4
10	stuffed green olives, sliced	10

To make the sauce, combine milk, margarine, flour, salt, and pepper in a saucepan. Cook and stir over medium-low heat until mixture thickens. Remove from heat, add the cheese, and stir until cheese melts. On 4 warmed plates, shape the cooked rice into 4 small nests. Place a poached egg in middle of each nest. Cover with sauce; top with olive slices. Serve immediately.

Yield: 4 servings

Exchange, 1 serving: 2 medium-fat meat, ½ low-fat milk
Each serving contains: Calories: 192, Carbohydrates: 7 g

Fair Island Eggs

These eggs look like little islands, hence the name.

4	onions, sliced	4
2 T.	low-calorie margarine	30 mL
1 c.	skim milk	250 mL
1 T.	all-purpose flour	15 mL
8	eggs, hard-cooked and sliced	8
½ c.	dry bread crumbs	125 mL

Brown onions in margarine and place in a layer on the bottom of a 9 in. (23 cm) square baking dish. Combine milk and flour in top of a double boiler; cook and stir until partially thickened. Season with salt and pepper to taste. Pour sauce over onions. Place sliced eggs on top of sauce. Sprinkle bread crumbs around the egg slices. Bake at 400°F (200°C) until crumbs are browned.

Yield: 8 servings

Exchange, 1 serving: 1 medium-fat meat, ½ bread
Each serving contains: Calories: 126, Carbohydrates: 6g

Eggs and Mushrooms

1 T.	olive oil	15 mL
2 T.	onion, minced	30 mL
1 T.	fresh parsley, minced	15 mL
2 c.	mushrooms, sliced	500 mL
½ c.	celery, sliced	125 mL
1 T.	all-purpose flour	15 mL
½ c.	Rhine wine	125 mL
6	eggs, hard-cooked and chopped	6
	salt and pepper to taste	

Heat olive oil in a nonstick skillet. Add onion and parsley; sauté for 2 minutes. Stir in the mushrooms and celery. Cover and cook over low heat for 10 minutes. Sprinkle flour over top of vegetables and mix well. Slowly stir in the wine. Cover and simmer for 5 minutes. Add the eggs, salt, and pepper. Cover and simmer for 5 more minutes, stirring.

Yield: 6 servings

Exchange, 1 serving: 1 medium-fat meat, ½ vegetable, ½ fat
Each serving contains: Calories: 106, Carbohydrates: 2 g

Shrimp-and-Egg Newburg

3 T.	low-calorie margarine	45 mL
1 qt.	skim milk	1 L
1 t.	salt	5 mL
6 oz.	Brilliant cooked frozen shrimp	180 g
¼ c.	Newburg Sauce	60 mL
2	egg yolks, uncooked	2
3	eggs, hard-cooked	3
3 c.	noodles, cooked	750 mL
10	bread slices, toasted	10
	paprika (optional)	
	fresh parsley (optional)	

Melt margarine in the top of a double boiler. Add 3 c. (750 mL) of the milk, the salt, shrimp, and Newburg Sauce. Combine egg yolks and remaining milk in a small bowl. Whip or beat to blend. Stir into shrimp mixture; cook and stir until thickened. Cut the hard-cooked eggs into quarters. Add to the sauce and heat. Serve on hot toast. If desired, garnish with paprika and parsley.

Yield: 10 servings

Exchange, 1 serving: 2 bread, ¾ medium-fat meat
Each serving contains: Calories: 224, Carbohydrates: 32 g

Creamy Scrambled Eggs

1 T.	low-calorie margarine	15 mL
3 oz.	cream cheese, softened	85 g
¼ c.	evaporated skim milk	60 mL
1 T.	sherry	15 mL
6	eggs	6
	salt and pepper to taste	

Coat a nonstick skillet with vegetable spray. Melt margarine in the skillet. Combine cream cheese, milk, and sherry in a bowl; beat to blend. Add eggs, one at a time, whipping until thoroughly blended. Season with salt and pepper. Pour into the heated skillet. Cook and stir over medium heat until eggs are cooked as desired.

Microwave: Melt margarine in a 2 qt. (2 L) baking dish. Beat remaining ingredients as described above. Pour into baking dish. Cook on medium for 4 minutes, stirring after 2 minutes. Return to microwave for 1½ minutes longer or until eggs are set but still slightly moist. Remove from microwave. Stir, cover, and allow to set for 2 minutes.

Yield: 6 servings

Exchange, 1 serving: 1 medium-fat meat, 1 fat
Each serving contains: Calories: 166, Carbohydrates: 3 g

Scrambled Eggs Primavera

2 T.	Mazola corn oil	30 mL
1 c.	zucchini, chopped	250 mL
½ c.	mushrooms, sliced	125 mL
¼ c.	green onion, thinly sliced	60 mL
4	eggs, lightly beaten	4
dash	dried basil	dash
4	English muffins, split and toasted	4
1	tomato, chopped	1
1 T.	parsley, chopped	15 mL

In a skillet, heat oil over medium-high heat. Add next 3 ingredients. Cook and stir for 2 minutes or until zucchini is crisp-tender. Reduce heat to medium low. Add eggs and basil. Cook and stir for 3 to 4 minutes or until eggs are set. Spoon onto muffin halves. Garnish with tomato and parsley.

Yield: 4 servings

Exchange, 1 serving: 2 bread, 1 lowfat milk, 1 vegetable
Each serving contains: Calories: 290, Carbohydrates: 33 g

Reprinted from "A Diet for the Young at Heart" by Mazola.

Italian-Style Scrambled Eggs

1 small	butternut squash, thinly sliced	1 small
1 small	onion, thinly sliced	1 small
3 T.	butter	45 mL
1 c.	meatless spaghetti sauce	250 mL
4	large eggs	4
2 T.	water	30 mL
	salt and pepper to taste	

In a medium skillet, lightly sauté squash and onion in 1 T. (15 mL) of the butter until onion is translucent. Add spaghetti sauce and season with salt and pepper; simmer 5 minutes and set aside. Beat together the eggs and water. In a large skillet, scramble eggs in remaining butter. Serve eggs topped with vegetable-sauce mixture.

Yield: 4 servings

Exchange, 1 serving: 1 bread, 1 vegetable, 1 medium-fat meat, 1 fat
Each serving contains: Calories: 213, Carbohydrates: 10 g

Spicy Scrambled Egg Enchiladas

8 oz.	tomato sauce	30 g
4 oz.	green chilies, diced and divided	120 g can
½ c.	Kretschmer regular wheat germ, divided	125 mL
2 T.	green onion, chopped	30 mL
1 T.	vegetable oil	15 mL
4	eggs	4
¼ t.	oregano, crushed	1 mL
dash	salt	dash
½ c.	Monterey Jack cheese, grated and divided	125 mL
4	flour or corn tortillas	4

Combine tomato sauce, half the chilies, 2 T. (30 mL) of the wheat germ and the green onion. Mix well. Heat oil in a skillet. Add eggs, remaining chilies and wheat germ, oregano and salt. Stir to combine, breaking up the eggs. Cook over medium–low heat for 2 to 2½ minutes until eggs are softly set. Stir in half the cheese. Remove from heat. Spread 2 T. (30 mL) of the sauce on a side of each tortilla. Divide egg mixture among tortillas and roll tip. Place seam side down on ovenproof baking dish. Top with remaining sauce and cheese. Bake at 450°F (230°C) for 10 to 12 minutes until thoroughly heated.

Yield: 4 servings

Exchange, 1 serving: 1 bread, 2 medium-fat meat
Each serving contains: Calories: 211, Carbohydrates: 18 g

With the courtesy of Kretschmer Wheat Germ/International Multifoods.

English Egg Muffins

2 T.	low-calorie margarine	30 mL
6	eggs, hard-cooked and chopped	6
1 T.	Dijon-style mustard	15 mL
1 T.	Worcestershire sauce	15 mL
1 T.	red wine vinegar	15 mL
1 T.	onion, finely chopped	15 mL
1 t.	fresh tarragon, chopped	5 mL
1 t.	fresh parsley	5 mL
	salt and pepper to taste	
4	English muffins, toasted	4

Melt margarine in a nonstick skillet. Combine the eggs, mustard, Worcestershire sauce, vinegar, onion, tarragon, parsley, salt, and pepper in the skillet; mix and stir until thoroughly heated. Spread on top of each toasted muffin half. Serve immediately.

Yield: 8 servings

Exchange, 1 serving: 1 bread, ¾ medium-fat meat, ⅓ fat
Each serving contains: Calories: 148, Carbohydrates: 14 g

Tomato-Cheese Quiche

6	eggs, beaten	6
9 in.	unbaked pie shell	23 cm
	salt and pepper to taste	
½ c.	cheddar cheese, shredded	125 mL
3	tomatoes	3

Pour eggs into pie shell. Sprinkle with salt and pepper. Top with cheese. Bake at 350°F (175°C) for 25 minutes or until partially set. Slice tomatoes; then slice each slice in half. Lay tomato slices around edge and in middle of the quiche. Place back in oven and bake for 15 to 20 minutes longer or until mixture is completely set.

Yield: 8 servings

Exchange, 1 serving: 1 medium-fat meat, 1 bread
Each serving contains: Calories: 152, Carbohydrates: 13 g

Eggs and Cheese Brunch

A quick and easy way to serve a group. This recipe is for one serving.

1	egg	1
1 t.	low-calorie margarine	5 mL
2 T.	farmer's cheese, cut or broken into small pieces	30 mL
	Salsa Sauce, warm	

In a bowl, whip the egg. Melt the margarine in a skillet. Add the egg and scramble. Top scrambled egg with cheese. Add small amount of water to skillet; cover. Cook over low heat until cheese melts. Remove to heated plate. Top with the sauce.

Yield: 1 serving

Exchange, 1 serving: 1 high-fat meat, ½ vegetable, 1⅓ fat
Each serving contains: Calories: 200, Carbohydrates: 3 g

Quick Eggs for Two

2	small potatoes, boiled, peeled, and sliced	2
1	small red onion, sliced and sautéed	1
2	eggs, hard-cooked and sliced	2
½ c.	mushrooms, sliced and sautéed	125 mL
	salt and pepper	

In the bottom of a nonstick skillet, layer the potatoes, onion, eggs, and then the mushrooms. Season with salt and pepper to taste. Add a small amount of water. Cover and simmer over low heat until heated. Lift out of skillet with a slotted spatula.

Microwave: Layer the ingredients in the order given above in 2 microwave dishes. Cover and cook on medium or reheat for 3 minutes or until hot.

Yield: 2 servings

Exchange, 1 serving: 1 bread, 1 medium-fat meat, ¼ vegetable
Each serving contains: Calories: 154, Carbohydrates: 15 g

Potato and Egg Casserole

You can have these ingredients ready the night before you plan to mix them.

6	potatoes, boiled, peeled, and sliced	6
6	eggs, hard-cooked and chopped	6
6	bacon slices, crisply fried	6
2 T.	fresh parsley, chopped	30 mL
	salt and pepper to taste	
½ c.	plain lowfat yogurt	125 mL

Place alternate layers of potatoes, eggs, and bacon in a greased baking dish. Sprinkle with parsley, salt, and pepper. With a fork, stir yogurt until loose and creamy. Pour yogurt over mixture in baking dish. Bake at 350°F (175°C) for 15 to 20 minutes or until golden brown and hot.

Yield: 6 servings

Exchange, 1 serving: 1 medium-fat meat, 1 bread, 1 fat
Each serving contains: Calories: 195, Carbohydrates: 17 g

Sweet Omelette

2	eggs	2
1 t.	granulated sugar replacement	5 mL
	vegetable cooking spray	
2 t.	Powdered Sugar Replacement	10 mL

Break eggs into bowl or cup, and beat with fork until blended. Beat in granulated sugar replacement. Coat small frying pan with vegetable spray. Heat until warm. Add eggs and cook them over low heat until lightly set. Run fork or spatula around edge of omelette. Tilt pan slightly to allow excess egg to seep under the pan. Continue cooking until firm. Fold in half; remove to heated serving plate. Sift 2 t. (10 mL) powdered sugar replacement over omelette.

Yield: 1 serving

Exchange with sugar replacement: 2 medium-fat meat
Each serving contains: Calories: 171, Carbohydrates: 10g

Exchange with fructose: 2 medium-fat meat
Each serving contains: Calories: 181, Carbohydrates: 10 g

Fillings for Sweet Omelette

Apple

1	small apple (peeled and sliced)	
½ t.	granulated sugar replacement	2 mL
¼ t.	cinnamon	1 mL
¼ t.	vanilla extract	1 mL

Combine apple slices with remaining ingredients. Toss to coat. When omelette is still slightly soft, spread apple mixture in center of eggs. Fold in half and cook until set.

Yield: 1 serving

Exchange, 1 serving: 1 fruit plus omelette
Each serving contains: Calories: 70 plus omelette, Carbohydrates: 44 g

Blueberry

½ c.	fresh blueberries, rinsed	125 mL
½ t.	almond extract	2 mL

When omelette is still slightly soft, spread blueberries in center of eggs. Sprinkle with almond extract. Fold in half and cook until set.

Yield: 1 serving

Exchange, 1 serving: 1 fruit plus omelette
Each serving contains: Calories: 40 plus omelette, Carbohydrates: 11 g

Flaming

1 T.	dark rum, heated	15 mL

Pour heated rum around sides of cooked omelette on serving dish. Ignite.

Yield: 1 serving

Exchange, 1 serving: Same as omelette
Each serving contains: Calories: Same as omelette, Carbohydrates: negligible

Fillings for Sweet Omelette (continued)

Berry-Cherry

5	strawberries, sliced	5
10	raspberries	10
4	Bing cherries, pitted and halved	4

When omelette is still slightly soft, spread fruit in center of eggs. Fold in half and cook until set.

Yield: 1 serving

Exchange, 1 serving: 1 fruit plus omelette
Each serving contains: Calories: 40 plus omelette, Carbohydrates: 14 g

Fruit Omelette

¼ c.	strawberries, sliced	60 mL
10	green grapes, cut in half	10
7	peaches, peeled and sliced	7
3	eggs	3
2 t.	granulated sugar replacement	10 mL
2 T.	farmer's cheese, shredded	30 mL
3 T.	lowfat blueberry yogurt	45 mL

Coat a nonstick skillet with vegetable spray. Add the fruits and gently sauté for 1 minute; remove from skillet. Respray the skillet. Combine eggs and granulated sugar replacement and beat well. Pour into the skillet and cook until set. Spread fruit over half of the eggs. Top with cheese. Fold eggs in half. Pour a small amount of water into the skillet. Cover and cook until cheese melts. Turn out onto a heated plate. Top with blueberry yogurt. Serve immediately.

Yield: 2 servings

Exchange, 1 serving: 1¾ medium-fat meat, 1¼ fruit
Each serving contains: Calories: 184, Carbohydrates: 13 g

Artichoke Omelette

2 t.	olive oil	10 mL
1 c.	artichoke hearts	250 mL
1 c.	mushrooms, sliced	250 mL
2 T.	tomato paste	30 mL
¼ c.	water	60 mL
1	garlic clove, minced	1
dash	red pepper	dash
	salt and pepper to taste	
1 T.	low-calorie margarine	15 mL
8	eggs, well beaten	8

Heat olive oil in a large skillet. Cut artichoke hearts in half. Sauté artichoke hearts and mushrooms in oil until lightly cooked. Stir in the tomato paste, water, garlic, red pepper, salt, and pepper. Cook until mixture thickens. (If using canned artichoke hearts, add to mixture at the end; cook just enough to heat.) Turn out into a bowl and keep warm. Melt margarine in the same skillet. Add the eggs and cook until firm. Turn out onto a heated platter. Top with the artichoke mixture; fold in half. Serve hot.

Yield: 8 servings

Exchange, 1 serving: 1 medium-fat meat, ½ vegetable, ⅓ fat
Each serving contains: Calories: 110, Carbohydrates: 3 g

Refrigerator Omelette

A good way to use leftover fresh vegetables.

1 c.	mixture of any of the following vegetables: celery, thinly sliced; mushrooms, sliced; onion, chopped; cherry tomatoes, quartered and seeded; garlic, minced; broccoli, finely chopped; cauliflower, finely chopped; green or red bell pepper, chopped	250 mL
2 T.	Swiss cheese, shredded	30 mL
3	eggs	3
1 T.	Butter Buds natural butter-flavored mix	15 mL
	salt and pepper to taste	

Coat a nonstick skillet with vegetable spray. Add the 1 c. (250 mL) mixed vegetables and sauté until crisp-tender; remove to a bowl. Respray the skillet. Combine the eggs, Butter Buds, salt, and pepper in a bowl; beat well. Pour into a skillet. Cook over low heat until almost set. Spread vegetables on half of the eggs. Top with Swiss cheese and fold in half. Pour a very small amount of water into the skillet. Cover and cook until cheese melts. Cut in half and place on 2 heated plates.

Yield: 2 servings

Exchange, 1 serving: 1¾ medium-fat meat, ½ vegetable
Each serving contains: Calories: 147, Carbohydrates: 3 g

Microwave Omelette

3	eggs, separated	3
½ c.	sour cream	125 mL
2 T.	green onion, sliced	30 mL
2 T.	tomato flesh	30 mL
1 T.	parsley, snipped	15 mL
½ c.	ham, cooked and diced	125 mL
	salt and pepper to taste	

Beat egg whites in a bowl until stiff; set aside. In another bowl, beat egg yolks until very thick and creamy; beat in the sour cream. Stir in the remaining ingredients. Season with salt and pepper to taste. Gently fold in the beaten egg whites. Place mixture in a 9- or 10 in. (23 or 25 cm) lightly greased pie pan; cover lightly with plastic wrap (make sure there is enough room for the eggs to expand). Cook in microwave on medium for 5 minutes, turning dish a half turn every minute. Allow to rest 1½ minutes before serving.

Yield: 6 servings

Exchange, 1 serving: 1 high-fat meat, 1 fat
Each serving contains: Calories: 169, Carbohydrates: negligible

Crab Egg Fu Yung

6	eggs, well beaten	6
2 c.	bean sprouts, washed and cleaned	500 mL
3 T.	onion, minced	45 mL
1 c.	crab meat, flaked	250 mL
	salt and pepper to taste	
1 T.	low-calorie margarine	15 mL
1½ c.	water	375 mL
3 T.	soy sauce	45 mL
1 T.	granulated sugar replacement	15 mL
1 T.	cornstarch	15 mL

In a bowl with the beaten eggs, add the bean sprouts, onion, crab meat, salt, and pepper; stir to mix. Melt margarine in a skillet; turn back and forth to coat entire bottom. Add the egg mixture. Cover and fry over low heat until bottom is set and firm. Carefully lift corner of eggs (try not to break them) and add a small amount of water under the egg. Cover and allow to cook over low heat until firm. Meanwhile, combine 1½ c. (375 mL) water in a saucepan with the soy sauce, sugar replacement, and cornstarch; mix to dissolve cornstarch. Cook and stir over medium heat until mixture is clear and thick. Carefully fold egg mixture in half. Gently turn out onto heated platter. Pour soy sauce mixture over the eggs. Serve immediately.

Yield: 6 servings

Exchange, 1 serving: 1½ medium-fat meat, ½ vegetable
Each serving contains: Calories: 125, Carbohydrates: 3 g

Breads and Cereals

Hot Cereal

Follow directions on side of package, or use these general directions. Any leftover cooked cereals can be frozen and thawed, or refrigerated and reheated.

To cook granular type cereals, such as farina, cornmeal, or brown flaked wheat:

½ c.	cereal	125 mL
2¼ c.	water	560 mL
½ t.	salt	2 mL

Pour cereal into top of a double boiler. Stir in the water and salt. Cover tightly. Place top of double boiler over simmering water. Cook for 7 to 10 minutes, if using quick-cooking granular cereal. Cook for 25 to 30 minutes, if using regular or long-cooking granular cereal.

To cook flaky cereals, such as rolled and flaked wheat or rolled oats:

4 c.	water	1 L
1 t.	salt	5 mL
1½ c.	cereal	375 mL

Combine water and salt in a saucepan; bring to a boil. Gradually sprinkle in the cereal. Bring back to the boil and reduce heat; cover and cook over low heat: Cook for 7 to 10 minutes, if using quick-cooking flaked cereal; cook for 20 to 30 minutes, if using regular or longer-cooking flaked cereal. Stir occasionally while cooking.

To cook whole grain or cracked cereals, such as barley, grits★, rice, or wheat:

4 c.	water	1 L
1 t.	salt	5 mL
¾ c.	cereal	190 mL

Combine water and salt in a saucepan; bring to the boil. Gradually sprinkle in the cereal. Bring back to the boil, reduce heat, cover, and cook over low heat: For rice, cook 35 to 45 minutes (wild rice takes longer). For other whole grain or cracked cereals, cook for 3½ to 4 hours.

Yield: ½ c. (125 mL)

Exchange, 1 serving: 1 bread
Each serving contains: Calories: 68, Carbohydrates: 15 g

*Although grits are granulated or ground, they must be cooked longer with more water than the normal granulated cereals, unless you are using the quick-cooking type.

Orange and Buttermilk Cereal

2 c.	graham flour	500 mL
1 t.	baking soda	5 mL
½ t.	salt	2 mL
2 T.	vegetable oil	30 mL
8 oz.	lowfat mandarin orange yogurt	240 g
1 T.	orange peel, freshly grated	15 mL
1 c.	buttermilk	250 mL

In order given, combine all ingredients in a large bowl; beat until well blended. Pour into a well-greased 8 in. (20 cm) baking pan. Bake at 325°F (165°C) for 30 to 40 minutes or until a toothpick inserted in middle comes out clean. Turn out onto a cooling rack. Break into large pieces and cool. To form the cereal: Break into medium-size pieces; place in a food processor and with a steel blade, chop into smaller pieces; or grind through a food grinder without the cutting knife, using just the large-hole blade. Spread pieces evenly on 2 cookie sheets. Toast for 25 to 30 minutes at 300°F (150°C). Change position of pans in the oven and stir cereal every 10 minutes; if you prefer a softer cereal, toast for less time.

Yield: 8 servings

Exchange, 1 serving: 1 bread
Each serving contains: Calories: 69, Carbohydrates: 14 g

Quick Homemade Cereal

2 c.	oatmeal	500 mL
1 c.	wheat germ	250 mL
⅓ c.	unsweetened coconut, shredded	90 mL
½ c.	brown sugar replacement	125 mL
¼ c.	low-calorie margarine, melted	60 mL
2 T.	liquid fructose	30 mL
2 T.	water	30 mL
¼ t.	salt	1 mL

Combine all ingredients in a large bowl; stir and fold to blend thoroughly. Spread mixture on a cookie sheet. Bake at 325°F (165°C) for 20 to 25 minutes, stirring or shaking pan occasionally to allow for even toasting of the cereal. Cool and store in a tightly sealed container. Cereal may be kept in the refrigerator, freezer, or on a kitchen shelf.

Yield: 10 servings

Exchange, 1 serving: 1 bread, 1 fat
Each serving contains: Calories: 125, Carbohydrates: 15 g

Oatmeal-Coconut Crunch

2 c.	oatmeal	500 mL
½ c.	unsweetened flaked coconut	125 mL
½ c.	dates, chopped	125 mL
½ c.	almonds, slivered	125 mL
1 T.	vanilla extract	15 mL
2 T.	granulated brown sugar replacement	30 mL
2 T.	granulated fructose	30 mL
3 T.	low-calorie margarine, melted	45 mL
3 T.	hot water	45 mL

Combine the oatmeal, coconut, dates, almonds, vanilla, brown sugar replacement, and fructose in a large bowl. Pour margarine and water over mixture and stir until completely moistened. Transfer to a well greased 13 × 9 × 2 in. (33 × 23 × 5 cm) baking pan. Pat down in bottom of pan. Bake at 350°F (175°C) for 20 minutes. Remove pan from oven and break cereal mixture into large pieces. Return to oven and bake for 5 to 7 more minutes or until crispy and toasty brown. Store in a tightly covered container on the kitchen shelf or freeze.

Yield: 8 servings

Exchange, 1 serving: ⅔ fruit, 2⅓ bread, 1 fat
Each serving contains: Calories: 123, Carbohydrates: 16 g

Crispy Golden Cereal

4 c.	oatmeal	1 L
2 c.	wheat germ	500 mL
1 c.	sesame seeds	250 mL
1 c.	walnuts, chopped	250 mL
½ c.	unsweetened flaked coconut	125 mL
¾ c.	vegetable oil	190 mL
½ c.	granulated brown sugar replacement	125 mL
¼ c.	water	60 mL
2 T.	vanilla extract	30 mL

Combine oatmeal, wheat germ, sesame seeds, walnuts, and coconut in a large bowl. In a blender, combine liquid shortening, brown sugar replacement, water, and vanilla. Beat until thoroughly mixed. Slowly pour liquid shortening mixture over cereal mixture; stir to coat cereal mixture completely. Spread out on cookie sheets. Bake at 350°F (175°C) for 1 hour. Stir frequently and reverse the oven position of pans after 30 minutes. Cool and store in tightly covered containers.

Yield: 20 servings

Exchange, 1 serving: 1 bread, 3 fat
Each serving contains: Calories: 215, Carbohydrates: 16 g

Wheat Germ Granola

3 c.	old-fashioned oatmeal	750 mL
1½ c.	wheat germ	375 mL
½ c.	almonds, chopped	125 mL
⅓ c.	sesame seeds	90 mL
¼ c.	vegetable oil	60 mL
⅓ c.	dietetic maple syrup	90 mL
1 c.	raisins	250 mL

Combine all ingredients except raisins, mixing well. Spread mixture evenly in a large shallow pan. Bake at 300°F (150°C) for 30 minutes, stirring every 10 minutes, until lightly toasted. Stir in the raisins. Cool completely. Store covered in a refrigerator.

Yield: 6½ cups (125 mL)

Exchange, ½ c. (125 mL): 1 bread, 1 fruit, 1 fat
Each serving contains: Calories: 147

Graham Cereal

3 c.	graham flour	750 mL
¼ c.	granulated brown sugar replacement	60 mL
¼ c.	dietetic maple syrup	60 mL
1 t.	baking soda	5 mL
1 t.	salt	5 mL
2 T.	low-calorie margarine, melted	30 mL
1½ c.	skim milk	375 mL
½ c.	water	125 mL

In the order given, combine all ingredients in a large bowl; beat until well blended. Pour into a well-greased 8 in. (20 cm) baking pan. Bake at 325°F (165°C) for 30 to 40 minutes or until a toothpick inserted comes out clean. Turn out onto a cooling rack. Break into large pieces and cool.

To form cereal: Break into small bits; place in a food processor and using a steel blade, chop into size pieces you prefer; or grind through a food grinder without the cutting knife, using just the small-hole blade. Spread pieces out evenly onto 2 cookie sheets. Toast for 25 to 30 minutes at 300°F (150°C). Reverse position of pans in the oven and stir cereal every 10 minutes; if you prefer a softer cereal, toast for less time. Cool before storing.

Yield: 12 servings

Exchange, 1 serving: 1 bread
Each serving contains: Calories: 68, Carbohydrates: 15 g

Carolina-Style Grits

1 c.	quick-cooking grits	250 mL
3 c.	water, boiling	750 mL
1 t.	salt	5 mL
8 oz.	sharp cheddar cheese, shredded	240 g
3 T.	low-calorie margarine	45 mL
dash	Tabasco sauce	dash

Stir grits into saucepan of boiling salted water. Cook on low heat for 5 minutes, stirring often. Pour into well-greased casserole. Add remaining ingredients. Stir until margarine melts. Cover and bake at 325°F (165°C) for 45 minutes to 1 hour. Serve warm.

Yield: 8 servings

Exchange, 1 serving: 1 high-fat meat, ⅔ bread
Each serving contains: Calories: 159, Carbohydrates: 10 g

Apricot and Oat Bran Softies

1 env.	unflavored gelatin	1 env.
1 T.	cold water	15 mL
¼ c.	water, boiling	60 mL
1 t.	vanilla extract	5 mL
dash	Tone's allspice	dash
¼ c.	dried apricots, cut in thin strips	60 mL
3½ c.	oat bran cereal	875 mL

Soften the gelatin in the cold water in a bowl. Add boiling water, vanilla, allspice, and apricot strips; stir to mix. Allow to cool to consistency of thick syrup. Add oat bran and blend until cereal is coated. Transfer to a plastic-lined 8 in. (20 cm) square pan and smooth the surface level in pan. Refrigerate until thoroughly set. Remove plastic liner with bar mixture to a cutting board. Cut into eight 2 × 4 in. (5 × 10 cm) bars.

Yield: 8 bars

Exchange, 1 bar: ¼ bread, ¼ fruit
Each serving contains: Calories: 55, Carbohydrates: 15 g

Wheat Softies

1 env.	unflavored gelatin	1 env.
⅓ c.	water	90 mL
¼ c.	chocolate chips	60 mL
3 c.	small shredded wheat biscuits	750 mL

In a saucepan, sprinkle gelatin over the water; stir to blend. Allow to soften for 3 minutes. Place over heat and bring to the boil and stir until gelatin is completely dissolved. Remove from heat and stir in the chocolate chips, mixing to dissolve the chips. Cool to a consistency of thick syrup. Crumble the shredded wheat biscuits into a bowl. Add the chocolate mixture, stirring until the cereal is thoroughly coated. Transfer to a plastic-lined 8 in. (20 cm) square pan and smooth the mixture in the pan. Refrigerate until thoroughly set. Remove plastic liner with the mixture to a cutting board. Cut into eight 2 × 4 in. (5 × 10 cm) bars or sixteen 2 × 2 in. (5 × 5 cm) squares.

Yield: 8 or 16 servings

Exchange, 1 serving (for 8 bars): 1⅓ bread
Each serving contains: Calories: 95, Carbohydrates: 21 g

Exchange, 1 serving (for 16 squares): ⅔ bread
Each serving contains: Calories: 47, Carbohydrates: 10 g

Graham Bars

2 c.	Graham Cereal	500 mL
2 T.	cornstarch	30 mL
¼ c.	warm water	60 mL
½ c.	raisins	125 mL
¼ c.	mini-chocolate chips	60 mL
1	egg, slightly beaten	1

Combine the cereal and cornstarch in a bowl; stir to coat cereal with cornstarch. Add water and stir until the cereal appears moistened. Allow to rest for 5 minutes. Add the remaining ingredients and stir to blend thoroughly. Transfer mixture to a well-greased 8 in. (20 cm) square baking pan; spread evenly with your palm, pressing tightly into bottom of pan. Bake at 350°F (175°C) for 15 minutes. Immediately cut into 12 bars while hot. Transfer bars to a cooling rack. Bars can be stored in the refrigerator or freezer.

Yield: 12 bars

Exchange, 1 bar: 1 bread, 1 fruit
Each serving contains: Calories: 110, Carbohydrates: 24 g

Cereal-Yogurt Bars

3 c.	Orange and Buttermilk Cereal	750 mL
2 T.	cornstarch	30 mL
2 T.	granulated fructose	30 mL
8 oz.	piña colada lowfat yogurt	240 g
⅓ c.	unsweetened coconut flakes	90 mL

Combine cereal, cornstarch, and fructose in a bowl. Stir to completely coat cereal. Heat the yogurt in a saucepan. Add yogurt all at once to the cereal mixture; stir to blend. Cover and allow to rest for 10 minutes. Stir in the coconut flakes. Transfer mixture to a well-greased 8 in. (20 cm) square baking pan. Spread evenly with the back of a wooden spoon, flattening mixture slightly into bottom of pan. Bake at 350° F (175°C) for 15 minutes. Immediately cut into 12 bars while hot. Transfer bars to cooling rack. Bars can be stored in the refrigerator or freezer.

Yield: 12 bars

Exchange, 1 bar: ¾ bread, ½ fat
Each serving contains: Calories: 70, Carbohydrates: 12 g

Toasted Oat Bars

3 env.	unflavored gelatin	3 env.
¾ c.	cold water	190 mL
½ c.	dates, chopped	125 mL
1 qt.	sweetened toasted oat cereal, slightly crushed	1 L
¼ c.	mini-chocolate chips	60 mL

Sprinkle gelatin over cold water in a saucepan. Allow to soften for 3 minutes. Cook and stir over medium heat until mixture is completely liquefied. Add the dates and cook and stir for 5 minutes. Remove from heat and cool to the consistency of thick syrup. Combine cereal and chocolate chips in large bowl. Pour gelatin mixture over cereal; fold to completely coat cereal. Transfer to two 8 in. (20 cm) greased baking dishes. Chill until set. Cut into 16 bars (8 per pan).

Yield: 16 bars

Exchange, 1 bar: 1 bread
Each serving contains: Calories: 64, Carbohydrates: 14 g

Orangeola Bars

1¼ c.	Health Valley Orangeola cereal	310 mL
¼ c.	Health Valley Sprouts 7 cereal	60 mL
⅓ c.	walnuts, finely ground	90 mL
2 T.	fresh or dried coconut, grated	30 mL
dash	ground or grated nutmeg	dash
2 T.	clover honey	30 mL
½ t.	vanilla	2 mL
2	egg whites, beaten stiff	2

In a mixing bowl, combine cereals, nuts, coconut, and nutmeg. Add honey and vanilla and mix thoroughly (it might be necessary to use your hands to do this). Then fold in egg whites and allow mixture to stand 2 to 3 minutes. Spread or press into greased 11 × 6½ × 2 in. (28 × 16.5 × 5 cm) baking pan. Bake in preheated 275°F (135°C) oven for 20 minutes. Remove from oven. Cut into 20 to 24 bars and transfer immediately to glass or china plate to cool.

Yield: 20 bars

Exchange, 1 bar: ⅔ bread
Each serving contains: Calories: 50, Carbohydrates: 10 g

Orange Pineapple-Nut Squares

Orangeola is a unique cereal made only by Health Valley. It gets its unusual flavor from sweet fruit and orange oil blended with oats.

2 c.	Health Valley Orangeola cereal, finely crushed	500 mL
½ t.	ground ginger	2 mL
4	egg yolks	4
2 T.	safflower oil	30 mL
¾ c.	milk	190 mL
½ c.	pecans, chopped	125 mL
1 c.	unsweetened crushed pineapple, drained	250 mL
4	egg whites	4

In a medium bowl, combine cereal and ginger. In a small bowl, beat egg yolks, then add oil and milk. Add to dry ingredients, then stir in nuts and pineapple. Beat egg whites until stiff and fold them into batter. Spoon batter into greased 8 in. (20 cm) square baking pan. Bake in preheated 350°F (175°C) oven for 30 to 35 minutes, until toothpick inserted in middle comes out dry.

Yield: 9 servings

Exchange, 1 serving: 2 bread, 1 fruit, 3 fat
Each serving contains: Calories: 315, Carbohydrates: 18 g

From Health Valley Foods.

Oatmeal-Coconut Crunch Bars

1 recipe	Oatmeal-Coconut Crunch	1 recipe
1 T.	cornstarch	15 mL
1 t.	baking powder	5 mL
2	eggs, slightly beaten	2
¼ c.	water	60 mL

Combine the crunch, cornstarch, and baking powder in a bowl; stir until mixture appears coated with cornstarch. In another bowl, whip eggs and water together. Pour over crunch mixture and stir until completely moistened. Transfer mixture to a well-greased 8 in. (20 cm) square baking pan. Pat evenly and firmly in bottom of pan. Bake at 350°F (175°C) for 20 minutes. Immediately cut into 12 equal bars. Cool slightly and remove bars from pan. Wrap bars in plastic wrap. Bars can be stored in the refrigerator or freezer.

Yield: 12 bars

Exchange, 1 bar: ½ fruit, ⅔ bread, ½ fat
Each serving contains: Calories: 83, Carbohydrates: 15 g

Rice Cereal Bars and Variations

2 env.	unflavored gelatin	2 env.
¼ c.	cold water	60 mL
2 t.	Tones clear imitation vanilla	10 mL
2 T.	granulated sugar replacement	30 mL
1	egg white	1
2 qts.	crisp rice cereal	2 L

Sprinkle gelatin over cold water in a small saucepan; allow to soften for 3 minutes. Cook and stir over low heat until gelatin dissolves; remove from heat. Stir in the vanilla and sugar replacement; cool slightly. Beat egg white until soft peaks form, Very slowly, trickle a small stream of gelatin mixture into egg white, beating until all gelatin mixture is blended. Beat at high speed until egg mixture is light and fluffy. Pour rice cereal into egg mixture; fold to completely blend and coat the cereal. Transfer to a 13 × 9 × 2 in. (33 × 23 × 5 cm) greased pan. Chill in refrigerator. Cut into 18 bars.

Yield: 18 bars

Exchange, 1 bar: ⅔ bread
Each serving contains: Calories: 49, Carbohydrates: 11 g

Optional additional ingredients

Add ½ c. (125 mL) mini-chocolate chips with the cereal.

Yield: 18 bars

Exchange, 1 bar: 1 bread
Each serving contains: Calories: 74, Carbohydrates: 14 g

Add ¾ c. (190 mL) chopped walnuts.

Yield: 18 bars

Exchange, 1 bar: ⅔ bread, ⅔ fat
Each serving contains: Calories: 82, Carbohydrates: 11 g

Add 1 c. (250 mL) unsweetened shredded coconut.

Yield: 18 bars

Exchange, 1 bar: ⅔ bread, ¼ fat
Each serving contains: Calories: 65, Carbohydrates: 11 g

Add ½ c. (125 mL) dried apricots, snipped fine.

Yield: 18 bars

Exchange, 1 bar: ⅔ bread, ½ fruit
Each serving contains: Calories: 68, Carbohydrates: 16 g

Add all of the above optional ingredients. Transfer mixture to 15½ × 10½ × 1 in. (39 × 25 × 3 cm) jelly roll pan. Chill until set. Cut into 25 bars, each approximately 3 × 2 in. (75 × 5 cm).

Yield: 25 bars

Exchange, 1 bar: 1 bread, 1½ fat
Each serving contains: Calories: 94, Carbohydrates: 16 g

Basic White Bread

There is nothing like homemade bread for breakfast.

1 pkg.	dry yeast	1 pkg.
¼ t.	granulated fructose	1 mL
¼ c.	warm water	60 mL
1 c.	boiling water	440 mL
¼ c.	dry milk solids	60 mL
2 T.	solid vegetable shortening	30 mL
1 T.	granulated sugar replacement	15 mL
2 t.	salt	10 mL
6 c.	all-purpose flour	1.5 L

Combine the yeast and fructose in a small bowl; stir to mix. Add the warm water and stir to blend; set aside. Pour boiling water into a large bowl. Add the milk solids, shortening, sugar replacement, and salt. Stir until shortening melts; cool to lukewarm (make sure it is not too hot or it will stop the yeast from working). Stir in half of the flour; beat to blend. Beat yeast mixture into the dough. Gradually add remaining flour. Turn out onto lightly floured surface and knead until smooth. Place dough in a well-greased bowl; turn once to coat both sides. Cover and allow to rise until double in size. Turn out onto lightly floured surface. Knead gently 10 times. (When used in other recipes, follow those directions at this point.) Form into 2 loaves. Place in well-greased loaf pans. Cover and allow to rise. Bake at 350°F (175°C) for 45 minutes or until done.

Yield: 2 loaves or 32 servings

Exchange, 1 serving: 1 bread
Each serving contains: Calories: 87, Carbohydrates: 16 g

Moist German-Style Potato Bread

Potato water

1	medium potato	1
1 c.	water	310 mL

Dough

1 pkg.	dry yeast	1 pkg.
2 c.	all-purpose flour	500 mL
1 c.	skim milk, scalded	250 mL
2 T.	solid vegetable shortening	30 mL
2 t.	salt	10 mL
4 c.	all-purpose flour	1 L

To make the potato water: Peel and cube the potato. Place in a saucepan and cover with the water; boil until potato is soft. Drain over a bowl and reserve the water. Mash the potato and add to drained water; cool to room temperature. Measure 1 c. (250 mL) potato water for this recipe; reserve any remaining potato water for another recipe.

To make the dough: Dissolve yeast in potato water. Set aside until yeast starts to become foamy. Beat in half of the flour until smooth. Cover and allow to rise until double in size. Pour scalded milk over shortening and salt in a bowl; stir until shortening melts. Set aside to cool. When cool, add milk-shortening mixture to the flour sponge. Gradually add the remaining flour. Knead on a lightly floured surface until smooth. Place in a well-greased bowl; turn once to coat both sides. Cover and allow to rise until double in size. Divide dough into 2 equal pieces. Twist into a small log. Place in well-greased bread pan. Cover and allow to rise again. Bake at 350°F (175°C) for 40 to 45 minutes or until browned and done.

Yield: 2 loaves or 32 servings

Exchange, 1 serving: 1 bread
Each serving contains: Calories: 91, Carbohydrates: 17 g

Wisconsin Rye Bread

2 pkg.	dry yeast	2 pkg.
2 c.	potato water,* lukewarm	500 mL
1 t.	caraway seed	5 mL
1 T.	salt	15 mL
1 c.	potatoes, cooked and diced	250 mL
2 c.	all-purpose flour	500 mL
4 c.	dark rye flour	1 L

Dissolve yeast in lukewarm potato water. Stir in remaining ingredients. Turn out onto lightly floured board and knead until smooth and elastic. Cover dough on board and allow to rise until double in size. Form into loaves or 32 buns. Place in well-greased loaf pans or baking sheets. Cover and allow to double in size. Brush with water. (If desired, sprinkle with coarse salt.) Bake at 375°F (190°C): for loaves, 1 hour or until done; for rolls, 40 to 45 minutes or until done.

Yield: 32 servings

Exchange, 1 serving: 1 bread
Each serving contains: Calories: 83, Carbohydrates: 17 g

*Read directions for potato water in Moist German-Style Potato Bread.

Herb Bread

This bread is delicious with flavored butters—and is a nice accompaniment to egg, meat, or vegetable dishes.

Herb mix

2 t.	salt	10 mL
1 t.	thyme	5 mL
1 t.	basil	5 mL
1 t.	marjoram	5 mL
1 t.	lemon rind, grated	5 mL
½ t.	paprika	2 mL
½ t.	dried parsley	2 mL
½ t.	onion flakes	2 mL
¼ t.	white pepper	1 mL

Dough

2 pkg.	dry yeast	2 pkg.
3 c.	water, lukewarm	750 mL
8 c.	all-purpose flour	2 L
½ c.	vegetable oil	125 mL

In a bowl, mix all ingredients for the herb mix; set aside.

To make the dough, dissolve the dry yeast in lukewarm water; allow to rest for 5 minutes or until foamy. Add 3 c. (750 mL) of the flour; beat until smooth. Beat in the herb mix; allow to rest for 5 minutes. Work in 4 c. (1 L) of the flour. Turn dough out onto lightly floured board; work in remaining flour. (If dough is too dry, add a small amount of water to your hands as you knead. Dough should be smooth and elastic.) Place dough in well-greased bowl; turn once to coat both sides. Cover and allow to double in size. Punch dough down; divide into 36 balls. Place in well-greased muffin tins. Cover and allow to rise again. Bake at 350°F (175°C) for 25 to 30 minutes or until done. (Tap the top of the loaf for doneness; sound should be hollow.) Be especially careful not to underbake.

Yield: 36 rolls

Exchange, 1 roll: 2 bread
Each serving contains: Calories: 135, Carbohydrates: 29 g

Quick Potato Bread

This loaf has the appearance and taste of homemade potato bread.

1 loaf	frozen white bread dough, thawed	1 loaf
¼ c.	potato flakes, dry	60 mL
	salt	

Pull the dough into small pieces. Dip each piece into the potato flakes, using about two-thirds of the flakes. Roll around and twist dough to incorporate the flakes into the dough. Form the pieces into a loaf. Place in a well-greased loaf pan. Using your fingers and palm of your hand, flatten the dough in the bottom of the pan; be sure to touch all sides and corners. Brush with boiling water; sprinkle remaining potato flakes on top. With the back of a spoon, press flakes into the dough. Salt the top, as desired. Cover and allow to rise until more than double in size. Bake at 350°F (175°C) for 30 minutes or until done and golden brown.

Yield: 16 servings

Exchange, 1 serving: 1 bread
Each serving contains: Calories: 70, Carbohydrates: 15 g

Poppy Seed Bread

Cut into small square shapes, which add a nice effect to a bread plate.

1 loaf	frozen bread dough, thawed	1 loaf
1 T.	poppy seed	15 mL

Pat the loaf of thawed dough into the bottom of a well-oiled 8 in. (20 cm) square baking pan. Brush with boiling water. Sprinkle poppy seed evenly over the top. Cover and allow to rise until over double in size. Bake at 350°F (175°C) for 25 to 30 minutes or until done and browned. Cut into 2 in. (5 cm) squares.

Yield: 16 servings

Exchange, 1 serving: 1 bread
Each serving contains: Calories: 69, Carbohydrates: 15 g

Caraway Rye Bran Bread

1 pkg.	active dry yeast	1 pkg.
¼ c.	warm water	60 mL
2 T.	granulated sugar replacement	30 mL
¾ t.	salt	4 mL
1 t.	orange peel, grated	5 mL
1 t.	caraway seeds	5 mL
1 c.	buttermilk, at room temperature	250 mL
2 c.	Kellogg's bran flakes cereal	500 mL
1 c.	rye flour	250 mL
1½ c.	all-purpose flour	375 mL
1 T.	milk	15 mL

In a large mixing bowl, dissolve yeast in warm water. Stir in sugar replacement, salt, orange peel, caraway seeds, and buttermilk. Stir in cereal and rye flour. Gradually mix in enough all-purpose flour to make a soft dough. Cover and let rest 15 minutes. On lightly floured surface, knead dough about 5 minutes or until smooth and elastic. Place in greased bowl, turning once to grease top. Cover loosely. Let rise in warm place until doubled.

Punch down the dough. Shape into a smooth, round ball. Sprinkle cornmeal lightly on a baking sheet or grease lightly. Place dough on baking sheet. Flatten slightly. Cut a large X across top of loaf with sharp knife. Cover and let rise in warm place until doubled. Brush loaf with milk. Bake at 350°F (175°C) about 35 minutes or until golden brown and loaf sounds hollow when tapped. Remove from baking sheet. Cool on rack.

Yield: 1 loaf, 16 slices

Exchange, 1 slice: 2 bread
Each serving contains: Calories: 140, Carbohydrates: 14 g

From Kellogg's Test Kitchens.

Whole Wheat Bran Bread

1 c.	all-purpose flour	250 mL
1 c.	whole wheat flour	250 mL
1 c.	Kellogg's All-Bran or Bran Buds cereal	250 mL
1 t.	salt	5 mL
1 pkg.	active dry yeast	1 pkg.
¾ c.	milk	190 mL
2 T.	molasses	30 mL
3 T.	margarine	45 mL
1	egg	1

Stir together the all-purpose flour and whole wheat flour. In the large bowl of your electric mixer, combine ½ c. (125 mL) of the flour mixture, the cereal, salt, and yeast. Set aside. In a small saucepan, heat milk, molasses and margarine until very warm. Gradually add to cereal mixture and beat for 2 minutes at medium speed with electric mixer, scraping bowl occasionally. Add egg and ¼ c. (60 mL) of the flour mixture. Beat 2 minutes at high speed. By hand, stir in enough remaining flour mixture to make a stiff dough. On lightly floured surface, knead dough about 5 minutes or until smooth and elastic. Place in greased bowl, turning once to grease top. Cover loosely. Let rise in warm place until doubled.

Punch down dough. Shape into a loaf. Place in greased 8 × 4 × 2 in. (20 × 10 × 5 cm) loaf pan. Cover and let rise in warm place until doubled. Bake at 375°F (190°C) about 25 minutes or until golden brown.

Yield: 1 loaf, 14 slices

Exchange, 1 serving: 1 bread, 1 fat
Each serving contains: Calories: 115, Carbohydrates: 21 g

From Kellogg's Test Kitchens.

Two Tone Bread

2 pkg.	dry yeast	2 pkg.
½ c.	warm water	125 mL
¼ c.	granulated sugar replacement	60 mL
⅓ c.	vegetable shortening, melted	90 mL
1 T.	salt	15 mL
2½ c.	2% milk, scalded and cooled	625 mL
5¼ c.	sifted Stone-Buhr all-purpose flour	1310 mL
3 T.	dark molasses	45 mL
2¼ c.	Stone-Buhr whole wheat flour	560 mL

Dissolve yeast in warm water. Add the granulated sugar replacement, shortening, salt, and milk. Mix until sugar replacement and salt are dissolved. Add about 3 c. (750 mL) of the all-purpose flour and beat well, about 5 minutes. Divide dough in half. To one half, stir in enough of the remaining all-purpose flour to make a moderately stiff dough. Turn onto lightly floured surface and knead until smooth and elastic, about 5 to 6 minutes. Place in well-greased bowl, turning once to grease surface; set aside.

To the remaining dough, stir in the molasses and whole wheat flour. Turn onto lightly floured surface. Knead until smooth and elastic, about 5 to 8 minutes, kneading in an additional 3 T. (45 mL) all-purpose flour to form a moderately stiff dough. Place in well-greased bowl, turning once to grease surface. Cover both doughs and let rise until doubled, about 1 to 1½ hours. Punch down. Cover and rest on lightly floured surface for 10 minutes. Separately, roll out half the light dough and half the dark, each to a 12 × 8 in. (30.5 × 20 cm) rectangle.

Place dark dough on top of light; beginning at short side roll up tightly. Repeat with remaining doughs. Place in 2 greased 9 × 5 in. (23 × 13 cm) loaf pans. Cover and let rise until doubled, about 45 to 60 minutes. Bake at 375°F (175°C) for 30 to 35 minutes or until done. Remove from pans and cool on wire rack.

Yield: 2 loaves or 32 slices

Exchange, 1 slice: 1 bread
Each serving contains: Calories: 69, Carbohydrates: 28 g

Based on a recipe from Arnold Foods Company, Inc.

No-Knead Whole Wheat Bread

3 c.	whole wheat flour	750 mL
1½ c.	uncooked quick-cooking or old-fashioned oats	375 mL
2 pkg.	active dry yeast	2 pkg.
1 T.	salt	15 mL
2½ c.	buttermilk	625 mL
½ c.	molasses	125 mL
⅓ c.	margarine	90 mL
2	eggs	2
2½ c.	all-purpose flour	625 mL
	vegetable oil	

Measure whole wheat flour into a large bowl. Add oats, undissolved yeast, and salt. In a saucepan, heat buttermilk, molasses and the margarine together until warm to the touch. Add warm liquid and eggs to ingredients in the bowl. Blend with electric mixer at low speed until well mixed, about 30 seconds. Beat at high speed for 3 minutes, scraping bowl occasionally. Stir in all-purpose flour with a wooden spoon. Cover and let rise in warm, draft-free place about 1 hour or until doubled. Punch down. Place in 2 greased 2 qt. (2 L) casseroles or ovenproof bowls. Brush dough lightly with oil. If crust browns too quickly, cover loosely with foil during last 5 to 10 minutes. Remove from pans immediately. Cool on rack.

Yield: 2 loaves or 40 servings

Exchange, 1 serving: 1 bread
Each serving contains: Calories: 73, Carbohydrates: 17 g

Herb Cornbread

1 pkg.	active dry yeast	1 pkg.
½ c.	warm water	125 mL
2 t.	celery seeds	10 mL
2 t.	ground sage	10 mL
dash	ground ginger	dash
13 oz. can	evaporated skim milk	390 g can
1 t.	salt	5 mL
2 T.	vegetable oil	30 mL
4 c.	all-purpose flour	1 L
½ c.	yellow cornmeal	125 mL

Dissolve yeast in water in a large mixer bowl. Blend in celery seeds, sage and ginger. Allow to stand at room temperature until mixture is bubbly. Stir in milk, salt, and oil. On low speed, beat in flour 1 c. (250 mL) at a time. Beat well after each addition. When mixture becomes too thick to beat with the mixer, stir in remaining flour and cornmeal with a spoon (dough should be heavy). Divide dough and place into 2 well-greased 1 lb. (500 g) coffee cans. (Dough may be frozen at this time for later use.) Cover and allow to rise until dough rises to top of can. Bake at 350°F (175°C) for 45 minutes. Serve warm.

Yield: 2 loaves or 28 servings

Exchange, 1 serving: 1 bread
Each serving contains: Calories: 70, Carbohydrates: 97 g

Quick Onion Bread

1 loaf	frozen bread dough	1 loaf	
1 pkg.	onion soup mix	1 pkg.	

Allow bread to thaw as directed on package. Roll dough out on unfloured board. Sprinkle half of soup mix over surface. Roll up jelly-roll style. Knead to work mix into dough; repeat with remaining soup mix. Form into loaf. Place in greased 9 × 5 in. (23 × 13 cm) loaf pan; cover. Allow to rise about 2 hours. Bake at 350°F (175°C) for 30 to 40 minutes, or until done.

Yield: 1 loaf or 14 slices

Exchange, 1 slice: 1 bread
Each serving contains: Calories: 80, Carbohydrates: 37 g

Fennel Bread

This loaf is especially good when served with ham.

1 loaf	frozen dark rye bread dough, thawed	1 loaf	
2 t.	fennel seed, crushed	10 mL	
2 t.	artificial bacon bits	10 mL	

Roll out the dough on an unfloured surface. Sprinkle with fennel seed and artificial bacon bits. Knead for 5 minutes. Form into a loaf and place in a greased bread pan; or make into rolls as described in Easy Rolls. Cover and allow to rise until more than double in size. Bake at 350°F (175°C) for 30 minutes or until done.

Yield: 16 servings

Exchange, 1 serving: 1 bread
Each serving contains: Calories: 60, Carbohydrates: 13 g

High Protein Bread

1 pkg.	dry yeast	1 pkg.
¼ c.	warm water	60 mL
5 c.	Stone-Buhr all-purpose flour	1 ¼ L
½ c.	dry milk	125 mL
⅓ c.	Stone-Buhr soy flour	90 mL
¼ c.	Stone-Buhr wheat germ	60 mL
3 T.	granulated sugar replacement	45 mL
1 T.	salt	15 mL
1 T.	vegetable oil	15 mL
1¾ c.	water	440 mL

Dissolve yeast in warm water. Combine dry ingredients in mixing bowl. Add dissolved yeast, oil and water, mixing well to blend. Knead dough until smooth and satiny. Place in well-greased bowl. Cover and allow to rise in a warm place for about 1½ hours. Punch down by plunging fist into the dough. Fold over edges of dough and turn it upside down. Cover and allow to rise again for 15 to 20 minutes. Shape into 2 loaves; place in greased 9 × 5 in. (33 × 13 cm) loaf pans. Cover and allow to stand about 1 hour in a warm place, or until dough rises and fills pans. Bake at 400°F (200°C) for 45 minutes or until done. Remove from pans and cool on wire rack.

Yield: 2 loaves or 32 slices

Exchange, 1 slice: 1 bread
Each serving contains: Calories: 71, Carbohydrates: 17 g

Based on a recipe from Arnold Foods Company, Inc.

Barley Flake Bread

¾ c.	boiling water	90 mL
½ c.	Stone-Buhr barley flakes, more for sprinkling pan	125 mL
3 T.	shortening	45 mL
¼ c.	light molasses	60 mL
2 t.	salt, more for sprinkling pan	10 mL
1 pkg.	dry yeast	1 pkg.
¼ c.	warm water	60 mL
1	egg, beaten	1
2¾ c.	sifted Stone-Buhr all-purpose flour	690 mL

Stir together boiling water, barley flakes, shortening, molasses, and salt. Cool to lukewarm. Sprinkle yeast on the warm water and stir to dissolve. Add yeast, egg, and 1¼ c. (310 mL) of the flour to the barley mixture. Beat with an electric mixer at medium speed for 2 minutes. With a spoon, beat and stir in remaining flour until batter is smooth.

Grease a 9 × 5 in. (33 × 13 cm) loaf pan and sprinkle lightly with barley flakes and salt. Spread batter in pan. With a floured hand. gently smooth top and shape the loaf. Cover and let rise until batter just reaches the top of the pan. about 1½ hours. Bake at 375°F (190°C) for 25 to 35 minutes or until done. Remove from pan and cool on rack before slicing.

Yield: 1 loaf or 16 slices

Exchange, 1 slice: 1 bread
Each serving contains: Calories: 73, Carbohydrates: 26 g

Based on a recipe from Arnold Foods Company, Inc.

Limpa-Style Rye Bread

1 loaf	**Wisconsin Rye Bread dough**	1 loaf
½ t.	**fennel seed**	2 mL
½ t.	**aniseed**	2 mL
2 T.	**fresh orange peel, grated**	30 mL

Cut or pull the dough into 16 pieces. Place fennel seed, aniseed, and orange peel in a small bowl; stir to mix. Roll each dough piece in the seasoning mixture and knead or work with your hands until mixture is well incorporated. Knead pieces into a large ball. Place dough ball on a lightly greased pie plate. Cover and allow to rise until at least double in size. Bake at 400°F (200°C) for 15 minutes; reduce heat to 350°F (175°C) for another 20 minutes or until done.

Yield: 16 servings

Exchange, 1 serving: 1 bread
Each serving contains: Calories: 60, Carbohydrates: 13 g

Granary Beer Bread

2 pkg.	**active dry yeast**	2 pkg.
½ c.	**warm water**	125 mL
1 c.	**dark or regular beer, at room temperature (without foam)**	250 mL
1	**egg, lightly beaten**	1
2 T.	**brown sugar replacement**	30 mL
3 T.	**margarine, melted**	45 mL
1½ t.	**salt**	7 mL
2 c.	**stone-ground whole wheat flour**	500 mL
1 c.	**wheat germ**	250 mL
1½ c.	**all-purpose flour**	375 mL
1 T.	**vegetable oil**	15 mL
1	**egg**	1
1 T.	**water**	15 mL

Dissolve yeast in warm water in a large bowl. Add beer, egg, sugar replacement, margarine and salt. Stir well to blend. Stir in whole wheat flour and wheat germ with a wooden spoon. Gradually stir in the all-purpose flour to make a soft dough that will leave the sides of the bowl. (Add a small amount of water if dough is too stiff.) Turn out onto floured board. Knead 5 to 10 minutes or until dough is smooth and elastic. Place dough in large, greased bowl, turning to coat all sides. Cover and allow to rise in a warm, draft-free place for 1½ to 2 hours or until doubled.

Punch dough down. Divide dough into 3 equal pieces. Shape each piece into a 16 in. (40 cm) rope. Braid ropes together. Shape into a ring and seal ends. Place in greased 9 in. (23 cm) springform or layer pan. Brush dough lightly with oil. Cover pan loosely with plastic wrap. Let rise for 1½ hours or until doubled. Brush dough with 1 egg beaten with 1 T. (15 mL) water. Bake at 350°F (175°C) for 40 to 50 minutes or until done. If crust browns too quickly, cover loosely with foil during the last 5 to 10 minutes. Remove from pan immediately. Cool on rack.

Yield: 1 loaf or 24 servings

Exchange, 1 serving: 1 bread
Each serving contains: Calories: 78, Carbohydrates: 9 g

Challah

1 pkg.	dry yeast	1 pkg.
¾ c.	warm water	190 mL
1 t.	salt	5 mL
¼ c.	sugar replacement	60 mL
2 T.	margarine, melted	30 mL
2	eggs, well beaten	2
3 c.	flour	750 mL
1 t.	skim milk	5 mL
	poppy seeds	

Soften yeast in warm water; allow to rest for 5 minutes. Add salt, sugar replacement, and margarine. Measure 1 T. (15 mL) of the beaten eggs. Place in cup and reserve. Add remaining eggs and 1 c. (250 mL) of the flour to yeast mixture; beat vigorously. Add remaining flour. Turn onto floured board and knead until smooth and elastic. Place in lightly greased bowl; cover. Allow to rise until double in size, about 1½ hours. Punch down; divide into thirds. Roll into 3 strips, 18 in. (45 cm) long, with the heel of the hand. Braid the 3 strips loosely, tucking under ends. Blend reserved beaten egg with 1 t. (5 mL) skim milk, carefully brush over braid. Sprinkle with poppy seeds; cover. Allow to rise until double in size, about 1½ hours. Bake at 350°F (175°C) for 1 hour, or until done.

Yield: 1 loaf or 18 slices

Exchange, 1 slice: 1 bread
Each serving contains: Calories: 70, Carbohydrates: 19 g

Potato Flake Bread

1 loaf	frozen white bread dough, thawed	1 loaf
½ c.	potato flakes, dried	125 mL
1	egg white	1
2 t.	water	10 mL

Press or roll dough as flat as possible. Combine egg white and water in a small cup; with a fork, beat until foamy. Lightly brush the flattened surface of the dough, reserving some egg liquid for later. Sprinkle ⅓ c. (90 mL) of the potato flakes over the moistened surface. Roll up jelly-roll style, turning in the side edges. Knead dough to incorporate the flakes into the dough. Form into a French-style loaf; place on a greased baking sheet. Cover and allow to rise until at least double in size. Lightly brush top of loaf with remaining egg mixture and sprinkle with remaining potato flakes. Bake at 350°F (175°C) for 22 to 25 minutes or until golden brown.

Yield: 16 servings

Exchange, 1 serving: 1 bread
Each serving contains: Calories: 72, Carbohydrates: 16 g

Banana Yeast Bread

Make bread in small loaf pans for a different look.

2	very ripe bananas	2
1 t.	solid vegetable shortening	5 mL
½ c.	boiling water	125 mL
¼ t.	banana flavoring	1 mL
⅓ c.	lukewarm water	90 mL
1 pkg.	dry yeast	1 pkg.
3 c.	all-purpose flour	750 mL

In a bowl, mash bananas almost to a purée. Combine boiling water and shortening in another bowl; stir to melt the shortening. Add to mashed bananas. Add banana flavoring and set aside until lukewarm. In a cup, dissolve yeast in lukewarm water. Stir into banana mixture. Add 1 c. (250 mL) of the flour and beat until smooth. Gradually add half of the remaining flour; continue beating to make a smooth sponge. Allow to rest for 10 minutes. Beat in remaining flour. Cover dough and allow to double in size. Turn into well-greased loaf pans. Cover and allow dough to just come to top of pans. Bake at 350°F (175°C) for 15 minutes or until loaf tops are rounded. Increase heat to 400°F (200°C) and bake for 30 to 40 minutes more. (Baking time may vary with the size pans you use.) Bread should be golden brown and sound hollow when you tap the top of the loaf. Brush lightly with small amount of low-calorie margarine. Cool on rack.

Yield: 16 servings

Exchange, 1 serving: 1 bread, ⅓ fruit
Each serving contains: Calories: 91, Carbohydrates: 19 g

Apricot Loaf

Adding a glaze of dissolved aspartame gives this loaf a nice glossy took, as well as helping to satisfy a sweet tooth.

1 c.	apricots	250 mL
2½ c.	flour	625 mL
2 t.	baking powder	10 mL
1 t.	baking soda	5 mL
dash	salt (optional)	dash
2 T.	grated orange rind	30 mL
¼ c.	sugar	60 mL
9 pkts.	concentrated acesulfame-K	9 pkts.
2	egg whites	2
⅔ c.	skim buttermilk	180 mL
⅔ c.	orange juice	180 mL
1 t.	vanilla extract	5 mL
¼ c.	unsweetened applesauce	60 mL

Glaze ingredients

1 t.	cornstarch	5 mL
¼ c.	water	60 mL
2 t.	measures-like-sugar aspartame	10 mL
½ t.	orange extract	2.5 mL

Snip the apricots into small pieces with a pair of scissors. Set aside. Combine the flour, baking powder, baking soda, salt, orange rind, sugar, and acesulfame-K in a bowl. Add the apricot pieces and stir to combine. In a separate container, beat the egg whites and combine with the buttermilk, orange juice, vanilla extract, and applesauce. Add the wet ingredients to the dry ones, stirring until just combined. Do not overmix. Pour into a 9 × 5-inch (23 × 13 cm) loaf pan that has been sprayed with non-stick vegetable cooking spray. Bake in a preheated 350°F (180°C) oven for 50 minutes.

Prepare the glaze as follows. Combine the cornstarch and water in a small saucepan. Heat over medium heat; stir with a wire whisk until thickened. Turn off the heat, stir in the aspartame and extract. As soon as the bread is out of the oven, turn it onto a plate. Use a toothpick to poke holes in the top. Mix the glaze and pour it over the top.

Yield: 20 servings

Exchange, 1 serving: 1 bread
Each serving contains: Calories: 83, Fiber: 0.8 g, Sodium: 52 mg,
Cholesterol: 0 mg, Carbohydrates: 18 g

Raisin Bread

1 pkg.	dry yeast	1 pkg.
¼ c.	warm water	60 mL
¾ c.	milk, scalded and cooled	180 mL
2 T.	sugar replacement	30 mL
1 t.	salt	5 mL
1	egg	1
2 T.	margarine, softened	30 mL
3¾ c.	flour	940 mL
1 c.	raisins	250 mL

Soften yeast in warm water; allow to rest for 5 minutes. Combine milk, sugar replacement, salt, egg, and margarine; mix thoroughly. Stir in yeast mixture. Add 1 c. (250 mL) of the flour. Beat until smooth, Mix in raisins. Blend in remaining flour. Knead for 5 minutes. Cover; allow to rise for 2 hours. Punch down; form into loaf. Place in greased 9 × 5 in. (23 × 13 cm) loaf pan; cover. Allow to rise for 1 hour. Bake at 400°F (200°C) for 30 minutes, or until loaf sounds hollow and is golden brown. Remove to rack.

Yield: 1 loaf or 14 slices

Exchange, 1 slice: 1 bread
Each serving contains: Calories: 68, Carbohydrates: 18 g

Spicy Prune Bread

2 c.	all-purpose flour, sifted	500 mL
2½ t.	baking powder	12 mL
½ t.	baking soda	2 mL
1 T.	salt	5 mL
1 t.	ground cinnamon	5 mL
½ t.	ground or grated nutmeg	2 mL
¼ t.	ground cloves	1 mL
1 c.	oatmeal	250 mL
¼ c.	buttermilk	310 mL
2 T.	vegetable oil	30 mL
1 c.	prunes, cooked, drained, pitted and diced	250 mL

Sift together the flour, baking powder, baking soda, salt, cinnamon, nutmeg and cloves. Stir in the oatmeal. Add buttermilk and oil; stir to completely blend. Fold in prunes. Spread into a well-greased 9 × 5 in. (23 × 13 cm) loaf pan. Bake at 350°F (175°C) for 1 hour or until done. Turn out on rack to cool.

Yield: 1 loaf or 16 servings

Exchange, 1 serving: 1 bread, ¼ fruit
Each serving contains: Calories: 85, Carbohydrates: 20 g

Peanut Butter Bread

1½ c.	all-purpose flour	375 mL
1 T.	baking powder	15 mL
½ t.	salt	2 mL
½ c.	sugar	125 mL
2 c.	Kellogg's bran flakes	500 mL
1⅓ c.	2% milk	440 mL
⅓ c.	peanut butter	90 mL
1	egg	1

Stir together flour, baking powder, salt and sugar. Set aside. Measure cereal and milk into large mixing bowl. Let stand 2 minutes or until cereal softens. Add peanut butter and egg. Beat well. Stir in flour mixture. Spread batter evenly in greased 9 × 5 × 3 in. (23 × 13 × 8 cm) loaf pan. Bake at 350°F (175°C) about 1 hour or until done. Cool 10 minutes before removing from pan. Cool completely before slicing.

Yield: 1 loaf or 15 slices

Exchange, 1 slice: 2 bread
Each serving contains: Calories: 135, Carbohydrates: 19 g

From Kellogg's Test Kitchens.

Mexican Seasoned Bread

1 loaf	Basic White Bread dough	1 loaf
4 t.	Mexican seasoning	20 mL
1	egg white	1
1 T.	water	15 mL

Cut or pull bread dough into 20 pieces. Place Mexican seasoning in a small bowl. Roll each dough piece into the seasoning. Knead or work with your hands until seasoning is well incorporated into the dough. Knead the pieces of dough into a large ball. Place on an 8 in. (20 cm) pie plate that has been lightly sprayed with vegetable spray. Cover and allow to rise until at least double in size. Combine egg white and water in a small bowl; with a fork, beat until foamy. Lightly brush surface of dough. Bake at 350°F (175°C) for 30 minutes or until dark brown.

Yield: 16 servings

Exchange, 1 serving: 1 bread
Each serving contains: Calories: 69, Carbohydrates: 15 g

Petite French Bread

Tuck these among muffins and other buns for a lavish bread display on your table.

1 recipe	**Basic White Bread dough**	1 recipe	
1	**egg white**	1	
1 t.	**water**	5 mL	

Divide dough into 30 balls. Roll each ball into a fingerlike form. Place on well-greased baking sheets about 2 in. (5 cm) apart. Cut small slashes across the tops. Cover and allow to double in size. Combine egg white and water in small bowl; beat with a fork to blend. Lightly brush the surface of each petite loaf with egg mixture. Bake at 400°F (200°C) for 15 minutes. Reduce heat to 350°F (175°C); bake until golden brown.

Yield: 30 servings

Exchange, 1 serving: 1 bread
Each serving contains: Calories: 90, Carbohydrates: 17 g

Easy Rolls

When frozen, these rolls come out perfect two to three weeks later. The directions include a quick variation for cloverleaf rolls.

1 loaf	**frozen white bread dough, thawed**	1 loaf	

Cut the bread dough lengthwise in half. Cut each half lengthwise in half. Cut each quarter strip in 4 equal pieces. Roll each piece into a ball. Flatten in the palm of the hand. Place balls in a well-greased baking sheet with the sides of the balls touching. Cover and allow to rise until more than double in size. Bake at 350°F (175°C) for 25 to 30 minutes or until browned.

For cloverleaf rolls: Divide each small piece (¼ of loaf) into 3 parts. Place the 3 parts in a well-oiled muffin tin. Cover and allow to rise until over double in size. Bake at 350°F (175°C) for 20 to 25 minutes or until done and golden brown.

Yield: 16 rolls

Exchange, 1 roll: 1 bread
Each serving contains: Calories: 69, Carbohydrates: 15 g

Semmel

These hard-crusted rolls, called semmel, are classic additions to any meal. They're especially good with soups and stews.

1 recipe	Moist German-Style Potato Bread	1 recipe	
1	egg yolk	1	
1 T.	ice water	5 mL	

Prepare the Moist German-Style Potato Bread. After the first rising, divide dough into 24 balls. Knead each ball and shape into a bun about 3 in. (75 cm) round by 1 in. (2.5 cm) high. Place about 2 in. (5 cm) apart on well-greased baking sheets. Cover and allow to rise slightly. Dip the handle of a wooden spoon into potato flour. Push spoon down across the middle of each roll, making a deep crease. Cover and allow to completely rise. Combine egg yolk and water in a small cup or bowl; blend with a fork. Lightly brush the top of each roll. Bake at 400°F (200°C) for 20 to 25 minutes until golden brown and top feels crispy hard.

Yield: 24 servings

Exchange, 1 serving: 1¾ bread
Each serving contains: Calories: 128, Carbohydrates: 29 g

Acorn Squash Rolls

The addition of acorn squash lends a unique twist to this "loaf of rolls."

1 c.	lukewarm water	250 mL
¼ c.	granulated sugar replacement	60 mL
1 T.	granulated fructose	15 mL
1 pkg.	dry yeast	1 pkg.
1 c.	acorn squash, cooked and mashed	250 mL
3 T.	vegetable oil	45 mL
2 t.	salt	10 mL
½ c.	dry milk powder	125 mL
4¼ c.	all-purpose flour	1.3 L

Combine the water, sugar replacement, fructose, and yeast in a large bowl; stir to dissolve yeast. Beat in the squash, oil, salt, and dry milk. Gradually, beat in as much flour as possible. Turn out onto a floured surface and knead remaining flour into dough. Knead until smooth and elastic. Allow to rise until double in size. Divide dough into 22 pieces. Roll each piece into a ball. Place, all together, in a well-greased rectangular loaf pan. Cover and allow to rise again. Bake at 400°F (200°C) for about 25 to 30 minutes or until done.

Yield: 22 servings

Exchange, 1 serving: 1¾ bread
Each serving contains: Calories: 114, Carbohydrates: 20 g

Country Cheese Rolls

1½ c.	skim milk, warmed	375 mL
¼ c.	low-calorie margarine, melted	60 mL
1 T.	granulated sugar replacement	15 mL
2 t.	salt	10 mL
1 t.	black pepper	5 mL
6½ c.	all-purpose flour	1.6 L
2 pkg.	dry yeast	2 pkg.
1 c.	water, lukewarm	250 mL
1 c.	cheddar cheese, grated	250 mL
1	egg white	1
1 t.	water	5 mL

In a large bowl, combine milk, margarine, sugar replacement, salt, pepper, and 2 c. (500 mL) of the flour; beat into a smooth paste. Dissolve yeast in the lukewarm water; set aside until foamy. Add the cheese and yeast to flour paste; beat until well blended. Beat in flour, 1 c. (250 mL) at a time, until dough is soft and comes away from the sides of the bowl. Knead dough on a floured surface, working in any remaining flour. Knead for about 10 minutes until smooth and elastic. Place dough in a well-oiled bowl; turn once to coat both sides. Cover with plastic wrap and set in a warm, draft-free place. Let rise for about 1 hour until double in size. Punch dough down; put on a floured surface and knead lightly. Divide the dough into 32 balls. Place balls in well-greased muffin tins. Combine the egg white and 1 t. (5 mL) of water in a cup; whip to mix. Brush over top of balls. Cover and allow to rise again. Bake at 375°F (190°C) for 20 to 25 minutes or until done.

Yield: 32 rolls

Exchange, 1 roll: 1 bread, ½ fat
Each roll contains: Calories: 110, Carbohydrates: 18 g

Cinnamon Rolls

Dough mixture

½ c.	skim milk	125 mL
2 t.	cider vinegar	10 mL
1 pkg.	dry yeast	1 pkg.
¼ c.	warm water	60 mL
⅓ c.	granulated sugar replacement	90 mL

or

2 t.	granulated fructose	10 mL
3 T.	solid shortening	45 mL
1	egg	1
½ t.	salt	2 mL
3 c.	all-purpose flour	750 mL

Cinnamon mixture

1 T.	margarine, melted	15 mL
⅓ c.	granulated sugar replacement	90 mL
	ground cinnamon	

Dough: Combine skim milk and vinegar in a large mixing bowl. Dissolve the yeast in the warm water. Add to skim milk mixture. Beat in sweetener of your choice, shortening, egg, and salt. Next, add 2 c. (500 mL) of the flour. Beat on low until the mixture is blended and smooth. Then add remaining flour and stir until all the flour is incorporated into the dough. Turn out onto a lightly floured surface; knead for 4 to 5 minutes until dough is smooth and elastic. Place in a greased bowl, turn dough over, cover, and allow to rise until double in size (about 1½ hours). Punch dough down and roll into a 12 × 9 in. (30 × 23 cm) rectangle.

Cinnamon mixture: Spread dough with melted margarine, mix the sugar replacement with desired amount of cinnamon, and sprinkle mixture on top of dough.

To assemble: Roll up, beginning at the 12 in. (30 cm) side. Tuck end of dough into the roll to seal. Cut into 18 slices. Place slightly apart in a 13 × 9 in. (33 × 23 cm) well-greased pan. Cover, and allow to rise until double in size (about 45 to 60 minutes). Bake at 375°F (190°C) for 25 to 30 minutes or until done.

Yield: 18 servings

Exchange, 1 serving: 1 bread
Each serving contains: Calories: 73, Carbohydrates: 13 g

Pecan Rolls

1 pkg.	dry yeast	1 pkg.
¼ c.	warm water	60 mL
½ c.	whole milk	125 mL
2 T.	margarine, softened	30 mL
½ c.	granulated sugar replacement	125 mL
or		
3 T.	granulated fructose	45 mL
1	egg	1
½ t.	salt	2 mL
2½ c.	all-purpose flour	625 mL
1 T.	margarine, melted	15 mL
⅓ c.	granulated sugar replacement	90 mL
	ground cinnamon	
½ c.	sugar-free maple-flavored syrup	125 mL
⅓ c.	ground pecans	90 mL

Dissolve the yeast in the warm water. Allow to rest for 2 minutes. Pour into a large mixing bowl. Add milk, softened margarine, the ½ c. of sugar replacement or the 3 T. of fructose, egg, salt, and 1½ c. (375 mL) of the flour, Beat on low to blend, then on high for 2 minutes. Stir in remaining 1 c. (250 mL) of flour. Transfer to a lightly floured surface; knead until smooth and elastic. Place in a greased bowl, turn dough over, and cover with plastic wrap and then a towel. Allow to rise until double in size. Punch dough down and roll into a 12 × 9 in. (30 × 23 cm) rectangle. Spread dough with melted margarine, mix the ⅓ c. (90 mL) of sugar replacement with desired amount of cinnamon, and sprinkle mixture on top of dough.

To assemble: Roll up, beginning at the 12 in. (30 cm) side. Tuck end of dough into the roll to seal. Cut into 18 slices. Pour sugarfree maple-flavored syrup in the bottom of a well-greased 13 × 9 in. (33 × 23 cm) pan. Sprinkle pecans over surface of syrup. Place slices of dough on top of the pecans. Then cover, and allow to rise until double in size (about 45 to 60 minutes). Bake at 375°F (190°C) for 25 to 30 minutes or until done.

Yield: 18 servings

Exchange, 1 serving: 1 bread
Each serving contains: Calories: 78, Carbohydrates: 16 g

Buttermilk Sticky Rolls

1 pkg.	dry yeast	1 pkg.
¼ c.	warm water	60 mL
¼ c.	buttermilk	190 mL
2 T.	margarine, softened	30 mL
½ c.	granulated sugar replacement	125 mL
or		
3 T.	granulated fructose	45 mL
1	egg	1
½ t.	salt	2 mL
3 c.	all-purpose flour	750 mL
1 T.	margarine, melted	15 mL
⅓ c.	granulated sugar replacement	90 mL
	ground cinnamon	
½ c.	sugar-free maple-flavored syrup	125 mL

Dissolve the yeast in the warm water. Allow to rest for 2 minutes. Pour into a large mixing bowl. Add buttermilk, softened margarine, sweetener, egg, salt, and 2 c. (500 mL) of the flour. Beat on low to blend, then on high for 2 minutes. Stir in remaining 1 c. (250 mL) of flour. Transfer to a lightly floured surface, and knead until smooth and elastic. Place in a greased bowl, turn dough over, and cover with plastic wrap and then a towel. Allow to rise until double in size. Punch dough down and roll into a 12 × 9 in. (30 × 23 cm) rectangle. Spread dough with melted margarine, mix the sugar replacement with desired amount of cinnamon, and sprinkle mixture on top of dough.

To assemble: Roll up, beginning at the 12 in. (30 cm) side. Tuck end of dough into the roll to seal. Cut into 18 slices. Pour sugar-free maple-flavored syrup in the bottom of a well-greased 13 × 9 in. (33 × 23 cm) pan. Place the cut slices of dough slightly apart on top of the syrup. Cover, and allow to rise until double in size (about 45 to 60 minutes). Bake at 375°F (190°C) for 25 to 30 minutes or until done.

Yield: 18 servings

Exchange, 1 serving: 1 bread
Each serving contains: Calories: 72, Carbohydrates: 12 g

Bran Batter Rolls

1 c.	Kellogg's All-Bran or Bran Buds cereal	250 mL
3 c.	all-purpose flour	750 mL
2 T.	sugar	30 mL
1½ t.	salt	7 mL
1 pkg.	active dry yeast	1 pkg.
1 c.	milk	250 mL
½ c.	water	125 mL
2 T.	margarine	30 mL
1	egg, lightly beaten	1
	poppy seeds (optional)	
	sesame seeds (optional)	

In the large bowl of your electric mixer, stir together the cereal, 1 c. (250 mL) of the flour, the sugar, salt, and yeast. Set aside. In a small saucepan, heat milk, water and margarine until warm. Add to cereal mixture. Reserve 1 T. (15 mL) of the egg. Add remaining egg to cereal mixture. Beat 30 seconds at low speed of electric mixer, scraping bowl constantly. Beat 3 minutes at high speed. By hand, stir in remaining flour to make a stiff batter. (Add a small amount of extra water if dough is too stiff.) Cover dough loosely. Let rise in warm place until doubled. Stir down the batter. Portion batter evenly into 16 greased 2½ in. (6.4 cm) muffin pan cups. Brush tops of rolls with reserved egg. Sprinkle with poppy or sesame seed, if desired. Bake at 400°F (200°C) for 18 to 20 minutes or until golden.

Yield: 16 rolls

Exchange, 1 roll: 1 bread, 1 fat
Each serving contains: Calories: 115, Carbohydrates: 7 g

From Kellogg's Test Kitchens.

Yeast Rolls

1 pkg.	dry yeast	1 pkg.
¼ c.	warm water	60 mL
2 T.	sugar replacement	30 mL
2 t.	salt	10 mL
1 T.	margarine, melted	15 mL
¾ c.	warm water	190 mL
3 ½ c.	flour	875 mL
1	egg, well beaten	1

Soften yeast in the ¼ c. (60 mL) warm water. Allow to rest for 5 minutes. Combine sugar replacement, salt, margarine, and the ¾ c. (190 mL) warm water; stir to mix. Add 1 c. (250 mL) of the flour; beat well. Blend in yeast mixture and the egg. Add remaining flour; mix well. Knead gently until dough is smooth; cover. Allow to rise for 1 hour. Punch down. Allow to rest for 10 minutes. Shape into 36 rolls. Place on greased cookie sheet or in greased muffin tins. Allow to rise until doubled in size, about 1½–2 hours. Bake at 400°F (200°C) for 20 to 25 minutes, or until golden brown.

Yield: 36 rolls

Exchange, 1 roll: 1 bread
Each serving contains: Calories: 68

Wheat Germ Croissants

3 c.	all-purpose flour	750 mL
1¼ c.	butter, softened	310 mL
2 pkg.	active dry yeast	2 pkg.
1 c.	warm water	250 mL
¾ c.	Kretschmer regular wheat germ	190 mL
1	egg	1
¼ c.	sugar	60 mL
¾ t.	salt	7 mL
1	egg	1
1 T.	water	15 mL

Beat ¼ c. (90 mL) flour and butter together until well blended. Spread into a 12 × 6 in. (30.5 × 15 cm) rectangle on waxed paper or foil. Refrigerate until firm, about 30 minutes. Dissolve yeast in warm water in large bowl. Add 2 c. (500 mL) flour, wheat germ, 1 egg, sugar and salt to dissolved yeast. Beat with electric mixer at medium speed for 1 minute. Gradually stir in remaining flour with wooden spoon to make a soft dough that leaves sides of bowl. (Add a small amount of extra water if dough is too stiff.) Turn out onto floured board. Knead 5 to 8 minutes until dough is smooth and elastic. Roll dough into a 14 in. (35 cm) square. Place refrigerated butter mixture on one side of rectangle. Fold dough over butter and pinch edges to seal. Roll into a 20 × 14 in. (51 × 35 cm) rectangle. Fold dough in thirds. Place on baking sheet. Refrigerate dough 10 minutes to firm the butter. Repeat rolling, folding, and refrigerating the dough 3 more times. lf butter begins to break through, sprinkle with flour to seal. Wrap and refrigerate dough for 2 to 3 hours after last folding.

Cut dough into thirds. Roll out each third separately and refrigerate remaining sections until ready to use. Roll the third of dough into a 20 × 14 in. (51 × 35 cm) rectangle. Cut crosswise into 4 equal pieces. Cut each piece diagonally to form 2 triangles. Roll up each triangle loosely, starting at 5 in. (13 cm) side and rolling towards the point. Place on ungreased baking sheets. Curve the dough rolls to form crescents. Cover loosely with plastic wrap. Let rise in warm draft-free place for 30 to 45 minutes until doubled. Brush dough with 1 egg, beaten with 1 T. water, just before baking. Bake at 350°F (175°C) for 18 to 22 minutes until golden. Serve warm if desired.

Yield: 2 dozen croissants

Exchange, 1 croissant: 1 bread
Each serving contains: Calories: 70, Carbohydrates: negligible

With the courtesy of Kretschmer Wheat Germ/International Multifoods.

Plain Yeast Kuchen Dough

1 pkg.	dry yeast	1 pkg.
¼ c.	lukewarm water	60 mL
1¾ c.	skim milk, scalded	440 mL
½ c.	granulated sugar replacement	125 mL
¼ c.	low-calorie margarine	60 mL
¼ c.	butter	60 mL
1 T.	lemon peel, freshly grated	15 mL
1 t.	salt	5 mL
1	egg, beaten	1
6 c.	all-purpose flour	1.5 L

To make the dough, dissolve the yeast in lukewarm water. In a bowl, combine the scalded milk, sugar replacement, margarine, butter, lemon peel, and salt; stir and cool to lukewarm. When cooled, beat in the egg. Stir in the yeast mixture. Add enough flour to make a soft dough (about 5 c. or 1.25 mL). Turn out on floured surface and knead in remaining flour until smooth and elastic. Cover tightly and allow to rise until double in size. Punch down and use as directed in recipe or form into desired shapes.

This dough can also be made into doughnuts and fried. To bake the kuchen, place on a well-greased baking sheet or 2 large pans. Bake at 375°F (190°C) until browned; baking time will vary, depending on size of loaves.

Yield: 32 servings

Exchange, 1 serving: 1 bread, ¼ fat
Each serving contains: Calories: 107, Carbohydrates: 17 g

Strawberry Kuchen

Crust

1 c.	all-purpose flour	250 mL
½ c.	low-calorie margarine	125 mL
1	egg yolk	1
1 T.	liquid sweetener	15 mL

Filling

2 c.	strawberries, sliced	500 mL
2	eggs, beaten	2
¼ c.	granulated sugar replacement	60 mL
2 t.	all-purpose flour	10 mL

To make the crust: Combine ingredients in a food processor or bowl. Cut into small pea-sized crumbs. Pat tightly into the bottom of a 13 × 9 in. (33 × 23 cm) pan.

For the filling: Combine all filling ingredients in a bowl and blend. Allow to rest for 10 minutes; stir again. Pour into the crust and spread evenly. Bake at 350°F (175°C) for 35 to 40 minutes or until filling is set.

Yield: 12 servings

Exchange, 1 serving: ⅔ bread, 1 fat
Each serving contains: Calories: 100, Carbohydrates: 10 g

Chocolate Raised Doughnuts

½ c.	skim milk	125 mL
1 pkg.	dry yeast	1 pkg.
¼ c.	warm water	1 mL
⅔ c.	granulated sugar replacement	180 mL
¼ c.	solid shortening	60 mL
2 T.	granulated fructose	30 mL
1	egg	1
½ t.	salt	2 mL
⅓ c.	unsweetened baking cocoa	90 mL
2½ c.	all-purpose flour	625 mL
	oil for deep-fat frying	

Pour skim milk in small saucepan. Bring to a boil, remove from heat, and allow to cool. Dissolve the yeast in the warm water. Combine skim milk, yeast mixture, granulated sugar replacement, shortening, fructose, egg, and salt in a large mixing bowl. Combine the cocoa with 1¼ c. (310 mL) of flour in another bowl. Stir to mix. Add to liquid mixture in bowl. Beat on low until mixture is blended and smooth. Add remaining flour and stir until all the flour is incorporated into the dough. Turn out onto a lightly floured surface; then knead for 4 to 5 minutes or until dough is smooth and elastic. Place in a greased bowl, turn dough over, cover, and allow to rise until double in size (about 1½ hours). Punch dough down and roll to about ½ in. (1.25 cm) thickness. Cut with floured doughnut cutter. Place doughnuts onto a greased cookie sheet or piece of waxed paper. Cover and allow to rise. Heat 2 to 3 in. (5 to 8 cm) of oil in deep fat fryer or heavy saucepan to 375°F (190°C). Heat a wide spatula in the oil. Gently slide spatula under a doughnut. Place doughnut in the hot oil, and fry about 2 minutes on each side. Remove from oil; drain on paper towels. Repeat with remaining doughnuts.

Yield: 18 servings

Exchange, 1 serving: ¾ bread
Each serving contains: Calories: 65, Carbohydrates: 14 g

Buttermilk Doughnuts

1 pkg.	dry yeast	1 pkg.
¼ c.	warm water	60 mL
1 c.	buttermilk, warmed	250 mL
1	egg	1
½ t.	salt	2 mL
2 T.	margarine, melted	30 mL
½ c.	granulated sugar replacement	125 mL
1 T.	granulated fructose	15 mL
3 c.	all-purpose flour	750 mL
	oil for deep-fat frying	

Dissolve yeast in warm water. Allow to rest for 5 minutes; then pour into a large mixing bowl. Add buttermilk, egg, salt, margarine, sugar replacement, fructose, and 2 c. (500 mL) of the flour. Beat on low until blended. Then beat on high for 2 minutes. Stir in remaining 1 c. (250 mL) of flour. Transfer dough to a floured surface. Knead until smooth and elastic. Transfer to a greased bowl; turn dough over. Cover with plastic wrap and then a towel. Allow to rise until double in size. Transfer to a lightly floured surface. Pat or roll dough to about ⅓ in. (8 mm) thickness. Cut with floured doughnut cutter. Allow to rest for 10 to 15 minutes. Heat about 3 in. (7.5 cm) of vegetable oil to 375°F (190°C) in a skillet or deep-fat fryer. Slide doughnuts into hot oil. Fry until golden brown, turning several times. Remove from oil and drain on paper towels.

Yield: 24 servings

Exchange, 1 serving: ¼ bread
Each serving contains: Calories: 63, Carbohydrates: 13 g

Dutch Doughnuts

1 pkg.	dry yeast	1 pkg.
¼ c.	warm water	60 mL
2	eggs	2
½ c.	skim milk	125 mL
¼ c.	whole milk	60 mL
1 t.	vanilla extract	5 mL
⅓ c.	granulated sugar replacement	90 mL
3 c.	all-purpose flour	750 mL
1 T.	baking powder	15 mL
1 t.	salt	5 mL
½ t.	ground cinnamon	2 mL
¼ t.	ground nutmeg	1 mL
	oil for deep-fat frying	

Dissolve yeast in warm water in a large bowl. Add eggs, skim and whole milk, vanilla, and sugar replacement. Beat until light and fluffy. Add 2 c. (500 mL) of the flour and the baking powder, salt, cinnamon, and nutmeg; beat on low until well blended. Stir in remaining flour. Transfer to floured surface. Roll dough to about 1 in. (8 mm) thickness. Cut with a floured doughnut cutter. Heat about 3 in. (7.5 cm) of vegetable oil to 375°F (190°C) in a skillet or deep-fat fryer. Slide doughnuts into hot oil. Fry until golden brown, turning several times. Remove from oil and drain on paper towels.

Yield: 24 servings

Exchange, 1 serving: ¼ bread
Each serving contains: Calories: 60, Carbohydrates: 12 g

Baked Orange Doughnuts

2 pkg.	yeast	2 pkg.
½ c.	warm water	125 mL
1 c.	orange juice	250 mL
⅓ c.	low-calorie margarine, melted and cooled	90 mL
¾ c.	granulated sugar replacement	190 mL
2 t.	salt	10 mL
1½ T.	orange peel	22 mL
2	eggs	2
3 c.	all-purpose flour	750 mL
	vegetable cooking spray	

Dissolve the yeast in warm water; set aside until it starts to bubble. In a large bowl, combine the yeast mixture, orange juice, margarine, sugar replacement, salt, orange peel, eggs, and 2 c. (500 mL) of the flour; beat on high speed for about 4 minutes. Gradually beat in the remaining flour. Transfer dough to a lightly floured surface and knead until smooth and elastic. Place dough in an oiled bowl; cover and allow to rise until doubled in size. Punch dough down. Roll out on a lightly floured surface until ¼ in. (6 mm) thick. Lift dough from surface and turn over; cover with a towel and allow to rest for 2 minutes. Cut dough with a doughnut cutter; place doughnuts on a greased baking sheet. Allow to rise until almost double in size. Bake at 350°F (175°C) for 10 minutes or until lightly browned. Coat immediately with the cooking spray.

Yield: 30 doughnuts

Exchange, 1 doughnut: 1 bread
Each serving contains: Calories: 60, Carbohydrates: 11 g

Raised Cherry-Yogurt Doughnuts

1 pkg.	dry yeast	1 pkg.
¼ c.	lukewarm water	60 mL
⅓ c.	skim milk, scalded	90 mL
8 oz.	cherry low-calorie yogurt	240 g
¼ t.	cherry flavoring	1 mL
3 c.	all-purpose flour	750 mL
	vegetable oil for frying	

Dissolve the yeast in lukewarm water; set aside. Combine the scalded milk, yogurt, and cherry flavoring in a large bowl; beat to blend. Add yeast mixture and half of the flour and beat until soft. Add ¾ c. (190 mL) more flour; mix until blended. Sprinkle remaining flour on a work surface. Knead dough on the floured surface until flour is incorporated and dough is smooth and elastic. Place in a greased bowl; turn once to coat both sides. Cover tightly with plastic. Refrigerate for 6 hours or overnight. Place dough on a very lightly floured surface. Roll until ½ in. (1.3 cm) thick. Cut with a doughnut cutter. Allow to rise for 30 to 45 minutes. Fry in vegetable oil that has been heated to 365°F (184°C). Turn and fry until lightly browned and done.

Yield: 18 doughnuts

Exchange, 1 doughnut: 1 bread
Each serving contains: Calories: 82, Carbohydrates: 19 g

Park Doughnuts

3	eggs, separated	3
¾ c.	granulated sugar replacement	190 mL
4½ c.	all-purpose flour	1.3 L
5 t.	baking powder	25 mL
1½ t.	salt	7 mL
1 c.	skim milk	250 mL
1 t.	nutmeg	5 mL
3 T.	vegetable oil	45 mL
	vegetable oil for frying	

In a bowl, beat the egg whites until stiff and dry. Beat the yolks into the egg whites, one at a time, until lemon colored. Gradually beat in the sugar replacement. In another bowl, sift flour, baking powder, and salt together twice. Add flour mixture alternately with the skim milk to the egg mixture, beating well after each addition. Add the nutmeg and the 3 T. (45 mL) oil. Turn out onto a lightly floured surface. Roll until 1½ in. (1.3 cm) thick and cut with doughnut cutter. Heat frying oil to 375°F (190°C). Drop in a few doughnuts at a time. Fry until puffed and golden brown. Remove with a slotted spoon and drain on paper towels.

Yield: 36 doughnuts

Exchange, 1 doughnut: 1 bread
Each serving contains: Calories: 74, Carbohydrates: 11 g

Cake Doughnuts

1 T.	granulated sugar	15 mL
4 T.	sugar replacement	60 mL
⅓ c.	buttermilk	80 mL
1	egg, well beaten	1
1 c.	flour	250 mL
⅛ t.	baking soda	1 mL
1 t.	baking powder	5 mL
dash each	nutmeg, cinnamon, vanilla extract, salt	dash each
	oil for deep-fat frying	

Combine sugars, buttermilk, and egg; beat well. Add remaining ingredients, except oil. Beat just until blended. Heat oil to 375°F (190°C). Drop dough from doughnut dropper into hot fat. Fry until golden brown, turning often. Drain.

Yield: 12 doughnuts

Exchange, 1 doughnut: 1 bread, 1 fat
Each serving contains: Calories: 130, Carbohydrates: 6 g

Golden Corn Coins

1 c.	yellow cornmeal	250 mL
1 t.	salt	5 mL
	boiling water	

Heat the oven to 450°F (230°C). Place a well-greased, rimmed cookie sheet in the oven. Combine the cornmeal, salt, and just enough boiling water to make a thick pancake-like batter. Carefully remove greased sheet from oven. Using a large serving spoon, quickly spoon batter onto the hot grease in 36 large fifty-cent size rounds. Place in oven and bake for 10 to 15 minutes or until lightly browned. Serve hot.

Yield: 36 coins

Exchange, 1 coin: ½ bread
Each serving contains: Calories: 13, Carbohydrates: 3 g

Chocolate Muffins

Great to make for people who need to be reminded to eat only a single portion. Make them, freeze them, and defrost as needed.

½ c.	unsweetened cocoa powder	125 mL
1 c.	flour	250 mL
1 t.	baking soda	5 mL
½ t.	baking powder	2 mL
pinch	salt (optional)	pinch
2 T.	sugar	30 mL
½ c.	fructose	125 mL
4 pkts.	concentrated acesulfame-K	4 pkts.
1 c.	nonfat buttermilk	250 mL
½ c.	prune purée	25 mL
2 t.	vanilla extract	10 mL
¼ t.	almond extract	1 mL
2	egg whites	2

Glaze

2 t.	unsweetened cocoa powder	10 mL
	hot water	
¼ c.	measures-like-sugar aspartame	60 mL

Sift the cocoa, flour, baking soda, baking powder, salt, sugar, fructose, and acesulfame-K together twice. Set aside. Use a food processor to combine the buttermilk, prune purée, vanilla, and almond extract. Add the dry ingredients and process briefly. Transfer to a mixing bowl. Beat the egg whites until stiff. Stir the egg whites into the batter.

Pour the batter into 18 muffin tin cups that have been coated with nonstick cooking spray. Bake in a preheated 325°F (160°C) oven for 20 minutes. Combine the glaze with a wire whisk. Pour a little glaze over each muffin.

Yield: 18 muffins

Exchange, 1 muffin: 1 bread
Each serving contains: Calories: 70, Carbohydrates: 22 g, Fiber: trace,
*   Sodium: 108 mg, Cholesterol: 0 mg*

Blueberry Muffins

Almost every doughnut shop, coffee bar and breakfast restaurant now sells blueberry muffins. A generous size of muffin has become the standard in restaurants and bakeries. However, the size specified in cookbooks, especially diabetic cookbooks, is a miniature version. We hope you won't be disappointed that we are calling for the old-fashioned small size. You can use a standard cupcake pan or paper liners.

1½ c.	flour	375 mL
1½ t.	baking powder	7 mL
¼ t.	baking soda	1 mL
1 T.	canola oil	15 mL
⅓ c.	egg substitute	90 mL
½ c.	nonfat buttermilk	125 mL
½ t.	vanilla extract	2 mL
2 T.	nonfat sour cream	30 mL
¼ c.	apple juice concentrate	60 mL
1 c.	blueberries (fresh or frozen without sugar and defrosted)	250 mL
3 T.	boiling water	45 mL
2 t.	concentrated aspartame	10 mL

Sift together the flour, baking powder, and baking soda. Set aside. Use a wire whisk to combine the oil, egg substitute, buttermilk, vanilla extract, sour cream, and apple juice concentrate. Stir the flour mixture into the wet mixture. Do not overmix. Stir in the blueberries. Pour into a muffin tin that has been coated with non-stick cooking spray.

Bake in a preheated 375°F (190°C) oven for 30 minutes. As soon as the muffins are out of the oven, combine the boiling water and aspartame to make a glaze. Use a toothpick to make holes in the tops of the muffins. Use a pastry brush to cover the tops with the glaze.

Yield: 12 muffins

Exchange, 1 muffin: 1 bread
Each serving contains: Calories: 90, Carbohydrates: 18 g, Fiber: trace, Sodium: 100 mg, Cholesterol: trace

Low-Calorie Lemon–Poppy Seed Muffins

These muffins are high in flavor and low in calories. They are great as a dessert or as a snack with coffee or tea.

1 c.	nonfat cottage cheese	250 mL
¼ c.	egg substitute	60 mL
¼ c.	flour	60 mL
1 t.	vanilla extract	5 mL
2 t.	lemon juice	10 mL
2 t.	grated lemon peel	10 mL
1 T.	sugar	15 mL
2 pkts.	concentrated acesulfame-K	2 pkts.
2 t.	poppy seed	10 mL
4 drops	yellow food coloring	4 drops
2	egg whites	2
⅛ t.	cream of tartar	.35 mL
3 T.	boiling water	45 mL
1 T.	measures-like-sugar aspartame	15 mL

Put the cottage cheese into a food processor or blender; process for a few minutes until very smooth. Add the egg substitute, flour, vanilla extract, lemon juice, lemon peel, sugar, acesulfame-K, poppy seed, and food coloring. Process until well combined. Use an electric mixer to beat the egg whites until they hold their peaks; add the cream of tartar and continue beating until soft. Add a small amount of the blended egg whites into the food processor and combine. Then pour the mixture from the food processor into another mixing bowl. Gently fold the rest of the beaten egg whites into the batter using a rubber spatula.

Pour approximately ¼ c. (60 mL) of batter into a muffin pan that has been sprayed with non-stick vegetable cooking spray. Bake in preheated 300°F (155°C) oven for 20 minutes. As soon as the muffins are out of the oven, combine the boiling water and aspartame to make the glaze. Use a fork to poke holes in the tops of the muffins. Pour the glaze into the holes.

Yield: 14 muffins

Exchange: free
Each serving contains: Calories: 29, Carbohydrates: 7 g, Fiber: trace, Sodium: 17 mg, Cholesterol: 1 mg

Orange Muffins

1 c.	orange juice	250 mL
1 T.	orange peel, grated	30 mL
½ c.	raisins, soaked	125 mL
⅓ c.	sugar replacement	80 mL
1 T.	margarine	30 mL
1	egg	1
¼ t.	salt	2 mL
1 t.	baking soda	5 mL
1 t.	baking powder	5 mL
½ t.	vanilla extract	2 mL
2 c.	flour	500 mL

Combine orange juice, orange peel, and raisins. Allow to rest for 1 hour. Cream together the sugar replacement, margarine, and egg. Add salt, baking soda, baking powder, and vanilla extract. Stir in orange juice mixture. Stir in enough of the flour to make a thick cake batter. Spoon into greased muffin tins, filling no more than two-thirds full. Bake at 350°F (175°C) for 20 to 25 minutes, or until done.

Microwave: Spoon into 6 oz. (180 mL) custard cups, filling two-thirds full. Cook on Low for 7 to 8 minutes. Increase heat to high for 2 minutes, until done.

Yield: 24 muffins

Exchange, 1 muffin: 1 bread
Each serving contains: Calories: 68, Carbohydrates: 18 g

Fresh Apple Muffins

2 T.	soft margarine	30 mL
2 T.	sugar replacement	30 mL
1	egg, beaten	1
1¼ c.	flour	310 mL
¼ t.	salt	2 mL
2 t.	baking powder	10 mL
6 T.	skim milk	90 mL
1 small	apple, peeled and chopped	1 small

Cream margarine and sugar replacement; add egg. Stir in remaining ingredients. Spoon into greased muffin tins, filling no more than two-thirds full. Bake at 400°F (200°C) for 25 minutes, or until done.

Yield: 12 muffins

Exchange, 1 muffin: 1 bread
Each serving contains: Calories: 72, Carbohydrates: 21 g

Popovers

1 c.	flour	250 mL
½ t.	salt	3 mL
2	eggs	2
1 c.	skim milk	250 mL

Sift flour and salt together; set aside. Beat eggs and skim milk; add to flour. Beat until smooth and creamy. Pour into heated greased muffin tins, filling half full or less. Bake at 375°F (190°C) for 50 minutes, or until popovers are golden brown and sound hollow. *Do not open oven for first 40 minutes.*

To make herb popovers: Add a ½ c. of finely chopped herbs (basil, rosemary, parsley, tarragon, thyme, or chives) and another ¼ t. salt to the batter just before baking.

Yield: 18 popovers

Exchange, 1 popover: ½ bread, ⅛ meat
Each serving contains: Calories: 44, Carbohydrates: 6 g

Scones

Scones are wonderful with a cup of tea or coffee. These low-fat scones are best served the same day they're baked. So they're perfect for a special brunch or meeting over coffee.

2 c.	flour	500 mL
1½ t.	baking powder	7 mL
1½ t.	baking soda	7 mL
dash	salt (optional)	dash
1½ T.	sugar	22 mL
3 pkts.	concentrated acesulfame-K	3 pkts.
2 t.	cinnamon	10 mL
3 T.	margarine or butter	45 mL
⅔ c.	nonfat yogurt, no sugar added	180 mL
2	egg whites	2

Combine in the bowl of a food processor the flour, baking powder, baking soda, salt, acesulfame-K, and cinnamon. Add the margarine cut into small pieces. Pulse the food processor off and on just long enough to combine; do not over-process. Add the yogurt and egg whites. Process very briefly. Turn this sticky dough out onto a lightly floured surface. Pat it out. Use a rolling pin to make a circle about ¾ inch (1.75 cm) thick and about 8 inches (20 cm) round. Cut into wedges as follows: Cut the circle in quarters, then cut each quarter into three sections. Place on a cookie sheet and bake in a preheated 425°F (220°C) oven for 15 minutes.

Yield: 12 scones

Exchange: 1 bread
Each serving contains: Calories: 110, Carbohydrates: 18 g, Fiber: trace, Sodium: 215 mg, Cholesterol: 0 mg

Scone Variations

Stir one of the following into flour mixture for Scones:

Apple

| 8 | chopped, dried apple halves | 8 |

Exchange, 1 scone: 1 bread, ¼ fruit
Each serving contains: Calories: 44, Carbohydrates: 160 g

Apricot

| 8 | chopped, dried apricot halves | 8 |

Exchange, 1 scone: 1 bread, ¼ fruit
Each serving contains: Calories: 44

Cranberry

| ¼ c. | chopped cranberries | 60 mL |

Exchange, 1 scone: 1 bread
Each serving contains: Calories: 34, Carbohydrates: 3 g

Dates

| 8 | chopped dates | 8 |

Exchange, 1 scone: 1 bread, ½ fruit
Each serving contains: Calories: 54, Carbohydrates: 4 g

Lemon

| 1 T. | grated lemon peel | 15 mL |

Exchange, 1 scone: 1 bread
Each serving contains: Calories: 34, Carbohydrates: negligible

Orange

| 1½ T. | grated orange peel | 25 mL |

Exchange, 1 scone: 1 bread
Each serving contains: Calories: 34, Carbohydrates: negligible

Peaches

| 8 | chopped dried peach halves | 25 mL |

Exchange, 1 scone: 1 fruit, ½ bread
Each serving contains: Calories: 54, Carbohydrates: 5 g

Raisin

| 4 T. | raisins | 60 mL |

Exchange, 1 scone: 1 bread, ¼ fruit
Each serving contains: Calories: 44, Carbohydrates: 3 g

Irish Scones

2 c.	all-purpose flour	500 mL
½ c.	solid vegetable shortening	125 mL
1 t.	baking soda	5 mL
1 t.	cream of tartar	5 mL
¼ t.	salt	1 mL
⅓ c.	currants	90 mL
¾ c.	skim milk	190 mL

In a food processor or bowl, combine the flour, shortening, baking soda, cream of tartar, and salt; cut into coarse crumbs. Mix in the currants. (If using a food processor, transfer mixture to a bowl.) Pour all of the milk into the mixture. Using a fork, gently stir until the dough holds together. Form into a ball and knead 10 to 12 times. Roll on a lightly floured surface to make a ½ in. (1.3 cm) thick circle. Cut into 10 wedges. Place wedges about 1 in. (2.5 cm) apart on an ungreased baking sheet. Bake at 400°F (200°C) for 12 to 15 minutes or until done.

Yield: 10 servings

Exchange, 1 serving: 1 bread, 2 fat, ½ fruit
Each serving contains: Calories: 192, Carbohydrates: 22 g

Bagels

1 loaf	Basic White Bread	1 loaf	
4 qts.	water	4 L	
1 T.	salt	15 mL	

Form dough into a square about ½ in. (1.3 cm) thick. Using a sharp knife, cut into 12 equal squares. Push your thumb through the middle of each square and roll around your fingers, forming a large doughnut shape. Work each into a uniform shape. Cover with a towel and let rise for 20 minutes. Pour the water into a deep pot; add the salt and stir. Bring to the boil and keep water just under the boiling point. Add bagels, one at a time; cook 4 or 5 at the same time, but do not overcrowd your pot. Simmer each bagel for 7 minutes; remove from water with a fork or slotted spoon. Place on a towel to drain and cool. Allowing space between each bagel, place on an unoiled baking sheet. Bake at 375°F (190°C) for 30 to 40 minutes or until brown.

Yield: 12 bagels

Exchange, 1 bagel: 1¼ bread
Each serving contains: Calories: 93, Carbohydrates: 20 g

Bread Sticks

Bread sticks are especially great when the meal has to be eaten from a plate on your lap. Bread sticks are easier to handle than a piece of bread or roll.

1 loaf	Basic White Bread dough	1 loaf	
1	egg yolk, beaten	1	
	sesame or poppy seeds (optional)		

Cut dough in half. Roll each half out into a rectangle on an unfloured surface. Cut into 40 strips. Roll each strip into a pencil shape. Place strips far apart on a lightly floured cookie sheet. Brush tops of sticks with beaten egg yolk. If desired, sprinkle with sesame or poppy seeds. Do not cover but allow to rise. Bake at 400°F (200°C) until brown and crisp. Serve hot or cold.

Yield: 40 servings

Exchange, 1 serving: ⅓ bread
Each serving contains: Calories: 26, Carbohydrates: 6 g

Melba Toast

½	loaf of bread, unsliced	½	

Cut the bread into the thinnest possible slices; remove the crusts and cut each slice in half. Place in a layer directly on the oven racks in a preheated oven. Bake at 250°F (120°C) for 10 minutes. Turn off the heat and allow the toasted slices to cool in the oven. Then store in a tightly sealed container in refrigerator or freezer.

Yield: 20 servings

Exchange, 1 serving: ½ bread
Each serving contains: Calories: 28, Carbohydrates: 6 g

Flour Tortillas

You can freeze these and use them as you want.

4 c.	all-purpose flour	1 L	
2 t.	salt	10 mL	
⅓ c.	lard	90 mL	
1 c.	warm water	250 mL	

Combine the flour, salt, and lard in a large bowl. With your fingers, work the flour and lard until well blended. Slowly add the water to form a stiff dough (if dough is too stiff, add small amounts of extra water); knead well. Tear dough into 36 equal pieces. Form each piece into a small ball. Cover and allow to rest for 20 minutes. Roll each piece into a 5 to 8 in. (12.5 to 20 cm) round. Use as directed in the recipe; or fry on a lightly greased grill or nonstick skillet. If you are going to freeze these tortillas, freeze each round between pieces of wax paper and then wrap securely in freezer wrap before frying.

Yield: 36 tortillas

Exchange, 1 tortilla: ¾ bread
Each serving contains: Calories: 57, Carbohydrates: 11 g

White Corn Tortillas

If you use this recipe to make the Toasted Tortillas in this chapter, roll the dough.

2 c.	harina de maiz blanco*	500 mL
1 t.	salt	5 mL
	boiling water	

Combine harina and salt in a bowl; stir to blend. Add just enough boiling water to make a very stiff dough. Allow to rest for 1½ hours.

Hand-shaping method: With moistened hands, pat the dough into 12 rounds, each with a 5 in. (12.5 cm) diameter. Lightly coat a nonstick skillet with vegetable spray. Fry tortillas until done; turn frequently.

Rolled method: Place dough between sheets of wax paper. Roll out thinly; cut into 5 in. (12.5 cm) rounds. Fry as directed above.

Yield: 12 tortillas

Exchange, 1 tortilla: ¾ bread
Each serving contains: Calories: 56, Carbohydrates: 10 g

*Harina de maiz blanco, a white cornmeal, is available in many large markets and in Hispanic shops.

Wheat Tortillas

2 c.	all-purpose flour	500 mL
1 t.	salt	5 mL
1 t.	baking powder	5 mL
½ c.	solid vegetable shortening	125 mL
	water	

In a food processor or bowl, combine the flour, salt, and baking powder. Add the shortening and blend until crumbled. Slowly add just enough water to make a soft dough. Remove to a lightly floured work surface and cover with pastry cloth. Allow to rest for half an hour. Roll out thinly; cut into 5 in. (12.5 cm) rounds. Fry on a lightly greased grill or skillet; turn frequently.

Yield: 18 tortillas

Exchange, 1 tortilla: ¾ bread
Each serving contains: Calories: 57, Carbohydrates: 12 g

Pita Bread

1 pkg.	dry yeast	1 pkg.
½ t.	sugar replacement	2 mL
1 t.	salt	5 mL
1 T.	liquid shortening	15 mL
1½ c.	warm water	375 mL
4 c.	flour	1000 mL

Dissolve yeast, sugar, salt, and liquid shortening in warm water. Add 3 c. (750 mL) of the flour; stir to mix well. (Dough should be fairly stiff; if not, add more flour.) Turn out onto floured surface; knead in remaining flour. (Dough will be very stiff.) Form into 15½ in. (40 cm) tube. Cut into 15 slices. Pat to make circles about 6 in. (15 cm) in diameter. Lay on lightly greased baking pans; cover. Allow to rise until almost doubled, about 1½–2 hours. Bake 475°F (245°C) for 10 to 12 minutes, or until lightly golden brown, puffed, and hollow. These freeze well.

Yield: 15 pita bread pockets

Exchange, 1 pocket: 1½ bread, ½ fat
Each serving contains: Calories: 70, Carbohydrates: 26 g

Puff-Cut Biscuits

2 c.	all-purpose flour	500 mL
3 t.	baking powder	15 mL
¾ t.	salt	4 mL
¼ c.	margarine, softened	60 mL
¾ c.	skim milk	190 mL

Pour flour into a bowl and add baking powder and salt; stir to blend. Using a fork, stir in margarine until mixture looks like coarse meal. Add milk. Stir with fork until all ingredients are moistened and mixture forms a ball. Turn out onto lightly floured board. Shape with hands into a 12 in. (30 cm) long roll. Cut into 12 pieces. Place pieces, cut side down, on ungreased baking sheet; flatten, if desired. Bake at 450°F (230°C) for 12 to 15 minutes.

Each serving contains: Carbohydrates: 17 g

Baking Powder Biscuits

1 c.	flour	250 mL
1 t.	baking powder	5 mL
½ t.	yeast	2 mL
½ t.	salt	2 mL
1 T.	liquid shortening	15 mL
6 T.	milk	90 mL
	vegetable cooking spray	

Combine all ingredients, except vegetable cooking spray; mix just until blended. Turn out on floured board. Roll out to a 1½ in. (1 cm) thickness. Cut into circles with floured 2 in. (5 cm) cutter. Place on baking sheet coated with vegetable cooking spray; cover. Allow to rest for 10 minutes. Bake at 450°F (230°C) for 12 to 15 minutes, or until lightly browned.

Yield: 10 biscuits

Exchange, 1 biscuit: 1 bread, 1½ fat
Each serving contains: Calories: 90, Carbohydrates: 10 g

Rice Fritters

2 c.	brown rice, cooked	500 mL
3	eggs, beaten	3
½ t.	vanilla extract	2 mL
½ t.	fresh lemon peel, finely grated	2 mL
⅓ c.	all-purpose flour	90 mL
⅓ c.	granulated sugar replacement	90 mL
1 T.	baking powder	15 mL
½ t.	salt	2 mL

With a wooden spoon, beat together rice, eggs, vanilla and lemon peel until thoroughly blended. Sift together the flour, sugar replacement, baking powder, and salt. Stir thoroughly into the rice mixture. Drop by spoonfuls into deep fat heated to 365°F (180°C). Fry until golden brown, turning if necessary.

Yield: 18 fritters

Exchange, 1 fritter: ½ bread
Each serving contains: Calories: 41, Carbohydrates: 13 g

Soya Crisps

1 c.	soya flour	250 mL
1 c.	chicken broth	250 mL
1 T.	liquid shortening	15 mL
1 t.	salt	5 mL

Blend soya flour and broth in saucepan until smooth. Bring gradually to a boil; remove from heat. Blend in liquid shortening and salt. Pour into large flat baking sheet to a depth of no more than ¼ in. (6 mm). Bake at 325°F (165°C) for 30 minutes. Cool slightly. Cut into 2¼ in. (6 cm) squares. Cut diagonally into triangles.

Yield: 80 chips

Exchange, 10 chips: 1 lean meat
Each serving contains: Calories: 50, Carbohydrates: negligible

Whole Wheat Pretzels

1½ c.	all-purpose flour	375 mL
1 pkg.	active dry yeast	1 pkg.
3 T.	instant nonfat dry milk	45 mL
1 T.	granulated sugar replacement	15 mL
1½ t.	salt	7 mL
1 T.	margarine	15 mL
1 c.	hot tap water	250 mL
1½ c.	stone-ground whole wheat flour	375 mL
1	egg white	1
1 T.	water	15 mL
	coarse salt	

Measure 1 c. (250 mL) of the all-purpose flour in a large bowl. Add the undissolved yeast, dry milk, sugar, and salt. Stir well to blend. Add margarine and hot water. Stir in the whole wheat flour. Gradually stir in remaining all-purpose flour to make a soft dough that leaves sides of the bowl. Add extra water, if needed. Turn out onto floured board. Knead 5 to 10 minutes or until dough is smooth and elastic. Cover and let rest 15 minutes on board.

Punch dough down. Roll into a 12 in. (30-cm) square. Cut into 24 strips. Roll each strip into a 14 in. (35 cm) long rope. Shape into pretzels. Place on greased baking sheets. Let stand, uncovered, 2 minutes. Brush dough with egg white mixed with 1 T. (15 mL) water. Sprinkle with coarse salt. Bake at 350°F (175°C) for 18 to 20 minutes until lightly browned. Immediately remove from baking sheet. Serve warm.

Yield: 24 pretzels

Exchange, 2 pretzels: 1 bread
Each serving contains: Calories: 80, Carbohydrates: 13 g

Cornbread Stuffing

6 T.	butter	90 mL
1 large	onion, chopped	1 large
1 c.	celery with tops, chopped	250 mL
1 t.	thyme	5 mL
1 t.	sage	5 mL
1 T.	salt	15 mL
1 t.	pepper	5 mL
6 c.	cornbread crumbs	1.5 L

Melt butter in medium saucepan. Add onion, celery, thyme, sage, salt, and pepper. Sauté over low heat for 3 to 4 minutes. Remove from heat. Add cornbread crumbs; toss to mix. Add water to moisten to stuffing consistency.

Yield: 6 c. (1500 mL)

Exchange, ½ c. (125 mL): 1 bread, 1 fat
Each serving contains: Calories: 125, Carbohydrates: 72 g

Prune-Apple Stuffing

1 c.	prunes, soaked and chopped	250 mL
1½ c.	apples, chopped	375 mL
½ c.	raisins	125 mL
1 t.	cinnamon	5 mL
½ t.	nutmeg	3 mL

Combine fruit and spices; mix thoroughly. Allow to rest for 10 minutes before using.

Yield: 3 c. (750 mL)

Exchange ¼ c. (60 mL): 1 fruit
Each serving contains: Calories: 60, Carbohydrates: 14 g

Herb-Seasoned Stuffing

1 lb.	loaf bread (2 to 3 days old)	500 g
½ c.	butter or margarine	125 mL
1 t.	thyme	5 mL
1 t.	sage	5 mL
1 t.	rosemary	5 mL
1 t.	dried lemon rind	5 mL

Remove crust from bread; cut bread into cubes. Melt butter or margarine in large skillet. Add seasonings; stir to mix. Add bread cubes. Toss or stir lightly to coat bread cubes. Pour onto baking sheet. Allow to dry by air or dry in very slow oven. These dried bread cubes are good as croutons; add salt and water to moisten when ready to use as stuffing.

Yield: 8 c. (2 L)

Exchange, ¼ c. (125 mL): 1 bread, 1 fat
Each serving contains: Calories: 11, Carbohydrates: 11 g

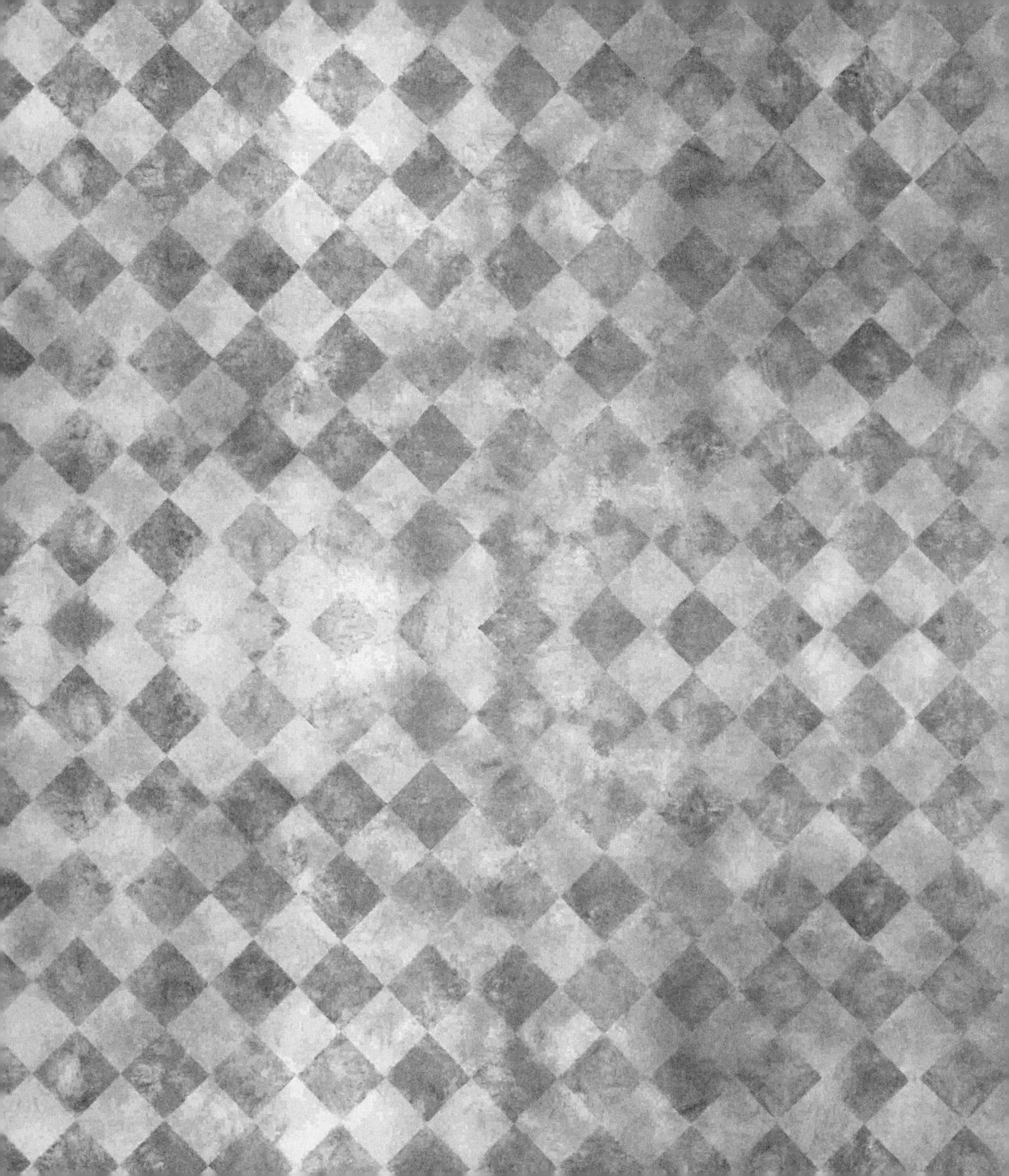

Soups

Chicken Broth

2 lb.	chicken, cut up	1 kg
½ med.	stalk celery, chopped	½ med.
8 to 10	green onions, chopped	8 to 10
2 T.	parsley, chopped	30 mL
2 t.	salt	10 mL
1 t.	thyme	5 mL
1 t.	marjoram	5 mL
½ t.	pepper	2 mL

Wash chicken pieces; place in large kettle. Cover with 2 qt. (2 L) water; bring to boil, cover and cook 1 hour or until chicken is tender. Add remaining ingredients; simmer 1 hour. Remove chicken; strain broth. Refrigerate broth overnight. Remove all fat from surface before reheating broth.

Yield: 2 qt. (2 L) broth

Exchange: negligible
Each serving contains: Calories: negligible, Carbohydrates: 1 g

Beef Broth

3 to 4 lb.	beef soup bones or chuck roast	1½ to 2 kg
½ stalk	celery, chopped	½ stalk
3	carrots, sliced	3
1 med.	onion, chopped	1 med.
½	green pepper, chopped	½
2	bay leaves	2
½ t. each	thyme, marjoram, paprika, pepper	2 mL each
2 t.	salt	10 mL

Place beef in large kettle; cover with 2 qt. (2 L) water. Bring to a boil, cover and cook 2 hours, or until meat is tender. Add remaining ingredients; simmer 1 hour. Remove beef; strain broth. Refrigerate broth overnight. Remove all fat from surface before reheating broth.

Yield: 2 qt. (2 L) broth

Exchange: negligible
Each serving contains: Calories: negligible, Carbohydrates: 2 g

Broth with Vegetables

Cook ½ c. (125 mL) vegetables or combination of vegetables in boiling salted water; drain. Add to hot broth just before serving.

Microwave: Add ½ c. (125 mL) vegetables (no water needed). Cook on High for 3 minutes. Add to hot broth just before serving.

Yield: ½ c. (125 mL)

Exchange, 1 serving: ½ vegetable
Each serving contains: Calories: 18, Carbohydrates: 12 g

Broth with Noodles

Cook ¼ c. (60 mL) noodles or broken spaghetti in boiling salted water; drain. Add to hot broth just before serving.

Microwave: Add ¼ c. (60 mL) noodles or pasta to 2 c. (500 ML) boiling salted water. Cook on High for 3 minutes. Hold 3 minutes. Drain. Add to hot broth just before serving.

Yield: ½ c. (125 mL)

Exchange, 1 serving: 1 bread
Each serving contains: Calories: 68, Carbohydrates: 24 g

Broth Orientale

2 T.	rice	30 mL
1½ c.	vegetable broth	375 mL
1 T.	celery, thinly sliced	15 mL
½ t.	onion, finely chopped	3 mL
1 T.	bean sprouts	5 mL
1	water chestnut, thinly sliced	1
	salt to taste	

Add rice to cold vegetable broth; bring to boil. Reduce heat; simmer 20 minutes. Add celery, onion, bean sprouts, and water chestnut; simmer 10 minutes. Add salt.

Microwave: Add rice to cold broth; heat to a boil. Cover. Hold 15 minutes. Add remaining ingredients, except salt. Cook 3 minutes. Hold 5 minutes. Add salt.

Yield: 1½ c. (310 mL)

Exchange, 1 serving: ⅛ bread, ⅛ vegetable
Each serving contains: Calories: 11, Carbohydrates: 22 g

Broth Italiano

⅛ c.	vermicelli, broken	30 mL
1 c.	broth	250 mL
1 oz.	thinly sliced prosciutto, shredded	30 g
⅛ t.	garlic powder	1 mL
⅛ t.	marjoram	1 mL
1 T.	Parmesan cheese, grated	15 mL

Cook vermicelli in boiling salted water; drain and rinse. Bring broth to boil. Add prosciutto, garlic powder, and marjoram. Simmer 5 minutes. Add vermicelli. Pour into bowl. Sprinkle Parmesan cheese over top.

Yield: 1¼ c. (310 mL)

Exchange, 1 serving: ½ bread, 1 medium-fat meat
Each serving contains: Calories: 107, Carbohydrates: negligible

Broth Madeira

Add 1 T. (15 mL) Madeira to 1 c. (250 mL) broth. Bring just to a boil. Garnish with lemon slice and fresh chopped parsley.

Microwave: Add 1 T. (15 mL) Madeira to 1 c. (250 mL) broth. Cook on High for 2 minutes. Garnish with lemon slice and fresh chopped parsley.

Yield: 1 c. (250 mL)

Exchange: negligible
Each serving contains: Calories: negligible, Carbohydrates: negligible

Vegetable Broth

1 c.	onion, chopped	250 mL
2 c.	carrots, diced	500 mL
1 c.	celery, chopped	250 mL
2 c.	spinach, cut in small pieces	500 mL
2 c.	tomato, peeled and chopped	500 mL
1	bay leaf	1
2 T.	parsley or parsley flakes	30 mL
½ t.	thyme	3 mL
1 blade	mace	1 blade
¼ t.	garlic or garlic powder	1 mL
1 T.	Worcestershire	15 mL
	salt to taste	

Place vegetables in large kettle. Cover with 2 to 3 qt. (2 to 3 L) water. Bring to boil; reduce heat and simmer for 2 hours. Stir frequently. Add seasonings. Simmer 1 hour. Strain. Add water to make 2 qt. (2 L).

Yield: 2 qt. (2 L) broth

Exchange: negligible
Each serving contains: Calories: negligible, Carbohydrates: 8 g

Tomato Beef Bouillon

2 T.	margarine	30 mL
¼ c.	onion, chopped	60 mL
46 oz.	tomato juice	1½ L
2 cans	beef broth or	2 cans
2½ c.	beef broth	625 mL
1	bay leaf	1
1 t.	salt	5 mL
½ t.	pepper	2 mL

Heat margarine in large saucepan. Add onion and cook until tender. Add tomato juice, beef broth (canned or homemade), bay leaf, salt, and pepper; beat thoroughly. *Do not boil.* Remove bay leaf. Ladle into warm bowls.

Yield: 8 servings, 1 c. (250 mL) each

Exchange, 1 serving: ¼ vegetable, 1 fat
Each serving contains: Calories: 58, Carbohydrates: 8 g

Added Touch: Top each serving with 1 t. (5 mL) grated American cheese.

Asian Minestrone

2 10¾ oz. cans	condensed chicken broth	2 300 g cans	
1	soup-can water	1	
2 oz.	uncooked spaghetti	60 g	
1 clove	garlic, minced	1 clove	
1 t.	ginger root, grated	5 mL	
1 c.	carrots, cut into julienne slices	250 mL	
1 c.	broccoli stems, thinly sliced, and small florets	250 mL	
	Wheat Germ Pork Balls (recipe follows)		
1 c.	fresh pea pods, halved	250 mL	
1 c.	fresh spinach, romaine lettuce or chard, chopped	250 mL	

Heat together broth and water in a large saucepan until the boiling point. Stir in spaghetti, garlic and ginger. Bring to a boil. Cover and simmer for 6 minutes. Add carrots and broccoli. Cover and simmer for 2 to 3 minutes until vegetables are crisp-tender. Add Wheat Germ Pork Balls, pea pods, and spinach, lettuce or chard. Heat thoroughly.

Wheat Germ Pork Balls

½ lb.	lean ground pork	250 g
¾ c.	Kretschmer regular wheat germ	190 mL
½ c.	water chestnuts, chopped	125 mL
2 T.	soy sauce	30 mL
2 T.	water	30 mL
1½ t.	ginger root, grated	7 mL
dash	black pepper	dash

For Wheat Germ Pork Balls, combine all ingredients. Shape into 24 balls. Place in a large, shallow baking pan. Bake at 400°F (200°C) for 20 minutes until lightly browned and thoroughly cooked. Cover and keep warm.

Note: ½ lb. (125 g) bulk pork sausage may be used instead of ground pork. Decrease soy sauce to 1 T. (15 mL) and increase water to 3 T. (45 mL).

Microwave: Prepare Wheat Germ Pork Balls as directed above. Place in 1½ qt. (1½ L) glass baking dish. Microwave on high for 6 to 8 minutes or until meat is no longer pink, rotating once. Set aside. Place broth and water in a 3 qt. (3 L) glass casserole. Microwave on high for 9 to 10 minutes or until liquid boils. Stir in spaghetti, garlic, and ginger. Microwave on high for 6 minutes. Add carrots and broccoli. Microwave on high for 2 to 3 minutes or until vegetables are crisp-tender and spaghetti is tender.

Add Wheat Germ Pork Balls, pea pods, and spinach. Microwave on high for 1½ to 2½ minutes or until pea pods are crisptender.

Yield: 6 servings

Exchange, 1 serving: 1 bread, 2 vegetable, 1 high-fat meat
Each serving contains: Calories: 219, Carbohydrates: 33 g

With the courtesy of Kretschmer Wheat Germ/International Multifoods.

Gazpacho

¼ c.	Mazola corn oil	60 mL	
½ c.	onion, finely chopped	125 mL	
1 clove	garlic, minced	1 clove	
1¼ c.	tomato, peeled and chopped	310 mL	
1 c.	green pepper, sliced into very thin strips	250 mL	
¼ c.	fresh parsley, chopped	60 mL	
dash	hot pepper sauce	dash	
¼ t.	dried basil	1 mL	
¼ t.	oregano	1 mL	
dash	black pepper	dash	
1	cucumber, halved lengthwise, seeded and very thinly sliced	1	
½ c.	chicken broth	125 mL	
½ c.	water	125 mL	
⅓ c.	dry white wine	90 mL	

In a small saucepan, heat oil over medium heat. Add onion and garlic. Cook, stirring, for 2 minutes. In large bowl, stir together onion mixture and remaining ingredients.

Yield: 4 servings

Exchange, 1 serving: 2 vegetable, 1½ fat
Each serving contains: Calories: 120, Carbohydrates: 10 g

"A Diet for the Young at Heart" by Mazola.

Cold Cucumber Soup

I happen to be a soup lover—so, a cold soup in summer is perfect.

2 large	cucumbers	2 large	
3 c.	water	750 mL	
2 T.	cornstarch	30 mL	
4	chicken bouillon cubes	4	
1 T.	white wine vinegar	15 mL	
1 T.	fresh dill, minced	15 mL	
½ c.	lowfat plain yogurt	125 mL	
	salt and pepper to taste		

Slice off ends of cucumbers; cut cucumbers into chunks. Combine 1 c. (250 mL) of the water and cucumber in blender or food processor. Mix together remaining water and cornstarch until blended. Combine cucumber and cornstarch mixtures in a large soup pot. Add bouillon cubes, vinegar, and dill. Simmer and stir over low heat until bouillon cubes dissolve and mixture is hot. Remove from heat and cool slightly. Refrigerate, covered, until chilled. Stir in yogurt. Season with salt and pepper. Refrigerate until serving time.

Yield: 4 servings

Exchange, 1 serving: ⅓ nonfat milk
Each serving contains: Calories: 31, Carbohydrates: 17 g

Spicy-Icy Tomato Soup

A cold soup with a snappy taste.

2 lbs.	tomatoes	1 kg
½ c.	onion, diced	125 mL
1 t.	garlic, minced	5 mL
4 oz. can	green chilies, drained and chopped	118 g can
3 T.	whole wheat, flour	45 mL
3 c.	chicken broth	750 mL
¼ t.	ground cumin	1 mL
¼ t.	ground coriander	1 mL
¼ t.	salt	1 mL
¼ t.	red pepper	1 mL
	fresh parsley sprigs	

Place tomatoes in blender or food processor and process until puréed. In a large saucepan or Dutch oven, heat oil and add onions, garlic, and chilies. Cook and stir until onions are soft. Add flour and cook 1 minute longer, stirring constantly. Gradually stir in puréed tomatoes and chicken broth. Add cumin, coriander, salt and red pepper. Bring mixture to a boil. Reduce heat, cover and simmer for about 25 minutes, stirring occasionally, to prevent sticking. Remove from heat; cool to room temperature. Pour into large bowl or storage container. Refrigerate until thoroughly chilled. When serving the soup, garnish each bowl with a parsley sprig.

Yield: 7 c. (1¾ L)

Exchange, 1 c. (250 mL): 2 vegetable, 1 fat
Each serving contains: Calories: 100, Carbohydrates: 7 g

Russian-Jewish Barley Soup

This recipe, given to me by my friend Sally Jordan, has been passed down through many generations of her family.

¾ c.	small lima beans	190 mL
4 qts.	water	4 L
1½ lbs.	neck or chuck soup bone	750 g
1 c.	celery, including leaves	250 mL
	salt and pepper to taste	
1	onion, chopped	1
1 c.	carrots, sliced	250 mL
1 c.	potatoes, diced	250 mL
½ c.	pearl barley	125 mL

Top of the stove method: Place lima beans in mixing bowl, cover with 2 c. (500 mL) boiling water; soak overnight. In large soup pot, place soup bone, celery, onion, and enough water to completely cover the bone. Season with salt and pepper. Bring to a boil, reduce heat and simmer until meat is very tender. Remove bone from soup pot and cut off all edible meat from the bone: return meat to the pot. Discard bone and membranes. Drain lima beans and add with the remaining ingredients to the soup pot. Adjust water to make 4 qts. (4 L) of soup. Taste and season with salt and pepper. Cover and simmer for 5 to 6 hours.

Slow cooker method: Place lima beans in mixing bowl. Cover with 2 c. (500 mL) boiling water: soak overnight. In a slow cooker, place soup bone, celery, onion and enough water to completely cover bone. Add salt and pepper to taste. Cook on low during the night (8 to 12 hours). In the morning, remove meat from bone, discard bone and membranes. Drain lima beans and add with remaining ingredients to slow cooker. Add enough water to make 4 qts. (4 L) of soup. Adjust salt and pepper to taste.

Yield: 4 qts. (4 L)

Exchange, 1 c. (250 mL): 1 bread, ½ medium-fat meat
Each serving contains: Calories: 98, Carbohydrates: 20 g

Tortilla Soup

Tortilla soup is a Mexican classic. Most tortilla soups contain cheese, some include meat. Tortilla chips take the place of bread croutons in this recipe. Aficionados who like the hot flavor of Mexican foods can add ½ t. (2 mL) cayenne pepper to the blender ingredients.

3	tomatoes, peeled and cut in half	3
1 med.	onion, coarsely chopped	1 med.
1 clove	garlic, minced	1 clove
2 T.	fresh parsley or coriander (cilantro), chopped	30 mL
15 oz. can	Health Valley tomato sauce	450 g can
¼ t.	honey	1 mL
2 13¾ oz. cans	Health Valley chicken broth	2 390 g cans
2 t.	Health Valley Instead of Salt all-purpose seasoning	5 mL
5½ oz. pkg.	Health Valley Buenitos tortilla chips	150 g pkg.
1 c.	cheddar cheese, grated	250 mL

In a blender, combine tomatoes, onion, garlic, parsley or coriander, tomato sauce, and honey. Cover and blend until nearly smooth. Pour into a large saucepan. Stir in the broth and seasoning; bring to a boil, cover and simmer for 20 minutes. Divide tortilla chips among 5 soup bowls, sprinkle with cheese and pour hot soup into the bowls over the cheese. Serve immediately.

Yield: 5 servings

Exchange, 1 serving: 1 bread, 2 vegetable, 1 high-fat meat, 1 fat
Each serving contains: Calories: 320, Carbohydrates: 34 g

From Health Valley Foods.

Meatball Vegetable Soup

10½ oz. can	condensed beef broth soup	300 g can
4 c.	water	1 L
3½ c.	whole peeled tomatoes, not drained	875 mL
1¾ c.	cooked red kidney beans, not drained	440 mL
2 med.	onions, sliced	2 med.
1 c.	carrots, sliced	250 mL
1 clove	garlic, finely chopped	1 clove
1	salt	5 mL
¼	pepper	1 mL
1	chili powder	5 mL
¾ c.	Kellogg's All-Bran cereal	190 mL
1	egg, slightly beaten	1
dash	black pepper	dash
1 lb.	lean ground beef	500 g
2 T.	vegetable oil	30 mL

In large saucepan or Dutch oven, combine 1 c. (250 mL) of condensed soup, the water and next 8 ingredients, cutting tomatoes into pieces with a spoon. Bring to a boil. Reduce heat and simmer, uncovered, 30 minutes. Slightly crush the cereal. Mix with egg, remaining condensed soup and pepper. Add ground beef, mixing until thoroughly combined. Shape into 1 in. (2.5 cm) meatballs. Brown meatballs in heated oil. Drain. Add meatballs to vegetable mixture. Simmer, covered, about 30 minutes longer.

Yield: 12 servings

Exchange, 1 serving: 1 bread, 1 medium-fat meat
Each serving contains: Calories: 150, Carbohydrates: 11 g

From Kellogg's Test Kitchens.

Louis's Seafood Chowder

3	tomatoes	3
⅓ c.	fresh green beans	90 mL
½ can	tomato soup	½ can
3 c.	water	750 mL
1 c.	celery, chopped	250 mL
1 c.	carrots, grated	250 mL
1 c.	mushrooms, sliced	250 mL
½ c.	cabbage, shredded	125 mL
½ c.	onion, chopped	125 mL
¼ c.	corn	60 mL
¼ c.	peas	60 mL
1 clove	garlic, finely chopped	1 clove
2 t.	salt	10 mL
½ t.	dried basil	2 mL
½ t.	parsley flakes	2 mL
¼ t.	dried marjoram	1 mL
¼ t.	ground red pepper	1 mL
½ lb.	sole, cut into bite-size pieces	250 g
4 oz.	small shrimp	120 g
4 oz.	crab meat, cut into bite-size pieces	120 g

Core but do not peel tomatoes; cut into medium-size pieces. Clean and snap beans. Combine tomato soup, water, and all vegetables in large saucepan. Add salt, basil, parsley flakes, sweet marjoram, and red pepper. Cover tightly and cook over low heat until tomatoes are soft. Add sole, shrimp, and crab. Cook until sole is firm but not broken. Serve in heated soup bowls.

Yield: 8 servings

Exchange, 1 serving: ½ bread, 1 medium-fat meat
Each serving contains: Calories: 99

Krupnik

This is an American version of a very filling Polish soup. It is very tasty and quick to make.

½ c.	pearl barley	125 mL
2 qts.	water	2 L
6	beef bouillon cubes	6
16 oz. box	Green Giant frozen mixed vegetables	457 g box
2½ oz. jar	Green Giant-frozen sliced mushrooms	72 g jar
3 med.	potatoes, diced	3 med.
1 T.	fresh parsley, chopped	15 mL
2 t.	dillseed	10 mL
2	egg yolks	2

Cook barley as directed on package. Meanwhile, heat water and bouillon cubes in large soup kettle until cubes are dissolved. Add frozen vegetables, mushrooms, potatoes, and 1 t. (5 mL) of the parsley and dillseed. Add the cooked barley. Beat egg yolks with a small amount of water. A little at a time, stir egg yolks into soup mixture. Pour into a large soup tureen. Garnish with the remaining parsley.

Yield: 6 servings

Exchange, 1 serving: 2 bread, ⅓ fat
Each serving contains: Calories: 165, Carbohydrates: 39 g

Vegetable Chowder

1 T.	Mazola corn oil	15 mL
1 med.	onion, sliced	1 med.
½ c.	celery, thinly sliced	125 mL
1 clove	garlic, minced	1 clove
2 c.	chicken broth	500 mL
16 oz. can	tomatoes, undrained and chopped	470 g can
1 c.	carrots, sliced	250 mL
1 t.	dried basil	5 mL
¼ t.	pepper	1 mL
20 oz. can	chick-peas, undrained	500 g can
12 oz. can	whole kernel corn, undrained	360 g can
1 c.	zucchini, sliced	250 mL

In 5 qt. (5 L) soup pot, heat oil over medium heat. Add onion, celery, and garlic. Cook, stirring, 5 minutes or until tender. Add next 5 ingredients. Cook about 25 minutes or until carrots are crisp-tender. Add remaining ingredients and cook 15 to 20 minutes.

Yield: 8 servings

Exchange, 1 c. (250 mL) serving: 3 bread, ½ vegetable, ½, lean meat
Each serving contains: Calories: 260

"A Diet-for the Young at Heart" by Mazola.

Fresh Pea Soup

A fast lunch.

1 t.	vegetable oil	5 mL
1 c.	onion, chopped	250 mL
1 c.	carrots, shredded	250 mL
4 c.	iceberg lettuce, shredded	1 L
4 c.	fresh peas, shelled	1 L
8 c.	chicken broth	2 L
1 t.	salt	5 mL
½ t.	black pepper	2 mL

In a large soup pot or Dutch oven, heat oil over medium heat. Stir in the onion and carrots. Cover and cook 5 minutes or until onion is translucent but not brown. Add remaining ingredients and bring to a boil. Cover, reduce heat and simmer 10 to 15 minutes, stirring occasionally, until peas are tender. Remove from heat. Pour 2 c. (500 mL) of the soup into blender container. Cover and blend on low until mixture is puréed. Stir into the soup in the pot. Serve hot. This soup freezes well for future use.

Yield: 10 c. (2½ L)

Exchange, 1 c. (250 mL): ¾ bread
Each serving contains: Calories: 46

Green Bean Soup

When green beans are abundant in the summer, try this quick soup.

3 c.	green beans, cleaned and snapped	750 mL
3 c.	chicken broth	750 mL
1 c.	carrots, cleaned and grated	250 mL
3	green onions with tops, trimmed and chopped	3
½ t.	salt	2 mL
⅓ c.	low-fat plain yogurt	90 mL

Combine beans and 1 c. (250 mL) of broth in saucepan or Dutch oven. Bring to boil, reduce heat and simmer until beans are tender. Remove from heat. Pour 1 c. (250 mL) of bean mixture into blender. Purée, return to pan. Add carrots, green onions, remaining broth, and salt to the soup. Simmer over low heat until mixture is hot. Remove from heat; stir in yogurt. Serve hot.

Yield: 6 servings

Exchange, 1 serving: 1 vegetable
Each serving contains: Calories: 29, Carbohydrates: 8 g

Broccoli Soup

Broccoli is a good source of potassium and vitamins A and C. Always cook (steam, simmer or stir-fry) broccoli briefly—it should be firm and a bright color when cooked.

15 oz. can	Health Valley potato soup	450 g can
13¾ oz. can	Health Valley chicken broth	390 g can
10 oz. pkg.	frozen broccoli spears, cut up	300 g pkg.
dash	ground or grated nutmeg	dash
½ t.	garlic powder	2 mL
½ L	Health Valley Instead of Salt all-purpose seasoning	2 mL

Heat potato soup and chicken broth together. Cut broccoli into ¾ in. (19 mm) pieces, add to the soup and cook 5 minutes. Add seasonings. Serve piping hot.

Yield: 6 servings

Exchange, 1 serving: ¼ bread, 1 vegetable, ½ fat
Each serving contains: Calories: 115, Carbohydrates: 9 g

From Health Valley Foods.

Lentil Soup

2 T.	Mazola corn oil	30 mL
1 c.	onion, sliced	250 mL
1 clove	garlic, minced	1 clove
4 c.	water	1 L
14½ oz. can	tomatoes	425 g can
1 c.	lentils, rinsed, drained	250 mL
2 T.	Worcestershire sauce	30 mL
1 c.	carrots, thinly sliced	250 mL
1 T.	lemon juice	15 mL
2 T.	fresh parsley, chopped	30 mL
	peel of small lemon, cut in very thin strips	

In 4 qt. (4 L) soup pot, heat oil over medium high heat. Add onion and garlic. Cook, stirring, 2 minutes or until tender. Add next 4 ingredients. Bring to a boil, reduce heat and simmer 1 to 1½ hours or until lentils are cooked. Add carrots and lemon juice during last 15 minutes. Garnish with parsley and lemon peel.

Yield: 6 c. (1½ L)

Exchange, 1 c. (250 mL) serving: 2 bread, 1 fat
Each serving contains: Calories: 180, Carbohydrates: 40 g

"A Diet for the Young at Heart" by Mazola.

Blanco Gazpacho

3	tomatoes, cut in chunks	3
1 large	cucumber, peeled and cut into 2 in. (5 cm) chunks	1 large
3 T.	onion, chopped	45 mL
1 slice	whole wheat bread	1 slice
2 c.	water	500 mL
½ c.	chicken broth	125 mL
2 T.	lemon juice	30 mL
1 clove	garlic	1 clove
1 T.	salt	5 mL
½ t.	black pepper	2 mL

Combine all ingredients in food processor fitted with the steel blade. Process on high speed, until mixture is smooth. Chill. Pour soup into bowls. Serve chilled. This soup freezes well for future use.

Yield: 4 c. (1 L)

Exchange, 1 c. (250 mL): 1 vegetable
Each serving contains: Calories: 40

Italian Stew

2 lbs.	stewing meat, cut in small pieces	1 kg
½ lb.	hot Italian sausage	250 g
2 c.	onions, diced	500 mL
1 T.	garlic, minced	30 mL
½ c.	dry red wine	125 mL
6 c.	eggplant, cut into 1 in. (2.5 cm) pieces	1½ L
4 c.	zucchini, cut into ½ in. (1.25 cm) pieces	1 L
2 c.	tomato sauce	500 mL
4	tomatoes, cut in chunks	4
2 t.	oregano	10 mL
1 t.	salt	5 mL
¼ t.	black pepper	1 mL
¼ t.	ground cinnamon	1 mL
1 c.	fresh parsley, chopped	250 mL

Place meats in a large soup pot or Dutch oven over medium heat. Cook and stir to brown the meat. When meat is browned, add onion and garlic and cook a few minutes longer, stirring until onion softens. Add wine: bring to a boil and simmer until most of the wine evaporates. Add eggplant, zucchini, tomato sauce, tomatoes, oregano, salt, pepper, and cinnamon. Bring to a boil, reduce heat and simmer 30 to 40 minutes, stirring occasionally. Skim off and discard any fat. Stir in the parsley. Ladle into hot bowls.

This stew freezes well for future use.

Yield: 11 c. (2¾ L)

Exchange, 1 c. (250 mL): 2 vegetable, 2 high-fat meat, 1 fat
Each serving contains: Calories: 295, Carbohydrates: 12 g

Crab Stew

10 oz. can	tomato soup	300 g can
1½ c.	water	375 mL
½ c.	crab meat, flaked	125 mL
½ c.	bamboo shoots	125 mL
½ c.	mushrooms, sliced	125 mL
½ c.	brown rice, cooked	125 mL
⅓ c.	celery, sliced	90 mL
¼ c.	chive, chopped	60 mL
	salt and pepper to taste	

Combine all ingredients in a saucepan. Cook over low heat, stirring occasionally, until vegetables are tender. Serve hot.

Yield: 4 servings

Exchange, 1 serving: ½ bread, ½ vegetable, ½ lean meat
Each serving contains: Calories: 79, Carbohydrates: 4 g

Savory Bean Stew

1 c.	dry Stone-Buhr soybeans	250 mL
1 qt.	water	1 L
⅓ c.	onion, chopped	90 mL
1 T.	margarine	15 mL
½ lb.	ground beef	250 g
4	tomatoes, cored but not peeled	4
	salt and pepper to taste	

Wash beans and combine with the water in a soup pot. Boil for 2 minutes. Cover and let stand for 1 hour. Simmer 1 to 1½ hours or until almost tender, adding water if necessary. In a casserole or pan, brown onion in margarine. Add beef, stir and cook slowly for a few minutes. Cut tomatoes into small pieces. Combine all the ingredients. Simmer until meat is tender and the flavors are blended, about 45 to 50 minutes. Season with salt and pepper.

Yield: 5 servings

Exchange, 1 serving: 1 bread, 1½ medium-fat meat, 1 vegetable
Each serving contains: Calories: 215, Carbohydrates: 9 g

With the compliments of Arnold Foods Company, Inc.

High Fiber Chili

1 lb.	lean ground beef	500 g
1 large	onion, sliced	1 large
½ c.	green pepper, chopped	125 mL
2 c.	Kellogg's bran flakes cereal	500 mL
1 c.	tomato sauce	250 mL
1¾ c.	cooked red kidney beans, not drained	440 mL
2 c.	whole peeled tomatoes, not drained	500 mL
½ c.	water	125 mL
1 T.	chili powder	15 mL
dash	garlic powder	dash
1 t.	salt	5 mL
1	bayleaf	1

In a large saucepan, cook beef, onion, and green pepper until meat is browned, stirring frequently. Drain off excess drippings. Stir in the remaining ingredients. Cover and simmer over low heat about 1 hour, stirring occasionally.

Yield: 6 servings

Exchange, 1 serving: 1 bread, 1 vegetable, 2 medium-fat meat
Each serving contains: Calories: 242, Carbohydrates: 32 g

From Kellogg's Test Kitchens.

Borscht

2 lbs.	chicken, cleaned	1 kg
4 qts.	water	4 L
5	tomatoes, quartered	5
5	beets, peeled and cut in strips	5
2	onions, sliced	2
2	potatoes, cubed	2
½ c.	dry lima beans	125 mL
2	celery stalks, diced	2
2	apples, sliced	2
1 t.	salt	5 mL
½ t.	lemon juice	2 mL
⅓ t.	pepper	½ mL
3	egg yolks, well beaten	3

Cut the chicken at the joints and the breasts into 4 pieces. Place chicken, water, vegetables, apples, salt, lemon juice, and pepper in a large soup pot. Simmer for 3 hours. Extra water may be added, if soup becomes too thick. (This should be done the night before and then reheated in the morning.) After the soup is warm, mix about 2 c. (500 mL) of the broth with the egg yolks. Gradually, stir the yolk mixture into the soup to blend.

To serve: Place a piece of chicken in the bottom of each heated bowl and top with soup.

Yield: 8 servings

Exchange, 1 serving: 2 lean meat, 1 bread, 1 vegetable
Each serving contains: Calories: 214, Carbohydrates: 22 g

Creamy Shrimp Bisque

1 c.	celery, sliced	250 mL
½ c.	white onion, chopped	125 mL
dash each	thyme, paprika, and basil	dash each
	salt and pepper to taste	
1 c.	water	250 mL
2 c.	frozen hash brown potatoes	500 mL
6 oz. pkg.	Brilliant cooked frozen shrimp	170 g pkg.
1 c.	2% milk	250 mL

Combine the celery, onion, seasonings, and water in a saucepan. Cook over medium heat until onion is tender. Stir in the potatoes; cover and simmer until potatoes are soft. Add the shrimp; cover and simmer for 3 minutes. Slowly add the milk. Cook and stir over low heat until mixture thickens (do not boil or milk will curdle).

Yield: 4 servings

Exchange, 1 serving: 1 bread, ½ lean meat, ¼ lowfat milk
Each serving contains: Calories: 123, Carbohydrates: 18 g

Country-Style Beef-Vegetable Soup

Another perfect soup for a cold day.

3 lbs.	beef soup bones	1½ kg
4½ qts.	water	4½ L
1 T.	salt	15 mL
1 qt.	cabbage, coarsely chopped	1 L
1½ c.	yellow onion, coarsely chopped	375 mL
1 c.	celery, sliced	250 mL
1 c.	potatoes, diced	250 mL
1	green pepper, chopped	1
6	tomatoes, chopped	6
6	carrots, sliced	6
10 oz. pkg.	lima beans, frozen	286 g pkg.
10 oz. pkg.	green beans, frozen	286 g pkg.
6 oz. can	tomato paste	180 g can
1 t.	black pepper	5 mL

Combine beef bones, water, and salt in large soup pot. Bring to the boil; reduce heat, cover, and simmer for 1 hour. Skim fat from the surface. Add the remaining ingredients; cover and simmer for 4 hours. Remove beef bones and allow to cool. Remove meat from bones and add to soup. Refrigerate soup until the next day. Remove all fat that is on the surface; reheat. Serve hot. This soup freezes well for future use.

Yield: 18 servings

Exchange, 1 serving: 1 vegetable, ⅓ bread, ⅓ lean meat
Each serving contains: Calories: 65 g, Carbohydrates: 10 g

Cheddar Cheese Soup

A creamy soup just for two.

1 c.	water	250 mL
1	chicken bouillon cube	1
¼ c.	onion, chopped	60 mL
¼ c.	celery, chopped	60 mL
2 t.	all-purpose flour	10 mL
1 t.	butter	5 mL
¼ t.	dry mustard	1 mL
1 c.	skim milk	250 mL
½ c.	cheddar cheese, grated	125 mL

In a saucepan, combine the water, bouillon cube, onion, celery, flour, butter, and mustard. Cook and stir until onion and celery are tender. Reduce heat and add the milk and cheese. Cook over low heat until cheese melts. Pour entire mixture into a blender; blend until smooth. (Be careful not to burn yourself.) Return mixture to pan and heat just to the simmering point. Serve in heated bowls.

Yield: 2 servings

Exchange, 1 serving: 1 high-fat meat, ½ nonfat milk, ½ fat
Each serving contains: Calories: 175, Carbohydrates: 7 g

Avgolemono

2 qt.	chicken broth	2 L	
3	eggs, separated	3	
	juice of 1 lemon		

Bring broth to a boil in saucepan. Beat egg whites until stiff. Add egg yolks. Beat slowly until mixture is a light yellow. Add lemon juice gradually, beating constantly. Pour small amount of chicken broth into egg mixture. Pour egg mixture into hot broth, beating constantly.

Yield: 8 servings, 1 c. (250 mL) each

Exchange, 1 serving: ¼ high-fat meat
Each serving contains: Calories: 27, Carbohydrates: 1 g

German Cabbage Soup

2 oz.	ground beef round	60 g
2 T.	onion, grated	30 mL
dash each	mustard, soy sauce, salt, pepper	dash each
1 T.	dry red wine	15 mL
1¼ c.	beef broth	300 mL
2 large	cabbage leaves, cut in pieces	2 large
½ med.	tomato, cubed	½ med.
½ t.	fresh parsley, chopped	2 mL

Combine ground round, onion, mustard, soy sauce, salt, and pepper; mix thoroughly. Form into tiny meatballs. Add wine to broth; bring to boil. Add meatballs to broth, one at a time. Bring to boil again. Cook meatballs 5 minutes; remove to soup bowl. Add cabbage and tomatoes to broth. Simmer 5 minutes. Pour over meatballs. Garnish with parsley.

Yield: 1½ c. (375 mL)

Exchange, 1 serving: 1 medium-fat meat, 1½ vegetable
Each serving contains: Calories: 55, Carbohydrates: 21 g

Ham and Split Pea Soup

2 lb.	meaty ham bone	1 kg
1	bay leaf	1
2 c.	dried green split peas	500 mL
1 c.	onions, chopped	250 mL
1 c.	celery, cubed	250 mL
1 c.	carrots, grated	250 mL
	salt and pepper to taste	

Cover ham bone and bay leaf with water. Simmer for 2 to 2½ hours. Remove bone and strain liquid. Refrigerate overnight. Remove lean meat from bone; set aside. Remove fat from surface of liquid. Heat liquid; add enough water to make 2½ qt. (2½ L). Add peas; simmer for 20 minutes. Remove from heat and allow to stand 1 hour. Add onions, celery, carrots, and lean pieces of ham. Add salt and pepper. Simmer for 40 minutes. Stir occasionally.

Yield: 10 servings

Exchange, 1 serving: ½ high-fat meat, 1 vegetable
Each serving contains: Calories: 204, Carbohydrates: 27 g

Cream of Chicken and Almond Soup

1 c.	chicken broth	250 mL
1	whole clove	1
1 sprig	parsley	1 sprig
½	bay leaf	½
pinch	mace	pinch
1 T.	celery, sliced	15 mL
1 T.	carrot, diced	15 mL
1 t.	onion, diced	5 mL
2 t.	stale bread crumbs	10 mL
½ oz.	chicken breast, cubed	15 g
1 t.	blanched almonds, crushed	5 mL
¼ c.	skim milk	60 mL
1 t.	flour	5 mL
	salt and pepper to taste	

Heat chicken broth, clove, parsley, bay leaf, and mace to a boil; remove from heat. Allow to rest 10 minutes; strain. Add celery, carrot, onion, bread crumbs, chicken, and almonds to seasoned chicken broth; simmer 20 minutes. Blend in skim milk and flour. Remove soup from heat; add milk mixture. Return to heat. Simmer (do not boil) 3 to 5 minutes. Add salt and pepper.

Yield: 1½ c. (375 mL)

Exchange, 1 serving: ½ lean meat, 1 vegetable, ¼ milk
Each serving contains: Calories: 89, Carbohydrates: 64 g

Crab Chowder

1 c.	milk	250 mL
1 t.	flour	5 mL
¼ c.	water	60 mL
¼ c.	cooked crabmeat, flaked	60 mL
3 T.	mushroom pieces	45 mL
3 T.	asparagus pieces	45 mL
	salt and pepper to taste	

Blend milk, flour, and water thoroughly; pour into saucepan. Add crabmeat, mushrooms, and asparagus. Cook over low heat until slightly thickened. Add salt and pepper.

Yield: 1 c. (250 mL)

Exchange, 1 serving: 1 milk, 1 vegetable, 1 lean meat
Each serving contains: Calories: 150, Carbohydrates: 29 g

Clam Chowder

1 slice	bacon	1 slice
1½ c.	fish or vegetable broth	375 mL
2 T.	carrot, diced	30 mL
1 T.	onion, diced	15 mL
1 T.	celery, diced	15 mL
1 large	tomato, diced	1 large
1 med.	potato, diced	1 med.
dash each	thyme, rosemary, salt, pepper	dash each
1 t.	flour	5 mL
¼ c.	water	60 mL
1 oz.	clams	30 g

Cook bacon until crisp; drain and crumble. Combine broth, carrot, onion, celery, tomato, potato, and seasonings. Simmer until vegetables are tender. Blend flour and water; stir into chowder. Reduce heat. Add clams and crumbled bacon. Heat to thicken slightly.

Microwave: Combine vegetables with broth and seasonings; cover. Cook on High for 4 minutes, or until vegetables are tender. Add flour-water mixture. Cook 30 seconds; stir. Add clams and bacon; stir. Cook 30 seconds. Hold 3 minutes.

Yield: 2 c. (500 mL)

Exchange, 1 serving: 1 lean meat, 1 fat, 1 vegetable, 1 bread
Each serving contains: Calories: 200, Carbohydrates: 40 g

Oyster Stew

1 t.	flour	5 mL
1 T.	celery, minced	15 mL
1 t.	salt	5 mL
dash each	Worcestershire sauce, soy sauce	dash each
1 T.	water	15 mL
1 oz.	oysters, with liquid	30 g
1 t.	butter	5 mL
1 c.	skim milk	250 mL

Blend flour, celery, seasonings, and water in saucepan; add oysters with liquid, and butter. Simmer over low heat until edges of oysters curl. Remove from heat; add skim milk. Reheat over low heat. Add extra salt if desired.

Yield: 1½ c. (375 mL)

Exchange, 1 serving: 1 lean meat, 1 milk, ¼ bread
Each serving contains: Calories: 220, Carbohydrates: 14 g

Bean Stew

1 T.	pinto beans	15 mL
1 T.	Northern beans	15 mL
1 T.	lentils	15 mL
1 c.	beef broth	250 mL
1 T.	carrot, sliced	15 mL
1 T.	hominy	15 mL
1 t.	onion, diced	5 mL
½ t.	green chilies, chopped	2 mL
dash each	garlic powder, oregano, salt, pepper	dash each

Boil beans and lentils in beef broth for 10 minutes, covered. Allow to stand 1 to 2 hours, or overnight. Place softened beans and remaining ingredients in baking dish. Bake at 350°F (175°C) for 45 minutes to 1 hour, or until ingredients are tender.

Microwave: Place beans and lentils in beef broth; cover. Cook on High for 5 minutes. Allow to stand 1 to 2 hours or overnight. Add remaining ingredients. Cook on Medium for 10 to 15 minutes, or until ingredients are tender.

Yield: 1½ c. (375 mL)

Exchange, 1 serving: 1 lean meat, 2 bread
Each serving contains: Calories: 225, Carbohydrates: 23 g

Zucchini Meatball Stew

1 oz.	ground beef	30 g
½ c.	ground zucchini	125 mL
1	onion, finely chopped	5 mL
1	egg	1
¼ c.	rice, uncooked	60 mL
dash each	oregano, cumin, garlic, salt, pepper	dash each
1 c.	beef broth	250 mL
1 large	tomato, diced	1 large
1 t.	parsley, chopped	5 mL
	salt and pepper to taste	

Combine ground beef, zucchini, onion, egg, rice, and seasonings; mix thoroughly. Shape into small meatballs. Combine beef broth, tomato, and parsley in saucepan; heat to boil. Drop meatballs into hot broth, one at a time. Cover and simmer 30 to 40 minutes. Add salt and pepper.

Microwave: Cook beef broth, tomato, and parsley on High for 3 minutes, covered. Drop meatballs into broth. Cook on High 5 minutes. Hold 10 minutes. Add salt and pepper.

Yield: 1¾ c. (430 mL)

Exchange, 1 serving: 2 medium-fat meat, 1 vegetable, 1 bread
Each serving contains: Calories: 203, Carbohydrates: 41 g

Pepper Pot

(Leftovers may be used)

2 oz.	lean pork, cut in 1 in. (2.5 cm) cubes	60 g
1 oz.	beef, cut in 1 in. (2.5 cm) cubes	30 g
1 oz.	chicken, cut in 1 in. (2.5 cm) cubes	30 g
¼ c.	carrot pieces	60 mL
¼ c.	onion slices	60 mL
¼ c.	celery pieces	60 mL
¼ c.	potatoes, cubed	60 mL
½ c.	water	125 mL
1 t.	flour	5 mL
dash each	curry powder, garlic powder, salt, pepper	dash each

Brown pork and beef cubes slowly in frying pan. Add chicken cubes for last few minutes; drain. Place meat, carrots, onions, celery, and potatoes in individual baking dish. Combine water, flour, and seasonings in screwtop jar; shake to blend well. Pour over meat mixture. Cover tightly and bake at 350°F (175°C) for 45 minutes to 1 hour, or until meat is tender and gravy has thickened.

Microwave: Reduce water to ¼ c. (60 mL). Cover. Cook on High for 10 minutes. Hold 5 minutes.

Yield: 1 serving

Exchange, 1 serving: 4 high-fat meat, 1 vegetable, 1 bread
Each serving contains: Calories: 418, Carbohydrates: 38 g

Stefado

1 stick	cinnamon	1 stick
1	bay leaf	1
5	whole cloves	5
12 oz.	beef roast, cubed	360 g
	salt and pepper to taste	
1 t.	margarine	5 mL
1½ c.	onions, sliced	375 mL
3 med.	tomatoes, peeled and cubed	3 med.
½ c.	red wine	125 mL
1 t.	brown sugar replacement	5 mL
2 T.	raisins	30 mL
1 c.	water	250 mL
1	garlic clove, crushed	1

Place cinnamon, bay leaf, and cloves in small cheesecloth bag. Combine with remaining ingredients in soup kettle; cook 1 to 1½ hours until meat is tender. Remove spice bag before serving.

Microwave: Same as above. Cook on High 15 to 20 minutes.

Yield: 3 servings, 1 c. (250 mL) each

Exchange, 1 serving: 4 high-fat meat, 1 vegetable
Each serving contains: Calories: 430, Carbohydrates: 33 g

Salads

Salade Niçoise

½ c.	Dia-Mel red wine vinegar salad dressing	125 mL
½ c.	Dia-Mel Italian salad dressing	125 mL
½ t.	dried dill	2 mL
½ t.	oregano	2 mL
dash	black pepper	dash
½	red or yellow onion, thinly sliced	½
3 oz.	marinated artichoke hearts, drained	90 g
1 c.	fresh green beans, cut and trimmed or frozen French-style green beans, thawed and drained	250 mL
2 small	Boston lettuce, torn into bite-size pieces	2 small
½	cucumber, sliced	½
2	tomatoes, cut in wedges	2
½ c.	mushrooms, sliced	125 mL
¼ c.	radishes, sliced	60 mL
½ c.	red pepper, sliced in thin strips	125 mL
1 med.	potato, cooked and sliced	1 med.
7 oz. can	tuna, packed in water, rinsed	200 g can
¼ c.	pitted black olives, sliced	60 mL
1	hard-cooked egg, chopped	1

Combine salad dressing with dill, oregano, and pepper. Marinate onion, artichoke hearts, and green beans in dressing mixture for 2 to 3 hours. Before serving, combine the marinated vegetables and dressing with the remaining ingredients except the hard-cooked egg. Toss to mix well. Garnish with the chopped egg.

Yield: 4 servings

Exchange, 1 serving: 2 lean meat, 3 vegetables
Each serving contains: Calories: 180, Carbohydrates: 38 g

For you from the Estee Corporation.

Poinsettia Salad

1 c.	Stone-Buhr brown rice, cooked	250 mL
7 oz. can	chunk-style tuna, drained	200 g can
½ c.	pecans, chopped	125 mL
⅓ c.	mayonnaise	90 mL
1 T.	lemon juice	15 mL
½ t.	Tabasco sauce	1 mL
1	canned whole pimiento	1
6	lettuce leaves	64

Cook rice according to package directions. Rinse with cold water and drain, well. Combine tuna, rice, pecans, mayonnaise, lemon juice, and Tabasco sauce. Toss lightly until well mixed. Press into 6 individual molds or use a ⅓ c. (90 mL) measure. Turn out each molded salad onto a lettuce leaf. Cut pimiento into petal shapes and arrange on salads to resemble poinsettias.

Yield: 6 servings

Exchange, 1 serving: 2 bread, 1 high-fat meat, 2 fat
Each serving contains: Calories: 335, Carbohydrates: 13 g

With the compliments of Arnold Foods Company, Inc.

Mushroom and Watercress Salad

This is a delightful new taste for most people.

3 c.	snow-white mushrooms, medium size	750 mL
2 T.	fresh lemon juice	30 mL
2 T.	white wine vinegar	30 mL
2 T.	olive oil	30 mL
¼ c.	water	90 mL
½ t.	salt	2 mL
¼ t.	dried tarragon, crushed	2 mL
¼ t.	ground basil	1 mL
1 c.	fresh watercress, chopped	250 mL

Clean and slice mushrooms, place in a medium bowl. Mix together the lemon juice, vinegar, oil, water, salt, tarragon, and basil. Pour dressing over mushrooms, mixing carefully to completely coat the mushrooms. Marinate overnight in the refrigerator. Just before serving, drain extra dressing from mushrooms, add watercress and toss to completely mix. Divide among 8 chilled salad plates.

Yield: 8 servings

Exchange, 1 serving: ½ vegetable, 1 fat
Each serving contains: Calories: 57, Carbohydrates: 2 g

Polynesian Cabbage Slaw

1 small	cabbage, shredded	1 small
8½ oz. can	pineapple chunks packed in juice	230 g can
1	orange, diced	1
¼ c.	green pepper, diced	60 mL
⅓ c.	Dia-Mel Thousand Island salad dressing	90 mL
⅓ c.	Dia-Mel French-style salad dressing	90 mL
⅓ c.	Dia-Mel catsup	90 mL

Drain pineapple chunks. In a large bowl, combine all ingredients and mix thoroughly. Chill before serving.

Yield: 6 servings

Exchange, 1 serving: 1 fruit, ½ vegetable
Each serving contains: Calories: 55, Carbohydrates: 33 g

For you from The Estee Corporation.

Old Time Carrot Slaw

A favorite slaw for your picnics.

⅓ c.	water	90 mL
2 T.	vegetable oil	30 mL
2 T.	white vinegar	30 mL
3 env.	aspartame sweetener	3 env.
½ t.	salt	2 mL
dash	black pepper	dash
3 c.	carrots, shredded	750 mL
8	ripe olives, sliced	8

Combine water, oil, vinegar, aspartame, salt and pepper. Stir to blend. Pour over carrots. Toss to completely coat. Garnish with olive slices. Cover tightly and chill thoroughly. Drain well before serving.

Yield: 6 servings

Exchange, 1 serving: 1 vegetable, 1 fat
Each serving contains: Calories: 73, Carbohydrates: 6 g

Sweet & Sour Slaw

2 med.	red onions	2 med.
4 c.	cabbage, finely shredded	1 mL
½ c.	cider vinegar	125 mL
1 t.	dry mustard	5 mL
1 t.	salt	5 mL
1 t.	celery seeds	5 mL
¼ t.	cornstarch	1 mL
⅓ c.	granulated sugar replacement	90 mL
2 T.	vegetable oil	30 mL

Thinly slice the onions and separate them into rings. In a large bowl, alternate layers of the cabbage and onion rings. In a small saucepan, combine vinegar, mustard, salt, celery seeds, and cornstarch. Stir to dissolve cornstarch. Cook over medium heat until mixture boils and is clear. Remove from heat, beat in sugar replacement and oil. Pour dressing over the cabbage. Cover tightly and refrigerate 8 hours or overnight, stirring occasionally. To serve, using a slotted spoon, lift salad out of the dressing.

Yield: 10 servings

Exchange, 1 serving: ½ fat
Each serving contains: Calories: 25, Carbohydrates: 23 g

Apple-Cabbage Slaw

¼ c.	Dia-Mel creamy Italian salad dressing	60 mL
¼ t.	prepared mustard	1 mL
dash	pepper	dash
2 c.	cabbage, shredded	500 mL
1 c.	unpared apple, thinly sliced	250 mL

In a medium bowl, combine salad dressing, mustard and pepper. Add cabbage and apple and toss lightly. Serve immediately.

Yield: 4 servings

Exchange, 1 serving: 1½ vegetable
Each serving contains: Calories: 35, Carbohydrates: 14 g

For you from **The Estee Corporation.**

Lemony Apple-Bran Salad

½ c.	lemon low-fat yogurt	125 mL
1 T.	fresh parsley, finely snipped	15 mL
2 c.	unpared red apples, cored and cubed	500 mL
½ c.	celery, thinly sliced	125 mL
½ c.	red grapes, halved and seeded	125 mL
½ c.	All-Bran or Bran Buds cereal	125 mL
6	lettuce leaves	6

Stir together yogurt, parsley, apples, celery and grapes. Cover and chill thoroughly. At serving time, stir in the cereal. Serve on lettuce leaves.

Yield: 6 servings

Exchange, 1 serving: 1 fruit, ½ bread
Each serving contains: Calories: 70, Carbohydrates: 22 g

From Kellogg's Test Kitchens.

Hot Bean Salad

2 c.	kidney beans, cooked and drained	500 mL
1 c.	celery, thinly sliced	250 mL
½ c.	sharp American cheese, diced	25 mL
¼ c.	sweet relish	60 mL
¼ c.	onions, coarsely chopped	60 mL
⅓ c.	low-calorie mayonnaise	90 mL
½ t.	salt	2 mL
⅓ c.	wheat germ	90 mL

Combine beans, celery, cheese, relish, onions, mayonnaise and salt in a large bowl. Stir to mix thoroughly. Spoon into 8 custard cups or baking dishes. Sprinkle wheat germ on top. Bake at 450°F (225°C) for 10 minutes or until bubbly.

Yield: 8 servings

Exchange, 1 serving: ⅔ bread, 1 lean meat
Each serving contains: Calories: 97, Carbohydrates: 27 g

Chilled Bean Salad

15½ oz. can	no-salt-added green beans	450 g can
15½ oz. can	no-salt-added wax beans	450 g can
1	red pepper, chopped	1
12	cherry tomatoes, cut in half	2
½ t.	dried dill	2 mL
½ t.	dried basil	2 mL
¼ c.	Dia-Mel red wine vinegar salad dressing	60 mL

Drain green and wax beans and combine with the red pepper and tomatoes. Add dillweed and basil to salad dressing; stir to combine. Pour dressing over vegetables and toss gently. Chill for several hours or overnight.

Yield: 6 servings

Exchange, 1 serving: 1½ vegetable
Each serving contains: Calories: 40, Carbohydrates: 10 g

For you from The Estee Corporation.

Vegetable-Bean Salad

8 oz. can	Featherweight cut green beans, drained	227 g can
8 oz. can	Featherweight cut wax beans, drained	227 g can
½ c.	green or red pepper, chopped	125 mL
¼ c.	onion, sliced	60 mL
½ c.	Featherweight Italian dressing	125 mL
6	lettuce leaves	6

In a medium bowl, combine all ingredients except the lettuce. Cover and marinate overnight in the refrigerator. Serve on lettuce.

Yield: 6 servings

Exchange, 1 serving: 1 vegetable
Each serving contains: Calories: 31, Carbohydrates: 7 g

Based on a recipe from Featherweight Brand Foods.

Wilted Lettuce Salad

2 T.	margarine	30 mL
¾ t.	paprika	3 mL
¼ t.	garlic salt	1 mL
1 T.	sesame seeds	15 mL
1 c.	All-Bran or Bran Buds cereal	250 mL
2 T.	Parmesan cheese, grated	30 mL
6	bacon slices	6
2 qts.	iceberg lettuce, torn into bite-size pieces	2 L
1	tomato, chopped	1
¼ c.	green onions, sliced	60 mL
½ t.	oregano	2 mL
¼ t.	pepper	1 mL
¼ c.	vinegar	60 mL
2 t.	sugar	10 mL

In a medium skillet, melt margarine over low heat. Stir in paprika, garlic salt and sesame seeds. Add cereal, stirring until well-coated. Cook, stirring constantly, 2 to 3 minutes or until cereal is crisp and lightly brown. Remove from heat. Add cheese, tossing lightly. Set aside.

Fry bacon until crisp. Drain, reserving 2 T. (30 mL) of the drippings. Crumble bacon into small pieces. Set aside. In a large bowl, toss lettuce with tomato, green onions, oregano, and pepper. Set aside. Combine reserved bacon drippings, vinegar, and sugar in a small saucepan. Bring to a boil. Pour over lettuce. Cover bowl about 1 minute. Portion salad into individual salad bowls. Sprinkle bacon and cereal mixture over each portion. Serve immediately.

Yield: 6 servings

Exchange, 1 serving: ½ bread, 2 vegetables, 2 fat
Each serving contains: Calories: 175, Carbohydrates: 18 g

From Kellogg's Test Kitchens.

Minted Brown Rice Salad

2½ c.	brown rice, cooked and hot	625 mL
⅓ c.	lemon juice	90 mL
2 T.	vegetable oil	30 mL
½ c.	fresh parsley, minced	125 mL
½ c.	fresh mint, minced	125 mL
¼ c.	green onions, thinly sliced	60 mL
½ c.	dates, finely chopped	125 mL
½ t.	salt	2 mL
2	oranges	2

Combine hot rice, lemon juice, oil, parsley, mint, onions, dates and salt in large bowl. Stir to completely blend. Cover and refrigerate until thoroughly chilled. Mound rice in a chilled, shallow serving dish. Peel oranges; slice crosswise. Decorate rice salad with the orange slices.

Yield: 6 servings

Exchange, 1 serving: 1 bread, 1 fruit, 1 fat
Each serving contains: Calories: 155, Carbohydrates: 22 g

Tabbouleh

½ c.	Stone-Buhr cracked wheat	125 mL
3 med.	fresh tomatoes, finely chopped	3 med.
1 c.	parsley, finely chopped	250 mL
1 c.	onion, finely chopped	250 mL
⅓ c.	fresh lemon juice	90 mL
2 t.	salt	10 mL
1 T.	vegetable oil	15 mL

Soak cracked wheat in cold water for about 10 minutes, drain. Wrap in cheese cloth and squeeze until dry. In large bowl, combine cracked wheat, tomatoes, parsley, onion, lemon juice, and salt; toss lightly with a fork. Marinate at least half hour before serving. Just before serving, stir in the oil.

Yield: 8 servings

Exchange, 1 serving: ⅔ bread, ½ fat
Each serving contains: Calories: 63, Carbohydrates: 15 g

With the compliments of Arnold Foods Company, Inc.

Tomatoes Vinaigrette

2 large	tomatoes, unpeeled and thinly sliced	2 large
2 T.	water	30 mL
1 T.	vegetable oil	15 mL
1 T.	red wine vinegar	15 mL
¼ t.	salt	1 mL
dash	dried basil	dash
dash	black pepper	dash
2 T.	chives, chopped	30 mL

Arrange tomato slices on 4 serving plates. Combine water, oil, vinegar, salt, basil and pepper in a bowl or jar. Stir to completely blend. Sprinkle tomato slices with dressing. Garnish with chive.

Yield: 4 servings

Exchange, 1 serving: ½ vegetable, ½ fat
Each serving contains: Calories: 42, Carbohydrates: 6 g

Mediterranean Eggplant Salad

A fast and interesting salad.

½ c.	long-grain brown rice	125 mL
1 med	eggplant	1 med
2 T.	vegetable oil	30 mL
1 t.	salt	5 mL
1 t.	ground cumin	5 mL
1 t.	ground cinnamon	5 mL
1 c.	celery, thinly sliced	250 mL
½ c.	green onion, thinly sliced	125 mL
2	tomatoes	2
8 large	lettuce leaves	8 large
8 oz.	lemon flavored yogurt	227 g

Prepare the rice as directed on package. Wash the eggplant and remove stem. Cut into 1 in. (2.5 cm) cubes. Heat the oil in a large skillet. Add eggplant and cook, stirring, until eggplant starts to brown. Add a small amount of water, cover tightly and reduce heat. Uncover pan in short intervals and stir, adding extra water, if needed. Cook until eggplant is tender. Drain any excess liquid. Remove from pan and stir in the salt, cumin and cinnamon. Carefully stir in the rice. Cool to room temperature. Add celery and green onion. Place in bowl, cover and refrigerate until completely chilled, about 2 hours or overnight. Place the lettuce leaves on 8 chilled salad plates. Divide salad equally among plates. Cut tomatoes into eighths; garnish each salad with 2 tomato wedges. Top with equal amounts of yogurt.

Yield: 8 servings

Exchange, 1 serving: 1 bread, 1 fat
Each serving contains: Calories: 109, Carbohydrates: 17 g

South-of-the-Border Salad Tray

This is a grand version of Pico de Gallo ("beak of the rooster") relish.

2 med	cucumbers	2 med
½ c.	cider vinegar	125 mL
2 T.	vegetable oil	30 mL
1 t.	salt	5 mL
1 large	white onion	1 large
3 large	oranges	3 large
1 large	avocado	1 large
1 T.	lemon juice	30 mL
½ c.	cold water	125 mL
	Bibb lettuce leaves	
½ t.	red pepper	2 mL

With a vegetable parer, peel lengthwise strips from each cucumber to make alternating green and white stripes. Cut off the ends and thinly slice the cucumbers into rounds; place in a large bowl. Add vinegar, oil, and salt. Mix and chill for at least 2 hours. (This can be made a day in advance.) To arrange salad, lift cucumbers from marinade, and save the marinade. Drain slightly. Peel onion and oranges and thinly slice lengthwise. Combine lemon juice and water in a small bowl. Peel and thinly slice the avocado; drop avocado slices into the lemon water to avoid discoloration. On a large platter or tray, arrange separate sections of cucumber, onion, orange and avocado slices. Garnish with lettuce leaves. Just before serving, combine reserved cucumber marinade with the red pepper. Pour over entire salad.

Yield: 12 servings

Exchange, 1 serving: ½ fruit, 1 fat
Each serving contains: Calories: 67, Carbohydrates: 10 g

Creamy Potato Salad

A family favorite.

2 lbs.	potatoes	1 kg
1½ t.	salt	7 mL
½ c.	green pepper, chopped	125 mL
¼ c.	onion, chopped	60 mL
¼ c.	wheat germ	60 mL
¼ c.	Dannon plain lowfat yogurt	60 mL
¼ c.	low-calorie mayonnaise	60 mL
1 t.	lemon juice	5 mL

Put potatoes and 1 t. (5 mL) of the salt into a large saucepan; add water to cover completely. Bring to a boil, cover and reduce heat. Simmer for 20 to 25 minutes or until potatoes are just tender. Do not overcook. Drain potatoes and rinse with cold water; peel. Cut potatoes into 1 in. (2.5 cm) pieces. Combine remaining ingredients, pour over hot potatoes. Stir gently to completely blend. Cover tightly and refrigerate until chilled.

Yield: 6 servings

Exchange, 1 serving: 1½ bread
Each serving contains: Calories: 128, Carbohydrates: 27 g

Plain Papaya Salad

2½ c.	papaya, diced	625 mL
2 c.	fresh pineapple, diced	500 mL
1 c.	celery, sliced	250 mL
2 T.	chives, chopped	30 mL
½ t.	salt	2 mL
6 large	lettuce leaves	6 large
6 T.	low-calorie mayonnaise	90 mL

Combine papaya, pineapple, celery, chive and salt in a large bowl: fold to blend. Serve on a large lettuce leaf. Top with 1 T. (15 mL) mayonnaise, divided among the servings.

Yield: 6 servings

Exchange, 1 serving: 1 fruit, ½ fat
Each serving contains: Calories: 69, Carbohydrates: 21 g

Cantaloupe-Strawberry Salad

A refreshing salad for summer.

2	cantaloupes	2
1 c.	fresh strawberries	250 mL
1 head	iceberg lettuce, cleaned	1 head
1 c.	Dannon lemon lowfat yogurt	250 mL

Cut cantaloupes into crosswise halves and remove seeds. Using a melon ball cutter, scoop the cantaloupes into balls. Tear lettuce into small pieces. Toss lettuce with yogurt in a large bowl. Arrange cantaloupe balls and strawberries in alternate circles on top of lettuce bed. Cover and chill thoroughly.

Yield: 8 servings

Exchange, 1 serving: 2 fruit
Each serving contains: Calories: 58, Carbohydrates: 23 g

Autumn Fruit Bowl

In these fruits you have the colors of a maple tree in autumn.

1	head romaine lettuce	1 head
2 c.	pineapple, cubed	500 mL
1	grapefruit, segmented	1
1	apple, sliced and dipped in lemon juice	1
1 c.	seedless red grapes	250 mL
1	orange, segmented	1

Combine fruits in a large bowl. Cover tightly and refrigerate until thoroughly chilled. Line a large salad bowl with romaine lettuce leaves; spoon in the fruit. Serve immediately or chill until serving time.

Yield: 12 servings

Exchange, 1 serving: 1 fruit
Each serving contains: Calories: 38, Carbohydrates: 14 g

Spinach-Orange-Chicken Salad

4 oz.	cooked chicken, cut in strips	125 g
2	oranges, peeled and segmented	2
¼ c.	red onion, thinly sliced	60 mL
4 c.	spinach, rinsed and torn into pieces	1 L
	Orange Salad Dressing (recipe follows)	

In a salad bowl, toss together the first 4 ingredients. Add dressing and toss to coat.

Orange Salad Dressing

2 T.	Mazola corn oil	30 mL
2 T.	orange juice	30 mL
2 T.	white wine vinegar	30 mL
½ t.	dry mustard	2 mL
¼ t.	ground ginger	1 mL
dash	salt and pepper	dash

Into a small jar with a tight-fitting lid, measure all the ingredients. Cover and shake well. Chill. Shake before serving. Makes about ⅓ c. (90 mL).

Yield: 4 servings

Exchange, 1 serving: 2 lean meat, 1 fat
Each serving contains: Calories: 160, Carbohydrates: 22 g

"A Diet for the Young at Heart" by Mazola.

Lemon Gazpacho Mold

1 pkg. (2 env.)	Featherweight lemon gelatin	1 pkg. (2 env.)
1 t.	Featherweight instant bouillon, beef flavor	5 mL
1 c.	boiling water	250 mL
2½ c.	Featherweight tomato juice	625 mL
2 t.	red wine vinegar	10 mL
1 t.	Worcestershire sauce	5 mL
¼ t.	hot pepper sauce	1 mL
1 c.	unpared cucumber, chopped	250 mL
½ c.	celery, chopped	125 mL
½ c.	tomato, seeded and chopped	125 mL
¼ c.	green pepper, chopped	60 mL
¼ c.	onion, finely chopped	60 mL
2 6½ oz. cans	Featherweight tuna, drained and flaked	2 190 g cans

Empty both envelopes of gelatin into a bowl. Add bouillon and boiling water; stir until dissolved. Add tomato juice, vinegar, Worcestershire and pepper sauces; stir well. Refrigerate until thickened. Add cucumber, celery, tomato, green pepper, onion, and tuna to the thickened gelatin; mix well. Turn mixture into a lightly oiled 5½ or 6 cup (1¼ or 1½ L) mold. Chill until firm. Unmold on a serving plate.

Yield: 6 servings

Exchange, 1 serving: 1½ lean meat, 1 vegetable
Each serving contains: Calories: 101, Carbohydrates: 20 g

Based on a recipe from Featherweight Brand Foods.

Classic Waldorf Salad

The always enjoyable fruit salad.

4 c.	cold water	1 L
⅓ c.	lemon juice	90 mL
2 c.	apple, thinly sliced	500 mL
1 c.	celery, thinly sliced	250 mL
½ c.	walnuts, coarsely chopped	125 mL
¼ c.	low-calorie mayonnaise	60 mL
2 T.	2% milk	30 mL

Combine water and lemon juice. Drop apple slices into lemon water; soak for 5 to 10 minutes. Drain apple pieces and pat with paper towel until slightly dry. Combine apple, celery, and walnuts in a bowl. In a cup, stir together the mayonnaise and milk; add to the apple mixture and toss to completely coat. Cover and chill thoroughly.

Yield: 6 servings

Exchange, 1 serving: 1 bread, 1½ fat
Each serving contains: Calories: 135, Carbohydrates: 14 g

Post-Holiday Turkey Salad

2 T.	vegetable oil	30 mL
2 T.	cider vinegar	30 mL
½ t.	curry powder	2 mL
½ t.	salt	2 mL
dash	white pepper	dash
½ t.	onion powder	2 mL
6 oz. pkg.	La Choy frozen pea pods, partially thawed	180 g pkg.
2 T.	pimientos, coarsely chopped	30 mL
½ c.	fresh mushrooms, sliced	125 mL
1½ c.	cooked turkey, cubed	375 mL
2 c.	iceberg lettuce, torn into pieces	500 mL
½ c.	celery, thinly sliced	125 mL

Shake together the oil, vinegar and seasonings in a jar with a tightfitting lid. Dry pea pods between paper towels to remove excess moisture. In medium bowl, combine pea pods, pimientos, mushrooms, and turkey. Add dressing; toss lightly. Cover: chill for about 1 hour, tossing once or twice. In a salad bowl, toss lightly the pea pod mixture with lettuce and celery.

Yield: 4 servings

Exchange, 1 serving: 2 lean meat, ½ fat
Each serving contains: Calories: 142, Carbohydrates: 6 g

Adapted from recipes from La Choy Food Products.

Gala Salad

14 oz. can	La Choy bean sprouts, rinsed and drained	420 g can
1 c.	fresh mushrooms, thinly sliced	250 mL
3 T.	lemon juice	45 mL
1 T.	sesame oil	15 mL
1 t.	liquid fructose	5 mL
1 t.	salt	5 mL
¼ t.	onion powder	1 mL
2 c.	cooked chicken, diced	500 mL
3 T.	pimiento, chopped	45 mL
1 T.	sesame seeds, toasted	15 mL
	crisp salad greens	

Cover bean sprouts with ice water; let stand for 30 minutes. Drain well. Place bean sprouts and mushrooms in mixing bowl. In another bowl, blend together lemon juice, oil, liquid fructose, salt, and onion powder. Add to vegetables; toss lightly. Chill. Just before serving, add chicken, pimiento and sesame seeds; toss lightly. Serve on crisp salad greens.

Yield: 4 servings

Exchange, 1 serving: 2 lean meat
Each serving contains: Calories: 120, Carbohydrates: 10 g

Adapted from a La Choy Food Products recipe.

Soy Chicken Salad

A lovely salad to serve on a hot July day.

2 c.	chicken, cooked and shredded	500 mL
½ c.	cucumber, sliced	125 mL
½ c.	alfalfa sprouts	125 mL
1	egg, hard-cooked and chopped	1
2 T.	lemon juice	30 mL
1 T.	vegetable oil	15 mL
2 t.	water	10 mL
2 t.	soy sauce	10 mL
½ t.	Dijon-style mustard	2 mL
dash	black pepper	dash

Combine chicken, cucumber, sprouts, and egg in a medium bowl. Cover tightly and refrigerate until serving time. To make the dressing, blend remaining ingredients. Just before serving, pour dressing over salad. Toss to completely coat the salad.

Yield: 3 c. (750 mL)

Exchange, 1 c. (250 mL): 2 lean meat, ½ vegetable
Each serving contains: Calories: 123, Carbohydrates: 2 g

Vegetable Aspic

2 env.	unflavored gelatin	2 env.
¼ c.	cold water	60 mL
3½ c.	fresh tomato, cut into wedges	875 mL
½ c.	celery leaves, finely chopped	125 mL
1 c.	white onion, chopped	250 mL
3 T.	fresh parsley, minced	45 mL
1	bay leaf	1
1 t.	salt	5 mL
¼ t.	pepper	1 mL
1 c.	celery, sliced	250 mL
1 c.	cabbage, shredded	250 mL

Soften gelatin in cold water; set aside. Combine tomato wedges, celery leaves, onions, parsley, bay leaf, salt, and pepper in a saucepan. Cook and stir over medium heat for 15 minutes. Pour small amount of tomato mixture into softened gelatin, then add to the saucepan. Cook and stir until gelatin is completely dissolved. Remove from heat. Discard bay leaf. Cool in refrigerator until mixture starts to thicken. Fold in celery and cabbage. Pour into slightly oiled mold or serving dish. Refrigerate until completely set.

Yield: 6 servings

Exchange, 1 serving: 1 vegetable
Each serving contains: Calories: 22, Carbohydrates: 10 g

Green Bean Salad

A favorite for many people. Fast and easy with a nice tang.

3 c.	green beans, cooked	750 mL
1 small	red onion, finely chopped	1 small
½ c.	radishes, sliced	125 mL
½ c.	low-calorie french dressing	125 mL
1½ c.	lettuce, finely shredded	375 mL

Combine beans, onions and radishes with the dressing. Divide shredded lettuce equally among 6 chilled serving dishes. With a slotted spoon, scoop equal amounts of bean salad onto the lettuce bed.

Yield: 6 servings

Exchange, 1 serving: 1 vegetable, ¼ fat
Each serving contains: Calories: 35, Carbohydrates: 10 g

Quick Bulgur Salad

A salad that also can be used as a stuffing for a pita sandwich.

⅓ c.	fresh lemon juice	90 mL
2 t.	fresh lemon peel, finely chopped	10 mL
2 T.	olive oil	30 mL
2 t.	salt	10 mL
¼ t.	black pepper, freshly ground	1 mL
1 c.	bulgur wheat	250 mL
1 c.	boiling water	250 mL
½ c.	fresh parsley, chopped	125 mL
½ c.	red onion, finely chopped	125 mL
2 c.	tomatoes, chopped	500 mL

Combine lemon juice, lemon peel, oil, salt, and pepper in a shaker bottle. Place bulgur in ovenproof bowl, add boiling water. Stir to blend. Cover tightly, allow to stand for 10 to 15 minutes or until all the water is absorbed. Toss with 2 forks to separate grains. Shake dressing and pour over bulgur; toss to thoroughly mix. Add remaining ingredients; toss again. Serve at room temperature.

Yield: 3 c. (750 mL)

Exchange, ½ c. (125 mL): 1 bread, 1 fat
Each serving contains: Calories: 125, Carbohydrates: 24 g

Marinated Potato Salad

¼ c.	Mazola corn oil	60 mL
¼ c.	green onion, thinly sliced	60 mL
2 T.	white wine vinegar	30 mL
2 T.	dry white wine	30 mL
1 T.	parsley, chopped	15 mL
½ t.	dried dill	2 mL
¼ t.	salt	1 mL
¼ t.	pepper	1 mL
2 lb.	red potatoes, cooked, sliced ¼ in. (6 mm) thick	1 kg

In a large bowl, stir together the first 8 ingredients. Add potatoes. Gently toss to coat potatoes. Cover; chill for several hours, tossing occasionally. If desired, salad may be served warm.

Yield: 6 servings

Exchange, 1 serving: 1½ bread, 2 fat
Each serving contains: Calories: 200, Carbohydrates: 15 g

"A Diet for the Young at Heart" by Mazola.

Chinese Salad

1 head	Bibb lettuce	1 head
1 head	Boston lettuce	1 head
2 stalks	Chinese cabbage	2 stalks
8 oz. can	water chestnuts	225 g can
8 oz. can	bamboo shoots	225 g can
1 c.	bean sprouts	250 mL
½ c.	Soy French Dressing	125 mL

Rinse lettuce and cabbage leaves. Break into bite-size pieces. Place in plastic bag or tightly covered container. Store in refrigerator 4 to 6 hours or overnight to crisp. Drain water chestnuts, bamboo shoots, and bean sprouts. Rinse with cold water. Drain thoroughly. Thinly slice the water chestnuts. Carefully pat greens dry with towel. Place in wooden bowl. Top with water chestnuts, bamboo shoots, and bean sprouts. Cover with Soy French Dressing. Toss lightly until all ingredients are coated.

Yield: 12 servings

Exchange, 1 serving: ½ vegetable
Each serving contains: Calories: 40, Carbohydrates: 14 g

Dandelion Salad

1 c.	young dandelion greens	250 mL
1 head	iceberg lettuce	1 head
2 T.	low-calorie Italian dressing	30 mL
2	tomatoes	2
1 small	cucumber	1 small
2 T.	low-calorie bleu cheese dressing	30 ML
1 T.	skim milk	15 mL

Rinse greens and lettuce. Pat dry with towel. Break into large pieces. Place in large plastic bag. Sprinkle with Italian dressing. Close tightly and store in refrigerator to crisp. Shake occasionally. Peel tomatoes and remove seeds; slice tomato flesh into strips. Peel cucumber; slice into ⅛ in. (3 mm) slices. Place greens, lettuce, tomatoes, and cucumber in wooden bowl. Blend bleu cheese dressing with skim milk. Cover salad with dressing. Toss to coat all ingredients.

Yield: 6 servings

Exchange, 1 serving: negligible
Each serving contains: Calories: negligible, Carbohydrates: 7 g

Added Touch: Top each serving with a few Garlic Croutons. Add exchange and calories for croutons.

Radish Salad

1 t.	salt	5 mL
1 t.	garlic powder	5 mL
1 t.	Dijon mustard	5 mL
1 T.	wine vinegar	15 mL
2 T.	liquid shortening	30 mL
2 t.	lemon juice	10 mL
1	watercress (small bunch)	1
½ head	iceberg lettuce	½ head
1 bunch	red radishes	1 bunch

Combine salt, garlic powder, Dijon mustard, vinegar, liquid shortening, and lemon juice in screwtop jar. Shake to blend. Coarsely chop watercress, lettuce, and radishes; place in salad bowl. Add dressing; toss to blend.

Yield: 6 servings

Exchange, 1 serving: 1 fat
Each serving contains: Calories: 60, Carbohydrates: negligible

Jean's Vegetable Salad

1 c.	asparagus, cut into 2 in. (5 cm) pieces	250 mL
1 c.	broccoli flowerets	250 mL
1 c.	cauliflowerets	250 mL
½ c.	celery, sliced	125 mL
½ c.	cucumber, scored and sliced	125 mL
1 c.	fresh mushrooms, sliced	250 mL
1 c.	green pepper, sliced	250 mL
½ c.	radishes, sliced	125 mL
10	pitted black olives, sliced	10
½ c.	low-calorie Italian dressing	125 mL

Combine all vegetables in large bowl. Cover with Italian dressing. Marinate overnight. Toss frequently.

Yield: 7 servings

Exchange, 1 serving: 1 vegetable
Each serving contains: Calories: 45, Carbohydrates: 9 g

Maude's Green Salad

½ head	iceberg lettuce	½ head
½ head	Boston lettuce	½ head
½ head	chicory	½ head
½ lb.	spinach	250 g
½ head	romaine lettuce	½ head
5 T.	low-calorie Italian dressing	75 mL
1 T.	Parmesan cheese	15 mL

Rinse and crisp the salad greens. Break iceberg lettuce into bite-size pieces. Carefully pat iceberg dry on towel. Place in large plastic bag. Add 1 T. (15 mL) Italian dressing. Shake lightly until all leaves are covered. Place in strip on medium platter or plate. Repeat with each green. Sprinkle lightly with Parmesan cheese.

Yield: 10 servings

Exchange: negligible
Each serving contains: Calories: negligible, Carbohydrates: negligible

German Potato Salad

6 slices	bacon, crispy fried	6 slices
1½ c.	cold water	375 mL
3 T.	flour	45 mL
1 med.	onion, chopped	1 med.
3 T.	sugar replacement	45 mL
¼ c.	vinegar	60 mL
6 med	boiled potatoes, sliced	6 med

Remove excess grease from bacon with paper towel. Break bacon into small pieces. Blend cold water and flour. Pour into saucepan. Add onion, sugar replacement, and vinegar. Heat, stirring, until thickened. Add bacon and potatoes while still warm from boiling and frying.

Yield: 8 servings

Exchange, 1 serving: 1 bread, 1 fat
Each serving contains: Calories: 113, Carbohydrates: 39 g

Swiss Salad

1 small head	iceberg lettuce	1 small head
1 head	romaine lettuce	1 head
¼ lb.	fresh spinach	125 g
1 large	cucumber	1 large
1	green pepper	1
1 c.	cherry tomatoes	250 mL
½ c.	low-calorie French dressing	125 mL

Rinse and wash greens. Drain thoroughly. Break into large pieces; place in plastic bag or tightly covered container. Store in refrigerator 4 to 6 hours or overnight to crisp. Score cucumber with tines of fork. Cut into ⅛ in. (3-mm) slices. Cut green pepper into thin rings. Cut cherry tomatoes in half. Just before serving, carefully pat greens dry on towel. Place greens in large wooden bowl; cover with French dressing. Toss greens lightly, coating all leaves with dressing. Top with cucumber, green pepper, and cherry tomatoes. Serve immediately.

Yield: 16 servings

Exchange, 1 serving: ½ vegetable
Each serving contains: Calories: 32, Carbohydrates: 43 g

Marinated Cucumbers

2 to 3	cucumbers, large	2 to 3
1 t.	salt	5 mL
1 t.	sugar replacement	5 mL
¼ c.	vinegar	60 mL
⅛ t.	pepper	1 mL

Score cucumbers with tines of fork. Cut into very thin slices. Sprinkle with salt. Chill 2 hours; drain well. Sprinkle with sugar replacement; add vinegar and pepper. Marinate 30 minutes or more before serving.

Yield: 6 to 8 servings

Exchange: negligible
Each serving contains: Calories: negligible, Carbohydrates: 4 g

Asparagus Salad

¼ lb.	spinach	125 g
1 head	romaine lettuce	1 head
10 spears	asparagus, raw	10 spears
½ head	red cabbage	½ head
½ c.	celery, sliced	125 mL
½	cucumber, peeled and sliced	½
½ c.	Lemon French Dressing	125 mL

Rinse greens. Break into bite-size pieces. Place in plastic bag or tightly covered container. Store in refrigerator 4 to 6 hours or overnight to crisp. Wash asparagus spears and cut into 2 in. (5 cm) pieces. Shred cabbage as for coleslaw; remove all hard pieces. Just before serving, carefully pat greens dry on towel. Place all ingredients in wooden bowl. Toss lightly to coat all ingredients with Lemon French Dressing.

Yield: 12 servings

Exchange, 1 serving: ½ vegetable
Each serving contains: Calories: 42, Carbohydrates: 7 g

Hot Green Pepper Salad

4	green peppers	4
1 T.	butter	15 mL
1 t.	oregano	5 mL
½ t.	thyme	2 mL
	salt and pepper to taste	
½ c.	mushroom pieces	125 mL

Rinse green peppers. Cut them into quarters. Melt butter in skillet. Add seasonings, green peppers, and mushrooms. Cook over low heat for 10 minutes. Serve immediately.

Yield: 4 servings

Exchange, 1 serving: 1 vegetable, 1 fat
Each serving contains: Calories: 60, Carbohydrates: 8 g

Shrimp and Green Bean Salad

2 c.	green beans	500 mL
2 c.	shrimp	500 mL
½ c.	mushrooms, thinly sliced	125 mL
¼ c.	Bay Salad Dressing	60 mL
	lettuce leaves	

Rinse and snap green beans. Cook in small amount of boiling salted water until crisp-tender. Drain and cool immediately in ice water; chill. Clean and devein shrimp, or use canned shrimp. Rinse thoroughly under cold water; chill. Combine green beans, shrimp, and mushrooms in bowl. Sprinkle with Bay Salad Dressing. Toss to coat. Chill thoroughly before serving. Serve on lettuce leaves.

Yield: 4 servings

Exchange, 1 serving: 1 lean meat, ½ vegetable
Each serving contains: Calories: 62, Carbohydrates: 20 g

Salmon Salad Plate

1 oz.	cold salmon, cooked	30 g	
½ small	tomato	½ small	
¼ c.	carrot sticks	60 mL	
¼	green pepper, sliced	¼	
¼ c.	eggplant sticks	60 mL	
1	egg, hard cooked	1	
1 T.	cottage cheese	15 mL	
	salt and pepper to taste		
	lettuce leaf		

Chill salmon. Peel tomato and remove seeds; slice tomato flesh into strips. Cook carrot, green pepper, eggplant, and tomato in boiling salted water until crisp-tender. (Remember, the carrots sticks may take more time to cook than the other vegetables.) Drain and chill. Cut egg in half lengthwise. Mash egg yolk with cottage cheese, salt, and pepper; stuff egg white halves. Arrange cooked salmon, vegetables, and stuffed eggs on crisp lettuce leaf.

Yield: 1 serving

Exchange, 1 serving: 2⅓ lean meat, 1 vegetable
Each serving contains: Calories: 193, Carbohydrates: 24 g

Waldorf Salad

1 c.	celery, sliced	250 mL
1 c.	seedless green grapes, halved	250 mL
1 c.	apple, diced	250 mL
4	dates, pitted and thinly sliced	4
½ c.	walnuts, chopped	125 mL
¼ c.	mayonnaise	60 mL
2 T.	dry white wine	30 mL
	lettuce leaves	

Place celery, grapes, apple, dates, and walnuts into bowl. Blend mayonnaise with wine; pour into bowl. Stir to blend with celery, fruit, and walnuts. Use slotted serving spoon to serve, shaking spoon slightly to remove excess dressing. Serve on crisp lettuce leaves.

Yield: 7 servings

Exchange, 1 serving: 2 fruit, ¼ vegetable, 1 fat
Each serving contains: Calories: 105

Herring Salad Plate

1 oz.	salted herring	30 g
½ small	onion, thinly sliced	½ small
¼ c.	beets, sliced	60 mL
	Italian or French dressing	
	lettuce leaf	

Soak herring overnight in water. Remove skin and bones. Cut into 1 in. (2.5-cm) pieces. Place herring, onion, and beets in glass bowl. Cover with dressing. Marinate 4 to 5 hours or overnight. Drain. (Keep liquid; it makes a very good salad dressing.) Arrange herring, onion, and beets on crisp lettuce leaf.

Yield: 2 servings

Exchange, 1 serving: ½ lean meat, 1 bread
Each serving contains: Calories: 50, Carbohydrates: 80 g

Lime Avocado Salad

1 pkg. (⅝ oz.)	low-calorie lime gelatin	1 pkg. (20 g)	
1½ c.	boiling water	375 mL	
3 oz.	cream cheese	90 g	
½ c.	low calorie whipped topping, prepared	125 mL	
½ c.	avocado, cubed	125 mL	
½ c.	unsweetened fruit cocktail	125 mL	
	vegetable cooking spray		
	shredded lettuce		

Dissolve gelatin in boiling water. Cool to consistency of beaten egg whites. Beat cream cheese; blend into gelatin mixture. Fold prepared whipped topping into gelatin mixture. Chill until quite firm. Fold in avocado and fruit cocktail. Pour into 1 qt. (1 L) ring mold coated with vegetable cooking spray. Chill until set. Serve on bed of shredded lettuce.

Yield: 8 servings

Exchange, 1 serving: ½ vegetable, ½ lean meat, 1 fat
Each serving contains: Calories: 78, Carbohydrates: 14 g

Cantaloupe Bowl

4	strawberries	4	
4	fresh pineapple cubes	4	
1 t.	sugar replacement	5 mL	
¼	6 in. (15 cm) cantaloupe	¼	

Sprinkle strawberries and pineapple with sugar replacement. Fill hollow of cantaloupe with fruit mixture.

Yield: 1 serving

Exchange, 1 serving: 2 fruit
Each serving contains: Calories: 90, Carbohydrates: 39 g

Grapefruit Salad

¼ c.	cranberries	60 mL	
1½ c.	grapefruit sections	375 mL	
1	apple, sliced	1	
2 T.	raisins	30 mL	
½ c.	orange juice	125 mL	
	lettuce leaves		

Prick cranberries with sharp fork. Combine with remaining ingredients, except lettuce. Marinate 4 to 6 hours or overnight, drain. Serve on crisp lettuce leaves.

Yield: 5 servings

Exchange, 1 serving: 1 fruit
Each serving contains: Calories: 40, Carbohydrates: 27 g

Cranberry Salad

1 pkg. (⅝ oz.)	low-calorie lemon gelatin	1 pkg. (20 g)	
1 T.	sugar replacement	15 mL	
1½ c.	boiling water	375 mL	
1	orange	1	
½ c.	cranberries	125 mL	
½ c.	celery, chopped	125 mL	
½ c.	apple, chopped	125 mL	

Dissolve gelatin and sugar replacement in boiling water. Cool to consistency of beaten egg whites. Grind orange (with peel) and cranberries; combine with celery and apple. Fold into gelatin mixture. Pour into mold or serving bowl. Chill until firm.

Yield: 8 servings

Exchange, 1 serving: 1 fruit
Each serving contains: Calories: 24, Carbohydrates: 17 g

Queen's Layered Gelatin

1 pkg. (⅝ oz.)	low-calorie strawberry gelatin	1 pkg. (20 g)
	vegetable cooking spray	
1 pkg. (⅝ oz.)	low-calorie lemon gelatin	1 pkg. (20 g)
3 oz.	cream cheese	90 g
1 c.	low-calorie whipped topping, prepared	250 mL
1 pkg. (⅝ oz.)	low-calorie orange gelatin	1 pkg. (20 g)
½ c.	unsweetened crushed pineapple, drained	125 mL
½ c.	carrot, grated	125 mL
	shredded lettuce	

Prepare strawberry gelatin as directed on package. Pour into 2 qt. (2-L) mold coated with vegetable cooking spray. Chill until firm. Prepare lemon gelatin as directed on package. Set until consistency of beaten egg whites. Whip cream cheese until light and fluffy. Fold into prepared whipped topping. Fold cream cheese topping into lemon gelatin. Pour over strawberry gelatin in mold. Chill until firm. Prepare orange gelatin as directed on package. Set until consistency of beaten egg whites. Fold in pineapple and carrot. Pour over lemon gelatin in mold. Chill until firm. Serve on bed of shredded lettuce.

Yield: 8 servings

Exchange, 1 serving: ½ vegetable, 1 fat
Each serving contains: Calories: 57, Carbohydrates: 36 g

Blueberry Salad

1½ c.	fresh or frozen blueberries	375 mL
2 t.	sugar replacement	10 mL
1 env.	unflavored gelatin	1 env.
2 t.	lemon juice	10 mL
1 c.	unsweetened crushed pineapple, drained	250 mL
1 c.	low-calorie whipped topping, prepared	250 mL

Place blueberries in saucepan. Sprinkle with sugar replacement. Allow to rest 30 minutes at room temperature; drain. Add enough boiling water to make 2 c. (500 mL). Sprinkle unflavored gelatin over surface. Stir to dissolve. Cook over low heat for 2 to 3 minutes. Allow to rest until cool. Add lemon juice. Remove ⅓ c. (90 mL) from blueberry mixture. Chill until set; reserve. Fold pineapple into remaining gelatin; chill until firm. Whip reserved gelatin until frothy. Fold in prepared whipped topping. Spread over blueberry gelatin. Chill until set.

Yield: 4 servings

Exchange, 1 serving: ½ fruit
Each serving contains: Calories: 24, Carbohydrates: 45 g

Cabbage-Pineapple Salad

3 c.	cabbage, shredded	750 mL
1 lb. can	unsweetened pineapple, diced	500 g can
2 T.	sugar replacement	30 mL
dash	salt	dash
½ c.	low-calorie whipped topping, prepared	125 mL

Combine cabbage and pineapple with juice, sugar replacement and salt. Stir to dissolve sugar. Allow to rest at room temperature for 1½ to 2 hours. Drain thoroughly. Fold topping into cabbage mixture.

Yield: 4 servings

Exchange, 1 serving: ½ fruit
Each serving contains: Calories: 28, Carbohydrates: 36 g

Fruit Bowl

¼ c.	cantaloupe balls	60 mL
⅛ c.	honeydew balls	30 mL
½ c.	watermelon balls	125 mL
¼ c.	fresh, unsweetened pineapple chunks	60 mL
	salt	
	low-calorie French dressing	
	lettuce	

Sprinkle each fruit with salt and French dressing. Combine all ingredients, except lettuce. Refrigerate 1 to 2 hours. Serve on small bed of lettuce.

Yield: 1 serving

Exchange, 1 serving: 1 fruit
Each serving contains: Calories: 40, Carbohydrates: 25 g

Fruit Salad

16 oz. can	unsweetened apricot halves	500 g can
16 oz. can	unsweetened pineapple chunks	500 g can
2 t.	lemon juice	10 mL
1 t.	cornstarch	5 mL
2 t.	sugar replacement	10 mL
1 t.	margarine	5 mL
1	apple, chopped	1
1	banana, sliced	
	low-calorie whipped topping	

Drain juice from apricots and pineapple into saucepan; add lemon juice and cornstarch. Cook over low heat to thicken. Remove from heat; add sugar replacement and margarine. Stir to blend; cool slightly. Combine all fruit in bowl. Pour sauce over fruit.

Yield: 6 servings

Exchange, 1 serving: 1 fruit
Each serving contains: Calories: 53, Carbohydrates: 29 g

Added Touch: Top each serving with a dab of whipped topping.

Apple Chicken Salad

1 c.	apple, diced	250 mL
1	lemon, juiced	1
3 c.	chicken, cooked and diced	750 mL
½ c.	celery, diced	125 mL
½ c.	seedless green grapes	125 mL
⅓ c.	low-calorie mayonnaise	90 mL
	lettuce leaves (optional)	

Combine the apple and lemon juice in a bowl. Toss to thoroughly coat apples with juice. Add the remaining ingredients except lettuce leaves; gently fold to mix. Place lettuce leaves either on individual chilled plates or in bottom and sides of chilled serving bowl or platter. Heap salad on the leaves.

Yield: 8 servings

Exchange, 1 serving: 2 lean meat, ½ fruit
Each serving contains: Calories: 84, Carbohydrates: 8 g

Bean Salad

Salad base

1 lb. can	green beans	500 g can
1 lb. can	wax beans	500 g can
1 lb. can	lima beans	500 g can
1 lb. can	red beans	500 g can

Dressing

½ c.	vegetable oil	125 mL
¼ c.	water	60 mL
1 T.	fresh parsley, snipped	15 mL
1 t.	salt	5 mL
1 t.	dry mustard	5 mL
½ t.	tarragon leaves	2 mL
½ t.	marjoram	2 mL
3 env.	Equal low-calorie sweetener	3 env.

Combine beans in a strainer or colander; drain thoroughly. Place in large glass bowl. Combine the dressing ingredients; stir to blend thoroughly. Pour over beans. Refrigerate, mixing 2 to 3 times a day. To serve, pour off dressing or serve salad with slotted spoon.

Yield: 20 servings

Exchange, 1 serving: 1 vegetable, ½ fat
Each serving contains: Calories: 45, Carbohydrates: 6 g

Individual Chef Salad

1 c.	salad greens	250 mL
½ oz.	turkey strips, cooked	15 g
½ oz.	ham strips, cooked	15 g
¼ oz.	Swiss cheese	8 g
½	tomato, chopped	½
1	egg, hard-cooked and quartered	1
1	wedge lemon	1
	salt and pepper to taste	

On a dinner plate or small platter, arrange the salad greens. Top with remaining ingredients.

Yield: 1 serving

Exchange, 1 serving: 1 high-fat meat
Each serving contains: Calories: 110, Carbohydrates: 3 g

Hors d'Oeuvres

Spicy Walnuts

Although nuts are high in calories, sometimes a spicy or sweet nut makes a nice addition to a salad or vegetable, particularly to entice those who wouldn't otherwise eat fresh or cooked vegetables. You might try using some of these on a salad with just a sweetened cider vinegar dressing.

2 c.	walnuts, broken into pieces	500 mL
½ c.	liquid sugar replacement	125 mL
¼ c.	water	60 mL
½ t.	orange rind, grated	2 mL
½ t.	lemon rind, grated	2 mL
¼ t.	ground cinnamon	1 mL
¼ t.	ground ginger	1 mL
dash each	ground clove, nutmeg and allspice	dash each

Combine all ingredients in a saucepan. Cook and stir until liquid has evaporated. Spread nuts on a tabletop or baking sheet. Cool. Store in refrigerator or freezer.

Yield: 2 c. (500 mL)

Exchange, 2 T. (30 mL): 2 fat
Each serving contains: Calories: 92, Carbohydrates: 2 g

Salted Garbanzo Beans

A nice evening snack instead of popcorn.

2 c.	Jack Rabbit garbanzo beans (chickpeas)	500 mL
1 qt.	water	1 L
¼ c.	salt	60 mL
	shortening or oil for frying	

Combine water and salt in a saucepan. Cook and stir over medium heat until salt is completely dissolved. Add garbanzo beans. Simmer for 10 minutes. Remove pan from heat, cover and allow garbanzo beans to soak overnight. Drain and spread garbanzo beans out in a single layer to dry at room temperature: or pat dry with a towel. In a deep fryer, heat shortening or oil to 350°F (175°C). Fry a few at a time for 6 to 8 minutes. Drain on a paper towel.

Yield: 3 c. (750 mL)

Exchange, ¼ c. (60 mL): 1 bread
Each serving contains: Calories: 67, Carbohydrates: 11 g

Stuffed Prunes

30 med	dried prunes	30 med	
30 halves	English walnuts	30 halves	

Wash prunes and soak overnight in water. Cook in the same water until prunes are semisoft but do not overcook. Drain thoroughly over a bowl. (You can refrigerate and use this liquid to sweeten other dishes or chill and serve it as a beverage.) Remove stones from prunes. Place a half walnut in the cavity of each prune. Set on a rack and allow to dry slightly. Store in the refrigerator.

Yield: 30 snacks

Exchange, 1 snack: ½ fruit, ⅓ fat
Each serving contains: Calories: 27, Carbohydrates: 8 g

Popcorn Variations

Popcorn is a very good fiber food. Here are a few variations you might like to try. I know each recipe makes a lot of popcorn, but popcorn freezes well after it is popped. All you have to do is store it in a freezer container.

3.5 oz bag	Pillsbury microwave frozen popcorn	99 g bag	
2 T.	any of the following seasonings or a combination: taco seasoning mix, creamy Italian salad dressing mix, sweet-and-sour Oriental seasoning mix, nacho cheese sauce mix, sloppy hot dog or hamburger seasoning mix	30 mL	

Pop the corn as directed on the package. Divide in half to make 4 c. (1 L) popped corn in each half. Sprinkle 1 T. (15 mL) of your chosen seasoning mix over the popped corn you plan to serve. Shake or toss with a fork to completely coat. Reserve the remaining popped corn for future use.

Yield: 4 c. (1 L)

Exchange, 1 c. (250 mL): 1 bread
Each serving contains: Calories: 65, Carbohydrates: 18 g

Salted Pumpkin Seeds

I like to make these from the seeds of the Halloween pumpkin.

2 c.	water	500 mL	
¼ c.	salt	60 mL	
2 c.	pumpkin seeds	500 mL	

Combine water and salt in a saucepan. Cook and stir until salt dissolves; cool. Add pumpkin seeds and soak overnight. Drain thoroughly. Pat seeds dry with a paper towel. Place on a cookie sheet. Bake at 300°F (150°C) until seeds are dry, about 1 hour.

Yield: 2 c. (500 mL)

Exchange, ¼ c. (60 mL): 2 fat
Each serving contains: Calories: 92, Carbohydrates: 6 g

Fruit Dip

8 oz.	plain low-calorie yogurt	240 g	Combine all ingredients. Whip until fluffy. Chill thoroughly.
4 T.	low-calorie preserves	60 mL	
½ t.	ground allspice	2 mL	**Yield: 1 c. (250 mL)**
½ t.	lemon juice	2 mL	

Exchange, 1 serving: 1 milk
Each serving contains: Calories: 192, Carbohydrates: 70 g

Onion Dip

4 oz.	plain low-calorie yogurt	120 g	Combine all ingredients. Chill thoroughly.
¼ c.	onions, finely chopped	60 mL	**Yield: ¾ c. (190 mL)**
1 t.	lemon juice	5 mL	
1 T.	parsley	15 mL	*Exchange, 1 serving: ½ milk, ½ vegetable*
dash each	hot pepper sauce, horseradish, salt, pepper	dash each	*Each serving contains: Calories: 72, Carbohydrates: 36 g*

Shrimp Dip

5 small	shrimp	5 small	Crush shrimp. Sprinkle with Worcestershire sauce and lemon juice. Combine yogurt and Chili Sauce. Add crushed shrimp; stir to blend. Chill.
½ t.	Worcestershire sauce	2 mL	
1 t.	lemon juice	5 mL	
4 oz.	plain low-calorie yogurt	120 g	**Yield: ¾ c. (190 mL)**
¼ c.	Chili Sauce	60 mL	

Exchange, 1 serving: 1 meat, ½ milk, ½ fruit
Each serving contains: Calories: 108, Carbohydrates: 31 g

Avocado Crisps

1	very ripe avocado	1	Peel and mash avocado. Add remaining ingredients. Beat until smooth. Spread thinly on crackers.
1 t.	lemon juice	5 mL	
1 t.	grated onion	5 mL	**Yield: 45 servings**
1 t.	onion salt	5 mL	
1 t.	paprika	5 mL	*Exchange, 5 servings: 1 bread, 1 fat*
½ t.	marjoram	2 mL	*Each 5 servings contain: Calories: 108, Carbohydrates: 5 g*
	thin crackers		

Stuffed Celery

2	5 in. (12 cm) stalks celery	2
1 T.	cream cheese, softened	30 mL
¼ t.	onion powder	1 mL
dash	paprika	dash
	salt and pepper to taste	

Thoroughly rinse and drain celery. Combine cream cheese, onion powder, and paprika. Blend until smooth and creamy. Add salt and pepper. Fill celery stalks. Chill.

Yield: 1 serving

Exchange, 1 serving: 1 fat
Each serving contains: Calories: 50, Carbohydrates: 7 g

Cheese Appetizers

4 oz.	Cheddar cheese, shredded	120 g
2 T.	margarine	30 mL
½ c.	flour	125 mL
1 t.	onion, grated	5 mL
½ t.	salt	2 mL
¼ t.	pepper	1 mL

Blend cheese and margarine until smooth. Add flour, onion, salt, and pepper. Stir until smooth. Shape dough into a roll, 1¼ in. (3.5 cm) in diameter. Wrap in plastic wrap or aluminum foil. Chill. Cut into ¼ in. (6 mm) slices. Bake at 400°F (200°C) for 8 minutes.

Yield: 24 servings

Exchange, 1 serving: ½ fat, ¼ bread
Each serving contains: Calories: 37, Carbohydrates: 3 g

Cucumbers in Yogurt

1	cucumber	1
1 small	onion	1 small
1 t.	salt	5 mL
½ t.	garlic powder	2 mL
1 t.	lemon juice	5 mL
½ t.	marjoram	2 mL
8 oz.	low-calorie yogurt	240 g

Peel and thinly slice cucumber and onion. Sprinkle with salt. Allow to rest 15 minutes. Drain and pat dry. Combine garlic powder, lemon juice, marjoram, and yogurt; mix thoroughly. Fold in sliced cucumber and onion. Chill.

Yield: 2 c. (500 mL)

Exchange, 1 serving: 1 milk
Each serving contains: Calories: 100, Carbohydrates: 62 g

Summer Chicken Canapés

4 oz.	ground cooked chicken	120 g
2 T.	margarine, softened	30 mL
¼ t.	dry mustard	2 mL
½ t.	meat tenderizer	2 mL
½ t.	salt	2 mL
⅛ t.	pepper	1 mL
¼ in. thick	cucumber slices	6 mm thick

Combine chicken, margarine, dry mustard, meat tenderizer, salt, and pepper. Mix thoroughly. Chill.

To make canapé: Place 1 t. (5 mL) of chicken mixture in center of cucumber slice.

Yield: 24 servings

Exchange, 2 servings: ½ fat
Each serving contains: Calories: 14, Carbohydrates: negligible

Garlic Bites

1 slice	white bread	1 slice
2 t.	low-calorie margarine	10 mL
¼ t.	garlic powder	2 mL

Remove crust from bread; cut bread into ¼ in. (6-mm) cubes. Melt margarine in small pan. Add garlic powder and heat until sizzling. Add bread cubes; sauté, tossing frequently until brown. Drain and cool.

Yield: 2 servings

Exchange, 1 serving: ½ bread, 1 fat
Each serving contains: Calories: 79, Carbohydrates: 7 g

Hors D'Oeuvre Spreads

Use one of following as a spread for 24 small crackers:

Anchovy

1 oz.	anchovy fillets	30 g
¼ c.	low-calorie margarine	60 mL

Rinse fillets in cold water; pat dry. Grind or chop fine; blend with margarine. Allow to rest.

Exchange, ¼ c. (60 mL): ½ fat, 1 meat
Each serving contains: Calories: 250

Caviar

2 T.	caviar	30 mL
¼ c.	low-calorie margarine	60 mL

Combine caviar and margarine. Refrigerate overnight.

Exchange, ¼ c. (60 mL): ½ fat, 1 meat
Each serving contains: Calories: 280

Crabmeat

2 T.	crabmeat	30 mL
¼ c.	low-calorie margarine	60 mL

Crush crabmeat; blend with margarine. Refrigerate overnight.

Exchange, ¼ c. (60 mL): ½ fat, ½ meat
Each serving contains: Calories: 230

Hors D'Oeuvre Spreads (continued)

Garlic

¼ t.	garlic	2 mL
dash	salt	dash
¼ c.	low-calorie margarine	60 mL

Blend ingredients together.

Exchange, ¼ c. (60 mL.): ½ fat
Each serving contains: Calories: 200, Carbohydrates: negligible

Herb

dash each	marjoram, oregano, chopped onion, salt, pepper	dash each
¼ c.	low-calorie margarine	60 mL

Blend ingredients together; allow to rest at room temperature 2 hours.

Exchange, ¼ c. (60 mL): ½ fat
Each serving contains: Calories: 200, Carbohydrates: negligible

Horseradish

1 T.	horseradish, grated	15 mL
1 t.	parsley, chopped	5 mL
¼ c.	low-calorie margarine	60 mL

Blend ingredients together; refrigerate overnight.

Exchange, ¼ c. (60 mL): ½ fat
Each serving contains: Calories: 200, Carbohydrates: negligible

Lemon

1 t.	lemon juice	5 mL
dash	salt	dash
¼ t.	parsley	2 mL
¼ c.	low-calorie margarine	60 mL

Blend ingredients together.

Exchange, ¼ c. (60 mL): ½ fat
Each serving contains: Calories: 200, Carbohydrates: negligible

Mustard

2 t.	Dijon mustard	10 mL
¼ c.	margarine	60 mL

Blend ingredients together.

Exchange, ¼ c. (60 mL): ½ fat
Each serving contains: Calories: 200, Carbohydrates: negligible

Note: Exchange and calorie figures above do not include crackers.

Spreads may be topped with 1 t. (5 mL):

Chicken	Salami	Crabmeat
Chicken liver	Sausage	Lobster
Ham	Tuna	

Exchange to add 6 crackers: 1 meat, plus cracker exchange

Bacon	Avocado

Exchange to add 5 crackers: 1 fat, plus cracker exchange

Cauliflower	Mushroom	Onion
Green pepper	Celery	Radish
Cucumber	Parsley	Tomato

Exchange: Only cracker exchange

Yield: ¼ c. (60 mL) spread for 24 crackers or ½ t. (3 mL) per cracker.

Exchange, 1 serving: ½ fat plus cracker exchange

Smoked Salmon Canapés

8 oz.	smoked salmon	240 g
3 oz.	cream cheese	90 g
½ t.	lemon juice	2 mL
1 t.	milk	5 mL
dash each	thyme, sage, salt, pepper	dash each

Place smoked salmon in blender. Blend until fine. Combine cream cheese, lemon juice, and milk. Stir to make a paste. Add seasonings. Mix well. Add salmon; blend thoroughly. Roll into 22 balls. Chill.

Yield: 22 servings

Exchange, 2 servings: 1 meat
Each serving contains: Calories: 34, Carbohydrates: negligible

Swiss Morsels

8 oz.	Swiss cheese, grated	240 g
4 oz.	ham, grated	120 g
2 T.	margarine, softened	30 mL
¼ t.	thyme	1 mL

Combine all ingredients; mix thoroughly. Shape 2 t. (10 mL) of mixture into a ball. Repeat with remaining mixture.

Yield: 34 servings

Exchange, 1 serving: ½ high-fat meat
Each serving contains: Calories: 51, Carbohydrates: negligible

Appetizer Meatballs

¾ lb.	ground beef	375 g
¼ lb.	ground pork	125 g
¾ c.	Stone-Buhr 4 grain cereal mates	190 mL
¼ c.	water chestnuts, finely chopped	60 mL
¼ t.	Worcestershire sauce	1 mL
½ c.	skim milk	125 mL
½ t.	garlic salt	2 mL
few drops	Tabasco sauce	few drops

Combine all ingredients and mix well. Shape into 75 small balls. In a nonstick pan, brown well over low heat. Place in chafing dish, add ½ c. (125 mL) warm water. Use toothpicks to serve.

Yield: 75 balls

Exchange, 5 balls: 1 medium-fat meat
Each serving contains: Calories: 70, Carbohydrates: 4 g

With the compliments of Arnold Foods Company. Inc.

Sesame Cheese Balls

3 oz. pkg.	cream cheese, softened	85 g pkg.	
¼ c.	blue cheese	60 mL	
¼ c.	dried beef, minced	60 mL	
dash	cayenne pepper	dash	
¼ c.	Stone-Buhr sesame seeds, toasted	60 mL	

Blend cheeses with dried beef and cayenne pepper. Shape into 20 small balls. Chill. Roll in sesame seeds.

Yield: 20 balls

Exchange, 1 ball: ½ fat
Each serving contains: Calories: 23, Carbohydrates: 2 g

With the compliments of Arnold Foods Company, Inc.

Spinach Crescents

½ c.	onion, finely chopped	125 mL
2 T.	cooking oil	30 mL
10 oz. pkg.	frozen chopped spinach, thawed and squeezed dry	300 g pkg.
¾ c.	Kretschmer regular wheat germ	190 mL
¾ c.	Parmesan cheese, grated	190 mL
½ c.	sour cream	125 mL
¼ c.	pine nuts	60 mL
½ t.	dried basil, crushed	2 mL
¾ t.	pepper	1 mL
dash	salt	dash
2 8 oz. pkg.	refrigerated crescent dinner rolls	2 240 g pkg.
1	egg white, beaten	1

Sauté onion in hot oil for 2 to 3 minutes until tender. Remove from heat. Add the remaining ingredients except crescent rolls and egg white. Mix the filling thoroughly. Separate crescent rolls into triangles. Cut each triangle in half lengthwise. Spread 1 T. (15 mL) of the filling, packed firmly, on each triangle. Roll up triangles, starting with the long end. Place on ungreased baking sheets. Brush with beaten egg white. Bake at 325°F (165°C) for 16 to 18 minutes until golden brown. Serve warm.

Yield: 32 appetizers

Exchange, 1 appetizer: ½ bread
Each serving contains: Calories: 30, Carbohydrates: 10 g

With the courtesy of Kretschmer Wheat Germ/Intentional Multifoods.

Spinach Dip

This dip has a very fresh flavor.

10 oz. pkg.	spinach, chopped	300 g pkg.
2 T.	onions, chopped finely	30 mL
8 oz.	Dannon plain lowfat yogurt	227 g
1 T.	mayonnaise	15 mL
½ t.	salt	2 mL
¼ t.	black pepper	1 mL

Stir all ingredients together until well blended.

Yield: 1½ c. (375 mL)

Exchange, 1¼ c. (60 mL): 1 fat
Each serving contains: Calories: 48, Carbohydrates: 10 g

Cheese Wafers

¾ c.	all-purpose-flour	190 mL
dash	cayenne pepper	dash
¼ c.	sesame seeds, toasted	60 mL
½ c.	margarine, softened	125 mL
2 c.	sharp cheddar cheese, shredded	500 mL
1 c.	All-Bran or Bran Buds cereal	250 mL

Stir together flour and pepper. Set aside. Measure sesame seeds into small shallow bowl. Beat margarine and cheese until very light and fluffy. Stir in the cereal. Add flour mixture, mixing until well combined. Drop by rounded teaspoonfuls into sesame seeds. Coat evenly. Place on ungreased baking sheets. Flatten with fork that has been dipped in flour. Bake at 350°F (175°C) for 12 minutes or until lightly browned around edges. Remove immediately from baking sheets. Cool on wire racks.

Yield: 5 dozen wafers

Exchange, 3 wafers: ½ bread, 1 medium-fat meat
Each serving contains: Calories: 120, Carbohydrates: 3 g

From Kellogg's Test Kitchens.

Cheesy Herb Crackers

⅔ c.	Kretschmer regular wheat germ	165 mL
⅓ c.	all-purpose flour	90 mL
½ t.	salt	2 mL
¾ c.	sharp cheddar cheese, grated	190 mL
¼ c.	margarine, softened	60 mL
1 T.	water	15 mL
2 T.	Kretschmer regular wheat germ	30 mL

Combine ⅔ c. (165 mL) wheat germ, flour and salt on waxed paper. Stir well to blend. Beat cheese and butter together until well-blended. Stir blended dry ingredients and water into cheese mixture. Mix well. Divide dough in half. Roll out each half on lightly floured, cloth- covered board to ¼ in. (4 mm) thickness. Cut with 2 in. (5 cm) cutter that has been dipped in flour. Place on ungreased baking sheets. Sprinkle lightly with the additional 2 T. (30 mL) wheat germ. Bake at 350° (175°C) for 8 to 10 minutes until very lightly browned. (Watch carefully to avoid overbrowning.) Remove from baking sheet. Cool on rack. Store in container with loosely fitting cover.

Yield: 4½ dozen crackers

Exchange, 4 crackers: 1 bread
Each serving contains: Calories: 68, Carbohydrates: 7 g

With the courtesy of Kretschmer Wheat Germ/International Multifoods.

Super Nachos

8 oz.	firm tofu (bean curd), drained and cut into 1 in. (2.5 cm) cubes	250 g
1½ c.	water	375 mL
¼ c.	onion, chopped	60 mL
2 cloves	garlic, minced	2 cloves
¾ c.	Health Valley Bellissimo pasta sauce	190 mL
dash	Tabasco sauce	dash
6 oz.	ground beef	180 g
½ c.	mushrooms, chopped	125 mL
2 t.	chili powder	10 mL
1 t.	paprika	5 mL
½ t.	ground cumin	2 mL
½ t.	oregano	2 mL
1 t.	Health Valley Instead of Salt steak & hamburger seasoning	5 mL
4	corn tortillas	4
4 oz.	cheddar cheese, grated	120 g
4 c.	lettuce, shredded	1 L
2 c.	tomatoes, diced	500 mL
1 c.	red pepper, chopped	250 mL
2 c.	green pepper, chopped	500 mL
	picante sauce	

In a small saucepan, combine tofu, 1 c. (250 mL) of the water, 2 T. (30 mL) of the chopped onion and garlic. Bring to a boil. Reduce heat and simmer 10 minutes. Drain off the water. Put the mixture in food processor. Add pasta sauce and process until smooth. Season with Tabasco sauce. Set aside.

Meanwhile, brown meat with chopped mushrooms and 1 T. (15 mL) of the chopped onions. Add seasonings and remaining water and simmer for 10 minutes or until water evaporates. On baking sheet, arrange tortillas in a single layer. Bake at 450°F (230°C) until crisp, about 4 minutes on each side. Preheat broiler. Spread on each tortilla ¼ of the tofu mixture, then ¼ of the seasoned beef, then ¼ of the grated cheese. Broil until cheese is bubbly, about 5 minutes. Place each tortilla on a separate plate. Surround each tortilla with ¼ of each vegetable: lettuce, tomatoes, onions, and red and green pepper. Serve picante sauce on the side.

Yield: 8 servings

Exchange, 1 serving: 1 bread, 1 high-fat meat
Each serving contains: Calories: 180, Carbohydrates: 12 g

From Health Valley Foods.

Party Starters

12	large mushrooms	12
dash	lemon juice	dash
2 T.	butter	30 mL
6½ oz. can	crab meat, drained and flaked	195 g can
¼ c.	La Choy water chestnuts, finely chopped	60 mL
1 T.	whole wheat bread crumbs	15 mL
1 T.	green onion, finely chopped	15 mL
1 t.	lemon juice	5 mL
1 t.	La Choy soy sauce	5 mL
1 T.	parsley, finely chopped	15 mL
1	egg, slightly beaten	1

Trim stems from mushrooms. Sprinkle caps with lemon juice. Finely chop the stems. Cook stems in butter for 2 minutes. Stir in the remaining ingredients, mixing well. Fill mushroom caps with mixture. Place in buttered 8 in. (20 cm) square pan. Bake at 350°F (175°C) for 20 minutes. Serve hot.

Yield: 12 appetizers

Exchange, 1 appetizer: ½ lean meat
Each serving contains: Calories: 29, Carbohydrates: 9 g

Hummus

1½ c.	chick peas, cooked and drained (liquid reserved)	375 mL
½ c.	tahini (ground sesame seeds)	125 mL
1 clove	garlic	1 clove
3 T.	lemon juice	45 mL
dash	cayenne pepper	dash
	chopped parsley for garnish	

In the bowl of a blender, combine chick peas, tahini, garlic, and lemon juice. Process until smooth. If mixture is too thick to blend well, add 1 T. (15 mL) of reserved chick pea cooking liquid. Sprinkle cayenne over top, garnish with parsley and serve with your favorite whole grain crackers.

Yield: 2 c. (500 mL)

Exchange, ¼ c. (60 mL): 1 medium-fat meat
Each serving contains: Calories: 80, Carbohydrates: 12 g

From Health Valley Foods.

Crunchy Bran Jumble

3 c.	Cracklin' Oat Bran cereal	750 mL
1 c.	salted peanuts	250 mL
1 c.	thin pretzel sticks	250 mL
⅓ c.	margarine, melted	90 mL
1 t.	Worcestershire sauce	5 mL
½ t.	seasoned salt	2 mL
1 T.	sesame seeds	15 mL

Measure cereal, peanuts and pretzels into 13 × 9 × 2 in. (33 × 23 × 5 cm) baking pan. Set aside. Stir together remaining ingredients. Pour over cereal mixture, stirring until well coated. Bake at 350°F (175°C) about 15 minutes. Do not stir. Cool in pan. Store in tightly covered container.

Yield: 5 cups (1¼ L)

Exchange, ¼ c. (60 mL) serving: 2 bread, 1½ fat
Each serving contains: Calories: 215, Carbohydrates: 20 g

From Kellogg's Test Kitchens.

Pizza Maria

60	Health Valley herb crackers	60
½ c.	Health Valley Bellissimo pasta sauce	125 mL
½ t.	Health Valley Instead of Salt vegetable seasoning	2 mL
½ t.	Health Valley Instead of Salt all-purpose seasoning	2 mL
1½ oz.	cheddar cheese, cut into ⅛ in. (3 mm) cubes	5 mL
	parsley sprouts for garnish	

Place crackers on cookie sheet. Mix pasta sauce with seasonings, drop ½ t. (1 mL) on each cracker, then top with 1 cheese cube. Bake at 400°F (200°C) for 5 minutes or until cheese melts. To serve, arrange on platter. Garnish with parsley sprigs. Serve at once.

Yield: 60 appetizer pizzas

Exchange, 2 appetizer pizzas: ½ bread
Each serving contains: Calories: 30, Carbohydrates: 5 g

From Health Valley Foods.

Spreads and Sauces

Raspberry Preserves

For this recipe, I substituted raspberries for Blueberry Preserves from The Complete Diabetic Cookbook *(Sterling Publishing Co., 1980). Preserves can also be made with blueberries and strawberries.*

1 c.	fresh or frozen unsweetened raspberries	250 mL
1 t.	low-calorie pectin	5 mL
1 t.	granulated sugar replacement	5 mL

Place raspberries in top of double boiler and cook over boiling water until soft and juicy. As they cook, crush berries against sides of double boiler. Add pectin and sugar replacement. Blend in thoroughly. Cook until medium thick.

Microwave: Place raspberries in glass bowl. Cook on High for 4 minutes until soft and juicy. Add pectin and sugar replacement. Blend thoroughly. Cook on High for 30 seconds.

Yield: ⅔ c. (180 mL)

Exchange, 2 T. (30 mL): ¼ fruit
Each serving contains: Calories: 7, Carbohydrates: 14 g

Wilted Relish

I like to serve this in a small serving bowl surrounded by Wasa crisp bread fiber. I cut each slice of the crisp bread into 6 cracker-type pieces.

1 c.	cabbage, finely chopped	250 mL
½ c.	cucumber, finely chopped	125 m
L½ c.	onion, finely chopped	125 mL
3 T.	salt	45 mL

Combine ingredients in a bowl or jar. Cover tightly. Shake well to cover vegetables with salt. Marinate at room temperature for at least 24 hours; shake several times. Drop mixture into a fine mesh strainer and thoroughly rinse with cool water. Place in bowl, cover tightly and refrigerate until completely chilled.

Yield: 1½ c. (250 mL)

Exchange: negligible
Each serving contains: Calories: negligible, Carbohydrates: 2 g

Hot South Seas Relish

1 c.	vinegar	250 mL
2 T.	chili powder	30 mL
1 t.	dry mustard	5 mL
dash	salt	dash
2	green tomatoes, chopped	2
1	green pepper, chopped	1
1 med	onion, chopped	1 med
½ t.	horseradish	2 mL

Heat vinegar, chili powder, mustard, and salt in a saucepan. Bring to boil and cook for 10 minutes. Place vegetables in bowl; pour hot sauce over entire mixture. Marinate at room temperature until cool. Serve or refrigerate.

Yield: 2 c. (500 mL)

Exchange, 1 T. (15 mL): negligible
Each serving contains: Calories: negligible, Carbohydrates: 1 g

Corn Relish

An old standby with lots of fiber.

1 c.	vinegar	250 mL
½ c.	granulated sugar replacement	125 mL
1 t.	dry mustard	5 mL
1 t.	salt	5 mL
¼ t.	turmeric	1 mL
2 c.	Green Giant whole kernel corn, drained	500 mL
¼ c.	cabbage, finely chopped	60 mL
½ c.	onion, chopped	125 mL
⅓ c.	red pepper, chopped	90 mL
¼ c.	green pepper, chopped	60 mL

Mix vinegar, sugar replacement, mustard, salt and turmeric in a saucepan; heat to the boiling point. Add vegetables. Boil until vegetables are tender. Pour into serving dish and refrigerate until completely chilled.

Yield: 3 c. (750 mL)

Exchange, ⅓ c. (90 mL): ½ bread
Each serving contains: Calories: 31, Carbohydrates: 31 g

Sweet and Sour Chutney

I like this Chutney with fowl or pork. It has a spicy bite to it.

3 c.	sour cherries	750 mL
3 c.	dark cherries	750 mL
2 c.	cider vinegar	500 mL
2 large	yellow onions, thinly sliced	2 large
1 c.	white raisins (sultanas)	250 mL
½ c.	fresh lemon juice	125 mL
3 T.	fresh ginger root, finely chopped	45 mL
½ t.	ground nutmeg	2 mL
½ t.	ground allspice	2 mL
¼ t.	ground red pepper	1 mL

Place cherries in a large enamel or glass saucepan. Crush slightly with a potato masher. Add remaining ingredients. Cook over medium heat until mixture boils. Reduce heat, simmer until mixture is very thick, about 2 to 4 hours. Stir occasionally to prevent sticking. Remove from heat; ladle into sterilized jars or freezer containers. Seal. Chutney keeps indefinitely in refrigerator or freezer.

Note: This recipe can be started on the burner and finished in a slow oven (275°F or 135°C). Or you can cook the mixture in a slow cooker on Low for 6 to 8 hours.

Yield: 4 c. (1 L)

Exchange, ¼ c. (60 mL): 2 fruit
Each serving contains: Calories: 78, Carbohydrates: 20 g

Tomato-Avocado Relish

This relish has a nice fresh flavor.

2 med.	tomatoes, chopped	2 med.
1	ripe avocado	1
½ t.	lemon juice	2 mL
	salt and pepper	

Place chopped tomatoes in a bowl. Peel avocado and chop into small pieces. Mix thoroughly with tomato. Stir in lemon juice. Place a plate or cover directly on top of tomato-avocado mixture. Weight the plate down into the mixture to be sure avocado is completely submersed in the liquid to prevent discoloration. Marinate for at least 6 hours. Drain thoroughly and chill. Before serving, sprinkle salt and pepper to taste.

Yield: 1 c. (250 mL)

Exchange, 1 T. (15 mL): 112 fat
Each serving contains: Calories: 26, Carbohydrates: 2 g

Apple-Grape Jelly

8 oz. bottle	baby apple-grape juice	237 g bottle	
4 t.	Slim Set jelling mix	20 mL	

Combine the juice and jelling mix in a medium saucepan. Using a wire whisk, whip until completely dissolved. Place pan over high heat and bring to the boil. Reduce heat and boil for 1 minute, stirring occasionally. Pour jelly into a serving dish or jar. Cool and refrigerate.

Yield: 1 c. (250 mL) or 15 servings

Exchange, 1 serving: ¼ fruit
Each serving contains: Calories: 9, Carbohydrates: 2 g

Peach and Clove Jelly

1 recipe	liquid from Peaches with Clove	1 recipe	
1 T.	Slim Set jelling mix	15 mL	
¼ t.	cider vinegar	1 mL	

Pour the liquid from Peaches with Clove into a measuring cup. Remove the cloves and add enough water to measure ¾ c. (190 mL). Pour into a small saucepan. Blend in the jelling mix and vinegar. Bring to the boil; reduce heat and boil for a minute. Pour into a clean glass jar or serving dish. Cool and refrigerate until jelled.

Yield: ⅔ c. (180 mL) or 10 servings

Exchange, 1 serving: negligible
Each serving contains: Calories: negligible, Carbohydrates: negligible

Fruit-Full Pineapple Preserves

If you like a lot of fruit in your preserves, this is the recipe for you.

20 oz. can	crushed pineapple, in its own juice	600 g can	
1 c.	apple juice	250 mL	
1 T.	Slim Set jelling mix	15 mL	

Drain pineapple by pouring contents of can into a strainer set over a large bowl. With the back of a spoon, push all of the juice out of the pineapple; reserve the pineapple. Pour pineapple juice into a medium saucepan. Add the apple juice; bring to the boil and reduce liquid to 1 c. (250 mL). Remove from heat and add the crushed pineapple and jelling mix. Stir thoroughly to dissolve jelling mix. Place pan back over heat and boil for 1 minute. Pour preserves into a serving dish or clean jars.

Yield: 2 c. (500 mL) or 30 servings

Exchange, 1 serving: ½ fruit
Each serving contains: Calories: 15, Carbohydrates: 4 g

Strawberry Jam

This soft jam is loaded with crushed strawberries.

¾ c.	boiling water	190 mL
½ lb.	frozen whole strawberries	250 g
2 T.	granulated sugar replacement	30 mL
4 t,	Slim Set jelling mix	20 mL
2	red food coloring drops (optional)	2

Pour boiling water over frozen strawberries in a medium saucepan. Allow to rest until strawberries thaw. With a wooden spoon, crush strawberries lightly on side of the saucepan. Using a potato masher or wire whisk, vigorously stir in the jelling mix and sugar replacement. Place sauce over high heat and bring to the boil; reduce heat but keep boiling, stirring, for 3 to 4 minutes. (Sugar replacement takes longer than sugar to form a jell.) Remove from heat and pour into jam jar or serving bowl.

Yield: 1⅔ c. (430 mL) or 20 servings

Exchange, 1 serving: negligible
Each serving contains: Calories: 3, Carbohydrates: 1 g

Mint Jelly

1 c.	apple juice	250 mL
⅓ c.	fresh mint leaves, crushed	90 mL
2 t.	lemon juice	10 mL
1	drop of green coloring	1
1 T.	Slim Set jelling mix	15 mL

Combine the apple juice and mint leaves in a saucepan. Boil for 2 minutes. Remove from heat and strain. Add the remaining ingredients. Stir thoroughly to dissolve jelling mix. Return to heat and boil for 1 minute. Strain into a serving dish or clean jar.

Yield: 1 c. (250 mL) or 15 servings

Exchange, 1 serving: ¼ fruit
Each serving contains: Calories: 8, Carbohydrates: 2 g

Orange Marmalade

1	orange	1	
¾ c.	water	190 mL	
2 T.	granulated sugar replacement	30 mL	
2 t.	Slim Set jelling mix	10 mL	

Peel the orange and chop the peel into small slivers. Pour the water in medium saucepan; add the slivers. Bring to the boil; reduce heat and simmer for 10 minutes. Squeeze the orange; pour the orange juice into a measuring cup. Add the orange peel, the cooking liquid and enough water to make 1 c. (250 mL). Pour the mixture back into the saucepan. Using a potato masher or wire whisk, add the jelling mix and sugar replacement, stirring until dissolved. Place the saucepan over high heat and bring to the boil; reduce heat but keep boiling and stirring for 2 to 3 minutes. Remove from heat and allow to rest to make sure it is going to jell; or pour into a jam jar or small bowl and allow to completely set.

Yield: ⅔ c. (180 mL) or 10 servings

Exchange, 1 serving: negligible
Each serving contains: Calories: 4, Carbohydrates: 1 g

Daiquiri Jelly

6 oz. can	frozen daiquiri mix, thawed	177 g can	
¼ c.	apple juice	60 mL	
½ c.	water	125 mL	
1 T.	granulated sugar replacement	15 mL	
2 T.	Slim Set jelling mix	30 mL	
1 T.	rum flavoring	15 mL	

Combine the daiquiri mix, apple juice, water, sugar replacement, and jelling mix in a saucepan. Stir until completely dissolved. Place saucepan over medium heat; cook and stir to the boiling point. Reduce heat and boil for a minute. Pour into glass jar or serving dish and allow to set.

Yield: 1½ c. (375 mL) or 22 servings

Exchange, 1 serving: ⅛ fruit
Each serving contains: Calories: 22, Carbohydrates: 5 g

Hot Tomato Jam

If you like hot jam, this one has a real kick.

1 c.	tomato juice	250 mL
½	bay leaf, crushed	½
½ t.	hot red pepperflakes	2 mL
⅛ t.	Tone's ground mace	½ mL
⅛ t.	onion, minced	½ mL
⅓ c.	apple juice	90 mL
4 t.	Slim Set jelling mix	20 mL

Combine the tomato juice, bay leaf, hot pepper, mace, and onion in a saucepan. Bring to the boil; reduce heat and simmer for 7 minutes. Remove bay leaf. Add apple juice and jelling mix. With a wire whisk, stir to dissolve jelling mix. Bring back to the boil and boil for a minute. Pour into serving dish or clean jar and allow to set.

Yield: 1 c. (250 mL) or 15 servings

Exchange, 1 serving: negligible
Each serving contains: Calories: 6, Carbohydrates: 1 g

Sweet Cherry Jam

1 c.	frozen sweet cherries, thawed	250 mL
½ c.	apple juice	125 mL
½ c.	water	125 mL
2 T.	granulated sugar replacement	30 mL
4 t.	Slim Set jelling mix	20 mL
¼ t.	unsweetened wild cherry drink mix	1 mL

Mash the sweet cherries with a potato masher. Pour cherries and cherry liquid into a saucepan. Add the remaining ingredients and stir to completely dissolve jelling mix. Place over medium heat and cook, stirring, until the mixture boils. Reduce heat and boil for a minute. Pour into a glass jar or serving dish and allow to set.

Yield: 1½ c. (375 mL) or 22 servings

Exchange, 1 serving: ¼ fruit
Each serving contains: Calories: 7, Carbohydrates: 2 g

Perfect Blueberry Jam

1 c.	apple juice	250 mL
1 c.	frozen blueberries	250 mL
2 t.	Slim Set jelling mix	10 mL

Pour apple juice over blueberries in a bowl. Cover and allow to sit at room temperature for at least 8 hours or overnight. Drain the blueberry liquid into a saucepan; reserve the blueberries. Add the jelling mix to the liquid; stir to dissolve. Place saucepan over medium heat; cook and stir until mixture boils. Reduce heat and boil for 1 minute. Remove saucepan from heat and stir in the berries. Return to heat and bring back to the boil. Stir and boil for 30 seconds. Pour into a glass jar or serving dish and allow to set.

Yield: 1½ c. (375 mL) or 22 servings

Exchange, 1 serving: ¼ fruit
Each serving contains: Calories: 10, Carbohydrates: 3 g

White Grape Jelly

1⅓ c.	white grape juice	340 mL
1 T.	Slim Set jelling mix	15 mL

In a saucepan, bring the juice to the boil; simmer until juice is reduced to 1 c. (250 mL). Remove from heat and add the jelling mix. Stir with a wire whisk to dissolve. Return to heat and boil for a minute. Pour in a serving dish or clean jar. Chill.

Yield: 1 c. (250 mL) or 15 servings

Exchange, 1 serving: ⅓ fruit
Each serving contains: Calories: 12, Carbohydrates: 3 g

Grapefruit-Grape Jelly

¾ c.	grapefruit juice	190 mL
⅓ c.	white grape juice	90 mL
2 t.	granulated fructose	10 mL
4 t.	Slim Set jelling mix	20 mL

Combine the juices and fructose in a saucepan. Simmer for 5 minutes; remove pan from heat. Add the jelling mix and stir to dissolve. Return to heat and bring to the boil; boil for a minute. Pour into a serving dish or clean jar and allow to set.

Yield: 1 c. (250 mL) or 15 servings

Exchange, 1 serving: ⅓ fruit
Each serving contains: Calories: 11, Carbohydrates: 3 g

Sour Cherry Jam

1 c.	frozen sour cherries, thawed	250 mL
¾ c.	water	190 mL
3 T.	granulated sugar replacement	45 mL
1 T.	Slim Set jelling mix	15 mL

Using a wire strainer, drain liquid of the sour cherries into a saucepan. With the back of a spoon, squeeze any remaining liquid from the cherries; reserve the cherries. Add remaining ingredients to the cherry liquid. Stir to completely dissolve the jelling mix. Place saucepan over medium heat; cook and stir until the mixture boils. Reduce heat and boil for a minute. Allow to cool for 5 minutes. Stir reserved cherries into the cherry syrup. Pour into glass jar or serving dish to set.

Yield: 1 c. (250 mL) or 15 servings

Exchange, 1 serving: ¼ fruit
Each serving contains: Calories: 7, Carbohydrates: 2 g

Red Currant Jelly

From the Diabetic Gourmet Cookbook *(Sterling Publishing Co., 1986).*

3 qts.	fresh currants	3 L
1 c.	water	250 mL
1 T.	fresh squeezed lemon juice	15 mL
3 to 4	red food coloring drops	3 to 4
½ c.	granulated sugar replacement	125 mL
1 pkg.	Slim Set fruit pectin	1 pkg.
	paraffin (optional)	

In a blender or food processor, crush the currants. Pour into a large saucepan. Add the water and bring to the boil. Reduce heat, cover, and simmer for 15 minutes; cool slightly. Pour mixture into jelly cloth or bag. Squeeze out juice into a large saucepan. Add the food coloring, sugar replacement, and jelling mix; stir to completely dissolve. Place over high heat and bring to the boil. Boil hard for 2 minutes, stirring constantly. Remove from heat and skim any foam from surface. Pour into jelly glasses, leaving ½ in. (1.25 cm) space at top for sealing. Seal with hot paraffin or sealing lid.

Yield: 4 c. (1 L) or 30 servings

Exchange, 1 serving: ¼ fruit
Each serving contains: Calories: 8, Carbohydrates: 1 g

Citrus Wine Sauce

This sauce has the tartness of lemons and limes, mellowed out by port wine.

1	orange	1
1	lemon	1
1	lime	1
½ c.	Red Currant Jelly	125 mL
1 c.	port wine	250 mL
1 t.	dry mustard	5 mL
1 t.	cornstarch	5 mL
½ t.	ginger	2 mL

Squeeze the juice from the orange, lemon, and lime; strain and set aside. Remove the white membrane from the fruit. Cut the skins of half of the orange, lemon, and lime into julienne strips. Place strips in a small saucepan and cover with water. Bring to the boil and simmer for 10 minutes; drain thoroughly. Set strips aside. Melt the currant jelly in the saucepan over low heat. Combine juices, wine, mustard, cornstarch, and ginger in a bowl. Stir until completely blended and the cornstarch dissolves. Add to the jelly in saucepan. Cook and stir until mixture is clear and slightly thickened. Add fruit strips and cook 2 minutes longer.

Yield: 2 c. (500 mL) or 15 servings

Exchange, 1 serving: ½ fruit
Each serving contains: Calories: 19, Carbohydrates: 4 g

Hot Barbecue Sauce

1 c.	canned tomato sauce	250 mL
¼ c.	lemon juice	60 mL
2	garlic cloves, minced	2
2 T.	soy sauce	30 mL
2 T.	steak sauce	30 mL
2 T.	chili powder	30 mL
1 T.	granulated brown sugar replacement	15 mL

Combine all ingredients in a saucepan. Cook and stir 10 minutes.

Yield: 1¼ c. (310 mL) or 10 servings

Exchange, 1 serving: ½ fruit
Each serving contains: Calories: 19, Carbohydrates: 5 g

Tomato Jam

¾ c.	tomato juice	190 mL
2	whole cloves	2
½	bay leaf, crushed	½
⅛ t.	onion, minced	½ mL
⅓ c.	apple juice	90 mL
4 t.	Slim Set jelling mix	20 mL

Combine the tomato juice, cloves, bay leaf, and onion in a saucepan. Bring to the boil; reduce heat and simmer for 3 minutes. Remove cloves and bay leaf. Add the apple juice and jelling mix. Stir with a wire whisk to dissolve the mix. Bring mixture back to the boil and boil for a minute. Remove from heat and pour into serving dish or clean jar.

Yield: 1 c. (250 mL) or 15 servings

Exchange, 1 serving: negligible
Each serving contains: Calories: 3, Carbohydrates: negligible

Blueberry Relish

½ c.	orange juice	125 mL
¼ c.	apple juice	60 mL
½ c.	small shallots, peeled	125 mL
1 t.	mustard seed	5 mL
¼ t.	Tone's ground nutmeg	1 mL
⅛ t.	Tone's ground cloves	½ mL
1 c.	blueberries	250 mL

In a saucepan, heat the juices, shallots, mustard seed, nutmeg, and cloves to the boiling point. Cover and simmer for 5 minutes. Remove from heat and cool to room temperature. Fold in the blueberries. Cover and chill thoroughly.

Yield: 8 servings

Exchange, 1 serving: ½ fruit
Each serving contains: Calories: 22, Carbohydrates: 5 g

Pear Relish

4	pears	4
2	lemons	2
1	orange	1
¼ c.	port	60 mL
¼ c.	granulated sugar replacement	60 mL
dash	ground ginger, nutmeg, and cloves	dash

Peel, core, and chop the pear. With a zester or sharp knife, cut peel strips from the lemons and orange; chop finely. Squeeze juice from the lemons and orange. Combine the juices, peels, and remaining ingredients in a saucepan. Bring to the boil, reduce heat, and simmer until pears are tender but still hold their shape. Refrigerate and chill thoroughly.

Yield: 12 servings

Exchange, 1 serving: 1 fruit
Each serving contains: Calories: 42, Carbohydrates: 10 g

Lemon-Herb Spread

½ c.	low-calorie margarine	125 mL
1 t.	lemon juice	5 mL
2 t.	lemon zest	10 mL
1 t.	chive, chopped	5 mL
½ t.	parsley, finely snipped	2 mL

In a bowl, cream the margarine. Very slowly beat in the lemon juice. Stir in the lemon zest, chive, and parsley. Refrigerate overnight.

Yield: ½ c. (125 mL) or 8 servings

Exchange, 1 serving: 1 fat
Each serving contains: Calories: 42, Carbohydrates: negligible

Orange Spread

This can be made with any of the available unsweetened soft-drink mixes. Orange Spread looks particularly nice on a holiday brunch table.

3 oz. pkg.	cream cheese	85 g pkg.
1 T.	skim milk	15 mL
1 env.	Equal low-calorie sweetener	1 env.
⅛ t.	orange unsweetened soft-drink mix	½ mL

Beat cream cheese and milk in a bowl until fluffy. Add the sweetener and soft-drink mix. Spoon into a serving dish.

Yield: 7 servings

Exchange, 1 serving: 1 fat
Each serving contains: Calories: 43, Carbohydrates: negligible

Bit o' Lemon

3 oz. pkg.	cream cheese	85 g pkg.
1 T.	lemon juice	15 mL
1 drop	yellow food coloring	1 drop
1 t.	lemon zest, chopped fine	5 mL
2 env.	Equal low-calorie sweetener	2 env.

In a bowl, whip the cream cheese, lemon juice, and food coloring until fluffy. Beat in the lemon zest and sweetener. Spoon into a serving dish.

Yield: 7 servings

Exchange, 1 serving: 1 fat
Each serving contains: Calories: 42, Carbohydrates: negligible

Chocolate-Flavored Spread

A chocolate lover's dream come true.

3 oz. pkg.	cream cheese	85 g pkg.
4 t.	skim milk	20 mL
2 T.	chocolate-flavored drink mix	30 mL
½ t.	cocoa, sifted	2 mL

Beat the cream cheese and skim milk in a bowl until fluffy. Slowly beat in the drink mix and cocoa.

Yield: 8 servings

Exchange, 1 serving: 1 fat
Each serving contains: Calories: 41, Carbohydrates: 2 g

Nutty Spread

2 T.	almonds	30 mL
3 oz. pkg.	cream cheese	85 g pkg.
2 t.	skim milk	10 mL
1 t.	vanilla extract	5 mL
1 t.	butternut flavoring	5 mL

Toast and crush the almonds; set aside. In a bowl, whip the cream cheese and skim milk until fluffy. Beat in the flavorings. Stir in the crushed almonds. Cover tightly and refrigerate overnight before serving.

Yield: 8 servings

Exchange, 1 serving: 1 fat
Each serving contains: Calories: 43, Carbohydrates: negligible

Norwegian Spread

3 oz. pkg.	cream cheese	85 g pkg.
1 T.	brandy flavoring	15 mL
¼ t.	ground cardamom	1 mL
¼ t.	lemon rind, grated	1 mL
2 env.	Equal low-calorie sweetener	2 env.

Whip the cream cheese and brandy in a bowl until fluffy. Beat in the cardamom, lemon rind, and sweetener. Spoon into a serving dish.

Yield: 7 servings

Exchange, 1 serving: 1 fat
Each serving contains: Calories: 45, Carbohydrates: 2 g

Vanilla Spread

This spread has a clean, fresh flavor.

3 oz. pkg.	cream cheese	85 g pkg.
4 t.	skim milk	20 mL
1 env.	Equal low-calorie sweetener	1 env.
2 in.	vanilla bean	5 cm

Whip cream cheese and skim milk in a bowl until fluffy. Beat in the sweetener. Pull the vanilla bean down the edge of a sharp knife; cut bean into 4 pieces. Bury the vanilla pieces in the whipped cheese. Cover tightly and refrigerate for at least 3 days. Remove vanilla bean before serving.

Yield: 7 servings

Exchange, 1 serving: 1 fat
Each serving contains: Calories: 42, Carbohydrates: negligible

Fresh Dill Mayonnaise

1	egg	1
2 T.	cider vinegar	30 mL
1 T.	chive, finely snipped	15 mL
2 t.	dillseed, crushed	10 mL
1 t.	Dijon-style mustard	5 mL
1 t.	salt	5 mL
1 c.	vegetable oil	250 mL

Break egg into a blender; add the vinegar, chive, dillseed, mustard, and salt. Whip on low speed until blended. Remove the hole cover in the blender lid. While blender is running, very slowly pour in the oil. Return hole cover to container top. Whip for 3 more minutes.

Yield: 1¼ c. (310 mL)

Exchange, ¼ c. (60 mL): 8 fats
Each serving contains: Calories: 385, Carbohydrates: negligible

Madeira Margarine

½ c.	low-calorie margarine	125 mL
2 T.	cream cheese	30 mL
1 T.	Madeira	15 mL

Cream the margarine and cream cheese in a bowl until fluffy. Very slowly beat in the Madeira. Refrigerate for at least 6 hours before serving.

Yield: ⅔ c. (180 mL) or 10 servings

Exchange, 1 serving: 1 fat
Each serving contains: Calories: 43, Carbohydrates: negligible

Garlic Margarine

I suggest using this spread at a late brunch when serving French bread and beef or ham.

4	garlic cloves	4
⅓ c.	water	90 mL
½ c.	low-calorie margarine	125 mL

Peel the garlic and boil in the water for 3 minutes; drain and crush. Meanwhile, cream the margarine in a bowl. Add the crushed garlic. Refrigerate overnight in a tightly covered glass container.

Yield: ½ c. (125 mL) or 8 servings

Exchange, 1 serving: 1 fat
Each serving contains: Calories: 42, Carbohydrates: negligible

Quick Tomato Sauce

1 c.	catsup	250 mL
½ c.	chili sauce	125 mL
2 T.	Worcestershire sauce	30 mL
1 T.	water	15 mL
1 t.	Dijon-style mustard	5 mL
1 t.	yellow mustard	5 mL
1 t.	cider vinegar	5 mL
½ t.	black pepper	2 mL
⅛ t.	mace	½ mL

Combine all ingredients in a bowl; stir to completely blend. Store in airtight container. Heat before using.

Yield: 1½ c. (375 mL) or 22 servings

Exchange, 1 serving: 1 vegetable
Each serving contains: Calories: 20, Carbohydrates: 5 g

Salsa

2 T.	olive oil	30 mL
1	garlic clove, chopped	1
3 T.	onion, chopped	45 mL
3	green chilies, chopped	3
3	medium tomatoes, peeled and chopped	3
1 t.	Tone's ground oregano	5 mL
	salt	

Heat the olive oil in a nonstick saucepan. Add the garlic, onion, and chilies. Cook until onion is translucent. Add the tomatoes, oregano, and salt to taste; stir to blend. Simmer for 10 minutes.

Yield: 6 servings

Exchange, 1 serving: ½ vegetable, 1 fat
Each serving contains: Calories: 60, Carbohydrates: 3 g

Newburg Sauce

Newburg sauce usually combines heavy cream and egg yolks, flavored with a wine. To cut calories and exchanges, I've developed this recipe for you.

¼ c.	sherry	60 mL
⅓ c.	evaporated skim milk	90 mL
⅓ c.	skim milk	90 mL
2 t.	cornstarch	10 mL
2	egg yolks, slightly beaten	2
¼ t.	salt	1 mL
⅛ t.	mace	½ mL
dash	white pepper	dash

Pour sherry in a small saucepan and heat to reduce to half the amount; set aside. Pour evaporated milk in the top of a double boiler. Heat over simmering water. Blend the skim milk and cornstarch in a cup; stir into the evaporated milk. Pour a small amount of warmed milk into the egg yolks; return the mixture to double boiler. Add salt, mace, and white pepper. Cook, stirring until thickened.

Yield: ¾ c. (190 mL) or 5 servings

Exchange, 1 serving: ⅓ lowfat milk
Each serving contains: Calories: 46, Carbohydrates: 4 g

Apple-Raisin Sauce

3	apples	3
½ c.	water	125 mL
¼ c.	raisins	60 mL
2 t.	cornstarch	10 mL

Peel, core, and chop the apples. Combine apples, water, and raisins in a saucepan. Heat to the boiling point. Remove pan from heat. Cover and allow to cool to room temperature. Stir in the cornstarch. Return pan to heat and cook until mixture is clear. Serve hot or cold.

Yield: 6 servings

Exchange, 1 serving: ¼ fruit
Each serving contains: Calories: 24, Carbohydrates: 8 g

Spanish Orange Sauce

1	slice bacon	1
1	onion slice, finely chopped	1
3	beef bouillon cubes	3
2 c.	water, boiling	500 mL
1 c.	orange juice	250 mL
¼ c.	port	60 mL

Fry bacon and onions in a skillet until brown; crumble the bacon. Dissolve bouillon in the boiling water. Add remaining ingredients to skillet. Heat to the boiling point and reduce liquid to 3 c. (750 mL). Serve hot.

Yield: 3 c. (750 mL) or 10 servings

Exchange, 1 serving: ½ fruit
Each serving contains: Calories: 20, Carbohydrates: 4 g

Sweet Barbecue Sauce

½ c.	Orange Marmalade	125 mL	
¼ c.	dry sherry	60 mL	
¼ c.	water	60 mL	
3 T.	soy sauce	45 mL	
2	garlic cloves, minced	2	
1 t.	Tone's ground ginger	5 mL	
1 t.	ground coriander	5 mL	

Combine all ingredients in a saucepan. Cook and stir over medium heat for 5 minutes.

Yield: 1¼ c. (310 mL) or 15 servings

Exchange, 1 serving: negligible
Each serving contains: Calories: 4, Carbohydrates: 1 g

Tomato Sauce

firm red tomatoes (or canned tomatoes without seasonings)

Quarter the tomatoes. Place in large kettle. Push down with hands or back of spoon to render some juice. Bake at 325°F (165°C) until soft pulp remains. Spoon into blender. Blend until smooth. Seal in sterilized jars or freeze.

Creole Sauce

28 oz. can	tomato	800 g can	
1 med.	onion (chopped)	1 med.	
1	green pepper	1	
1 t.	paprika	5 mL	
¼ t.	marjoram	2 mL	
	salt and pepper to taste		

Combine all ingredients and cook over low heat for 25 minutes.

Yield: 2 c. (500 mL)

Exchange, 1 serving: 1 vegetable
Each serving contains: Calories: 25, Carbohydrates: 9 g

Italian Tomato Sauce

6	tomatoes, peeled and cubed	6	
¼ c.	green pepper, chopped	60 mL	
¼ c.	onion, chopped	60 mL	
2 T.	parsley, chopped	30 mL	
1 T.	lemon juice	15 mL	
dash each	oregano, marjoram, thyme, crushed bay leaf, horseradish	dash each	
	salt and pepper to taste		

Combine all ingredients in blender. Whip until smooth. Add enough water to make 2 c. (500 mL).

Yield: 2 c. (500 mL)

Exchange, 1 serving: 2 vegetable
Each serving contains: Calories: 10, Carbohydrates: 7 g

Chili Sauce

28 oz. can	tomatoes	800 g can
1 med.	apple	1 med.
1 med.	onion	1 med.
1 small	green pepper	1 small
1 c.	wine vinegar	250 mL
½ c.	sugar replacement	125 mL
1 T.	salt	15 mL
½ t.	ground clove	3 mL
½ t.	cinnamon	3 mL
½ t.	nutmeg	3 mL

Mash tomatoes; pour into kettle. Grind together apple, onion, green pepper, and vinegar. Add to kettle; cook until thick. Remove from heat. Add sugar replacement and seasonings. Return to heat; cook 5 minutes, stirring constantly.

Yield: 2 c. (500 mL)

Exchange, ½ c. (125 mL): 1 fruit
Each serving contains: Calories: 45, Carbohydrates: 14 g

Variations for Italian Dressing

To ½ c. (125 mL) low calorie Italian dressing, add:

Anchovy

Mash 1 oz. (30 g) anchovy fillets.

Exchange: 1 meat

Bacon

Grind 1 T. (15 mL) Bacos; allow to mellow several hours.

Exchange: ½ fat

Parmesan

Add 1 T. (15 mL) Parmesan cheese; allow to mellow several hours.

Exchange: ⅛ meat

Tomato

Add 1 T. (15 mL) tomato purée.

Wine

Add 1 T. (15 mL) dry white or red wine.
Each serving contains: Calories: 24, Carbohydrates: negligible

Variations for French Dressing

To ½ c. (125 mL) low calorie French dressing, add:

Avocado

Mash avocado to make 2 T. (30 mL).

Exchange: 1 fat

Cheese

Mash bleu cheese or Roquefort cheese to make 2 T. (30 mL).

Exchange: ¼ meat

Egg

Crumble 1 hard-cooked egg yolk; combine with dash of hot pepper sauce.

Exchange: 1 meat

Lemon

Add 1 T. (15 mL) lemon juice.

Soy Sauce

Add 1 T. (15 mL) soy sauce.
Each serving contains: Calories: 100, Carbohydrates: 0 g

Variations for Bleu Cheese Dressing

To ½ c. (125 mL) low calorie bleu cheese dressing, add:

Anchovy

Mash 1 oz. (30 g) anchovy fillets.

Exchange: 1 meat

Bacon

Grind 1 T. (15 mL) Bacos; allow to mellow several hours.

Exchange: ½ fat

Chive

Chop chives to make 2 T. (30 mL); allow to mellow several hours.

Herb

Combine 1 t. (5 mL) each ground parsley, chives, and marjoram.

Each serving contains: Calories: 56, Carbohydrates: 0 g

Salad Dressing

1½ c.	cold water	375 mL
¼ c.	vinegar	60 mL
1½ t.	salt	7 mL
1 t.	yellow mustard	5 mL
2 T.	flour	30 mL
1	egg, well beaten	1
¼ c.	sugar replacement	60 mL
2 t.	margarine	10 mL

Combine cold water, vinegar, salt, mustard, flour, and egg in top of double boiler. Stir to blend. Cook until thick. Remove from heat. Add sugar replacement and margarine. Stir to blend.

Yield: 1 c. (250 mL)

Exchange, 2 T. (30 mL): ½ vegetable, ½ fat
Each serving contains: Calories: 31, Carbohydrates: 16 g

Sweet Yogurt Dressing

1 c.	low-calorie yogurt	250 mL
½ t.	mace	2 mL
2 t.	sugar replacement	10 mL
dash	salt	dash
½ c.	low-calorie whipped topping, prepared	125 mL

Drain yogurt; beat until smooth and fluffy. Add mace, sugar replacement, and salt. Beat until blended. Fold in prepared whipped topping. Place in refrigerator until ready to serve. Good on fruit or gelatin salads.

Yield: 1 c. (250 mL)

Exchange, 1 serving: 1 milk
Each serving contains: Calories: 100, Carbohydrates: 8 g

Herb Yogurt Dressing

1 c.	low-calorie yogurt	250 mL
2 T.	vinegar	30 mL
1 t.	onion, grated	5 mL
1 t.	celery seeds	5 mL
1 t.	dry mustard	5 mL
1 t.	salt	5 mL
½ t.	thyme	2 mL
	salt and pepper to taste	

Beat yogurt until smooth. Add remaining ingredients; blend well. Cover. Allow to rest at least 1 hour before serving.

Yield: 1 c. (250 mL)

Exchange, 1 serving: 1 milk
Each serving contains: Calories: 86, Carbohydrates: 2 g

Bay Salad Dressing

3 T.	liquid shortening	45 mL
½ c.	onion, finely chopped	125 mL
2 T.	fresh parsley, finely chopped	30 mL
2 T.	celery with leaves, finely chopped	30 mL
1	bay leaf	1
dash each	thyme, mace, rosemary	dash each
2 T.	white wine	30 mL
1 c.	yogurt	250 mL
2 T.	skim milk	30 mL
	salt and pepper to taste	

Heat liquid shortening in small skillet. Add onion, parsley, celery, and seasonings. Cook over very low heat, stirring constantly, for 15 minutes. *Do not allow vegetables to burn.*

Set aside to cool. Add wine; stir to mix. Allow to rest 30 minutes. Strain, reserving liquid. Beat yogurt with skim milk. Continue beating, adding wine liquid. Add salt and pepper. Blend.

Yield: 1½ c. (375 mL)

Exchange, ¼ c. (60 mL): ½ vegetable, ½ fat
Each serving contains: Calories: 44, Carbohydrates: 5 g

Tangy Barbecue Sauce

1 c.	Chili Sauce	250 mL
2 T.	lemon juice	30 mL
1 T.	Worcestershire sauce	15 mL
1 t.	horseradish	5 mL
1 t.	Dijon mustard	5 mL
1 T.	brown sugar replacement	15 mL
dash each	hot pepper sauce, soy sauce, salt, pepper	dash each

Combine all ingredients; stir to blend well.

Yield: 1 c. (250 mL)

Exchange, 1 serving: 2 fruit
Each serving contains: Calories: 90, Carbohydrates: 16 g

Hollandaise Sauce

1	egg yolk	1
1 T.	evaporated (regular or skim) milk	15 mL
⅛ t.	salt	1 mL
dash	cayenne pepper	dash
1 T.	lemon juice	15 mL
1 T.	margarine	15 mL

In the top of a double boiler, heat egg yolk, evaporated milk, salt, and cayenne pepper until thick. Place over hot water. Beat lemon juice into egg mixture until thick and creamy. Remove double boiler from heat. Add margarine, 1 t. (5 mL) at a time. Beat until margarine is melted and blended in.

Yield: ½ c. (125 mL)

Exchange, 1 serving: ½ high-fat meat, 3 fat
Each serving contains: Calories: 213, Carbohydrates: 0 g

White Sauce

2 T.	margarine	30 mL
1½ T.	flour	25 mL
¼ t.	salt	1 mL
1 t.	Worcestershire sauce	5 mL
1 c.	skim milk	250 mL

Melt margarine. Add flour, salt, and Worcestershire sauce. Blend thoroughly. Add skim milk. Cook until slightly thickened.

Yield: 1 c. (250 mL)

Exchange, ½ c. (125 mL): 1 bread, ½ high-fat meat
Each serving contains: Calories: 190, Carbohydrates: 19 g

Orange Sauce

½ t.	cornstarch	2 mL
2 T.	cold water	30 mL
½ c.	orange juice concentrate	125 mL
2 t.	unsweetened orange drink mix	10 mL

Dissolve cornstarch in cold water. Add orange juice concentrate and drink mix. Cook over low heat until slightly thickened. Use as glaze on poultry or pork.

Yield: ½ c. (125 mL)

Exchange, 1 serving: 1 fruit
Each serving contains: Calories: 52, Carbohydrates: 14 g

Teriyaki Marinade

⅓ c.	soya sauce	80 mL
2 T.	wine vinegar	30 mL
2 T.	sugar replacement	30 mL
2 t.	salt	10 mL
1 t.	ginger, powdered	5 mL
½ t.	garlic powder	2 mL

Blend well.

Each serving contains: Carbohydrates: 8 g

Beverages

Old-Fashioned Hot Chocolate

2 oz.	baking chocolate	60 g
1 c.	water	250 mL
dash	salt	dash
3 c.	skim milk	750 mL
2 T.	liquid sugar replacement	30 mL

Cook chocolate and water over low heat until chocolate is melted. Add salt and cook for 2 minutes. Gradually stir in milk and stir constantly. When mixture is piping hot, remove from heat and add liquid sugar replacement. Beat until frothy. Serve in warmed mugs.

Yield: 4 servings

Exchange, 1 serving: ¾ nonfat milk, 2 fat
Each serving contains: Calories: 130, Carbohydrates: 28 g

Cinnamon-Chocolate Drink

Perfect to drink on a cold winter night.

4 c.	skim milk	1 L
2 oz.	semisweet chocolate	60 g
2	cinnamon sticks	2
1 t.	vanilla	5 mL

Combine milk, semisweet chocolate and cinnamon sticks in saucepan. Cook and stir over low heat until chocolate melts. Remove from heat and stir in vanilla. Remove cinnamon sticks. Serve in warmed mugs.

Yield: 4 servings

Exchange, 1 serving: 1 high-fat milk
Each serving contains: Calories: 170, Carbohydrates: 24 g

Instant Drink Mix

2 c.	dry milk	500 mL
¼ c.	cocoa	60 mL
4 pkg.	aspartame sweetener	4 pkg.

Combine all ingredients in electric blender. Blend at high speed to thoroughly mix.

Cold: Pour ice water into a tall glass. Add 3 T. (45 mL) instant drink mix and stir briskly to dissolve completely.

Hot: Place 3 T. (45 mL) of instant drink mix in a cup. Add hot water and stir to dissolve.

Yield: 1½ c. (375 mL)

Exchange, 3 T. (45 mL): 3¾ lowfat milk
Each serving contains: Calories: 62, Carbohydrates: 28 g

If milk is used, add milk exchange and calories.

Instant Banana Shake

1	ripe banana	1
3 T.	Instant Drink Mix	45 mL
1 c.	2% milk	250 mL

Slice banana into a bowl and beat until creamy. Beat in drink mix. Add milk and mix thoroughly. Serve at once.

Yield: 2 servings

Exchange, 1 serving: ¾ lowfat milk, 1 fruit
Each serving contains: Calories: 143, Carbohydrates: 35 g

Instant Ice Cream Soda

So-o-o-o good.

3 T.	Instant Drink Mix	45 mL
¼ c.	cold water	60 mL
½ c.	vanilla ice cream, softened	125 mL
½ can	cold diet soda	½ can

Combine drink mix and water in a tall glass, stir to completely blend. Add ice cream and fill with diet soda.

Yield: 1 serving

Exchange, 1 serving: 1 bread, 1 lowfat milk
Each serving contains: Calories: 200, Carbohydrates: 44 g

Mocha Drink

1 c.	water	250 mL
2 T.	instant coffee	30 mL
2 oz.	baking chocolate	60 g
dash	salt	dash
3 c.	skim milk	750 mL
5 pkg.	granulated sugar replacement	5 pkg.

Combine water, instant coffee, baking chocolate and salt in saucepan. Cook and stir over low heat until chocolate melts. Gradually add milk, stirring constantly. When piping hot, remove from heat. Stir in sugar replacement. Serve in cups or mugs. (Optional: Top each cup with 1 T. (15 mL) prepared nondairy whipped topping.)

Yield: 4 servings

Exchange, 1 serving: ¾ nonfat milk, 2 fat
Each serving contains: Calories: 130, Carbohydrates: 17 g

Exchange, 1 serving with topping: ¾ no-fat milk, 2 fat
Each serving contains: Calories: 138, Carbohydrates: 17 g

Crème de Cacao-Cola

My personal favorite after-dinner drink.

1 T.	crème de cacao	15 mL
¾ c.	diet cola soda	190 mL
	ice	

Combine all ingredients in glass, stir to blend.

Yield: 1 drink

Exchange, 1 serving: ¼ bread
Each serving contains: Calories: 15, Carbohydrates: 11 g

Chocolate Eggnog

1	egg, beaten (see note below)	1
3 T.	Chocolate Whipped Topping	45 mL
dash	salt	dash
¾ c.	skim milk	190 mL
¼ t.	vanilla extract	2 mL

Combine all ingredients in tall glass or mixing bowl. Beat to blend. Serve at once.

Yield: 1 serving

Exchange, 1 serving: 1 medium-fat meat, ¾ medium-fat milk
Each serving contains: Calories: 175, Carbohydrates: 45 g

Note: For a creamier eggnog: Separate egg and beat yolk with all the ingredients. Beat egg white separately until stiff. Then fold egg white into eggnog mixture.

Vanilla Shake

As good as the ones in your favorite fast-food restaurant.

½ c.	skim milk	125 mL
1 c.	frozen fat-free non-dairy whipped topping	250 mL
1 T.	vanilla extract	15 mL
½ c.	crushed ice	125 mL

Place all the ingredients in a blender or food processor. Process at the highest speed until liquefied. Serve immediately.

Yield: 1 serving

Exchange, 1 serving: 1½ starch/bread
Each serving contains: Calories: 165, Total fat: 0 g, Carbohydrates: 26 g, Protein: 4 g, Sodium: 67 mg, Cholesterol: 2 mg

Apple-Cider Raisin Delight

1½ c.	water	375 mL
1½ c.	apple cider	375 mL
1 c.	raisins	250 mL
1 c.	chopped apples	250 mL
3 T.	lemon juice	45 mL
1 T.	low-calorie margarine	15 mL
1 t.	cinnamon	5 mL
½ t.	salt	2 mL
3 T.	cornstarch	45 mL

Reserve ½ c. (125 mL) of the water. Combine the remaining 1 c. (250 mL) of water with the apple cider, raisins, apples, lemon juice, margarine, cinnamon, and salt in a saucepan. Bring to a boil. Now combine the reserved ½ c. (125 mL) of water with the cornstarch. Pour into the apple mixture. Cook and stir until thick. Cool slightly. Transfer to a serving dish. Cool completely.

Yield: 12 servings

Exchange, 1 serving: 1¼ fruit
Each serving contains: Calories: 72, Carbohydrates: 18

Pineapple-Mint Drink

If you don't have a fresh pineapple, use canned pineapple packed in its own juice. Drain it first.

½ c.	water (or drained pineapple juice)	125 mL
1 c.	pineapple, cut into pieces	250 mL
3 whole	oranges, seeded and chopped	3 whole
1 c.	crushed ice	250 mL
½ t.	mint extract	3 mL

Put all the ingredients into a blender or food processor. Blend at the highest speed until the ice is liquefied.

Yield: 6 servings

Exchange, 1 serving: ¾ fruit
Each serving contains: Calories: 44, Total fat: 0.2 g, Carbohydrates: 1 g, Protein: 0.7 g, Sodium: 2 mg, Cholesterol: 0 mg

Chocolate Frappé

A wonderful chocolaty taste. My daughter Anna loves this drink.

1 env.	hot chocolate mix, no sugar added	1 env.	
3 T.	hot water	45 mL	
1 c.	skim milk	250 mL	
1 c.	crushed ice	250 mL	

In a small bowl, combine the hot chocolate mix and water until a smooth paste forms. Put the milk and crushed ice into a food processor or blender. Using a rubber scraper, pour the chocolate paste over the milk and ice mixture. Process at the highest speed until the ice is liquefied. Serve in tall glasses.

Yield: 2 servings

Exchange, 1 serving: 1 milk
Each serving contains: Calories: 73, Total fat: 0.7 g, Carbohydrates: 1 g, Protein: 5 g, Sodium: 147 mg, Cholesterol: 2 mg

Butter-Almond Frappé

Do you like butter-almond ice cream? This is a wonderful substitute!

1 c.	frozen fat-free non-dairy whipped topping	250 mL	
½ t.	butter extract	3 mL	
½ t.	almond extract	3 mL	
1 c.	crushed ice	250 mL	

Put all the ingredients into a food processor or blender. Blend at the highest speed until the ice is liquefied.

Yield: 1 serving

Exchange, 1 serving: 1 fruit
Each serving contains: Calories: 125, Total fat: 0 g, Carbohydrates: 20 g, Protein: 0 g, Sodium: 7 mg, Cholesterol: 0 mg

Virgin Piña Colada

This is thick and frothy; imagine yourself sitting beside a pool in the tropics sipping it.

1 c.	frozen fat-free nondairy whipped topping	250 mL	
2 T.	crushed pineapple in juice, drained	30 mL	
1 t.	rum extract	5 mL	
1 t.	coconut extract	5 mL	
1 c.	crushed ice	250 mL	

Place all the ingredients in a food processor or blender. Process at the highest speed until the ice is liquefied.

Yield: 1 serving

Exchange, 1 serving: 1½ fruit
Each serving contains: Calories: 40, Total fat: 0 g, Carbohydrates: 30 g, Protein: 0.1 g, Sodium: 7 mg, Cholesterol: 0 mg

Icy Eggnog

Terrific for holiday get-togethers. Serve in punch cups sprinkled with nutmeg or cinnamon.

3 c.	skim milk	750 mL
¾ c.	egg substitute, liquid	185 mL
1 T.	sugar	15 mL
2 pkgs.	sugar substitute	2 pkgs.
1 t.	vanilla extract	5 mL
1 c.	crushed ice	250 mL

Put all the ingredients in a blender or food processor and process at the highest speed until the ice is liquefied.

Yield: 8 servings

Exchange, 1 serving: ½ milk
Each serving contains: Calories: 60, Total fat: 1 g, Carbohydrates: 6 g, Protein: 6 g, Sodium: 91 mg, Cholesterol: 2 mg

Orange Banana Smoothie

As good as it can be. Use sweet oranges and remove the white skin.

2	oranges, peeled and cut into chunks	2
1	ripe banana, peeled and sliced	1
½ c.	skim milk	125 mL
1 pkg.	aspartame sweetener	1 pkg.
¼ t.	almond extract	2 mL
3	ice cubes	3

Put all the ingredients into a blender or food processor. Blend at the highest speed until smooth. Pour into four glasses. Serve cold.

Yield: 4 servings

Exchange, 1 serving: 1 starch/bread
Each serving contains: Calories: 69, Total fat: 0.3 g, Carbohydrates: 16 g, Protein: 2 g, Sodium: 17 mg, Cholesterol: 1 mg

Strawberry Smoothie

I've used frozen berries in this with excellent results.

1 c.	skim milk	250 mL
¾ c.	fresh or sugar-free whole frozen strawberries	185 mL
1 pkg.	sugar substitute	1 pkg.
½ t.	lemon extract	3 mL
1 c.	crushed ice	250 mL

Put all the ingredients in a blender or food processor. Blend at the highest speed until the ice is liquefied.

Yield: 4 servings

Exchange, 1 serving: 1 vegetable
Each serving contains: Calories: 31, Total fat: 0.2 g, Carbohydrates: 5 g, Protein: 2 g, Sodium: 35 mg, Cholesterol: 1 mg

Raspberry Frappé

Raspberry extract makes all the difference. Buy it at a specialty food shop since supermarkets carry only the most ordinary flavors.

1 c.	raspberry sugar-free soda	250 mL
⅓ c.	plain yogurt	80 mL
1 pkg.	sugar substitute	1 pkg.
1 t.	raspberry extract	5 mL
½ T.	vanilla extract	7.5 mL

Put all the ingredients into a blender or food processor. Blend or process at the highest speed until the ice is liquefied.

Yield: 1 serving

Exchange, 1 serving: 1 vegetable; ½ fat
Each serving contains: Calories: 63, Total fat: 2 g, Carbohydrates: 5 g, Protein: 3 g, Sodium: 39 mg, Cholesterol: 10 mg

Mocha Frappé

As self-indulgent as those high-fat fancy coffee drinks.

1 env.	sugar-free hot chocolate mix	1 env.
3 T.	hot coffee	45 mL
1 c.	skim milk	250 mL
1 c.	crushed ice	250 mL

Put all the ingredients into a food processor or blender. Process at the highest speed until the ice is liquefied.

Yield: 1 serving

Exchange, 1 serving: 1 milk
Each serving contains: Calories: 86, Total fat: 0.4 g, Carbohydrates: 12 g, Protein: 8 g, Sodium: 134 mg, Cholesterol: 4 mg

Chocolate Mint Dessert Drink

2 c.	lowfat ice cream	500 mL
2 T.	chocolate flavoring or extract	30 mL
2 T.	mint flavoring or extract	30 mL
1 T.	chunky peanut butter	15 mL
4	fresh mint sprigs (optional)	4

Combine the ice cream, flavorings, and peanut butter in a blender. Blend until smooth and creamy. Pour into four wine glasses. If desired, garnish each with a mint sprig.

Yield: 4 servings

Exchange, 1 serving: 1 lowfat milk
Each serving contains: Calories: 116, Carbohydrates: 15 g

Tropical Punch

1 c.	mango nectar	250 mL
1 c.	unsweetened pineapple juice	250 mL
¾ c.	guava nectar	190 mL
¼ c.	lime juice	60 mL
6½ c.	cracked ice	1625 mL

Mix juices in a large pitcher. Combine 1 c. (250 mL) of the punch with 2 c. (500 mL) of the cracked ice in a blender. Blend until smooth. Pour into two glasses, Repeat procedure with remaining punch in batches.

Yield: 6 servings

Exchange, 1 serving: 1 fruit
Each serving contains: Calories: 69, Carbohydrates: 17 g

Party Pineapple Punch

2	bananas	2
3 c.	unsweetened pineapple juice	750 mL
6 oz. can	orange juice concentrate	178 g can
3 c.	cold water	750 mL
2 T.	lemon juice	30 mL
5 env.	aspartame sweetener	5 env.
1 bottle (1 qt.)	diet lemon-lime soda	1 bottle (1 L)

Cut bananas into chunks and place in a blender. Add 1 c. (250 mL) of the pineapple juice and orange juice concentrate. Blend until smooth. Transfer to large bowl. Add the remaining 2 c. (500 mL) of the pineapple juice and the cold water, lemon juice, and aspartame sweetener. Stir to completely mix. Pour into a large metal baking pan. Place in freezer and allow to freeze into a slush. Scoop into a punch bowl. Pour the lemon-lime soda down the sides of the bowl. Stir gently to mix. Serve in small punch cups.

Yield: 24 servings

Exchange, 1 serving: ⅔ fruit
Each serving contains: Calories: 39, Carbohydrates: 9 g

Double-Raspberry Cooler

1½ c.	cracked ice	375 mL
1½ c.	fresh or frozen unsweetened raspberries	190 mL
4	thin slices of lemon	4
6 T.	low-calorie raspberry syrup	90 mL
2 c.	sparkling water	500 mL

Divide cracked ice and raspberries equally among four glasses. Add one lemon slice, 1½ T. (21 mL) raspberry syrup, and ½ c. (125 mL) sparkling water to each glass. Serve with spoons so that the fruit can be muddled.

Yield: 4 servings

Exchange, 1 serving: ¾ fruit
Each serving contains: Calories: 43, Carbohydrates: 10 g

Mango Cooler

1 lb.	mango	500 g
½ c.	fresh lemon juice	125 mL
1 T.	rum flavoring	15 mL
1 T.	granulated fructose	15 mL
or		
6 env.	aspartame sweetener	6 env.
3 c.	cracked ice	750 mL

Peel, pit, and chop mango. Place mango pieces in a blender and process to a purée. Add lemon juice, rum flavoring, and sweetener of your choice. Then add the cracked ice and blend until smooth. Pour into chilled glasses.

Yield: 4 servings

Exchange, 1 serving: 1 fruit
Each serving contains: Calories: 50, Carbohydrates: 12 g

Cranberry Grapefruit Cooler

3 c.	unsweetened pink grapefruit juice	3 c.
2½ c.	low-calorie cranberry juice cocktail	625 mL
2 T.	granulated sugar replacement	30 mL
or		
5 env.	aspartame sweetener	5 env.
3 c.	cracked ice	750 mL
6	thin slices of lime	6

Combine pink grapefruit juice, cranberry juice, and sweetener of your choice in a large pitcher. Stir to dissolve sweetener. Divide the cracked ice equally among six glasses. Pour juice mixture into glasses. Garnish each glass with a slice of lime. This makes a perfect dessert drink after a barbecue dinner on a warm night.

Yield: 6 servings

Exchange, 1 serving: 1 fruit
Each serving contains: Calories: 63, Carbohydrates: 16 g

Strawberry Slush

1½ c.	frozen, unsweetened whole strawberries	375 mL
½ c.	buttermilk	125 mL
1 T.	granulated fructose	15 mL

Allow strawberries to thaw slightly. Reserve one or two of the larger strawberries. Combine buttermilk and fructose in a blender or food processor. With the motor running, gradually add the strawberries (keeping top of blender covered to prevent splashing). Process into a slush. Pour into a decorative glass. Cut reserved strawberries into medium-sized pieces. Stir into strawberry slush.

Yield: 1 serving

Exchange, 1 serving: 1 fruit, ½ skim milk
Each serving contains: Calories: 105, Carbohydrates: 21 g

Orange Sipper

1½ c.	buttermilk	375 mL
⅓ c.	orange juice concentrate, undiluted	90 mL
2 T.	granulated sugar replacement	30 mL
1 t.	vanilla extract	5 mL
3	ice cubes	3

Combine buttermilk, orange juice concentrate, sweetener of your choice, and vanilla. Blend until completely mixed. With blender running, drop ice cubes, one at a time, into the liquid. Blend until smooth. (Extra amount of drink can be frozen for later use. Place in freezer container. Allow to thaw slightly before using, then process in blender.)

Yield: 4 servings

Exchange, 1 serving: ⅓ skim milk, ½ fruit
Each serving contains: Calories: 87, Carbohydrates: 17 g

Peach Slush

1½ c.	frozen, unsweetened peach slices	375 mL
½ c.	skim milk	125 mL
3 env.	aspartame sweetener	3 env.
1	fresh mint sprig (optional)	1

Allow peach slices to thaw slightly. Pour milk into a blender or food processor. With the motor running, gradually add the peach slices (keeping top of blender covered to prevent splashing). Process into a slush. Blend in aspartame sweetener. Pour into a decorative glass. If desired, garnish with a sprig of mint.

Yield: 1 serving

Exchange, 1 serving: 1½ fruit, ½ skim milk
Each serving contains: Calories: 143, Carbohydrates: 30 g

Peach Smoothie

1¼ c.	nonfat plain yogurt	310 mL
1 lb.	ripe peaches	500 g
2 T.	fresh lemon juice	30 mL
2 T.	liquid fructose	30 mL
¼ t.	vanilla extract	1 mL

Divide 1 c. (250 mL) of the yogurt among 8 to 10 sections of an ice-cube tray. Freeze hard (at least 4 to 5 hours). Peel, pit, and slice peaches. Combine peach slices and lemon juice in a blender. Process until almost a purée. Add the remaining ¼ c. yogurt and the liquid fructose and vanilla. Process into a purée. Add frozen yogurt cubes and process until smooth. Pour into four decorative glasses.

Yield: 4 servings

Exchange, 1 serving: 1 fruit, ½ skim milk
Each serving contains: Calories: 81, Carbohydrates: 16 g

Strawberry Yogurt Nog

1½ c.	fresh or frozen unsweetened strawberries	375 mL
1½ c.	skim milk	375 mL
8 oz.	nonfat plain yogurt	227 g
1 t.	vanilla extract	5 mL
1 t.	strawberry flavoring	5 mL
6 env.	aspartame sweetener	6 env.
or		
1 T.	granulated fructose	15 mL
3	ice cubes	3

(If you are using fresh strawberries, you might want to set four aside for garnish.) Combine strawberries, milk, yogurt, vanilla extract, strawberry flavoring, and sweetener of your choice in a blender. Process until smooth. With the motor running, add ice cubes, one at a time, through the feed tube in the lid. Blend until smooth, Pour into decorative red wine glasses. (Cut reserved fresh strawberries into a fan. Lay on top of nog.)

Yield: 4 servings

Exchange, 1 serving: 1 skim milk
Each serving contains: Calories: 76, Carbohydrates: 10 g

Black-Raspberry Tofu Cream

1 c.	fresh or frozen black raspberries	250 mL
½ c.	skim milk	125 mL
1 t.	vanilla extract	5 mL
3 env.	aspartame sweetener	3 env.
½ pkg. (10.5 oz.)	firm tofu	½ pkg. (297 g)

Combine black raspberries and skim milk in a blender. Process until smooth. Add vanilla and aspartame sweetener. Process to mix. Add tofu. Process until smooth. Pour into two white wine glasses.

Yield: 2 servings

Exchange, 1 serving: 1 skim milk, 1 medium-fat meat
Each serving contains: Calories: 157, Carbohydrates: 14 g

Banana Yogurt Nog

1	banana	1
1½ c.	skim milk	375 mL
8 oz.	nonfat plain yogurt	227 g
2 t.	vanilla extract	10 mL
4 env.	aspartame sweetener	4 env.
or		
1½ T.	granulated sugar replacement	21 mL
3	ice cubes	3

Combine banana, milk, yogurt, vanilla extract, and sweetener of your choice in a blender. Process until smooth. With the motor running, add ice cubes, one at a time, through the feed tube in the lid. Blend until smooth. Pour into decorative red wine glasses.

Yield: 4 servings

Exchange, 1 serving: 1 skim milk
Each serving contains: Calories: 86, Carbohydrates: 14 g

Banana Tofu Cream

½ c.	skim milk	125 mL
1	banana	1
1 t.	vanilla extract	5 mL
3 env.	aspartame sweetener	3 env.
½ pkg. (10.5 oz.)	firm tofu	½ pkg. (297 g)
	ground nutmeg	

Combine skim milk and banana in a blender. Process until smooth. Add vanilla and aspartame sweetener. Process to mix. Add tofu. Process until smooth. Pour into two white wine glasses. (A champagne flute can also be used.) Sprinkle surface with nutmeg.

Yield: 2 servings

Exchange, 1 serving: 1½ skim milk, 1 fat
Each serving contains: Calories: 122, Carbohydrates: 18 g

Hot Cider

2 c.	apple cider	500 mL
2 (3 in.)	cinnamon sticks	2 (7.5 cm)
½ t.	whole cloves	2 mL
⅛ t.	ground nutmeg	½ mL
2 env.	aspartame sweetener	2 env.
2 t.	rum flavoring	10 mL

In a small saucepan, heat the apple cider, cinnamon sticks, whole cloves, and nutmeg until boiling. Reduce heat and simmer gently for 5 to 6 minutes. Remove from heat; then remove cinnamon sticks and whole cloves. Stir in aspartame sweetener and rum flavoring. Pour into two preheated cups or mugs. (To preheat mugs: Pour boiling or very hot water into mugs, allow to stand for 1 to 2 minutes, then pour out hot water and fill with drink.)

Yield: 2 servings

Exchange, 1 serving: 1 fruit
Each serving contains: Calories: 100, Carbohydrates: 13 g

Coffee and Cream

1 env. (2 c.)	nondairy whipped topping powder	1 env. (2 c.)
3 T.	lemon juice	45 mL
2 T.	water	30 mL
4 env.	aspartame sweetener	4 env.
1 T.	instant coffee powder	15 mL
2 c.	cracked ice	500 mL
1 c.	diet ginger ale	250 mL

Combine whipped-topping powder, lemon juice, water, aspartame sweetener, and instant coffee powder in a blender. Process until foamy. Add ice and process using the off/on switch until smooth. Add ginger ale and process on low until blended.

Yield: 6 servings

Exchange, 1 serving: 1 fat, ¼ fruit
Each serving contains: Calories: 62, Carbohydrates: 6 g

Quick Cappuccino

3 c.	hot strong coffee*	750 mL
3 c.	scalded skim milk	750 mL
12 env.	aspartame sweetener	12 env.
	unsweetened cocoa powder	

Pour scalded milk into a blender. Place hot pad over blender cover to protect yourself against burning. Process the milk until frothy. Pour ½ c. (500 mL) of the strong coffee into each of six cups or mugs. Pour ½ c. (500 mL) of the hot milk into each of the cups. Stir two envelopes of aspartame sweetener into each cup. Sprinkle with a small amount of unsweetened cocoa. Serve immediately.

Yield: 6 servings

Exchange, 1 serving: ½ lowfat milk
Each serving contains: Calories: 50, Carbohydrates: 6 g

*To brew strong coffee, use double the amount of coffee that you would normally use.

Prince Alex After-Dinner Drink

2 T.	water	30 mL
2 T.	lowfat ice cream	30 mL
1 T.	liquid nondairy creamer	15 mL
1 t.	chocolate flavoring	5 mL
	ground nutmeg	

Shake ingredients (except nutmeg) with ice cubes in a shaker jar. Place one ice cube into a chilled cocktail glass. Strain mixture over ice cube in glass. Dust with nutmeg.

Yield: 1 serving

Exchange, 1 serving: negligible
Each serving contains: Calories: negligible, Carbohydrates: negligible

Cranberry-Apple Fizz

1½ c.	cranberry fruit cocktail	375 mL
3 c.	apple juice	750 mL
16 oz.	seltzer	500 mL
14	lemon slices	14

Combine cranberry cocktail and apple juice in a pitcher or glass container. Chill thoroughly. just before serving, add the seltzer water. Pour into glasses filled with ice. Garnish each with a lemon slice.

Yield: 14 servings

Exchange, 1 serving: 1 fruit
Each serving contains: Calories: 43, Carbohydrates: 10 g

Pineapple-Strawberry Juice

Serving fruit juices in combination makes a delightful difference.

2 c.	pineapple juice	500 mL	Combine the juices and chill.
2 c.	strawberry juice	500 mL	**Yield: 4 c. (1 L) or 8 servings**

Exchange, 1 serving: 1½ fruit
Each serving contains: Calories: 58, Carbohydrates: 16 g

Lemonade Tea

Perfect for a hot summer day.

6 oz. can	frozen lemonade	177 mL can	Prepare lemonade as directed on the can. Add to iced tea. Stir to blend. To serve, pour over ice in a glass. You
1 qt.	iced tea	1 L	may garnish the glass with a lemon slice or mint leaves.

Yield: 10 servings

Exchange, 1 serving: 1 fruit
Each serving contains: Calories: 42, Carbohydrates: 11 g

Barley Water

An old English breakfast drink.

1 qt.	water	1 L	Peel and squeeze the lemons; reserve the juice. Combine the water barley and lemon peel in saucepan.
¼ c.	pearl barley	60 mL	Bring to the boil, reduce heat, and simmer slowly for
2	lemons	2	2 to 2½ hours. Strain and cool to room temperature.
4 env.	Equal low-calorie sweetener	4 env.	Add the reserved lemon juice and Equal low-calorie sweetener. Stir to blend. Chill thoroughly. This drink may be served with or without ice.

Yield: 1 qt. (1 L) or 8 servings

Exchange, 1 serving: negligible
Each serving contains: Calories: negligible, Carbohydrates: 2 g

Premium Juice

An absolutely lovely color for any table.

2 c.	pink grapefruit juice	500 mL	Combine the juices and chill.
2 c.	pineapple juice	500 mL	**Yield: 6 c. (1.5 L) or 12 servings**
2 c.	orange juice	500 mL	

Exchange, 1 serving: 1½ fruit
Each serving contains: Calories: 44, Carbohydrates: 14 g

Tomato Breakfast Juice

6 oz. can	tomato juice	170 mL can	Combine all the ingredients in a glass. Stir to blend.
½ t.	lemon juice	2 mL	
dash	Worcestershire sauce	dash	
dash	hot pepper sauce	dash	
dash	salt	dash	
1 env.	Equal low-calorie sweetener	1 env.	

Yield: 1 serving

Exchange, 1 serving: 1 fruit
Each serving contains: Calories: 37, Carbohydrates: 9 g

Fresh Lime Cooler

⅓ c.	lime juice, freshly squeezed	90 mL	Combine all the ingredients in a blender or shaker. Blend on slow speed or shake until well blended and foamy. Pour into a glass.
½ c.	ice, finely crushed	125 mL	
2 env.	Equal low-calorie sweetener	2 env.	
1	egg white	1	

Yield: 1 serving

Exchange, 1 serving: negligible
Each serving contains: Calories: 17, Carbohydrates: 2 g

Mulled Cider

1 qt.	apple cider	1 L	Combine the ingredients in a saucepan. Bring just to the boiling point; reduce heat and simmer for 3 minutes. Strain and serve.
7	whole cloves	7	
2 in. piece	cinnamon stick	5 cm piece	

Yield: 6 servings

Exchange, 1 serving: 2 fruit
Each serving contains: Calories: 80, Carbohydrates: 20 g

Rose Tea

A delightful flavor and aroma.

1 c.	rose petals	250 mL	Press rose petals and vanilla bean in a tea strainer or gauze bag; cover securely. Place in a teapot. Pour boiling water into a pot. Cover and steep to the desired strength.
1 in.	vanilla bean	2.5 cm	
3 c.	water, boiling	750 mL	

Yield: 3 servings

Exchange, 1 serving: negligible
Each serving contains: Calories: negligible, Carbohydrates: negligible

Hot Tomato Cocktail

2 c.	tomato juice	500 mL	
3 T.	lemon juice	45 mL	
¼ t.	ground nutmeg	1 mL	
⅛ t.	ground ginger	½ mL	
dash	hot pepper sauce	dash	

Combine all ingredients in a saucepan. Heat just to the boiling point and serve.

Yield: 4 servings

Exchange, 1 serving: 1 vegetable
Each serving contains: Calories: 22, Carbohydrates: 5 g

Spiced Cranberry-Apple Juice

½ c.	water	125 mL
1	cinnamon stick, broken	1
¼ t.	ground nutmeg	1 mL
¼ t.	orange peel	1 mL
2 c.	cranberry juice cocktail	500 mL
1 c.	apple juice	250 mL
1 T.	lemon juice	15 mL

Combine the water, cinnamon stick pieces, nutmeg, and orange peel in small saucepan. Heat to boiling point and boil for 3 minutes. Remove from heat; allow to cool to room temperature. Remove cinnamon and orange peel. Combine juices and spiced water. Chill thoroughly or serve hot.

Yield: 3¼ c. (810 mL) or 6 servings

Exchange, 1 serving: 1¾ fruit
Each serving contains: Calories: 75, Carbohydrates: 19 g

Mulled Grape Juice

1 qt.	grape juice	1 L
1 c.	water	250 mL
4 in.	cinnamon stick	10 cm
10	whole cloves	10
⅓ c.	lemon juice	90 mL

Combine the grape juice, water, cinnamon stick, and cloves in a saucepan. Bring to the boil, reduce heat, and simmer very slowly for 12 minutes. Remove cinnamon stick and cloves. Add the lemon juice. Stir and serve.

Yield: 8 servings

Exchange, 1 serving: 2 fruit
Each serving contains: Calories: 82, Carbohydrates: 21 g

Quick Morning Cocoa

¼ c.	cocoa	60 mL
¼ t.	salt	1 mL
½ c.	water	125 mL
3½ c.	skim milk	875 mL
2 T.	granulated sugar replacement	30 mL
3 env.	Equal low-calorie sweetener	3 env.

Combine the cocoa and salt in a saucepan. Stir in water. Cook over low heat until mixture is well blended. Slowly stir in the milk and granulated sugar replacement. Cook and stir over low heat for 2 more minutes. Remove from heat. Cool slightly. Stir in the Equal low-calorie sweetener.

Yield: 4 servings

Exchange, 1 serving: ¾ medium-fat milk, ½ bread
Each serving contains: Calories: 128, Carbohydrates: 19 g

Demitasse

1 qt.	water	1 L
¾ c.	freshly and finely ground coffee	190 mL
3 T.	granulated sugar replacement	45 mL

Combine water and coffee in saucepan. Bring to the boil and allow to boil hard for 1 minute. Remove from heat and allow froth to settle. Stir in sugar replacement. Place back on the stove and bring to the boil. Remove from heat; allow mixture to settle. Place back on the stove and again bring to the boil. Pour some of the froth into each of 12 demitasse cups. Pour in the remaining coffee. Serve hot.

Yield: 12 servings

Exchange, 1 serving: negligible
Each serving contains: Calories: negligible, Carbohydrates: negligible

Spiced Coffee

For each cup served, repeat this recipe.

¾ c.	brewed coffee	190 mL
dash	ground nutmeg	dash
	cinnamon stick	

Combine the coffee and nutmeg in a cup. Stir with a cinnamon stick. Leave cinnamon stick in the cup to serve.

Yield: 1 serving

Exchange, 1 serving: negligible
Each serving contains: Calories: negligible, Carbohydrates: negligible

Espresso

Use this recipe for each cup of espresso.

1 T.	dark coffee	15 mL
¾ c.	water	190 mL
	lemon rind (optional)	
	Equal low-calorie sweetener (optional)	

Brew as you would in any coffee maker. Serve with a twist of lemon and the sweetener, if desired. (If you have an espresso maker, use machine directions.)

Yield: 1 serving

Exchange, 1 serving: negligible
Each serving contains: Calories: negligible, Carbohydrates: negligible

Coffee Mocha

1 oz.	unsweetened chocolate	30 g
12 c.	skim milk	125 mL
¼ c.	evaporated skim milk	60 mL
¼ c.	water	60 mL
3 c.	hot strong coffee, brewed	750 mL
3 T.	granulated sugar replacement	45 mL

Melt the chocolate with skim milk in top of a double boiler. With an electric beater, beat in the evaporated milk and water. Beat until smooth and well blended. Add coffee and sugar replacement. Serve hot.

Yield: 5 servings

Exchange, 1 serving: ¾ medium-fat milk
Each serving contains: Calories: 65, Carbohydrates: 7 g

Café au Lait

⅓ c.	hot strong coffee, brewed	90 mL
⅓ c.	skim milk	90 mL

Pour the coffee and milk simultaneously into a heated cup.

Yield: 1 serving

Exchange, 1 serving: ⅓ nonfat milk
Each serving contains: Calories: 27, Carbohydrates: 4 g

Apricot Morning Drink

16 oz. can	Featherweight water pack apricot halves	454 g can
1½ c.	skim milk	375 mL
3	eggs	3
1	vanilla extract	5 mL
½ t.	Featherweight liquid sweetener	2 mL
	ground cinnamon	

Combine all ingredients except the cinnamon in a blender and cover. Blend at medium speed 30 seconds. Pour into glasses and sprinkle apricot drink with cinnamon.

Yield: 3 servings

Exchange, 1 serving: 1 fruit, 1 high-fat meat, ½ nonfat milk
Each serving contains: Calories: 191, Carbohydrates: 16 g

Based on a recipe from Featherweight Brand Foods.

THESE DESSERTS ARE GOOD ENOUGH FOR EVERYONE!

We offer this section as a help to people with diabetes, people who want to enjoy delicious desserts while keeping their blood sugar under control. Desserts pose the most dietary challenges for diabetics and their families—but sweets and delicious desserts can be prepared to suit the needs of diabetics without sacrificing taste!

Our philosophy is that recipes should be so delicious that everyone in the family is served the same dessert. The idea of serving the same dish to everyone began years ago with cooking classes and a book we did for people who needed to restrict their sodium or salt. We noticed that in some families everyone was served "regular" (high-sodium) tasty foods, everyone except the person on the special diet, who was served rather unpalatable "low sodium" foods. In other families where everyone was served the same low sodium foods, an effort was made to see that the food was truly delicious. Our experience has been overwhelmingly the same: People make more of an effort to see that foods are delicious when everyone eats the same thing.

We believe that it is quite feasible to serve desserts that are good for diabetics and acceptable to other people too. We offer here a collection of recipes with little or no sugar or other concentrated sweets, and with as little fat as possible. We have been troubled by real-life scenes in which everyone is served some tempting dessert—everyone, that is, except the diabetic. "We're having chocolate cake and ice cream tonight—except for Tom. (He's diabetic.) Here's your apple, Tom."

What's wrong with this scene? First of all, it's not very considerate of Tom's feelings. Who among us wants to hear the people closest to us remind us that we are different? Second, we have seen chocolate cakes and such lead diabetic friends off their diets. We can add a third reason for serving the same dessert to everyone: Those of us who are fortunate enough not to have diabetes still have coronary arteries. We do not need the saturated fat, cholesterol, and calories associated with classic dessert ingredients (heavy cream, chocolate, cream cheese, egg yolks).

In our recipes we make much use of cocoa, nonfat cream cheese, skim milk, nonfat ricotta cheese, nonfat cottage cheese, and egg whites or egg substitutes. If any non-diabetic cooks reading this introduction need one more reason to serve everyone the same dessert, here it is: People who are related to a diabetic are at a higher genetic risk for developing diabetes themselves as they get older. People with a genetic predisposition to diabetes are unwise to let themselves become overweight. Although we non-diabetics may be able to better tolerate concentrated sweets, we don't need them. Getting into the habit of stocking our kitchens with low-calorie, low-fat, low-sugar ingredients can make it easier to keep the extra pounds off.

WHAT ABOUT FATS?

On the issue of which fats to buy, there may not be a simple answer. Butter or margarine? Both have problems. The problems with butter have been well publicized: Butter has saturated fat and cholesterol. But recently margarine has come under increasing attack. British medical experts in November 1994 issued a warning against margarine's trans fatty acids and against hydrogenated polyunsaturated fats. Some researchers have linked vegetable oils with an increased risk of cardiovascular heart disease.

IS MARGARINE HEALTHIER THAN BUTTER?

Some medical and nutritional experts would say that it is, while others disagree. Your information may vary, depending on what country you live in. Some people use neither butter nor margarine. They use olive oil in cooking. They may also use a non-stick cooking spray. We have a friend who keeps a little sign to himself on his toaster: "Use jelly, stupid." In our recipes we say "margarine or butter." You decide after talking to your physician, dietitian, or diabetic educator. We call for as little fat as possible. But for cookies or flour-based pie crust, either use a little fat or just don't make the recipe. We suggest saving richer confections that require more than one fat exchange for special occasions, for everyone.

HONEST READING OF DIETARY INFORMATION

In our recipes we tell you, among other things, how many calories and grams of fat a recipe has, and what the diabetic exchanges are per serving. Please be aware, however, that stated portions in all recipes today, ours included, are for very small portions. Portion sizes have been standardized; these standard portions are smaller than what many people eat in real life. A serving of cake is listed as one-twelfth or even one-twentieth of the cake. "Nice" portions are likely to be twice that size. If you eat a generous portion, you need to double (or sometimes triple) the nutritional values and diabetic exchanges.

SOME RECIPES ARE HEALTHIER THAN OTHERS

In this cookbook, we give you a range of recipes. Fresh fruit is a classic healthy dessert. Many people with diabetes make it a habit to save one fruit exchange to have as their dessert. Many of our fruit-based recipes cost few calories and one fruit exchange. We also offer recipes for richer desserts that cost more calories and exchanges, in which case you may need to plan your eating to save enough fat and starch exchanges for dessert.

DESSERTS ARE EXPECTED TO TASTE SWEET

Human beings like the natural sweet taste of sugar (sucrose), honey, maple syrup, molasses, corn syrup, etc. These are all caloric sweeteners. We'll discuss non-caloric sweeteners a little later. Sugar is not the only caloric sweetener that can raise your blood sugar. Labels on food products often brag that they contain no sugar. But they may contain other ingredients that raise your blood sugar. Some "no sugar" cookbooks make great use of sweet fruit juice concentrates. Frozen grape juice concentrate adds a nice, sweet taste to foods, but many diabetics who check their blood sugar find it acts just like sugar. That's why it gives such a nice, sweet taste. Apple juice concentrate also adds sweetness.

You will need to test your own blood sugar to see how your body reacts.

Fructose is a fruit sugar; it can be found in the "diet" section of most large food stores. Some diabetics whose blood sugar is under good control find that fructose causes less of a blood sugar rise than sucrose. Also, since it is sweeter, you can use less in cooking. But we know diabetics in good control who find that fructose plays havoc with their blood sugar. When you test your blood sugar, you will learn how fructose or fruit juice concentrates affect you as an individual.

Diabetics traditionally were told to avoid sugar completely. But more recently researchers have found that diabetics can tolerate small amounts of sugar when they take it in at the same time as other foods.

Some recipes call for a very small amount of sugar. In cake recipes, for example, sugar does more than just add sweetness. Its bulk is necessary for the cake to rise up and be light and tender and, well, cake-like. A cake made with no sugar or with a relative like fructose will not have the tenderness, color, or texture of cake. One-twelfth of a cake made with a very small amount of sugar contains very little sugar indeed.

Sorbitol and its relative mannitol are caloric sweeteners that are used in manufacturing commercial products. Sorbitol is found in some "diabetic" products such as candy bars. Sorbitol has distinct drawbacks: First, it gives many people diarrhea. Secondly, it has calories. Third, its presence in a confection often makes it necessary to add fat for creaminess. So a product with sorbitol is not necessarily good for a person with diabetes.

You can now buy many jelly substitutes or fruit spreads made without sugar. Some are made with saccharin. With others, the first ingredient listed may be a sweet juice concentrate, which can raise your blood sugar. Read carefully all labels that brag about having no sugar added. Ask your dietitian or diabetic educator about any products that confuse you. And, of course, test your blood sugar to know how different products affect you.

Alcohol is another ingredient where professional advice is needed. Although people with diabetes traditionally have been advised not to drink at all, newer research says that some can drink limited amounts of non-sweet drinks at the same time that other foods are eaten. In a few recipes we have used very small amounts of liqueurs to add flavor to cooked dishes. The longer the cooking, the more alcohol cooks out, leaving just a nice flavor.

NON-CALORIC SWEETENERS

Can we admit that sugar substitutes can taste awful? Many people find the taste of saccharin bitter. We didn't find anyone, diabetic or not, who liked the taste of saccharin brown sugar substitute. It's simple enough for a recipe to call for brown sugar substitute but that

AMOUNT OF ARTIFICIAL SWEETENERS TO SUBSTITUTE FOR SUGAR

SUGAR	ACESULFAME-K	ASPARTAME	SACCHARIN
2 t.	1 pkt.	1 pkt. or ¼ t.	1 pkt. or ¼ t.
1 T.	1¼ pkt.	1½ pkt. or ½ t.	1⅓ pkt. or ⅓ t.
¼ cup	3 pkt.	6 pkt. or 1¾ t.	3 pkt. or 1⅛ t.
⅓ cup	4 pkt.	8 pkt. or 2½ t.	4 pkt. or 1¼ t.
½ cup	6 pkt.	12 pkt. or 3½ t.	6 pkt. or 2 t.
⅔ cup	8 pkt.	16 pkt. or 5 t.	8 pkt. or 2½ t.
¾ cup	9 pkt.	18 pkt. or 5¼ t.	9 pkt. or 3½ t.
1 cup	12 pkt.	24 pkt. or 7¼ t.	12 pkt. or 4 t.

Please keep in mind that aspartame must be added after cooking. We like to store our aspartame in little covered containers with a vanilla bean. We do this with Equal Measure® (the concentrated form) and NutraSweet Spoonful® (the measures-like-sugar type.)

doesn't mean the finished dish will taste the same as it would with brown sugar.

The three major sugar substitutes available in the United States are saccharin (Sweet'n Low®, Sugar Twin®, Sprinkle Sweet®), aspartame (Equal®, Equal Measure®, NutraSweet® or NutraSweet Spoonful®), and acesulfame-K (Sweet One®). The subject of sugar substitutes is quite confusing because of all the brand names and different formulations. We offer two charts. The first will help you know which ingredient our recipes call for without using brand names. It will also help you in shopping. The second chart will help you adapt your old recipes to the use of artificial sweeteners.

In our recipes we call for specific non-caloric sweeteners. We have found that in many cases a particular one works better than the others for specific recipes. Note carefully whether a recipe (ours or anyone else's) calls for a product that is substituted cup for cup with sugar. We use the phrase "measures-like-sugar saccharin" to refer to products such as Sugar Twin® that are substituted, cup for cup with sugar. We use the phrase "measures-like-sugar aspartame" to refer to products such as NutraSweet Spoonful®. Most artificial sweetener products, however, are formulated to require much safer amounts. We use the words "saccharin," " aspartame," or "acesulfame- K" for these concentrated products.

We hope readers will find our dessert recipes helpful. If you are diabetic and also the cook, we hope our book will make your life easier. Why not just serve the same dessert to everyone in your family? You do not have to add an explanation. It's just chocolate cake or Grape-Nuts Pudding. For those of you readers who are not diabetic but are cooking for people who are, we hope these recipes will give you ideas on how to satisfy a sweet tooth safely. Although we clearly are not in charge of the other person's diabetes, we can do things that help. Cooking appropriate foods—especially desserts—is one good way.

Karin Cadwell, Ph.D., R.N.
Edith White, M. Ed.

Pastry Basics

Pastry Cups

1	egg	1	
dash	salt	dash	
½ c.	skim milk	125 mL	
1 t.	vanilla extract	5 mL	
½ c.	flour	125 mL	
	oil for deep-fat frying		

Combine egg and salt in mixing bowl; beat to blend thoroughly. Add milk, vanilla and flour, beating just to blend until smooth. Heat rosette iron in hot deep fat (365°F or 180°C), and shake off excess oil. Dip into batter to within ¼ in. (6 mm) of top of iron. Return to hot oil; cover iron completely with oil. Fry until golden brown. Drain on absorbent paper.

Yield: 10 pastry cups

Exchange, 1 pastry cup: ⅓ bread
Each serving contains: Calories: 34, Carbohydrates: 6 g

Individual Meringue Nests

Use these with almost anything—fruits, puddings, custards, or ice cream.

4	egg whites	4	
dash	salt	dash	
¼ t.	cream of tartar	1 mL	
½ c.	granulated sugar replacement	125 mL	
1 T.	white vinegar	15 mL	
1 T.	white vanilla extract	15 mL	

Beat egg whites, salt and cream of tartar into soft peaks. Gradually add granulated sugar replacement, vinegar and vanilla. Beat until mixture forms stiff peaks. Cover cookie sheet with parchment or plain paper. Draw eight 4 in. (10 cm) circles; divide meringue evenly among circles. Using the back of a spoon, shape into nests. Bake at 250°F (120°C) for 45 to 50 minutes. Turn off heat an allow to dry in oven for about 1 hour.

Yield: 8 servings

Exchange, 1 serving: negligible
Each serving contains: Calories: negligible, Carbohydrates: 13 g

Cream Puff Pastry

1 c.	water	250 mL
¼ c.	margarine	60 mL
dash	salt	dash
1 c.	flour	250 mL
4	eggs	4

Combine water, margarine and salt in medium saucepan. Cook and stir over high heat until boiling; reduce heat. Add flour and cook and stir over medium heat until mixture comes clean from sides of pan and forms ball in center. Remove from heat; cool slightly. With spoon, electric beater or food processor, add eggs, one at a time. Beat after each addition until batter is smooth and glossy.

For Cream Puffs: Drop tablespoonfuls onto lightly greased baking sheets. Bake at 425°F (220°C) for 15 minutes; reduce heat to 350°F (175°C) and bake 25 minutes longer, or until puffs are free of moisture beads. (Puff pastry will collapse if removed from oven early.) Remove from oven. Remove tops or cut into sides to allow hot air to escape; cool completely.

For Éclairs: Spoon pastry batter into pastry bag fitted with ½ in. (1.25 cm) tube. Shape batter into 1 × 4 in. (2 × 10 cm) strips. Bake as for cream puffs.

Fillings: Fill with flavored creams or puddings.

Yield: 10 puffs or éclairs

Exchange, 1 puff or éclair: ⅔ full-fat milk plus filling exchange
Each serving contains: Calories: 114 plus filling calories, Carbohydrates: 10 g

Phyllo Dough

Greek phyllo dough is low in fat and calories and it's easy to use to make pie shells, individual tarts, napoleons, or turnovers. Most grocery stores sell frozen packages. Defrosted dough may be kept in the refrigerator for a few weeks.

To use phyllo, bring the dough to room temperature. Arrange two surfaces to work on, one for the current sheet and one to store the balance. Take out sheets of phyllo only as needed.

While working on one, be careful to keep the others moist. Phyllo dough dries out quickly when uncovered, so have all the equipment and ingredients ready before taking the dough out of the package. Using plastic wrap, cover the sheets you are not currently using. A large, clean, plastic-wastebasket-size bag works better than two narrow sheets of plastic wrap. Place a damp dish towel over the plastic, taking care that the towel does not touch the dough and cause it to fall apart. Discard any problem sheets.

Instructions accompanying phyllo suggest covering each layer with softened butter. But using a butter-flavored non-stick cooking spray works well.

Yield: a sheet of dough is one serving

Exchange, 1 serving: 2 breads
Each serving contains: Calories: 180, Carbohydrates: 10 g, Fiber: 1 g, Sodium: 120 mg, Cholesterol: 0 mg

Phyllo Top Crust for a 9 In. (23 cm) Pie

Phyllo dough can be used to make an attractive top crust with few calories and little fat. Put your choice of pie filling into a pie pan with no bottom crust.

| 4 sheets | phyllo dough | 4 sheets |
| | butter-flavored non-stick cooking spray | |

Place one large sheet of dough on a dry surface. Spray lightly with non-stick cooking spray. Put a second sheet on top. Place a 9 inch (23 cm) metal pie pan face-up in the center of the top layer of the double layer of dough. Spray again. Use scissors to cut away any dough that sticks out more than one inch (2.5 cm) around the edge of the pan. Carefully lift this dough up over the top of the filled pie shell. Use scissors to cut off excess dough, more than one inch (2.5 cm) around edge. Use your fingers to form the edge into a fluted pie shell. Spray lightly with non-stick cooking spray. Bake in a preheated 375°F (190°C) oven for seven minutes or until nicely browned.

Each serving contains: Carbohydrates: 5 g

Tart Shells

Phyllo pastry tarts may be available in your supermarket, if not, use this recipe.

Put four sheets of phyllo dough on a work surface. Cut a few inches from one side to form squares. Cut each of these squares into four pieces, making 16 small squares.

Take one square and lay it flat. Coat it with non-stick cooking spray. Place another square on top of it, cattycorner, forming an eight-pointed star. Carefully press it to the inside or outside of a tart pan or custard cup that has been sprayed with non-stick cooking spray. Press the dough against the inside of a 6 oz (188 g) custard cup to make a tart shell that can hold ½ c. (120 mL) of filling. Leave the cup in place to protect the delicate shell.

Repeat to make seven other shells. Place them on a cookie sheet, not touching. Bake in a preheated 375°F (190°C) oven for 8–9 minutes. When the dough is golden brown, remove turnovers from the oven and let cool for a few minutes. Carefully lift the phyllo shells from the custard cups or the tart pan and allow to finish cooling on a wire rack. Before serving, fill with your choice of filling. Good choices include fresh or frozen berries, defrosted (sprinkled with a little aspartame or acesulfame-K, if desired); pudding (vanilla or chocolate, no-sugar, no-fat, instant mixes or other recipes, such as the ones in the pudding chapter); a thin layer of vanilla pudding plus fruit; sugar-free, fat-free frozen yogurt.

These tarts are not good finger food. As they are so thin, they shatter easily. But eaten with a fork or spoon, they are elegant and seem self-indulgent despite their low calories and low fat.

Each serving contains: Carbohydrates: 3 g

Margarine Pastry

1¼ c.	all-purpose flour	310 mL	
dash	salt	dash	
½ c.	Mazola regular or salted margarine	125 mL	
2 T.	cold water	30 mL	

Mix the flour and salt. With pastry blender or 2 knives, cut in the margarine until fine crumbs form. Sprinkle cold water over mixture while tossing with the fork to blend well. Press dough firmly into a ball with your hands.

Yield: 8 tarts

Exchange, 1 tart: 2 bread, 1 fat
Each serving contains: Calories: 158, Carbohydrates: 18 g

"A Diet For the Young at Heart" by Mazola.

Napoleon Pastry

4 sheets	phyllo dough	4 sheets

If you are unfamiliar with how to work with phyllo dough, first read the general instructions elsewhere in this book (see Index).

Take one sheet of phyllo dough and spread it flat; coat with butter-flavored non-stick vegetable cooking spray. Fold the dough in half and spray it again. Fold it again; the sheet is now one-quarter of its original size. Using scissors, cut it into four pieces. You now have four small pieces, each of which is four layers thick. Carefully lift each onto a cookie sheet that has been sprayed with non-stick vegetable cooking spray. Make as many sections as you need. Plan to stack the dough four pieces high for a super napoleon; in this case, one sheet of phyllo makes one napoleon, with fillings. Bake in a preheated 375°F (1 90°C) oven for approximately six minutes. The dough should be lightly browned but not burnt. Use a pancake turner to lift each piece off, and place each on a wire rack to cool. Store in an airtight container. The analysis is for a four-layer napoleon, unfilled. Be sure to add the extra calories and exchanges for the fillings.

Yield: 4 napoleons

Exchange, 1 napoleon: 2 breads
Each serving contains: Calories: 180, Carbohydrates: 10 g, Fiber: 1 g, Sodium: 120 mg, Cholesterol: 0 mg

Wheat Germ Single-Crust Pastry

1 c.	all-purpose-flour	25 mL
2 T.	Kretschmer wheat germ	30 mL
½ t.	salt	2 mL
6 T.	vegetable shortening	90 mL
2–3 T.	cold water	30–45 mL

Combine flour, wheat germ and salt in bowl. Stir well to blend. Cut in shortening with pastry blender until mixture looks like coarse meal. Add water a little at a time, mixing lightly with fork. Shape dough into a firm ball. Refrigerate, it desired, for easier handling and to prevent shrinkage. Roll out into a 12 in. (30.5 cm) circle on a lightly floured cloth-covered board. Place loosely in 9 in. (23 cm) pie plate. Fold edge under. Press into upright rim. Flute as desired. Prick entire surface of pastry bottom and sides with fork before baking. Bake at 475°F (250°C) for 8 to 10 minutes until lightly browned. Cool on rack.

Yield: 9 in. (23 cm) piecrust or 8 servings

Exchange, 1 serving: 2 bread
Each serving contains: Calories: 135, Carbohydrates: 7 g

With the courtesy of Kretschmer Wheat Germ/International Multifoods.

100% Whole Wheat Pastry

1 c.	whole wheat flour	250 mL
½ t.	salt	2 mL
6 T.	vegetable shortening	90 mL
2–3 T.	cold water	30–40 mL

Measure flour into a bowl and add salt. Stir to blend. Cut in half the shortening with a pastry blender until mixture looks like coarse meal, then the remaining shortening until particles are the size of small peas. Add water a little at a time, mixing lightly with a fork. Shape dough into a firm ball with hands. Flatten with your palm. Refrigerate, if desired, for easier handling and to prevent shrinkage. Roll out into a 12 in. (30.5 cm) circle on lightly floured cloth-covered board. Place loosely in 9 in. (23 cm) pie pan. Fold edge under. Press to make an upright rim. Flute edge, as desired. Prick entire surface of bottom and sides with a fork before baking pastry. Bake at 425°F (220°C) for 10 to 12 minutes. Cool on rack.

Yield: 9 in. (23 cm) piecrust or 8 servings

Exchange, 1 serving: 2 bread
Each serving contains: Calories: 133, Carbohydrates: 11 g

Rye Pastry

1¼ c.	medium rye flour	310 mL
1 t.	granulated sugar replacement	5 mL
½ t.	baking powder	2 mL
½ t.	salt	2 mL
⅓ c.	vegetable shortening	90 mL
3–4 T.	cold water	45–60 mL

Measure flour into a bowl and add the sugar, baking powder and salt. Stir well to blend. Cut in the shortening until mixture looks like coarse meal. Add water a little at a time, mixing lightly with fork. With your hands, shape dough into a firm ball. Roll into a 12 in. (30.5 cm) circle on lightly floured, cloth-covered board. Place loosely in a 9 in. (23 cm) pie pan. Fold edge under. Press to make an upright rim. Flute edge. Prick bottom and sides with a fork before baking pastry. Bake at 425°F (220°C) for 8 to 10 minutes. Cool on rack.

Yield: 9 in. (23 cm) pie crust or 8 servings

Exchange, 1 serving: 1 bread, 1½ fat
Each serving contains: Calories: 132, Carbohydrates: 13 g

Low-Calorie Pastry

¾ c.	zwieback crumbs	190 mL
3 T.	unsalted margarine, melted	45 mL

Combine crumbs with margarine. Press into a 9 in. (23 cm) pie pan. Bake at 350°F (175°C) for 8 minutes. Cool thoroughly.

Yield: 8 servings

Exchange, 1 serving: 1 fat, ½ bread
Each serving contains: Calories: 80, Carbohydrates: 16 g

Pastries, Strudels, and Roll-Ups

Pastry with Chocolate Cheese Filling

Cake

1¾ c.	flour	440 mL
1 pkg.	dry yeast	1 pkg.
⅓ c.	sour cream	90 mL
¼ c.	margarine	60 mL
2 T.	water	30 mL
3 T.	granulated sugar replacement	45 mL
dash	salt	dash
1	egg	1

Filling

3 oz. pkg.	cream cheese	110 g pkg.
2 T.	granulated sugar replacement	30 mL
1	egg yolk	1
1 T.	sour cream	15 mL
1 oz.	baking chocolate, melted	30 g
1 T.	vanilla extract	5 mL

Topping

1	egg white, beaten	1
1 t.	granulated sugar replacement	5 mL

Sift flour and mix with the dry yeast in a large bowl. In a saucepan, blend together the sour cream, margarine, water, sugar replacement, salt and egg. Heat until warm, stirring constantly. Stir in the flour and mix into a soft dough. Knead the dough on a lightly floured surface. Place in a greased bowl and allow to rise until doubled in size.

Combine the filling ingredients and beat until thoroughly blended. Turn dough out onto lightly floured surface and knead a few times. Roll dough out into a 9 × 16 in. (23 × 40 cm) rectangle. Spread the cheese filling evenly over the dough and roll up from the longer edge to make a 16 in. (40 cm) roll. Place, seam side down, on greased cookie sheet. Set in a warm place for 45 minutes or until dough has doubled in size. Brush with topping of beaten egg white mixed with sugar replacement. Bake at 325°F (165°C) for 25 to 30 minutes or until golden brown. Remove from oven and serve warm.

Yield: 15 servings

Exchange, 1 serving: ¾ bread, ¾ fat
Each serving contains: Calories: 130, Carbohydrates: 17 g

Viennese Ruffles au Chocolat

Absolutely great—and look at the exchange and calorie counts.

⅔ c.	flour, sifted	165 mL
2 T.	cocoa	30 mL
½ t.	salt	2 mL
3 T.	granulated sugar replacement	45 mL
⅓ c.	white wine	90 mL
6	egg whites, stiffly beaten	6
	Powdered Sugar Replacement	

Combine flour, cocoa, salt and sugar in large mixing bowl; beat in white wine to make a medium batter. Fold stiffly beaten egg whites into mixture. Pour batter into a pastry bag with a large, plain or fluted, tube. Squeeze batter into hot, deep fat (365°F or 180°C) and fry until delicately browned. Drain on absorbent paper, such as paper toweling. Sprinkle with powdered sugar replacement.

Yield: 30 ruffles

Exchange, 1 ruffle: ¼ bread
Each serving contains: Calories: 15, Carbohydrates: 6 g

Butterscotch-Chocolate Charlotte Russe

1 env.	unflavored gelatin	1 env.
¼ c.	cold water	60 mL
1 c.	skim evaporated milk	250 mL
1 T.	butter	15 mL
1 oz.	baking chocolate	30 g
⅓ c.	granulated brown sugar replacement	60 mL
1½ c.	skim milk	375 mL
2	eggs, separated	2
dash	salt	dash
¼ t.	vanilla extract	1 mL
12	ladyfingers	12

Soften gelatin in cold water; set aside. Pour skim evaporated milk into freezer tray and place in freezer to thoroughly chill until edges are slightly frozen. Melt butter and baking chocolate in top of double boiler. Add brown sugar replacement and cook until well blended. Add milk. Heat and stir until warm. Pour over well-beaten egg yolks, stirring constantly. Add salt and return to top of double boiler. Cook over hot water, stirring constantly, until mixture coats a spoon. Remove from heat and add softened gelatin. Stir until dissolved. Chill until mixture begins to thicken. Beat egg whites until stiff and fold into the cooled chocolate mixture. In chilled mixing bowl, combine vanilla extract and slightly frozen evaporated milk and beat until stiff. Fold into mixture. Pour into a decorative mold lined with separated ladyfingers. Chill until firm. Unmold onto a serving plate.

Yield: 8 servings

Exchange, 1 serving: 1 low-fat milk, ⅔ fat
Each serving contains: Calories: 112, Carbohydrates: 24 g

Chocolate Charlotte Russe

1 env.	unflavored gelatin	1 env.
3 T.	cold water	45 mL
1 oz.	baking chocolate	30 g
¼ c.	boiling water	60 mL
¼ c.	granulated sugar replacement	60 mL
dash	salt	dash
1¾ c.	skim evaporated milk	440 mL
1 t.	vanilla extract	5 mL
10	ladyfingers	10

Soften gelatin in cold water for 5 minutes. Melt baking chocolate in top of double boiler; add boiling water and cook slowly, stirring constantly, to a smooth and thick paste. Add sugar replacement, salt and ¼ c. (190 mL) of the evaporated milk. Cook and stir 5 minutes longer. Remove from heat and add softened gelatin, stirring until gelatin is dissolved. Cool. Place remaining evaporated milk in a freezer tray and freeze until thoroughly chilled and edges are slightly frozen. When chocolate mixture begins to thicken and cool, whip slightly frozen milk until stiff and fold into cooled chocolate mixture with the vanilla. Line a decorative mold with the ladyfingers and pour the chocolate mixture into the mold. Chill until firm; unmold onto a serving plate.

Yield: 8 servings

Exchange, 1 serving: ⅔ bread, ½ fat
Each serving contains: Calories: 81, Carbohydrates: 22 g

Quick Chocolate Pastries

1 recipe	Pastry Cups	1 recipe
1 pkg.	low-calorie chocolate pudding mix	1 pkg.
2 c.	skim milk	500 mL
1 t.	unflavored gelatin	5 mL
1 t.	cinnamon	5 mL
1	egg white	1
1 c.	nondairy whipped topping	250 mL

Prepare pastry cups as directed in recipe. Cool completely. Combine pudding mix and milk in saucepan; add gelatin and cinnamon. Cook and stir as directed on package until pudding is very thick. Cool. Beat egg white until very stiff. Fold into pudding mixture. Refrigerate until completely set. Fill pastry cups. Turn nondairy whipped topping into decorative pastry tube. Decorate tops of pastries.

Yield: 10 servings

Exchange, 1 serving: ¾ bread
Each serving contains: Calories: 67, Carbohydrates: 19 g

Mizithropeta

1 c.	dry cottage cheese	250 mL
2 T.	granulated sugar replacement	30 mL
½ t.	vanilla extract	2 mL
½ t.	lemon rind, grated	2 mL
1	egg	1
10	phyllo leaves	10
¼ c.	butter, melted	60 mL
1	egg white, slightly beaten	1
4 t.	Powdered Sugar Replacement	20 mL
2 t.	cinnamon	10 mL

Combine cottage cheese, granulated sugar replacement, vanilla, lemon rind, and the whole egg in bowl. Stir to completely blend. Cut each phyllo leaf into three pieces and fold each piece in half. Combine melted butter and slightly beaten egg white in cup, beating with fork to blend. Brush each folded phyllo piece lightly with butter mixture. Place heaping 1 T. (15 mL) of cheese mixture in center of each piece, and fold phyllo leaves into triangular shape. Lightly brush top of triangle with butter mixture, and place on lightly greased cookie sheets. Bake at 350°F (175°C) for 10 to 12 minutes, or until lightly browned. Remove to cooling rack; cool. Combine powdered sugar replacement and cinnamon in cup, stir to mix, and sprinkle over triangles.

Yield: 30 triangles

Exchange, 2 triangles: ⅓ low-fat milk
Each serving contains: Calories: 68, Carbohydrates: 5 g

Royal Pastry

½ lb.	phyllo leaves	225 g
¼ c.	butter, melted	60 mL
1	egg white, slightly beaten	1
5	eggs, separated	5
3 T.	granulated sugar replacement	45 mL
1 t.	rum flavoring	5 mL
½ t.	cinnamon	2 mL
¼ t.	nutmeg	1 mL
1 c.	walnuts, finely ground	250 mL
½ c.	bread crumbs, finely ground	125 mL

Place one-sixth of the phyllo leaves on lightly greased 9 × 13 in. (23 × 33 cm) baking dish. Combine melted butter and the slightly beaten egg white in cup; beat with fork to blend. Brush phyllo leaves lightly with some of the butter mixture. Repeat entire procedure 2 more times, using a total of half of the phyllo leaves. Beat the 5 egg yolks with sugar replacement until light, thick and lemon-colored. Add rum flavoring, cinnamon, nutmeg, walnuts, and bread crumbs; fold to mix. Beat the 5 egg whites until stiff and then fold into walnut mixture. Spread evenly over phyllo leaves in baking dish. On towel, brush one-third of remaining phyllo leaves with melted butter mixture. Lay on top of walnut mixture. Repeat 2 more times with remaining phyllo leaves. Bake at 350°F (175°C) for 40 to 45 minutes, or until golden brown. While warm, score into 4 slices on short side and 6 slices on long side to form 24 squares. Score each square into a triangle.

Yield: 48 triangles

Exchange, 1 triangle: ½ fruit, ½ high-fat meat
Each serving contains: Calories: 64, Carbohydrates: 5 g

Mutzenmandein

2 c.	flour	500 mL
2 t.	baking powder	10 mL
¼ c.	granulated sugar replacement	60 mL
3	eggs	3
1 t.	rum extract	5 mL
½ t.	almond extract	2 mL
⅓ c.	cold margarine	90 mL
2 T.	water	30 mL
	oil for deep-fat frying	

Combine flour and baking powder in sifter; sift twice. Pour into large bowl, pushing flour mixture up the sides of the bowl, and add sugar replacement, eggs and flavorings to center well. Push and work flour into egg mixture. Add cold margarine and work into crumbs. Add water, only if needed to make smooth, firm dough. Chill slightly. Roll out ½ in. (1 cm) thick on lightly floured board, and cut into 2 × 1 in. (5 × 2 cm) rectangles. With sharp knife, cut each rectangle lengthwise into small strips. Fry in hot, deep fat (365°F or 180°C) until golden brown. Remove with slotted spoon to absorbent paper.

Yield: 32 pastries

Exchange, 1 pastry: ⅓ bread, ½ fat
Each serving contains: Calories: 50, Carbohydrates: 2 g

Basic Roll-Up Recipe

Use this for all the "jelly-roll" style recipes that follow. It's easy to do.

1 c.	cake flour, sifted	250 mL
1 t.	baking powder	5 mL
3 large	eggs	3 large
¼ c.	sugar	60 mL
3 pkgs.	acesulfame-K	3 pkgs.
⅓ c.	water	80 mL
1 t.	vanilla extract	5 mL

Spray a 15 × 10 × 1 in. (37 × 25 × 3 cm) jelly-roll pan; line the bottom with waxed paper; spray the paper. Sift the flour and baking powder together. With an electric mixer, beat the eggs in a medium bowl until thick and creamy and light in color. Gradually add the sugar and the acesulfame-K, beating constantly until the mixture is very thick. Stir in the water and vanilla. Fold in the flour mixture. Spread the batter evenly in the prepared pan.

Bake at 375°F (190°C) for 12 minutes or until the center of the cake springs back when lightly pressed. Loosen the cake around the edges with a knife. Invert the pan onto a clear tea towel, and peel off the waxed paper. Starting at the short end, roll up the cake and towel together. Place the roll seam-side-down on a wire rack and cool completely. When cool unroll carefully and assemble with filling. With a sharp knife, score the places where the slices will be, so they are even.

Yield: 10 servings

Exchange, 1 serving: 1 starch/bread
Each serving contains: Calories: 82, Total fat: 2 g, Carbohydrates: 14 g, Protein: 3 g, Sodium: 56 mg, Cholesterol: 64 mg

Fresh Strawberry Roll-Up

This recipe is a great alternative to Strawberry Shortcake—wonderful in the summer.

1 recipe	Basic Roll-Up Recipe	1 recipe	
2 c.	frozen low-fat non-dairy whipped topping	500 mL	
2 c.	fresh strawberries, hulled and quartered	500 mL	

Prepare the Basic Roll-Up Recipe. Cool and unroll. Stir the non-dairy whipped topping and the strawberries together. Spread this filling evenly on the roll. Starting from the short end, roll up the cake by lifting the cake with the end of the towel. Place the roll seam-side-down on a serving plate.

Yield: 10 slices

Exchange, 1 serving: 1 starch/bread, 1 fat
Each serving contains: Calories: 124, Total fat: 4 g, Carbohydrates: 19 g, Protein: 3 g, Sodium: 56 mg, Cholesterol: 64 mg

Chocolate Roll-Up

If you love chocolate, this will be a favorite.

1 recipe	Basic Roll-Up Recipe	1 recipe	
1 pkg.	sugar-free low-fat no-cook chocolate pudding mix	1 pkg.	
1½ c.	skim milk	375 mL	
2 T.	crème de cacao (optional)	30 mL	
½ c.	white topping (optional)	125 mL	

Prepare the Basic Roll-Up Recipe. Cool and unroll. Put the pudding mix in a mixing bowl. Add the skim milk and crème de cacao, if desired. Whip until thickened. Spread the pudding on the roll. Roll up the cake from the short end. To start rolling, lift the cake with the end of the towel. When rolled, place the roll seam-side-down on a serving plate. Optional: Top each slice with a dollop of your favorite white topping.

Yield: 10 slices

Exchange, 1 serving: 1 fruit, ½ lean meat
Each serving contains: Calories: 96, Total fat: 2 g, Carbohydrates: 17 g, Protein: 5 g, Sodium: 97 mg, Cholesterol: 65 mg

Peach Melba Roll-Up

Since there is no fresh fruit, you can make this "off the shelf" anytime.

1 recipe	Basic Roll-Up Recipe	1 recipe
1 recipe	Vanilla Tart Filling	1 recipe
15 oz.	sliced peaches in juice, drained	425 g can

Prepare the Basic Roll-Up Recipe. Cool and unroll. Prepare the tart filling and then spread it evenly on the cooled roll. Arrange the peach slices all over the surface and roll up the cake from the short end. To start rolling, lift the cake with the end of the towel. When rolled, place the roll seam-side down on a serving plate.

Yield: 10 slices

Exchange, 1 serving: 1½ starch/bread; ½ fat
Each serving contains: Calories: 164, Total fat: 5 g, Carbohydrates: 26 g, Protein: 5 g, Sodium: 110 mg, Cholesterol: 92 mg

Banana Walnut Roll-Up

1 recipe	Basic Roll-Up Recipe	1 recipe
1 recipe	Vanilla Tart Filling	1 recipe
3 small	ripe bananas, peeled and sliced	3 small
¼ c.	chopped walnuts	60 mL

Prepare the Basic Roll-Up Recipe. Cool and unroll. Prepare the tart filling and then stir the bananas and walnuts into it. Spread the filling evenly on the cooked roll and roll up the cake from the short end. To start rolling, lift the cake with the end of the towel. When rolled, place the roll seam-side-down on a serving plate.

Yield: 10 slices

Exchange, 1 serving: 2 starch/bread, 1 fat
Each serving contains: Calories: 195, Total fat: 7 g, Carbohydrates: 29 g, Protein: 6 g, Sodium: 108 mg, Cholesterol: 92 mg

Raisin Apple Spiral

1 pkg.	active dry yeast	1 pkg.
¾ c.	milk, warmed	190 mL
¼ c.	margarine, softened	60 mL
½ t.	salt	2 mL
2¼ c.	all-purpose flour	560 mL
1 c.	wheat germ	250 mL
1	egg	1
1 recipe	Raisin Apple Filling	1 recipe
	vegetable oil for brushing dough	
1	egg	1
1 T.	water	15 mL
⅓ c.	Powdered Sugar Replacement	90 mL
¼ t.	orange rind, grated	1 mL
3 t.	orange juice	15 mL

Raisin Apple Filling

1 c.	apple, chopped	250 mL
½ c.	raisins	125 mL
2 T.	butter	30 mL
½ c.	walnuts, chopped	125 mL
2 T.	orange rind, grated	30 mL
¼ t.	ground cinnamon	1 mL
¼ t.	ground or grated nutmeg	1 mL
dash	ground cloves	dash
dash	salt	dash

In a large bowl, dissolve the yeast in warm milk. Add margarine and salt, stirring until margarine almost melts. Stir in 1 c. (250 mL) of the flour, wheat germ, and egg. With an electric mixer, beat at medium speed for 2 minutes. Scrape bowl occasionally. With wooden spoon, gradually stir in just enough remaining flour to make a soft dough which leaves sides of bowl. Cover and allow to rise in warm, draft-free place about 1 hour or until doubled. Roll on floured board into a 24 × 4 in. (61 × 10 cm) strip. Spread the Raisin Apple Filling across middle of strip. To seal, lift dough and pinch lengthwise edges together with seam-side down, coil loosely, snail fashion. Place on greased baking sheet with space between to allow for rising. Brush dough lightly with oil. Cover and allow to rise about 1 hour or until doubled. Brush with 1 egg mixed with the water just before baking. Bake at 350°F (175°C) for 20 to 25 minutes until golden. Immediately remove from baking sheet. Cool slightly on rack. Combine powdered sugar replacement and orange rind and gradually add orange juice, beating until smooth. Drizzle on bread. Serve warm.

Combine apple, raisins and butter in a small saucepan. Cover and simmer over low heat for 10 minutes. Remove from heat and stir in the remaining ingredients. Cool.

Yield: 1 coffeecake or 24 servings

Exchange, 1 serving: 1 bread, 1 fat
Each serving contains: Calories: 112, Carbohydrates: 18 g

Squash or Pumpkin Roll

A variation on the traditional jelly roll, this one has a cream-cheese filling and a lovely, moist cake.

3	eggs	3
¼ c.	sugar	125 mL
3 pkts.	concentrated acesulfame-K	3 pkts.
1 t.	lemon juice	5 mL
¾ c.	canned squash or pumpkin	190 mL
¾ c.	flour	190 mL
1 t.	baking powder	5 mL
1 t.	ginger	5 mL
2 t.	cinnamon	10 mL
½ t.	nutmeg	2 mL
1 c.	chopped walnuts	250 mL

Filling

6 oz.	nonfat cream cheese	185 mL
4 T.	margarine or butter	60 mL
½ t.	butter-flavored extract	2 mL
½ t.	vanilla extract	2 mL
2 T.	sugar	30 mL
4 pkts.	concentrated acesulfame-K	4 pkts.

Beat eggs at high speed for 5 minutes until they are thick and light in color. Gradually add sugar, acesulfame-K, lemon, and squash. Sift the flour, baking powder, and spices all together and fold into the mixture. Mix well. Spread into a 10-in. (25 cm) jelly-roll pan lined with wax paper coated well with non-stick cooking spray. Spread nuts over the top. Bake at 375°F (190°C) for 12 minutes, until a toothpick inserted comes out clean. Turn onto a dish towel. Roll up with the towel in between. Cool.

To make the filling, whip together the cream cheese, margarine, and butter and vanilla extracts. Slowly add the sugar and acesulfame-K. Unroll the cake. Spread filling over the entire cake. Reroll and chill.

Yield: 20 slices

Exchange, 1 serving: ½ bread + 1 fat
Each serving contains: Calories: 111, Carbohydrates: 14 g, Fiber: 0.88 g, Sodium: 98 mg, Cholesterol: 42 mg

Traditional Cream Puffs

These look and taste like the cream puffs sold in bakeries.

1 recipe	Cream Puff Pastry	1 recipe
1 recipe	Vanilla Tart Filling	1 recipe
1 recipe	Chocolate Glaze or Napoleon Fudge Topping	1 recipe

Prepare the puff pastry, tart filling, and one of the toppings. Bake the cream puffs. Assemble by putting tart filling inside the puffs, covering with the tops, and drizzling with Chocolate Glaze or Napoleon Fudge.

Yield: 12 Traditional Cream Puffs

Exchange, 1 serving: 1 starch/bread, 2 fat
Each serving contains: Calories: 176, Total fat: 10 g, Carbohydrates: 15 g, Protein: 5 g, Sodium: 78 mg, Cholesterol: 94 mg

Light Chocolate Cream Puffs

Very impressive, and easier than pie!

1 recipe	Cream Puff Pastry	1 recipe
1 recipe	Chocolate Pudding	1 recipe
1 recipe	Chocolate Glaze or Napoleon Fudge Topping	1 recipe

Prepare the cream puffs from the puff pastry, make the Chocolate Pudding, and the glaze or fudge topping. Assemble the cream puffs by putting the pudding inside the pastry and drizzling the glaze or fudge topping over the top.

Yield: 12 Light Chocolate Cream Puffs

Exchange, 1 serving: 2 vegetable, 3 fat
Each serving contains: Calories: 139, Total fat: 15 g, Carbohydrates: 11 g, Protein: 4 g, Sodium: 62 mg, Cholesterol: 71 mg

Light Mocha Cream Puffs

1 recipe	Cream Puff Pastry	1 recipe
1 recipe	Mocha Tart Filling	1 recipe
1 recipe	Chocolate Glaze or Napoleon Fudge Topping	1 recipe

Prepare the cream puff pastry and the mocha filling. Bake the cream puffs. Assemble by putting the filling inside the cream puffs. Drizzle chocolate glaze or fudge topping over the top of the cream puffs.

Yield: 12 Light Mocha Cream Puffs

Exchange, 1 serving: 2 vegetable, 1½ fat
Each serving contains: Calories: 125, Total fat: 8 g, Carbohydrates: 10 g, Protein: 4 g, Sodium: 40 mg, Cholesterol: 71 mg

Strawberry Cream Puffs

An easy alternative to strawberry shortcake and very pretty.

1 recipe	Cream Puff Pastry	1 recipe
3 c.	fresh strawberries, or frozen whole strawberries without sugar	750 mL
1 c.	frozen low-fat non-dairy whipped topping	250 mL

Make and bake the cream puffs. Put ¼ c. (60 mL) strawberries in each puff. Put the top back on. Add a dollop of whipped topping to the top.

Yield: 12 Strawberry Cream Puffs

Exchange, 1 serving: 1 starch/bread; 1½ fat
Each serving contains: Calories: 142, Total fat: 7 g, Carbohydrates: 12 g, Protein: 3 g, Sodium: 22 mg, Cholesterol: 71 mg

Banana Cream Puffs

If you have bananas, all the rest of the ingredients are "on the shelf." I love this for unexpected guests.

1 recipe	Cream Puff Pastry	1 recipe	
1 recipe	Vanilla Tart Filling	1 recipe	
4 med	bananas, peeled and sliced	4 med	
3 t.	lemon juice	15 mL	
1 c.	frozen low-fat nondairy whipped topping	250 mL	

Prepare the cream puffs and Vanilla Tart Filling. Bake the cream puffs. Put the banana slices into a medium mixing bowl. Pour the lemon juice over the bananas and toss to distribute the lemon juice evenly. Add the pudding and mix. Spoon this pudding mixture into the cream puffs. Put the cream puff tops on and add a dollop of white topping.

Yield: 12 Banana Cream Puffs

Exchange, 1 serving: 1½ starch/bread, 2 fat
Each serving contains: Calories: 216, Total fat: 10 g, Carbohydrates: 24 g, Protein: 5 g, Sodium: 66 mg, Cholesterol: 94 mg

Cream Puffs with Raspberry Sauce

The raspberry sauce is striking against the light colors of the Puffs and filling and adds a contrasting flavor and texture, too.

1 recipe	Cream Puff Pastry	1 recipe	
1 recipe	Vanilla Tart Filling	1 recipe	
1 recipe	Raspberry Sauce	1 recipe	

Prepare the cream puffs, tart filling, and Raspberry Sauce. Bake the cream puffs. Fill them with the filling and put the tops back on. Spoon the sauce over the puffs.

Yield: 12 Cream Puffs with Raspberry Sauce

Exchange, 1 serving: 1 starch/bread, 1 vegetable, 2 fat
Each serving contains: Calories: 199, Total fat: 10 g, Carbohydrates: 20 g, Protein: 5 g, Sodium: 71 mg, Cholesterol: 94 mg

New Zealand Cream Puffs

Kiwis are ready to eat when they yield to gentle pressure. Eat them at their sweetest.

1 recipe	Cream Puff Pastry	1 recipe	
4	kiwi fruit, peeled and chopped	4	
2 c.	fresh strawberries, hulled and sliced	500 mL	
2 c.	frozen low-fat non-dairy whipped topping, thawed	500 mL	

Prepare the cream puffs according to the directions. When ready to assemble, put the chopped kiwis and sliced strawberries in a bowl. Add the whipped topping and fold the mixture together. Spoon the fruit mixture into the cream puffs. Put the tops back on and serve immediately.

Yield: 12 New Zealand Cream Puffs

Exchange, 1 serving: 1 starch/bread, 2 fat
Each serving contains: Calories: 167, Total fat: 9 g, Carbohydrates: 16 g, Protein: 4 g, Sodium: 23 mg, Cholesterol: 71 mg

Icy Peach Cream Puffs

Only the puffs are prepared ahead of time for this. Prepare them in the morning and refrigerate the peaches. Assemble everything after serving dinner.

1 recipe	Cream Puff Pastry	1 recipe	
3 c.	sugar-free low-fat vanilla ice cream or frozen yogurt	750 mL	
30 oz.	canned peaches packed in juice, drained, chopped and chilled	850 g	

Prepare the basic cream puff recipe. Bake the puffs. When ready to serve, put ½ c. (60 mL) ice cream in each puff. Distribute the chopped peaches over the ice cream. Put on the tops and serve immediately.

Yield: 12 Icy Peach Cream Puffs

Exchange, 1 serving: 1½ starch/bread, 1 fat
Each serving contains: Calories: 172, Total fat: 8 g, Carbohydrates: 22 g, Protein: 4 g, Sodium: 39 mg, Cholesterol: 71 mg

Frozen Chocolate Cream Puffs

Prepare these ahead of time and freeze them. I move them to the refrigerator just as I'm putting dinner on the table. They are perfect for dessert.

1 recipe	Cream Puff Pastry	1 recipe	
3 c.	cold skim milk	750 mL	
2 pkgs.	sugar-free chocolate pudding mix	2 pkgs.	

Prepare the basic cream puffs. Bake them. In a medium mixing bowl, beat together the skim milk and the pudding mix with an electric mixer until thick. Scoop the pudding into the cream puffs. Put the tops on and freeze. When frozen, put them in plastic bags until you are ready to use them.

Yield: 12 Frozen Chocolate Cream Puffs

Exchange, 1 serving: 1 milk, 1½ fat
Each serving contains: Calories: 141, Total fat: 8 g, Carbohydrates: 12 g, Protein: 6 g, Sodium: 90 mg, Cholesterol: 72 mg

Frozen Raspberry Cream Puffs

These make-ahead cream puffs are perfect to freeze and eat one at a time.

1 recipe	Cream Puff Pastry	1 recipe	
1 recipe	Raspberry Filling for Raspberry Cream Pie	1 recipe	

Prepare the basic cream puffs and the filling for the raspberry cream pie. Bake the puffs. Spoon the filling into the cream puffs, put on the tops, and freeze them. After they are frozen, put them in plastic freezer bags. Remove from the freezer at the beginning of dinner and they will be ready by dessert time.

Yield: 12 Frozen Raspberry Cream Puffs

Exchange, 1 serving: 1 starch/bread, 2 fat
Each serving contains: Calories: 156, Total fat: 9 g, Carbohydrates: 15 g, Protein: 3 g, Sodium: 49 mg, Cholesterol: 71 mg

Turnovers

A turnover is a piece of pastry wrapped around a filling, usually fruit-based. When you use phyllo dough for the pastry, you get a turnover with a relatively low cost in calories and exchanges, depending on the filling you choose. One sheet of phyllo dough makes a large turnover. Half would be considered a serving. Phyllo dough with fruit filling in it is best eaten on the day it is baked.

4 sheets	phyllo dough	4 sheets
1 c.	filling	250 mL

Follow the general directions for phyllo dough. Spread out one large sheet, coat with butter-flavored non-stick vegetable cooking spray. Fold the dough into thirds the long way. Spray again. Put ¼ c. (60 mL) filling on the dough about 2 inches (5 cm) from the bottom. Using your fingers, fold the dough up and over the filling; then press down gently. Fold this filled section up towards the plain dough. Fold it up again, as if you were folding a flag. Continue until all the dough has been folded up over the filling. Use your fingers to be sure it is scaled at the edges. Spray the dough again. Put the turnover on a cookie sheet that has been sprayed with non-stick vegetable cooking spray. Repeat with the other three turnovers, or as many as you want. Bake in a preheated 375°F (190°C) oven for 10 minutes.

Yield: 4 turnovers (filling counted separately)

Exchange, 1 serving: 1 bread
Each serving contains: Calories: 72, Carbohydrates: 17 g, Fiber: trace, Sodium: 120 mg, Cholesterol: 0 mg

Apple Turnovers

Need something to serve in a pinch? These turnovers can be made in only 10 minutes and are quite tasty.

2 slices	bread (crust removed)	2 slices
1	apple, peeled, cored and sliced thin	1
1 t.	lemon juice	5 mL
¼ t.	cinnamon	1 mL
1 pkt.	concentrated acesulfame-K	1 pkt.

Roll the bread thin with a rolling pin. Microwave the other ingredients until the apple is tender. The length of time will depend on the type of apple and the power of the oven. I start with 10 seconds on medium and adjust from there. The key is, you don't want the apple mushy. Place half the mixture on each piece of bread. Fold the bread diagonally to form a triangle. Moisten the edges of the bread and press the sides of the turnover together with fork. Lightly spray both sides with vegetable cooking spray. Place on a cookie sheet coated with non-stick vegetable cooking spray. Bake at 425°F (220°C) for about 7 minutes or until brown.

Yield: 2 turnovers

Exchange, 1 serving: 1 bread + ½ fruit
Each serving contains: Calories: 95, Carbohydrates: 11 g, Fiber: 2 g, Sodium: 102 mg, Cholesterol: 1 mg

Strawberry Turnovers

¼ t.	cornstarch	2 mL	
1 T.	water	15 mL	
½ c.	Strawberry Topping	125 mL	
1	dough for Basic Pie Shell	1	
	Vanilla Gloss		

Blend cornstarch and water. Add to Strawberry Topping. Cook over low heat until very thick. Roll pie dough thin. Cut into eight 4 in. (10 cm) squares. Place 1½ t. (7 mL) of the strawberry mixture into center of each square. Fold each square into a triangle; press sides securely together to seal. Bake at 400°F (200°C) for 9 to 11 minutes, or until golden brown. Brush with Vanilla Gloss.

Microwave: Use microwave only for strawberry filling. Blend cornstarch and water. Add to Strawberry Topping. Cook on High for 30 seconds, or until very thick. Proceed as above.

Yield: 8 turnovers

Exchange, 1 turnover: 1 bread
Each serving contains: Calories: 180, Carbohydrates: 20 g

Hawaiian Napoleon

3 piles	phyllo dough napoleon rectangles	3 piles	
¼ c.	sugar-free vanilla pudding made with skim milk	60 mL	
1 T.	pineapple, crushed, in juice	15 mL	
1 t.	coconut flakes	25 mL	
1 t.	Strawberry-Kiwi Glaze	25 mL	

Bake sheets of phyllo according to the general instructions at the beginning of this chapter. Cut the pile of four sprayed sheets into 16 rectangles. Bake in a preheated 375°F (190°C) oven for 8 minutes. Three of these rectangular piles are used to make each napoleon.

Place one cooked and cooled four-layer rectangular stack on a dessert plate. Spread on the vanilla pudding. Place a second rectangular pile on top of the vanilla pudding. Top this layer with the crushed pineapple. Sprinkle on the coconut. Add the last layer of phyllo. Smooth on the Strawberry Kiwi Glaze.

Yield: 1 Hawaiian Napoleon

Exchange, 1 serving: 1 fruit, ⅓ starch/bread
Each serving contains: Calories: 105, Total fat: 1 g, Carbohydrates: 21 g, Protein: 1 g, Sodium: 248 mg, Cholesterol: 0 mg

Strawberry Kiwi Glaze

Glaze Hawaiian Napoleons with this.

¼ c.	lemon juice	60 mL
¼ c.	water	60 mL
1 T.	cornstarch	15 mL
2 t.	strawberry-kiwi Crystal Light mix	10 mL

In a small saucepan, mix together the lemon juice, water, and cornstarch. Stir until smooth. Heat over medium heat until the mixture begins to boil. Stirring constantly, lower heat and cook until mixture turns from milky to opaque and thickens. Set aside to cool. Stir in strawberry-kiwi mix. Blend well. Add a few drops of water if the mixture becomes too thick to spread evenly.

Yield: ½ cup of glaze-25 servings (1 t. [5 mL] per serving)

Exchange, 1 serving: free
Each serving contains: Calories: 2, Total fat: 0 g, Carbohydrates: 1 g, Protein: 0 g, Sodium: 0 mg, Cholesterol: 0 mg

Washington's Birthday Napoleon

For each napoleon prepare the following.

3 piles	phyllo dough napoleon rectangles (4 deep)	3 piles
¼ c.	sugar-free vanilla pudding, made with skim milk	60 mL
2	maraschino cherries, finely chopped	2
1 t.	fruit-only cherry preserves	5 mL
½ t.	Cherry Glaze	3 mL

Bake sheets of phyllo according to the general instructions at the beginning of this chapter. Cut the pile of four sprayed sheets into 16 rectangles. Bake in a preheated 375°F (190°C) oven for 8 minutes. Three of these rectangular piles are used to make each napoleon.

Arrange one phyllo dough rectangle on a dessert plate. Put the vanilla pudding in a small bowl. Add the maraschino cherries. Mix well. Spread the cherry preserves gently onto the phyllo rectangle. Cover with a second rectangle. Pile the vanilla pudding on this layer. Spread to the edges. Put the last rectangle on top. Frost the top layer with Cherry Glaze.

Yield: 1 Washington's Birthday Napoleon

Exchange, 1 serving: 1 fruit
Each serving contains: Calories: 86, Total fat: 0.9 g, Carbohydrates: 16 g, Protein: 0.9 g, Sodium: 243 mg, Cholesterol: 1 mg

Cherry Glaze

This can be refrigerated and reheated when needed.

¼ c.	sugar-free cherry preserves	60 mL
1 t.	Kirschwasser (cherry liqueur)	5 mL

Put the cherry preserves into a small saucepan. Add the cherry liqueur and mix well with a fork or wire whisk. Heat gently, stirring constantly. Cool.

Yield: 12 servings

Exchange, 1 serving: free
Each serving contains: Calories: 13, Total fat: 0 g, Carbohydrates: 0 g, Protein: 0 g, Sodium: 3 mg, Cholesterol: 0 mg

Mocha Napoleon

For each napoleon prepare the following.

3 piles	phyllo dough napoleon rectangles (4 deep)	3 piles
¼ c.	Mocha Tart Filling (recipe follows)	60 mL
1 t.	seedless, no-sugar-added raspberry jam	5 mL
¼ c.	frozen low-fat nondairy whipped topping	60 mL
1 t.	Mocha Glaze	5 mL

Bake sheets of phyllo according to the general instructions at the beginning of this chapter. Cut the pile of four sprayed sheets into 16 rectangles. Bake in a preheated 375°F (190°C) oven for 8 minutes.

Arrange one phyllo rectangle on a dessert plate. Spread the Mocha Tart Filling on top of the phyllo. Put a second phyllo rectangle on a flat surface such as a tabletop. Carefully spread the raspberry jam on this rectangle and then place this, jam-side-up, on the previous layer. Spread the non-dairy whipped topping on top of the jam. Top this layer with the last rectangle. Smooth the Mocha Glaze on the top.

Yield: 1 Mocha Napoleon

Exchange, 1 serving: 1 fruit, ½ high-fat meat
Each serving contains: Calories: 122, Total fat: 3 g, Carbohydrates: 18 g, Protein: 3 g, Sodium: 146 mg, Cholesterol: 1 mg

Mocha Tart Filling

For a sharper coffee taste, use instant espresso coffee powder.

1 pkg.	sugar-free chocolate pudding mix*	1 pkg.
1½ c.	skim milk	375 mL
3 t.	instant coffee powder	15 mL

Combine all the ingredients in a saucepan. Bring to a boil and cook, stirring constantly until pudding has thickened.

Yield: Enough for 6 napoleons

Exchange, 1 serving: 1 vegetable
Each serving of filling contains: Calories: 24, Total fat: 0.1 g, Carbohydrates: 4 g, Protein: 2 g, Sodium: 68 mg, Cholesterol: 1 mg

*4 serving size

Mocha Glaze

Drizzle over napoleons for a coffee-chocolate accent.

2 T.	cocoa powder	30 mL
2 t.	instant coffee powder	10 mL
2 T.	hot water	30 mL
2 T.	fat-free cream cheese	30 mL
2 t.	aspartame sweetener	10 mL

Stir together the cocoa powder and instant coffee powder. Add the hot water and mix together until the mixture is smooth and evenly moist. Beat in the cream cheese and sweetener until smooth.

Yield: 15 servings

Exchange, 1 serving: free
Each serving contains: Calories: 5, Total fat: 0.1 g, Carbohydrates: 0.9 g, Protein: 0.3 g, Sodium: 9 mg, Cholesterol: 0 mg

Chocolate Glaze

Add a little extra milk to get the right consistency if this is too thick.

2 T.	cocoa powder	30 mL
2 T.	skim milk	30 mL
2 T.	fat-free cream cheese	30 mL
2 t.	aspartame sweetener	10 mL

Combine the cocoa powder and skim milk in a small bowl until the mixture is moistened. Using a fork, beat in the cream cheese. The mixture will be smooth. Add in the aspartame and mix well.

Yield: enough for 15 napoleons

Exchange, 1 serving: free
Each serving of filling contains: Calories: 5, Total fat: 0.1 g, Carbohydrates: 0.9 g, Protein: 0.4 g, Sodium: 10 mg, Cholesterol: 0 mg

Hot Fudge Napoleon

For each napoleon, prepare the following:

3 piles	phyllo dough napoleon rectangles (4 deep)	3 piles
¼ c.	sugar-free vanilla low-fat ice cream or frozen yogurt	60 mL
2 T.	sugar-free vanilla pudding made with skim milk	30 mL
2 T.	frozen low-fat nondairy whipped topping, thawed	30 mL
5 t.	Napoleon Fudge Topping	25 mL
1	fresh cherry or maraschino cherry	1

Bake sheets of phyllo according to the general instructions at the beginning of this chapter. Cut the pile of four sprayed sheets into 16 rectangles. Bake in a preheated 375°F (190°C) oven for 8 minutes.

Arrange one phyllo rectangle on a dessert plate. Put the ice cream onto the rectangle and cover with another phyllo rectangle. In a small bowl, combine the pudding and whipped topping with a fork. Spread this onto the phyllo rectangle. Lay the last rectangle on the top of the pile. Top the napoleon with the hot Napoleon Fudge Topping and the cherry.

Yield: 1 Hot Fudge Napoleon

Exchange, 1 serving: 1 starch/bread, 1 fat
Each serving contains: Calories: 160, Total fat: 5 g, Carbohydrates: 18 g, Protein: 3 g, Sodium: 260 mg, Cholesterol: 5 mg

Napoleon Fudge Topping

Rich and creamy, this topping tastes like the kind from the nicest bakeries.

2 T.	cocoa powder, unsweetened	30 mL
1 t.	canola oil	5 mL
2 t.	skim milk	10 mL
2 t.	aspartame sweetener	10 mL
½ t.	vanilla extract	3 mL
⅛ t.	butter extract	1 mL

Put the cocoa powder in a small saucepan. Add the canola oil and skim milk. Heat gently over a low flame, stirring constantly, until the mixture is blended and heated. Remove from heat. Stir in the aspartame and extracts and mix well. Spoon while still warm over the top of the napoleon.

Yield: enough for 2 napoleons

Exchange, 1 serving: 1 starch/bread
*Each serving of topping contains: Calories: 90, Total fat: 3 g, Carbo-
hydrates: 12 g, Protein: 2 g, Sodium: 160 mg, Cholesterol: 0 mg*

Berry Good Napoleon

For each napoleon, prepare the following:

3 piles	phyllo dough napoleon rectangles (4 deep)	3 piles
2	fresh strawberries or frozen whole strawberries, defrosted, diced	2
6	fresh raspberries or frozen whole raspberries, defrosted, diced	6
2 T.	lemon filling for Berry Good Napoleons	30 mL
¼ c.	sugar-free vanilla pudding made with skim milk	60 mL
2 T.	frozen low-fat nondairy whipped topping, thawed	30 mL

Bake sheets of phyllo according to the general instructions at the beginning of the chapter. Cut the pile of four sprayed sheets into 16 rectangles. Bake in a preheated 375°F (190°C) oven for 8 minutes.

Arrange one phyllo rectangle on a dessert plate. Mix the strawberries and raspberries together in a small bowl. Mash lightly with a fork. Set aside. Spread the lemon filling on the phyllo rectangle. Top with another rectangle. In another bowl, mix together the pudding and whipped topping. Do this gently with a fork. Spread the pudding on the rectangle. Top with the third rectangle. Spoon the fruit over the top.

Yield: 1 Berry Good Napoleon

Exchange, 1 serving: 1 starch/bread
*Each serving contains: Calories: 102, Total fat: 2 g, Carbohydrates:
17 g, Protein: 2 g, Sodium: 248 mg, Cholesterol: 0 mg*

Lemon Filling

Light and lemony.

1 T.	cornstarch	15 mL
2 T.	water	30 mL
⅓ c.	fresh lemon juice	80 mL
7 pkgs.	acesulfame-K	7 pkgs.
¼ c.	egg substitute	60 mL
2 t.	vanilla extract	10 mL

Put the cornstarch and water into a small saucepan and mix to dissolve the cornstarch. Add the lemon juice and acesulfame-K. Cook gently, stirring constantly until the mixture thickens. In another pan, heat the egg substitute. Spoon some of the lemon mixture into the eggs. Mix well. Now combine in the rest of the lemon mixture and the vanilla extract. Cook over low heat for a minute or two. Cool.

Yield: 1 cup: enough for 8 Berry Good Napoleons

Exchange, 1 serving: free
Each serving of filling contains: Calories: 14, Total fat: 0.3 g, Carbohydrates: 2 g, Protein: 0.1 g, Sodium: 14 mg, Cholesterol: 0 mg

Phyllo Strudel

You won't believe how easy strudel is until you try.

Read the directions for phyllo dough in Pastry Basics. Layer four sheets, spraying each from edge to edge with non-stick cooking spray. Don't cut them into napoleon rectangles. Leave one in. (2.5 cm) free of filling at each edge. Spoon the filling, leaving one in. (2.5 cm) clear from the left edge along the short side. Roll from the right side. The filling will roll up into the inside.

Put the roll on an ungreased cookie sheet with the seam down and tuck the ends under. Brush with melted butter. Bake in a preheated 325°F (165°C) oven for 25–30 minutes. Cool before slicing. Best if sliced with an electric knife or a very sharp serrated knife.

Yield: 10 slices

Exchange, 1 serving: ½ fat
Each serving contains: Calories: 33, Total fat: 2 g, Carbohydrates: 4 g, Protein: 1 g, Sodium: 48 mg, Cholesterol: 3 mg

Date Strudel

½ c.	dates, cut up	125 mL
1 c.	water	250 mL
1 T.	cornstarch	15 mL
¼ c.	margarine	60 mL
⅓ lb.	phyllo leaves	150 g
	fine bread crumbs	

Combine dates, water, and cornstarch in saucepan. Cook and stir until very thick; remove from heat. Melt margarine. Place two phyllo leaves, side by side, on a lightly dampened, lightly bread-crumbed cloth. Brush leaves lightly with melted margarine. Lay a second leaf on top of each leaf. Brush each layer lightly with melted margarine. Repeat using all of the leaves. Place date filling 2 in. (5 cm) in from long edges. Fold long edges in over the filling. Fold over the ends. Roll up dough, jelly-roll fashion. Score top into 10 pieces with a sharp knife or scissors and place on greased cookie sheet. Bake at 350°F (175°C) for 25 minutes, or until lightly browned.

Yield: 10 pieces

Exchange, 1 piece: 1 bread, ½ fat
Each serving contains: Calories: 100, Carbohydrates: 16 g

Apple Walnut Strudel

2	apples	2
⅓ c.	walnuts, chopped	90 mL
¼ t.	lemon juice	1 mL
¼ c.	margarine	60 mL
⅓ lb.	phyllo leaves	150 g
	bread crumbs	

Peel, core and chop apples. Combine apples, walnuts, and lemon juice in mixing bowl; fold to mix. Melt margarine. Place 2 phyllo leaves on a lightly dampened, lightly bread-crumbed cloth. Brush leaves lightly with melted margarine. Lay a second leaf on top of each leaf. Brush each layer lightly with melted margarine. Repeat using all the leaves. Place apple filling 2 in. (5 cm) in from long edges. Fold long edges in over the filling. Fold over the ends. Roll up dough, jelly-roll fashion. Score top into 10 pieces with a sharp knife or scissors and place on greased cookie sheet. Bake at 350°F (175°C) for 25 minutes, or until lightly browned.

Yield: 10 pieces

Exchange, 1 piece: ½ bread, 1 fat
Each serving contains: Calories: 108, Carbohydrates: 18 g

Cherry Strudel Filling

No one will believe this is low-calorie, it's so yummy.

1 lb.	sweet cherries, pitted	450 g
¼ c.	almonds, chopped	60 mL
2 T.	sugar	30 mL

Combine all ingredients. Roll and bake in phyllo sheets as directed previously.

Yield: filling for 10 servings

Exchange, 1 serving: ½ starch/bread, ½ fat
Each serving of filling contains: Calories: 63, Total fat: 2 g, Carbohydrates: 1 g, Protein: 1 g, Sodium: 0 mg, Cholesterol: 0 mg

Prune Filling for Strudel

When I make this strudel, everyone asks what the filling is made of. No one ever guesses prunes.

1 c.	prunes, pitted	250 mL
½ c.	unsweetened apple juice	125 mL
2 t.	lemon peel	10 mL

In a small saucepan, cover the prunes with the juice. Bring to a boil over medium heat. Let stand 10 minutes. Pour off any unabsorbed liquid. Purée in a blender or food processor. Mix in the lemon peel. Roll and bake in phyllo sheets as directed previously.

Yield: filling for 10 servings

Exchange, 1 serving: ⅔ fruit
Each serving of filling contains: Calories: 44, Total fat: 0.1 g, Carbohydrates: 11 g, Protein: 1 g, Sodium: 1 mg, Cholesterol: 0 mg

Apricot Filling for Strudel

A little sweet and tangy.

1 c.	dried apricots	250 mL
½ c.	orange juice	125 mL
2 t.	orange rind	10 mL

Put the apricots into a small saucepan. Cover with orange juice. Bring to a boil. Let stand 10 minutes. Pour out any unabsorbed liquid. Puree in a food processor or blender. Mix in the orange rind. Roll and bake in phyllo sheets as directed previously.

Yield: filling for 10 servings

Exchange, 1 serving: ⅔ fruit
Each serving of filling contains: Calories: 44, Total fat: 0.1 g, Carbohydrates: 11 g, Protein: 0.7 g, Sodium: 2 mg, Cholesterol: 0 mg

Cream Cheese Pastries

Without the new fat-free dairy products, this recipe would have too much fat.

4 T.	butter or margarine	60 mL
8 oz	fat-free cream cheese	225 g
2 T.	sugar	30 mL
4 pkgs.	acesulfame-K sugar substitute	4 pkgs.
1 large	egg or equivalent egg substitute, lightly beaten	1 large
1½ c.	flour	375 mL
1 t.	baking powder	5 mL
½ t.	butter extract	3 mL
½ c.	fat-free sour cream	125 mL

In a large mixing bowl, cream the butter and cream cheese together until soft and creamy. Blend in the sugar and acesulfame-K. Blend in the egg. In another bowl, sift together the flour and baking powder. In a small bowl mix together the butter extract and sour cream. In the large mixing bow containing the butter and cream cheese, alternately add the flour mixture and the sour cream mixture. Blend thoroughly. Make a ball and wrap it in plastic wrap. Refrigerate until chilled. Roll dough on a lightly floured board until it is about ⅛ in. (3 mm) thick. Use cookie cutters to cut the dough into shapes. Place cookies on a baking sheet that has been coated with non-stick cooking spray. Bake in a preheated 400°F (200°C) oven for 8–10 minutes.

Yield: 90 (small) pastry cookies

Exchange, 1 serving: free
Each serving contains: Calories: 17, Total fat: 0.6 g, Carbohydrates: 2 g, Protein: 1 g, Sodium: 23 mg, Cholesterol: 4 mg

Cookies

Cookies present an inherent challenge in diabetic cooking. Without fat, cookies don't hold together. Without sugar, cookies don't have a nice light texture, don't rise up, and don't brown nicely. We present a collection of excellent cookie recipes with a minimum of sugar and the balance of sweetening added with artificial sweeteners.

Our best hint for serving cookies is to count out the appropriate number and then serve them on a small, decorative plate. When the cookies are presented, make it look like a special occasion. Serve tea from a pretty teapot in pretty teacups. Or serve the cookies with a cup of coffee, dietetic hot chocolate, or a glass of skim milk. Again, make snack time special by using nice napkins and place mats. For many people this helps satisfy a need to feel nurtured and loved.

Did you ever just stand up in the kitchen and munch cookies as you leaned against the counter? We've probably all done this when we were hungry or otherwise needy. It's all too easy to take in many too many calories and exchanges this way. So serve your cookies or squares or scones on a decorative plate and enjoy.

For some classic recipes, we offer a choice, because some people like their brownies rich and fudgy, while others prefer cakelike ones.

Walnut Roll-Up Cookies

1 pkg.	active dry yeast	1 pkg.
¼ c.	warm water	60 mL
2 c.	flour	500 mL
¼ c.+ 2 T.	fat-free fruit-based butter-and-oil replacement	90 mL
2 T.	oil replacement	30 mL
1 large	egg or equivalent egg substitute, lightly beaten	1 large
3 oz.	fat-free cream cheese	80 g
2 T.	sugar	15 mL
1 t.	orange peel, grated	5 mL
1 t.	orange extract	5 mL
½ c.	walnuts, finely ground	125 mL

In a small mixing bowl, combine the yeast and warm water. In a large mixing bowl, combine the flour and butter replacement. Beat in the egg. Add the yeast and mix just until blended. On a lightly floured board, roll out the dough into two 13 × 9 in. (33 × 22 cm) rectangles. In a mixing bowl, beat the cream cheese until light and fluffy. Add the sugar, orange peel, and the orange extract. Beat well. Spread half the cream cheese mixture on each rectangle. Sprinkle with walnuts. Starting at the long side, roll up the rectangles. Place each roll on a cookie sheet that has been coated with nonstick vegetable cooking spray. Put the seam side down. Bake in a preheated 375°F (190°C) oven for 20–25 minutes. Cool. Cut into 1 in. (2.5 cm) slices.

Yield: 24 cookies

Exchange, 1 cookie: 1 starch/bread
Each serving contains: Calories: 73, Total fat: 2 g, Carbohydrates: 12 g, Protein: 3 g, Sodium: 14 mg, Cholesterol: 9 mg

No-Bake Coconut Surprise

An easy treat to whip together and store in the refrigerator.

1 (8 oz.) pkg.	nonfat cream cheese	1 (250 mL) pkg.
1 pkt.	concentrated acesulfame-K	1 pkt.
1 T.	walnuts, chopped	15 mL
1 t.	orange extract	5 mL
¼ c.	toasted flaked coconut	60 mL

Beat the cheese with acesulfame-K until light and fluffy; add the walnuts and the extract. Shape into 20 balls, each about ½ t. Roll each in coconut. Chill.

Yield: 20 cookies

Exchange, 1 cookie: ½ meat
Each serving contains: Calories: 33, Fiber: trace, Sodium: 54 mg, Cholesterol: 1.6 mg

Cookie Cutter Cookies

Children and adults love cookies cut into shapes. If you like sprinkles, try dusting these with Crystal Light as they come out of the oven.

1 c.	margarine or butter	350 mL
¼ c.	sugar	60 mL
6 pkts.	concentrated acesulfame-K	6 pkts.
2½ c.	flour	625 mL
1 t.	baking soda	5 mL
1 t.	cream of tartar	5 mL
1 t.	vanilla extract	5 mL
1 t.	almond extract	5 mL
1	egg or equivalent egg substitute	1

Cream the margarine and sugar. Stir in the rest of the ingredients one at a time in the order listed. Form the dough into a ball, wrap it in plastic wrap, and refrigerate it for at least two hours. Cut the dough into thirds. Roll each third ⅛ in. (5 mm) thick on a lightly floured board. Cut the dough into shapes with the cookie cutters. Place the cookies onto ungreased cookie sheets. Bake at 400°F (200°C) for 5–8 minutes.

Yield: 100 small cookies

Exchange, 1 cookie: ½ fat
Each serving contains: Calories: 29, Carbohydrates: 3 g, Fiber: trace, Sodium: 13 mg, Cholesterol: 0 mg

Cinnamon Crescents

These cookies look very fancy when they are made up. They are yummy too!

1 c.	margarine or butter	250 mL
2 c.	flour, sifted	500 mL
1	egg yolk	1
¼ c.	nonfat sour cream	190 mL
3 T.	sugar	45 mL
3 pkts.	concentrated acesulfame-K	3 pkts.
¾ c.	finely chopped walnuts	190 mL
2 t.	cinnamon	30 mL
1	egg white, slightly beaten in 1 T. (15 mL) water	1

Cut the margarine into the flour until the mixture resembles coarse crumbs. Stir in the egg yolk and sour cream. Form a ball. Cover with plastic wrap and chill for two hours. Combine the sugar, acesulfame-K, walnuts, and cinnamon. Divide the dough into fourths. Roll each into an 11 in. (28 cm) circle. Sprinkle with a quarter of the sugar mixture. Cut into 16 wedges. Roll up the wedges, starting at the widest end. Place the rolls on an ungreased cookie sheet. Brush with egg white and water. Bake in a 350°F (180°C) oven for 20 minutes or until golden brown. Cool on wire racks.

Yield: 48 cookies

Exchange, 1 cookie: ½ bread + ½ fat
Each serving contains: Calories: 70, Carbohydrates: 4 g, Fiber: trace, Sodium: 6.6 mg, Cholesterol: 6.2 mg

Snickerdoodles

New research has indicated that the smell of cinnamon baking is all aphrodisiac! These cookies may be the way to his (or her) heart.

1 c.	margarine or butter	250 mL
¼ c.	sugar	60 mL
6 pkts.	concentrated acesulfame-K	6 pkts.
2	eggs	2
1 t.	vanilla extract	5 mL
2⅔ c.	flour, sifted	690 mL
2 t.	cream of tartar	10 mL
1 t.	baking soda	5 mL
Coating		
2 T.	sugar	30 mL
1 t.	cinnamon	5 mL

Beat the margarine until light. Add the sugar and acesulfame-K and beat until fluffy. Beat in the eggs and vanilla. Sift together the flour, cream of tartar, and baking soda. Add this to the margarine mixture.

Combine the sugar and cinnamon in a separate bowl. With floured hands, shape the dough into small balls about 1 inch (2.5 cm) apiece and roll each one in the sugar-cinnamon mixture. Place each 2 inches (5 cm) apart on an ungreased baking sheet. Bake at 400°F (200°C) for 8–10 minutes. Cool on wire racks.

Yield: 6 dozen cookies

Exchange, 1 cookie: ½ fat
Each serving contains: Calories: 44, Carbohydrates: 5 g, Fiber: trace, Sodium: 18 mg, Cholesterol: 7.6 mg

Swedish Ginger Snaps

These treats are called "pepparkakor" in Swedish, and for Christmas are cut into hearts, stars and other Christmas shapes.

⅓ c.	molasses	90 mL
1 t.	ginger	5 mL
1 t.	cinnamon	5 mL
½ t.	ground cloves	2 mL
6 pkts.	concentrated acesulfame-K	6 pkts.
¼ T.	baking soda	3 mL
⅔ c.	margarine or butter	180 mL
⅔ c.	nonfat sour cream	180 mL
¼ c.	egg substitute (or 1 egg)	60 mL
5 c.	sifted flour	1.25 L

In a saucepan, bring the molasses and spices to a boil. Remove from the heat and add the acesulfame-K, baking soda, and margarine. Stir until the margarine melts. Add the sour cream, egg substitute, and flour and mix thoroughly. Turn out onto lightly floured board and knead into a ball. Wrap in plastic wrap and refrigerate two hours or more. Roll a manageable amount of dough on a lightly floured board to a thickness of ¼ in. (55 mm) and cut with cookie cutters. Place on a cookie sheet coated with nonstick cooking spray. Bake at 325°F (160°C) for 8–10 minutes.

Yield: 250 very thin cookies

Exchange: free
Each serving contains: Calories: 13, Carbohydrates: 2 g, Fiber: trace, Sodium: 12 mg, Cholesterol: trace

Dream Cookies

½ c.	margarine or butter	125 mL
¼ c.	sugar	60 mL
6 pkts.	concentrated acesulfame-K	6 pkts.
½ c.	nonfat cream cheese	125 mL
2 t.	vanilla extract	10 mL
1 t.	baking powder	5 mL
2 c.	flour, sifted	500 mL
20	blanched almonds, halved	20

Brown the margarine slightly in a frying pan. Let it cool and transfer it to a bowl. Add the sugar, acesulfame-K, and cream cheese. Beat until smooth and blended. Add the vanilla and baking powder. Mix well. Add the flour and mix. The dough will be crumbly. Using your hands, roll the dough into smooth balls about the size of walnuts. Place each on a cookie sheet sprayed with non-stick cooking spray. Put half an almond on the top of each ball. Bake in a 250°F (120°C) oven until golden brown, about half an hour.

Yield: 40 cookies

Exchange, 1 cookie: ½ bread + ½ fat
Each serving contains: Calories: 51, Carbohydrates: 6 g, Fiber: trace, Sodium: 12 mg, Cholesterol: trace

Amaretto Dreams

These fragile cookies are much like the ones that come in fancy packages at the grocery store. They are easy to make and much less expensive.

¼ c.	margarine	125 mL
2 t.	Amaretto	10 mL
1 t.	almond extract	5 mL
2	egg whites	2
8 t.	fructose	40 mL
¼ c.	flour	125 mL
⅓ c.	blanched almonds, ground	90 mL

In a small saucepan, melt the margarine; stir in the Amaretto and almond extract. Set aside to cool. In a medium bowl, beat the egg whites until soft peaks form; beat in the fructose, then fold in the flour; beat in the margarine mixture. Mix the almonds into the batter. Drop by small teaspoonfuls onto baking sheets coated with non-stick vegetable cooking spray, spacing mounds well apart. Using a fork dipped in cold water, flatten each mound with a crisscross pattern to make a thin round. Bake in batches in a preheated 450°F (230°C) oven for 5 minutes or until lightly browned around the edges.

Once the cookies are removed from the oven, quickly place them over a rolling pin to give them a gently curved shape.

Yield: 46 cookies

Exchange: free
Each serving contains: Calories: 23, Carbohydrates: 1 g, Fiber: trace, Sodium: 2.3 mg, Cholesterol: 0 mg

Thumb Cookies

Cute and yummy. One of the easiest cookies to make.

1	egg or egg substitute, beaten	1
2 T.	skim milk	30 mL
1½ c.	flour	375 mL
2 T.	sugar	30 mL
3 pkts.	concentrated acesulfame-K	3 pkts.
2 t.	baking powder	10 mL
½ c.	margarine or butter	125 mL
1 t.	vanilla extract	5 mL
2 T.	fruit-only raspberry or strawberry jam	30 mL

In a large bowl, beat together the egg and milk. Remove 1 T. and set it aside to be used later. Sift together the dry ingredients. Add the flour mixture, margarine, and vanilla extract to the egg mixture. Mix until thoroughly blended. Roll into balls the size of walnuts. Place the balls on ungreased cookie sheets. Press a thumbprint into the top of each. Fill with jam. Brush the cookies with the egg-and-milk mixture that was set aside previously. Bake at 350°F (180°C) for 10–15 minutes.

Yield: 42 cookies

Exchange, 1 cookie: ½ bread
Each serving contains: Calories: 45, Carbohydrates: 5 g, Fiber: trace, Sodium: 47 mg, Cholesterol: trace

Walnut Spice Kisses

This is a meringue cookie and it's easy to make. When the weather is damp, meringue tends to be sticky. They are crisp if the humidity is low.

1	egg white	1
2 dashes	salt	2 dashes
2 T.	sugar	30 mL
2 pkts.	concentrated acesulfame-K	2 pkts.
1 t.	cinnamon	5 mL
⅛ t.	nutmeg	.5 mL
⅛ t.	cloves	.5 mL
1 c.	finely chopped walnuts	250 mL
30	walnut halves	30

Beat the egg white until stiff. Gradually beat in the salt. In another bowl, mix the sugar and acesulfame-K with the spices. Beat this into the egg white mixture. Fold in the chopped walnuts. Drop by teaspoonful onto a cookie sheet coated with non-stick cooking spray. Top each cookie with a walnut half. Bake at 250°F (120°C) for 35–40 minutes.

Yield: 30 cookies

Exchange, 1 cookie: ½ fat
Each serving contains: Calories: 32, Carbohydrates: 1 g, Fiber: trace, Sodium: 2 mg, Cholesterol: 0 mg

Peanut Butter Cookies

As good as Grandma used to make.

2 T.	margarine or butter	30 mL
½ c.	peanut butter	125 mL
¼ c.	sugar	60 mL
3 pkts.	concentrated acesulfame-K	3 pkts.
1	egg or egg substitute, beaten	1
2 c.	flour	500 mL
4 t.	baking powder	20 mL
⅓ c.	milk	90 mL

Cream the margarine thoroughly, add the peanut butter and cream together, then blend in the sugar and acesulfame-K. Add the beaten egg. Mix and sift the dry ingredients and add them alternately to the creamed mixture with the milk. Roll into small balls and place on a baking sheet coated with non-stick cooking spray. Flatten with the bottom of a glass dipped in flour. Then, using a fork, make criss-cross impressions in each cookie. Bake in a 400°F (200°C) oven for 7 minutes.

Yield: 70 cookies

Exchange: free
Each serving contains: Calories: 27, Carbohydrates: 4 g, Fiber: trace, Sodium: 37 mg, Cholesterol: 0 mg

Coconut Kisses

If you love coconut, you'll love these easy-to-make cookies.

¼ t.	salt	1 mL
1/2 c.	egg whites	125 mL
¼ c.	sugar	60 mL
6 pkts.	concentrated acesulfame-K	6 pkts.
½ t.	vanilla extract	2 mL
2½ c.	shredded coconut	625 mL

Add the salt to the egg whites and beat until foamy. Gradually beat in the sugar and acesulfame-K. Beat until the egg whites are stiff. Fold in the vanilla extract and coconut.

Drop by teaspoonfuls onto cookie sheets coated with non-stick cooking spray. Leave about 2 inches (3 cm) between cookies for spreading. Bake in a 325°F (160°C) oven for 20 minutes. The cookies will be light brown. Cool on wire racks.

Yield: 50 cookies

Exchange: free
Each serving contains: Calories: 22, Carbohydrates: 4 g, Fiber: trace, Sodium: 10 mg, Cholesterol: 0 mg

Crisp Oat Cookies

Crisp cookies that store well.

⅓ c.	margarine or butter	90 mL
⅓ c.	nonfat cream cheese	90 mL
¼ c.	sugar	90 mL
3 pkts.	concentrated acesulfame-K	3 pkts.
3 c.	oatmeal	750 mL

Beat together the margarine, cream cheese, sugar, and acesulfame-K. Mix in the oatmeal until well blended. Roll the dough into small balls. Place each ball on a cookie sheet sprayed with non-stick cooking spray. Flatten the balls crosswise with a fork. Bake in a 350°F (180°C) oven until light brown, about 8 minutes.

Yield: 50 cookies

Exchange, 1 cookie: ½ bread
Each serving contains: Calories: 67, Carbohydrates: 5 g, Fiber: trace, Sodium: 7 mg, Cholesterol: trace

Pecan Tea Cookies

These cookies are rolled into balls, so they are fast to make. Everyone will love them.

2 c.	finely chopped pecans	500 mL
1 c.	margarine	250 mL
2 T.	sugar	30 mL
2 pkts.	concentrated acesulfame-K	2 pkts.
2 c.	flour	500 mL
1 t.	vanilla extract	5 mL
1 T.	water	15 mL

Mix all the ingredients together. Chill for half an hour. Shape into small balls. Place on a cookie sheet coated with non-stick cooking spray. Bake in a 350°F (180°C) oven for 12–13 minutes until light brown.

Yield: 80 cookies

Exchange, 1 cookie: 1 fat
Each serving contains: Calories: 50, Carbohydrates: 3 g, Fiber: trace, Sodium: trace, Cholesterol: 0 mg

Fun Form Cookies

All kids like form cookies and chocolate makes them better.

⅓ c.	margarine, softened	90 mL
½ c.	liquid fructose	125 mL
1	egg, slightly beaten	1
1 t.	rum flavoring	5 mL
2 c.	all-purpose flour	500 mL
2 t.	baking powder	10 mL
¼ t.	salt	1 mL
1 oz.	baking chocolate, melted	30 g

Combine margarine and fructose in mixing bowl, beat until smooth and creamy. Add egg and rum flavoring and beat well. Sift flour, baking powder and salt together. Stir into creamed mixture. Divide dough in half. To one half of dough, work in the melted chocolate. Combine white and chocolate doughs and work with your hands to slightly mix doughs. Wrap in plastic wrap and refrigerate overnight. Roll out to ⅛ in. (3 mm) thickness. Cut into 2 in. (5 cm) decorative shapes. Place on ungreased cookie sheets. Bake at 400°F (200°C) for 8 to 10 minutes.

Yield: 72 cookies

Exchange, 1 cookie: ¼ bread, ¼ fat
Each serving contains: Calories: 26, Carbohydrates: 4 g

Chocolate Chewies

A chocolate-covered raisin cookie.

1½ oz.	baking chocolate	45 mL
½ c.	butter	125 mL
2 T.	boiling water	30 mL
¼ c.	chopped raisins	60 mL
3	eggs	3
⅓ c.	granulated sugar replacement	90 mL
¾ c.	flour	190 mL
½ t.	baking powder	2 mL
½ t.	salt	2 mL
dash	nutmeg	dash

Melt chocolate and butter in top of double boiler over simmering water. In a small bowl, pour boiling water over raisins. Set aside and stir occasionally to plump the raisins. Beat eggs and sugar replacement until light and fluffy; add chocolate mixture. Sift together the flour, baking powder, salt and nutmeg. Blend into creamed mixture. Fold in plumped raisins with water. Chill at least 2 hours. Drop by teaspoonfuls onto greased cookie sheets. Bake at 350°F (175°C) for 10 to 12 minutes.

Yield: 24 cookies

Exchange, 1 cookie: ⅓ bread, 1 fat
Each serving contains: Calories: 72, Carbohydrates: 8 g

Cornflake Macaroons

A favorite at bake sales.

2	egg whites	2
½ c.	granulated sugar replacement	125 mL
3 T.	sorbitol	45 mL
2 c.	cornflakes, unsweetened	500 mL
⅓ c.	mini chocolate chips	90 mL
½ c.	grated coconut, unsweetened	125 mL
½ t.	vanilla extract	2 mL

Beat egg whites until they are stiff enough to hold their shape but not until they lose their shiny appearance. Carefully, fold in remaining ingredients. Drop by teaspoonfuls onto a well-greased cookie sheet. Bake at 350°F (175°C) for 10 to 15 minutes or until done. Remove macaroons immediately with a spatula.

Yield: 24 cookies

Exchange, 1 cookie: ¼ bread, ¼ fat
Each serving contains: Calories: 27, Carbohydrates: 8 g

Cocoa Drops

1 c.	vegetable shortening, softened	250 mL
½ c.	granulated brown sugar replacement	125 mL
2	eggs	2
1¼ c.	skim milk	310 mL
2½ t.	vanilla extract	12 mL
4 c.	cake flour	1 L
1 t.	salt	5 mL
3 t.	baking powder	15 mL
¾ c.	cocoa	190 mL

Mix shortening and brown sugar replacement together. Add eggs and beat well. Combine milk and vanilla extract. Sift dry ingredients together and add alternately with milk to the batter. Drop by teaspoonfuls onto a greased cookie sheet. Bake at 350°F (175°C) for 10 to 12 minutes.

Yield: 120 cookies

Exchange, 1 cookie: ⅓ bread, ⅓ fat
Each serving contains: Calories: 30, Carbohydrates: 6 g

Rich Teas

A cookie to serve at parties.

½ c.	vegetable shortening, softened	125 mL
¼ c.	granulated sugar replacement	60 mL
1	egg, beaten	1
1 t.	vanilla extract	5 mL
½ t.	salt	2 mL
5 T.	skim milk	75 mL
2 c.	cake flour, sifted	500 mL
1½ oz.	baking chocolate	45 g

Cream shortening and sugar replacement. Add beaten egg, vanilla extract, salt and milk. Blend thoroughly and add half of the sifted flour. When well mixed, add melted chocolate and remaining flour. Mold with cookie press on cold, ungreased cookie sheet. Bake at 350°F (175°C) for 12 to 15 minutes.

Yield: 72 cookies

Exchange, 1 cookie: ¼ bread, ⅓ fat
Each serving contains: Calories: 27

Fructose Chocolate-Oatmeal Cookies

Freeze batches of these for Christmas.

2½ c.	cake flour	625 mL
1 t.	baking powder	5 mL
¼ t.	baking soda	1 mL
½ t.	salt	2 mL
1 t.	cinnamon	5 mL
1 c.	vegetable shortening, softened	250 mL
½ c.	liquid fructose	125 mL
2	eggs, beaten	2
2 oz.	baking chocolate, melted	60 g
1½ c.	oatmeal	375 mL

Sift cake flour, baking powder, baking soda, salt and cinnamon together. Cream shortening and fructose. Add beaten eggs, melted chocolate and oatmeal. Mix thoroughly. Add sifted dry ingredients. Drop from a teaspoon onto a greased cookie sheet. Bake at 325°F (165°C) for 15 to 20 minutes.

Yield: 66 cookies

Exchange, 1 cookie: ¼ bread, ½ fat
Each serving contains: Calories: 53, Carbohydrates: 7 g

Banana Cookies

2¼ c.	flour	560 mL
2 t.	baking powder	10 mL
½ t.	salt	2 mL
¼ t.	baking soda	1 mL
⅓ c.	vegetable shortening, softened	90 mL
⅓ c.	granulated sugar replacement	90 mL
⅓ c.	cocoa	90 mL
2	eggs, beaten	2
½ t.	vanilla extract	2 mL
4	bananas, mashed	4

Sift dry ingredients together. Cream shortening, sugar replacement and cocoa thoroughly; add eggs and vanilla extract. Beat well. Add mashed bananas alternately with dry ingredients. Drop by teaspoonfuls onto greased cookie sheet. Bake at 350°F (175°C) for 12 to 15 minutes.

Yield: 60 cookies

Exchange, 1 cookie: ⅓ bread, ½ fat
Each serving contains: Calories: 36, Carbohydrates: 9 g

Walnut Wheels

A different chocolate walnut cookie.

⅓ c.	butter softened	90 mL
½ c.	granulated sugar replacement	125 mL
1	egg	1
1 oz.	baking chocolate, melted	30 g
1 T.	warm water	15 mL
1 t.	vanilla extract	5 mL
⅔ c.	cake flour, sifted	180 mL
½ t.	baking powder	2 mL
¼ t.	salt	1 mL
24	walnut halves	24

Cream butter until light and fluffy, then beat in sugar replacement. Beat in egg, chocolate, warm water, and vanilla extract. Stir in cake flour, baking powder, and salt. Drop by teaspoonfuls onto greased baking sheet. Garnish each cookie with a walnut half. Bake at 350°F (175°C) for 8 to 10 minutes.

Yield: 24 cookies

Exchange, 1 cookie: 1¼ bread, ½ fat
Each serving contains: Calories: 40, Carbohydrates: 8 g

Chocolate Kisses

2	egg whites	2
dash	salt	dash
⅛ t.	cream of tartar	½ mL
3 T.	granulated sugar replacement	45 mL
2 oz.	semisweet chocolate	60 g
¼ c.	walnuts, finely chopped	60 mL
1 t.	vanilla extract	5 mL

Beat egg whites until foamy, then add salt and cream of tartar. Continue beating until eggs are stiff but not dry. Add sugar replacement, beating thoroughly. Cut or grate chocolate into very small pieces. Fold in chocolate, walnuts and vanilla extract. Drop from a teaspoon onto ungreased heavy paper. Bake at 300°F (150°C) for 20 to 25 minutes. Remove from paper while slightly warm.

Yield: 18 kisses

Exchange, 1 kiss: ½ fat
Each serving contains: Calories: 28, Carbohydrates: 4 g

German Crinkles

2 c.	flour	500 mL
2 t.	baking powder	10 mL
½ t.	salt	2 mL
½ c.	vegetable shortening, softened	125 mL
⅔ c.	granulated sugar replacement	160 mL
2 t.	vanilla extract	10 mL
2	eggs, slightly beaten	2
1½ oz.	baking chocolate, melted	45 mL
⅓ c.	skim milk	90 mL
1¼ c.	hazelnuts, finely ground	60 mL

Sift together flour, baking powder, and salt. Set aside. Cream shortening, sugar replacement, and vanilla extract. Beat in eggs and melted chocolate. Alternately, add flour mixture with milk to creamed mixture. Blend in hazelnuts. Chill 4 hours. Form into balls. Place on greased cookie sheet with space for cookies to spread. Bake at 350°F (175°C) for 12 to 15 minutes. Cool slightly; remove from pan.

Yield: 50 cookies

Exchange, 1 cookie: ¼ bread, ½ fat
Each serving contains: Calories: 47, Carbohydrates: 8 g

Scottish Melts

3	eggs, beaten	3
½ c.	granulated sugar replacement	125 mL
¼ t.	salt	1 mL
3 T.	shortening, melted	45 mL
1 oz.	baking chocolate, melted	30 g
1 T.	vanilla extract	15 mL
3 c.	oatmeal	50 mL

Beat eggs, add sugar replacement gradually and beat well with each addition. Add salt, shortening, chocolate, vanilla extract and the oatmeal. Drop by teaspoonfuls onto greased cookie sheet. Bake at 325°F (165°C) for 17 to 25 minutes. Remove from pan while still warm.

Yield: 106 cookies

Exchange, 4 cookies: ¼ bread, ½ fat
Each serving contains: Calories: 40, Carbohydrates: 1 g

Citrus Cookies

8 oz. box	no-sugar chocolate cake mix	226 g box
4 t.	lemon peel, freshly grated	20 mL
2 t.	orange peel, freshly grated	10 mL
3 T.	orange juice	45 mL
1	egg white	1

Combine all ingredients in mixing bowl and beat at medium speed until mixture is smooth. Drop by teaspoonfuls onto greased cookie sheet. Bake at 350°F (175°C) for 8 to 10 minutes. Remove from pan immediately.

Yield: 60 cookies

Exchange, 1 cookie: ¼ bread
Each serving contains: Calories: 15, Carbohydrates: 3 g

Filbert Balls

8 oz. box	no-sugar chocolate cake mix	226 g box
1	egg yolk	1
2 t.	vanilla extract	10 mL
1	egg white	1
1	water	5 mL
½ c.	filberts, finely ground	125 mL

Combine cake mix, egg yolk, water and vanilla extract in mixing bowl; beat until smooth. Refrigerate until easy to handle. Form dough by teaspoon into balls. Dip balls in mixture of beaten egg white and water; shake off excess. Then roll in ground filberts. Place on greased cookie sheet. Bake at 350°F (175°C) for 10 to 12 minutes.

Yield: 60 cookies

Exchange, 1 cookie: ¼ bread, ¼ fat
Each serving contains: Calories: 22, Carbohydrates: 3 g

Buttermilk Oat Crisps

8 oz. box	no-sugar chocolate cake mix	226 g box
1 c.	oatmeal	250 mL
½ c.	buttermilk	125 mL
½ c.	margarine, melted	125 mL

Combine ingredients in mixing bowl. Stir until dry ingredients are just moistened. Knead dough on very lightly floured board until mixture is completely blended. Roll out ⅛ in. (3 mm) thick. Cut into 2 × 4 in. (5 × 10 cm) rectangular strips. Place on ungreased cookie sheet. Bake at 400°F (200°C) for 6 to 8 minutes.

Yield: 54 cookies

Exchange, 1 cookie: ¼ bread, ½ fat
Each serving contains: Calories: 34, Carbohydrates: 4 g

Sour Cream Drops

8 oz. box	no-sugar chocolate cake mix	226 g box
1	egg	1
⅓ c.	sour cream	90 mL

Combine all ingredients; mix to blend thoroughly. Chill at least 4 hours. Drop by teaspoonfuls onto greased cookie sheet. Bake at 350°F (175°C) for 8 to 12 minutes. Cool slightly; remove from pan.

Yield: 24 cookies

Exchange, 1 cookie: ½ bread, ½ fat
Each serving contains: Calories: 47, Carbohydrates: 7 g

Truffles

7 oz. box	no-sugar white frosting mix	200 g box
2 T.	cocoa	30 mL
2	egg yolks	2
1 T.	brandy flavoring	15 mL

Beat egg yolks until light and slightly thick. Add frosting mix, cocoa and brandy flavoring. Stir until completely blended. If needed, add water to make a workable paste. Shape dough into small balls. Place on waxed paper and let firm several hours in refrigerator.

Yield: 36 pieces

Exchange, 1 piece: ¼ bread, 12 fat
Each serving contains: Calories: 38, Carbohydrates: 8 g

Chocolate-Cherry Drops

8 oz. box	no-sugar chocolate cake mix	226 g box
1 T.	low-calorie cherry preserves	15 mL
2 t.	cherry flavoring	10 mL
2 T.	water	30 mL

Combine all ingredients in mixing bowl; stir until completely blended. Drop by teaspoonfuls onto greased cookie sheet. Bake at 350°F (175°C) for 10 to 12 minutes.

Yield: 60 cookies

Exchange, 1 cookie: ¼ bread
Each serving contains: Calories: 15, Carbohydrates: 3 g

Pecan Balls

A real seller at church fairs.

8 oz. box	no-sugar chocolate cake mix	226 g box
1 T.	cornstarch	15 mL
¼ c.	pecans, finely ground	60 mL
3 T.	water	45 mL

Combine all ingredients in mixing bowl and stir to blend thoroughly. Cover bowl tightly; chill until firm. Roll in your palms into small, marble-size balls. Place on ungreased cookie sheet. Bake at 350°F (175°C) for 10 to 12 minutes.

Yield: 40 cookies

Exchange, 1 cookie: ⅓ bread, 1¼ fat
Each serving contains: Calories: 31, Carbohydrates: 5 g

Pineapple Queens

4½	sweet cherries	4½
8 oz. box	no-sugar chocolate cake mix	226 g box
¼ c.	crushed pineapple and unsweetened juice	60 mL

Drain cherries and pat dry. Cut each cherry into 8 slices, a total of 36 slices. In mixing bowl, combine cake mix and pineapple with its own juice. Stir to completely blend. Drop by teaspoonfuls onto greased cookie sheet. Top each cookie with a cherry slice. Bake at 350°F (175°C) for 10 to 12 minutes.

Yield: 36 cookies

Exchange, 1 cookie: ⅓ bread
Each serving contains: Calories: 26, Carbohydrates: 5 g

Bachelor Buttons

¾ c.	low-calorie margarine	190 mL
½ c.	granulated brown sugar replacement	125 mL
¼ c.	granulated sugar replacement	60 mL
¼ c.	liquid fructose	60 mL
1 T.	water	15 mL
1	egg	1
2 c.	all-purpose flour	500 mL
1 t.	baking soda	5 mL
¼ t. each	ginger, cinnamon, salt	1 mL each
1 t.	vanilla extract	5 mL
½ c.	chopped walnuts	125 mL

Cream together the margarine, both sugar replacements, fructose, and water until light and fluffy. Add egg and beat well. Combine flour, baking soda, ginger, cinnamon, and salt. Add to the creamed mixture and mix well. Next, stir in vanilla and nuts. Cover. Chill for several hours or overnight. Then form dough into 1 in. (2.5 cm) balls. Place on lightly greased cookie sheets about 2 in. (5 cm) apart. Gently press each cookie with a fork. Bake at 350°F (175°C) for 15 to 17 minutes. Allow cookies to cool slightly on cookie sheet before removing.

Yield: 42 cookies

Exchange, 1 cookie: ⅓ starch/bread, ½ fat
Each serving contains: Calories: 51, Carbohydrates: 6 g

Melted Chocolate Cookies

¾ c.	semisweet chocolate chips	190 mL
1½ c.	all-purpose flour	375 mL
1 t.	baking soda	5 mL
½ t.	salt	2 mL
½ c.	low-calorie margarine, softened	125 mL
⅓ c.	granulated fructose	90 mL
1 t.	vanilla extract	5 mL
1	egg	1

Melt chocolate chips in a microwave oven or over simmering water. Cool to room temperature. Combine flour, baking soda, and salt in a bowl. Stir to blend. In a medium-size mixing bowl, beat margarine and fructose until smooth. Beat in vanilla and egg. Continue beating at least 2 more minutes. Add melted chocolate chips and beat well. Then gradually beat in flour mixture. Drop batter by teaspoonfuls onto an ungreased cookie sheet. Bake at 375°F (190°C) for 8 minutes. (Cookies will be soft.) Allow to cool on pan for 2 to 3 minutes; then move to rack. These are crisp chocolate cookies. If you prefer softer cookies, try putting a slice of apple in your cookie tin with the baked cookies.

Yield: 48 cookies

Exchange, 1 cookie: ½ starch/bread
Each serving contains: Calories: 42, Carbohydrates: 6 g

Chocolate-Coconut Drops

⅓ c.	margarine	90 mL
2 T.	granulated brown sugar replacement	30 mL
1 t.	vanilla extract	5 mL
2	eggs	2
1½ c.	flour	375 mL
½ c.	cocoa	125 mL
½ t.	salt	2 mL
1 t.	baking soda	5 mL
⅓ c.	skim milk	90 mL
½ c.	unsweetened coconut, grated	125 mL

Cream together margarine and brown sugar replacement. Beat in vanilla and eggs until light and fluffy. Sift flour, cocoa, salt, and baking soda together; add alternately with milk to creamed mixture. Stir until well blended. Fold in coconut. Drop by teaspoonfuls onto lightly greased cookie sheets. Bake at 375°F (190°C) for 10 to 12 minutes.

Microwave: Place 6 to 8 cookies on waxed paper. Cook on Low for 3 to 4 minutes, or until tops are set. Cool.

Yield: 40 cookies

Exchange 1 cookie: ¼ bread, ½ fat
Each serving contains: Calories: 39, Carbohydrates: 5 g

Hermit Cookies

½ c.	shortening	125 mL
3 T.	granulated brown sugar replacement	45 mL
1	egg	1
1½ c.	flour, sifted	375 mL
1 t.	baking powder	5 mL
1 t.	cinnamon	5 mL
¼ t.	salt	1 mL
¼ t.	baking soda	1 mL
¼ t.	nutmeg	1 mL
¼ t.	cloves, ground	1 mL
⅓ c.	skim milk	90 mL
⅓ c.	raisins, chopped	90 mL
¼ c.	walnuts, chopped	60 mL

Cream together shortening and brown sugar replacement. Add egg; beat until light and fluffy. Combine flour, baking powder, cinnamon, salt, baking soda, nutmeg and cloves in sifter; add alternately with milk to creamed mixture. Fold in raisins and walnuts. Drop by teaspoonfuls onto lightly greased baking sheets, 2 to 3 in. (5 to 7 cm) apart. Bake at 350°F (175°C) for 12 to 15 minutes.

Yield: 48 cookies

Exchange, 1 cookie: ⅓ fruit, ½ fat
Each serving contains: Calories: 40, Carbohydrates: 5 g

Fruit Cookies

½ c.	margarine	60 mL
4 t.	granulated sugar replacement	20 mL
2	eggs	2
2 c.	flour, sifted	500 mL
½ t.	baking soda	2 mL
¼ t.	salt	1 mL
½ t.	nutmeg	2 mL
¼ c.	hot apple juice	60 mL
¼ c.	raisins, chopped	60 mL
¼ c.	currants	60 mL

Cream together margarine and sugar replacement. Add eggs; beat until fluffy. Combine flour, baking soda, salt, and nutmeg in sifter; add alternately with hot apple juice to creamed mixture. Fold in raisins and currants. Allow to rest 15 minutes. Drop by teaspoonfuls onto lightly greased cookie sheet, 2 to 3 in. (5 to 7 cm) apart. Bake at 350°F (175°C) for 12 to 15 minutes.

Yield: 60 cookies

Exchange, 1 cookie: ½ fruit
Each serving contains: Calories: 27, Carbohydrates: 5 g

Cinnamon Cookies

2	eggs	2
2 T.	water	30 mL
5 t.	granulated sugar replacement	25 mL
1 t.	cinnamon	5 mL
1½ c.	flour	375 mL
½ t.	baking soda	2 mL
¼ t.	salt	1 mL

Beat eggs and water until light and fluffy. Beat in sugar replacement and cinnamon. Combine flour, baking soda and salt in sifter; sift half of the dry ingredients over egg mixture. Fold to completely blend. Repeat with remaining dry ingredients. Drop by teaspoonfuls onto greased cookie sheets, 2 to 3 inches (5 to 7 cm) apart. Bake at 375°F (190°C) for 10 to 12 minutes.

Yield: 20 cookies

Exchange, 1 cookie: 1½ bread
Each serving contains: Calories: 41, Carbohydrates: 8 g

Carrot Cookies

½ c.	margarine	125 mL
1 T.	granulated brown sugar replacement	15 mL
2 t.	granulated sugar replacement	10 mL
1	egg	1
2 T.	water	30 mL
1 t.	vanilla extract	5 mL
1 c.	cooked carrots, mashed	250 mL
2 c.	flour	500 mL
½ t.	salt	2 mL
2 t.	baking powder	10 mL

Cream together margarine and sugar replacements. Add egg, water, and vanilla, beating until light and fluffy, and beat in carrots. Combine flour, salt, and baking powder in sifter. Sift dry ingredients into carrot mixture; stir to blend completely. Drop by teaspoonfuls onto lightly greased cookie sheets. Bake at 375°F (190°C) for 10 to 12 minutes.

Microwave: Place 6 to 8 cookies on waxed paper. Cook on Low for 3 to 4 minutes, or until tops are set.

Yield: 50 cookies

Exchange, 1 cookie: ½ vegetable
Each serving contains: Calories: 35, Carbohydrates: 5 g

Chocolate Chip Cookies

¼ c.	margarine	60 mL
1 T.	granulated fructose	15 mL
1	egg	1
3 T.	water	45 mL
1 t.	vanilla extract	5 mL
¾ c.	flour	190 mL
¼ t.	baking soda	1 mL
¼ t.	salt	1 mL
½ c.	small semisweet chocolate chips	125 mL

Cream together margarine and fructose; beat in egg, water, and vanilla. Combine flour, baking soda, and salt in sifter. Sift dry ingredients into creamed mixture, stirring to blend thoroughly. Stir in chocolate chips. Drop by teaspoonfuls onto lightly greased cookie sheet, 2 in. (5 cm) apart. Bake at 375°F (190°C) for 8 to 10 minutes.

Yield: 30 cookies

Exchange, 1 cookie: ½ fruit, ½ fat
Each serving contains: Calories: 41, Carbohydrates: 5 g

Christmas Melt-Aways

3	egg whites, beaten stiff	3
2 T.	granulated sugar replacement or granulated fructose	30 mL
½ t.	cream of tartar	2 mL
¼ t.	salt	1 mL
2 t.	green mint flavoring	10 mL

Beat sugar replacement, cream of tartar, salt and flavoring into egg whites. Drop by teaspoonfuls onto lightly greased cookie sheets. Bake at 325°F (165°C) for 10 minutes. Remove from pan right away.

Yield: 36 cookies

Exchange, 6 cookies with sugar replacement: negligible
Each serving contains: Calories: 10

Exchange, 6 cookies with fructose: ¼ fruit
Each serving contains: Calories: 22, Carbohydrates: 1 g

Walnut Kisses

3	egg whites, beaten stiff	3
2 T.	granulated sugar replacement or granulated fructose	30 mL
2 T.	cake flour, sifted	30 mL
⅓ c.	walnuts, chopped fine	90 mL
½ t.	vanilla extract	2 mL

Beat sugar replacement into stiff egg whites. Sprinkle flour over egg white mixture; gently fold flour into egg whites with wire whisk or wooden spoon. Fold in walnuts and vanilla. Drop by teaspoonfuls onto lightly greased cookie sheets. Bake at 325°F (165°C) for 10 minutes. Remove from pan immediately.

Yield: 36 cookies

Exchange, 6 cookies with sugar replacement: ⅓ milk
Each serving contains: Calories: 63

Exchange, 6 cookies with fructose: ½ milk
Each serving contains: Calories: 78, Carbohydrates: 1 g

Popcorn Drops

2 c.	unsalted popped corn	500 mL
3	egg whites	3
½ t.	baking powder	2 mL
¼ t.	salt	1 mL
¼ t.	cream of tartar	1 mL
2 T.	granulated sugar replacement	30 mL

Place popped corn in food processor or food grinder; grind into kernel-size pieces. Beat egg whites until frothy and add baking powder, salt, and cream of tartar. Beat into stiff peaks. Add sugar replacement, beating until well blended. Fold popcorn pieces into stiffly beaten egg whites. Drop by teaspoonfuls onto lightly greased cookie sheets. Bake at 350°F (175°C) for 12 to 14 minutes, or until lightly browned.

Yield: 36 cookies

Exchange, 6 cookies: negligible
Each serving contains: Calories: 16, Carbohydrates: 1 g

Pineapple Drops

¼ c.	margarine	60 mL
1 T.	granulated brown sugar replacement	15 mL
1 T.	granulated sugar replacement	15 mL
1	egg	1
1 t.	pineapple flavoring	5 mL
1¼ c.	flour, sifted	310 mL
½ t.	baking powder	2 mL
¼ t.	baking soda	1 mL
½ c.	unsweetened crushed pineapple, with juice	125 mL

Cream together margarine and sugar replacements. Add egg and pineapple flavoring, beating until fluffy. Combine flour, baking powder, and baking soda in sifter. Add alternately with crushed pineapple (and juice) to creamed mixture, mixing thoroughly. Drop by teaspoonfuls onto lightly greased cookie sheets, 2 to 3 in. (5 to 7 cm) apart. Bake at 375°F (190°C) for 10 to 12 minutes.

Yield: 36 cookies

Exchange, 1 cookie: ⅓ fruit
Each serving contains: Calories: 29, Carbohydrates: 5 g

Fattegmand

2	eggs	2
1 T.	granulated sugar replacement	15 mL
3 T.	evaporated skim milk	45 mL
¼ t.	salt	1 mL
2 c.	flour	500 mL
	oil for deep-fat frying	

Combine all ingredients, except oil; mix just until blended. Roll out on lightly floured surface and form into 70 thin strips. Fry in deep fat, heated to 365°F (180°C), until golden brown. Remove to absorbent paper.

Yield: 70 cookies

Exchange, 2 cookies: ⅓ bread
Each serving contains: Calories: 28, Carbohydrates: 3 g

Walnut Party Cookies

½ c.	margarine, soft	125 mL
2 T.	granulated sugar replacement	30 mL
dash	salt	dash
1 t.	vanilla extract	5 mL
1½ c.	cake flour, sifted	375 mL
24	walnut halves	24

Combine margarine, sugar replacement, salt and vanilla in medium mixing bowl. Beat until light and fluffy. Stir in cake flour and refrigerate dough for at least 1 hour. Form dough into 24 small balls, place on ungreased cookie sheet and press walnut half into top of each cookie ball. Bake at 350°F (175°C) for 20 minutes, or until done.

Microwave: Place 6 to 8 cookie balls in circle on waxed paper; press walnut half into top of each. Cook on Low for 5 to 6 minutes.

Yield: 24 cookies

Exchange, 1 cookie: ½ fruit, 1 fat
Each serving contains: Calories: 55, Carbohydrates: 7 g

Cinnamon Nut Balls

1¼ c.	flour	310 mL
1 t.	baking powder	5 mL
⅛ t.	salt	1 mL
½ c.	margarine, soft	125 mL
3 T.	granulated sugar replacement	45 mL
1	egg, beaten	1
1 t.	vanilla extract	5 mL
2 t.	cinnamon	10 mL
½ c.	walnuts, finely chopped	125 mL

Sift together flour, baking powder, and salt. Beat margarine, sugar replacement, egg, and vanilla until creamy. Add flour mixture, stirring to mix completely. Refrigerate 1 hour. Shape level tablespoonfuls of cookie dough into balls and roll each one in mixture of cinnamon and walnuts. Place on greased cookie sheets 2 in. (5 cm) apart. Bake at 375°F (190°C) for 12 to 15 minutes. Remove from pan immediately.

Yield: 30 cookies

Exchange, 1 cookie: ⅓ bread, 1 fat
Each serving contains: Calories: 60, Carbohydrates: 6 g

Kaiser Cookies

3 T.	margarine	45 mL
1 T.	granulated sugar replacement	15 mL
1 t.	vanilla extract	5 mL
1	egg	1
1 c.	flour, sifted	250 mL
⅔ c.	water	160 mL

Beat margarine until fluffy. Add sugar replacement, vanilla and egg, beating until well blended. Add flour and water alternately to margarine mixture, beating to a thin batter. Lightly grease krumkake or kaiser iron. Place 1 T. (15 mL) of batter in center of iron, close lid, cook on both sides until golden brown, and remove from iron. Cool on rack.

Yield: 16 cookies

Exchange, 1 cookie: ⅓ fruit, ½ fat
Each serving contains: Calories: 50, Carbohydrates: 7 g

Raisin Spice Cookies

8 oz. pkg.	sugar-free yellow cake mix	226 g pkg.
3 T.	water	45 mL
1 t.	ground cinnamon	5 mL
¼ t.	ground nutmeg	1 mL
⅛ t.	ground cloves	½ mL
⅓ c.	raisins	90 mL

Use a vegetable spray to lightly grease the cookie sheets. Combine cake mix, water, and spices in a small bowl. Beat thoroughly Stir in raisins. Drop by teaspoonfuls about 2 in. (5 cm) apart onto the greased cookie sheets. Bake at 350°F (175 °C) for 10 to 12 minutes.

Yield: 30 cookies

Exchange, 1 cookie: ⅓ bread
Each serving contains: Calories: 33, Carbohydrates: 7 g

Macaroons

8 oz. pkg.	sugar-free white cake mix	226 g pkg.
1	egg white	1
1 t.	coconut flavoring	5 mL
2 T.	water	30 mL
¾ c.	unsweetened flaked coconut	190 mL

Use a vegetable spray to lightly grease the cookie sheets. Combine cake mix, egg white, coconut flavoring, and water in a small bowl. Beat at low speed until mixture is thoroughly blended. Blend in the flaked coconut. Drop by teaspoonfuls about 2 in. (5 cm) apart onto the greased cookie sheets. Bake at 375°F (190°C) for 9 to 11 minutes. Allow cookies to cool slightly on sheets before removing.

Yield: 40 cookies

Exchange, 1 cookie: ⅓ bread, ¼ fat
Each serving contains: Calories: 35, Carbohydrates: 4 g

Gingerbread Cookies

8 oz. pkg.	sugar-free yellow cake mix	226 g pkg.
½ t.	ground ginger	2 mL
¼ t.	ground nutmeg	1 mL
3 T.	Cary's Sugar-Free Maple-Flavored Syrup	45 mL
2 t.	water	10 mL

Use a vegetable spray to lightly grease the cookie sheets. Combine cake mix, ginger, and nutmeg in a small bowl. Stir to mix. Beat in maple syrup and water. Drop by teaspoonfuls about 2 in. (5 cm) apart onto the greased cookie sheets. Bake at 375°F (190°C) for 9 to 11 minutes.

Yield: 30 cookies

Exchange, 1 cookie: ⅓ bread
Each serving contains: Calories: 30, Carbohydrates: 5 g

Chocolate Sour Cream Cookies

8 oz. pkg.	sugar-free chocolate cake mix	226 g pkg.
3 T.	sour cream	45 mL
1 t.	water	5 mL

Use a vegetable spray to lightly grease the cookie sheets. Combine cake mix, sour cream, and water in a small bowl. Beat thoroughly. Drop from a teaspoon onto the greased cookie sheets. Bake at 350°F (175°C) for 9 to 10 minutes.

Yield: 30 cookies

Exchange, 1 cookie: ⅓ bread
Each serving contains: Calories: 33, Carbohydrates: 5 g

Apple Cookies

1	Granny Smith apple, peeled and chopped	1
8 oz. pkg.	sugar-free white cake mix	226 g pkg.

Use a vegetable spray to lightly grease the cookie sheets. Place apple in a microwave-safe bowl. Cover and cook on High for 2 minutes, stirring after 1 minute. Uncover and continue cooking on Medium until apple mixture is very thick and tender. Cool. Stir in cake mix. Drop from a teaspoon about 2 in. (5 cm) apart onto the greased cookie sheets. Bake at 375°F (190°C) for 8 to 10 minutes.

Yield: 30 cookies

Exchange, 1 cookie: 1⅓ bread
Each serving contains: Calories: 36, Carbohydrates: 6 g

Brandy Lizzies

8 oz. pkg.	sugar-free yellow cake mix	226 g pkg.
1	egg white	1
2 T.	water	30 mL
1 t.	brandy flavoring	5 mL
1 c.	quick-cooking oatmeal	250 mL
½ c.	raisins, chopped	125 mL
¼ c.	pecans, chopped	60 mL

Combine cake mix, egg white, water, and brandy flavoring in a small bowl. Beat thoroughly. Stir in dry oatmeal, raisins, and pecans. Chill for 2 hours. Use a vegetable spray to lightly grease the cookie sheets. Drop from a teaspoon onto the greased cookie sheets. Bake at 350°F (175°C) for 9 to 10 minutes.

Yield: 40 cookies

Exchange, 1 cookie: ⅓ bread, ¼ fat
Each serving contains: Calories: 36, Carbohydrates: 6 g

Raisin Oatmeal Cookies

1 c.	all-purpose flour	250 mL
1 t.	ground cinnamon	5 mL
½ t.	baking powder	2 mL
½ t.	baking soda	2 mL
¼ t.	salt	1 mL
½ c. (1 stick)	solid margarine, softened	125 mL (1 stick)
2 T.	granulated fructose	30 mL
1 large	egg	1 large
1 t.	vanilla extract	5 mL
1 c.	granulated sugar replacement	250 mL
1¼ c.	quick-cooking oatmeal	310 mL
½ c.	raisins	125 mL

Combine flour, cinnamon, baking powder, baking soda, and salt in a bowl. Stir to mix. Combine margarine, fructose, egg, and vanilla in a mixing bowl. Beat until thoroughly blended. Beat in sweetener. Gradually add flour mixture. Beat until blended. Meanwhile, combine oatmeal and raisins in a bowl. Work with your fingers or a spoon to separate the raisins and coat them with the oatmeal. Beat into cookie mixture. Drop by tablespoonfuls onto an ungreased cookie sheet. Bake at 375°F (190°C) for 10 to 12 minutes. Cool slightly on cookie sheet; then move to cooling rack.

Yield: 36 cookies

Exchange, 1 cookie: ½ bread, ¼ fat
Each serving contains: Calories: 61, Carbohydrates: 7 g

Carob Cookies

1¼ c.	all-purpose flour	310 mL
⅓ c.	powdered carob	90 mL
½ t.	baking soda	2 mL
¼ t.	salt	1 mL
½ c.	margarine, softened	125 mL
½ c.	granulated fructose	125 mL
1	egg	1
1 t.	vanilla extract	5 mL

Combine flour, carob, baking soda, and salt in mixing bowl, In another mixing bowl, cream margarine and fructose. Next, beat in egg and vanilla extract. Then gradually beat in flour mixture. Drop onto an ungreased cookie sheet. Bake at 350°F (175°C) for 10 to 12 minutes. Allow to cool on cookie sheet for 2 minutes before removing to a cooling rack.

Yield: 36 cookies

Exchange, 1 cookie: ¼ bread, ⅓ fat
Each serving contains: Calories: 45, Carbohydrates: 4 g

Carob Chip Cookies

1½ c.	all-purpose flour	375 mL
¾ t.	baking powder	4 mL
½ t.	salt	2 mL
¾ c.	margarine, softened	190 mL
½ c.	granulated fructose	125 mL
1	egg	1
1 t.	vanilla extract	5 mL
½ c.	unsweetened carob minichips	125 mL

Combine flour, baking powder, and salt in mixing bowl. In another mixing bowl, cream margarine and fructose; then beat in egg and vanilla extract. Gradually beat flour mixture into creamed mixture. Stir in carob chips. Drop onto an ungreased cookie sheet. Bake at 375°F (190°C) for 8 to 10 minutes. Allow to cool on cookie sheet for 2 minutes before removing to a cooling rack.

Yield: 36 cookies

Exchange, 1 cookie: ¼ bread, ½ fat
Each serving contains: Calories: 43, Carbohydrates: 4 g

Pecan Cookies

8 oz. pkg.	light cream cheese	227 g pkg.
3 T.	granulated fructose	45 mL
1 t.	vanilla extract	5 mL
1	egg	1
1	egg white	1
1 c.	all-purpose flour	250 mL
½ t.	baking soda	2 mL
½ t.	baking powder	2 mL
⅓ c.	sugar-free white frosting mix	90 mL
48	pecan halves	48
¼ c.	sugar-free white frosting mix	60 mL
1 T.	water	15 mL

Combine cream cheese, fructose, and vanilla in a mixing bowl. Beat until fluffy. Beat in egg and egg white. Beat at least 3 minutes. Combine flour, baking soda, baking powder, and the ⅓ c. (90 mL) of white frosting mix in a bowl. Stir to mix. (Break up any lumps in frosting mix.) Gradually beat flour mixture into cream-cheese mixture. Cover with plastic wrap and refrigerate at least 3 hours or until completely chilled. Drop by teaspoonfuls onto an ungreased cookie sheet. Bake at 325°F (165°C) for 15 to 20 minutes. Remove from pan immediately. Press one pecan half into the middle of each cookie. Combine the ¼ c. (60 mL) of white frosting mix and water in a cup. Stir to blend into a glaze. Add extra water if needed. Lightly brush a glaze on each cookie. Move to cooling rack.

Yield: 48 cookies

Exchange, 1 cookie: ⅓ bread, ¼ fat
Each serving contains: Calories: 30, Carbohydrates: 4 g

Applesauce Spice Cookies

2 c.	cake flour	500 mL
1 t.	baking powder	5 mL
½ t.	baking soda	2 mL
½ t.	ground cinnamon	2 mL
¼ t.	ground cloves	1 mL
¼ t.	ground nutmeg	1 mL
¼ t.	salt	1 mL
½ c. (1 stick)	solid margarine	125 mL (1 stick)
2 T.	granulated fructose	30 mL
1 large	egg	1 large
¾ c.	granulated sugar replacement	190 mL
1 c.	unsweetened applesauce	250 mL

Sift cake flour, baking powder, baking soda, cinnamon, cloves, nutmeg, and salt into a bowl. Combine margarine and fructose in a mixing bowl. Beat until creamy. Beat in egg and sweetener. Add flour mixture alternately with applesauce to creamed mixture, beginning and ending with flour mixture. Drop on a well-greased cookie sheet. Bake at 375°F (190°C) for 12 to 15 minutes.

Yield: 36 cookies

Exchange, 1 cookie: ⅓, bread, ½ fat
Each serving contains: Calories: 57, Carbohydrates: 4 g

Chocolate Thins

¼ c.	solid margarine, softened	60 mL
4 t.	granulated sugar replacement	20 mL
1	egg	1
2 T.	unsweetened cocoa powder	30 mL
1 t.	vanilla extract	5 mL
1 c.	all-purpose flour	250 mL
1 t.	baking powder	5 mL
¼ t.	baking soda	1 mL
dash	salt	dash
2 T.	water	30 mL

Combine margarine, sugar replacement, egg, cocoa, and vanilla in a mixing bowl or food processor. With an electric mixer or steel blade, process until creamy. Add flour, baking powder, baking soda, salt, and water. Mix well. Shape dough into two balls. Wrap each ball in plastic wrap and refrigerate at least 2 hours or overnight. Roll out dough to ⅛ in. (3 mm) thickness on a lightly floured surface. Cut with a 2½ in. (6.25 cm) round cookie cutter and place on ungreased cookie sheets. Bake at 350°F (175°C) for 8 to 10 minutes.

Yield: 30 cookies

Exchange, 1 cookie: ¼ bread, ¼ fat
Each serving contains: Calories: 22, Carbohydrates: 2 g

Hazelnut Cookies

8 oz. pkg.	light cream cheese	227 g pkg.
3 T.	granulated fructose	45 mL
1 t.	vanilla extract	5 mL
1	egg	1
1	egg white	1
1 c.	all-purpose flour	250 mL
½ t.	baking soda	2 mL
½ t.	baking powder	2 mL
⅓ c.	hazelnuts, finely ground	90 mL

Combine cream cheese, fructose, and vanilla in a mixing bowl. Beat until fluffy. Beat in egg and egg white. Beat at least 3 minutes. Combine flour, baking soda, and baking powder in a bowl. Stir to mix. Gradually beat flour mixture into cream-cheese mixture. Stir in ground hazelnuts. Cover with plastic wrap and refrigerate at least 3 hours or until completely chilled. Drop by teaspoonfuls onto an ungreased cookie sheet. Bake at 325°F (165°C) for 15 to 20 minutes. Remove from pan and place on cooling rack immediately.

Yield: 48 cookies

Exchange, 1 cookie: ⅛ bread, ½ fat
Each serving contains: Calories: 34, Carbohydrates: 2 g

Vanilla Wafers

¼ c.	solid margarine, softened	60 ml
4 t.	granulated sugar replacement	20 mL
1	egg	1
1 T.	vanilla extract	15 mL
1 c.	all-purpose flour	250 mL
1 t.	baking powder	5 mL
¼ t.	baking soda	1 mL
dash	salt	dash
2 T.	water	30 mL

Combine margarine, sugar replacement, egg, and vanilla in a mixing bowl or food processor. With an electric mixer or steel blade, process until creamy. Add flour, baking powder, baking soda, salt, and water. Mix well. Shape dough into two balls. Wrap each ball in plastic wrap and refrigerate at least 2 hours or overnight. Roll out dough to ⅛ in. (3 mm) thickness on a lightly floured surface. Cut with a 2½ in. (6.25 cm) round cookie cutter and place on ungreased cookie sheets. Bake at 350°F (175°C) for 8 to 10 minutes.

Yield: 30 cookies

Exchange, 1 cookie: ¼ bread, ¼ fat
Each serving contains: Calories: 21, Carbohydrates: 2 g

Lemon Sandwich Cookies

Cookie

½ c.	solid margarine	125 mL
½ c.	granulated sugar replacement	125 mL
2	eggs	2
1 T.	lemon juice	15 mL
1 t.	vanilla extract	5 mL
1½ c.	all-purpose flour	375 mL
¼ t.	baking soda	1 mL
dash	salt	dash

Filling

⅓ c.	sugar-free white frosting-mix powder	90 mL
1 t.	grated lemon peel	5 mL
1 T.	hot lemon juice	15 mL
	yellow food coloring	

Combine margarine, sweetener, eggs, lemon juice, and vanilla in a mixing bowl. Beat to blend. Stir in flour, baking soda, and salt. Work into a soft, smooth dough. Divide dough in half. Shape each half into a 7 × 1½ in. (17.5 × 3.75 cm) roll. Wrap in plastic wrap and chill for 8 hours or overnight. Cut each roll into approximately ¼ in. (3 mm) slices, or cut 48 slices from each roll. Place on ungreased cookie sheet. Bake at 400°F (200°C) for 5 to 6 minutes or until edges begin to brown. Cool completely before filling.

Combine frosting-mix powder, lemon peel, hot lemon juice, and yellow food coloring in a small bowl. Beat with a small wire whisk or fork until smooth. Put cookies together in pairs with filling.

Yield: 48 cookies

Exchange, 1 cookie: ⅓ bread, ⅓ fat
Each serving contains: Calories: 41, Carbohydrates: 4 g

Fancies

3	eggs	3
1 c.	granulated sugar replacement	250 mL
3 T.	granulated fructose	45 mL
½ t.	salt	2 mL
3 T.	melted shortening	45 mL
1 T.	vanilla extract	15 mL
3 c.	quick-cooking oatmeal	750 mL

Beat eggs until lemon-colored. Gradually beat in sugar replacement and fructose. Beat in salt, melted shortening, and vanilla. Beat well. Beat in oatmeal. Drop teaspoonfuls onto a greased cookie sheet. Bake at 325°F (165°C) for 17 to 20 minutes or until done. Move from pan to cooling rack while still warm.

Yield: 110 tea cookies

Exchange, 1 cookie: ⅛ bread
Each serving contains: Calories: 13, Carbohydrates: 2 g

Christmas Bells

¼ c. (½ stick)	solid margarine	60 mL (½ stick)	
¼ c.	solid vegetable shortening	60 mL	
½ c.	granulated sugar replacement	125 mL	
1	egg	1	
1 t.	vanilla extract	5 mL	
1½ c.	all-purpose flour	375 mL	
¼ t.	baking soda	1 mL	
dash	salt	dash	
	red or green food coloring		

Combine margarine, shortening, sweetener of your choice, egg, and vanilla in a mixing bowl. Beat to blend. Stir in flour, baking soda, and salt. Transfer about two-thirds of the dough to another bowl, and color with several drops of food coloring. (The dough will be stiff. Work dough with a spoon or fork; then knead dough to incorporate the coloring completely.) Shape colored dough into a 10 × 1½ in. (25 × 3.75 cm) roll. Knead remaining uncolored dough until soft. Roll out on a lightly floured surface into a 11 × 6 in. (27.5 × 15 cm) rectangle. Lightly brush surface with water. Wrap uncolored dough around the colored dough roll. Do not wrap the ends of the roll. Cut away any excess dough from seam edge and side edges. Reserve cut-away dough. Dampen edge of dough along 10 in. (25 cm) side of roll. Press edges of dough together to tighten. Carefully roll entire cookie roll to secure the doughs together. Wrap in plastic wrap. With the handle of a wooden spoon or your hands, carefully form the dough into a bell by pressing the top of the roll together slightly and leaving the lower half flared and curved like the bottom of a bell. Refrigerate at least 8 hours or overnight. Cut roll into about ⅛ in. (3 mm) slices. Place cookies on ungreased cookie sheets. Form a very small amount of the reserved dough into a ball to make the clapper for the bell. Place clapper on the bottom edge of bell. Bake at 375°F (190°C) for 7 to 8 minutes or until edges are lightly browned. Move cookies to cooling rack.

Yield: 60 cookies

Exchange, 1 cookie: ⅛ bread, ½ fat
Each serving contains: Calories: 29, Carbohydrates: 2 g

Chocolate Fruit Drops

1 T.	margarine, melted	15 L
1 oz.	unsweetened baking chocolate, melted	28 g
¼ c.	granulated fructose	60 mL
1	egg, slightly beaten	1
½ c. + 2 T.	all-purpose flour	155 mL
½ t.	cream of tartar	2 mL
¼ t.	baking soda	1 mL
⅓ c.	unsweetened dried mixed fruit*	90 mL

Combine melted margarine and chocolate in a bowl. Add fructose and egg. Stir until completely mixed. Add flour, cream of tartar, and baking soda. Stir until blended. Stir in dried fruit. Drop small balls of the cookie dough onto an ungreased cookie sheet. Bake at 350°F (175°C) for 10 minutes. Remove from cookie sheet immediately.

Yield: 24 cookies

Exchange, 1 cookie: ⅓ bread
Each serving contains: Calories: 27, Carbohydrates: 4 g

*Unsweetened dried mixed fruit can be bought at health food stores.

Apple Raisin Cookies

⅓ c.	unsweetened applesauce	90 mL
1	egg	1
1 t.	vanilla extract	5 mL
1 c.	all-purpose flour	250 mL
2 T.	granulated sugar replacement	30 mL
1 t.	baking powder	5 mL
½ c.	diced apple	125 mL
¼ c.	chopped raisins	60 mL

Combine applesauce, egg, and vanilla in a medium-size bowl. Beat with a fork until thoroughly blended. Thoroughly stir in flour, sugar replacement, and baking powder. Stir in apple pieces and chopped raisins. Spray cookie sheet lightly with a vegetable-oil spray. Drop cookie dough on the greased cookie sheet. Bake at 350°F (175°C) for 10 to 12 minutes. Cookies will be white; don't try to brown them. Remove from cool sheet, and cool.

Yield: 24 cookies

Exchange, 1 cookie: ⅓ bread
Each serving contains: Calories: 30, Carbohydrates: 5 g

Oatmeal Mounds with Raisins

1 T.	margarine, melted	15 mL
¼ c.	granulated fructose	60 mL
¼ c.	apple juice	60 mL
1	egg	1
½ t.	vanilla extract	2 mL
1 c.	all-purpose flour	250 mL
½ t.	cream of tartar	2 mL
¼ t.	baking soda	1 mL
1 c.	quick-cooking oatmeal	250 mL
⅓ c.	raisins	90 mL
2 qt.	boiling water	2 L

Combine melted margarine and fructose in a medium-size bowl. Stir to blend. Add apple juice, egg, and vanilla extract. With a fork, beat until thoroughly mixed. Beat in flour, cream of tartar, and baking soda. Stir in oatmeal. Place raisins in a strainer, and pour boiling water over the raisins. Drain, pat raisins dry, and chop them. Stir raisins into cookie mixture. Drop in mounds on an ungreased cookie sheet. Bake at 350°F (175°C) for 10 to 12 minutes or until very lightly browned. Remove from cookie sheet immediately. Cool on rack.

Yield: 30 cookies

Exchange, 1 cookie: ½ bread
Each serving contains: Calories: 45, Carbohydrates: 9 g

Spicy Hermits

1 T.	margarine, melted	15 mL
¼ c.	granulated fructose	60 mL
¼ c.	hot water	60 mL
2 T.	instant-coffee powder	30 mL
1	egg, slightly beaten	1
1⅓ c.	all-purpose flour	340 mL
½ t.	cream of tartar	2 mL
¼ t.	baking soda	1 mL
½ t.	ground cinnamon	2 mL
¼ t.	ground nutmeg	1 mL
¼ t.	ground cloves	1 mL
¼ c.	chopped raisins	60 mL

Stir melted margarine. Add fructose, hot water, and coffee powder. Stir until completely mixed. Beat in egg, Add flour, cream of tartar, baking soda, and spices. Stir until blended. Stir in raisins. Drop cookie dough onto an ungreased cookie sheet. Bake at 350°F (175°C) for 10 to 12 minutes. Remove from cookie sheet immediately.

Yield: 30 cookies

Exchange, 1 cookie: ⅓ bread
Each serving contains: Calories: 28, Carbohydrates: 6 g

Fairy Drops

⅓ c.	unsweetened applesauce	90 mL
2	egg whites	2
1 t.	vanilla extract	5 mL
½ t.	almond flavoring	2 mL
1 c.	all-purpose flour	250 mL
2 T.	granulated sugar replacement	30 mL
1 T.	ground cardamom	15 mL
½ t.	cream of tartar	2 mL
¼ t.	baking soda	1 mL

Combine applesauce, egg whites, vanilla, and almond flavoring in a medium-size bowl. Beat with a fork until thoroughly blended. Combine flour, sugar replacement, cardamom, cream of tartar, and baking soda in a sifter. Sift onto a piece of waxed paper; pour back into sifter and sift again. Pour flour mixture back into sifter, and sift directly into the applesauce mixture. Beat with a fork until well blended. Mixture will be sticky. Cover and chill for at least one hour or until needed. Spray cookie sheet lightly with a vegetable-oil spray. Drop cookie dough onto the greased cookie sheet. Bake at 375°F (190°C) for 12 to 15 minutes. Remove from cookie sheet and cool.

Yield: 24 cookies

Exchange, 1 cookie: ⅓ bread
Each serving contains: Calories: 20, Carbohydrates: 4 g

Chocolate Oatmeal Cookies

1 T.	margarine, melted	15 L
1 oz.	unsweetened baking chocolate, melted	28 g
¼ c.	granulated fructose	60 mL
1	egg, slightly beaten	1
½ c.	all-purpose flour	125 mL
3 T.	quick-cooking oatmeal	45 mL
½ t.	cream of tartar	2 mL
¼ t.	baking soda	1 mL

Stir melted margarine and chocolate until blended. Add fructose and egg. Stir until completely mixed. Add flour, oatmeal, cream of tartar, and baking soda. Stir until blended. Drop small balls of the cookie dough onto an ungreased cookie sheet. Bake at 350°F (175°C) for 10 minutes. Remove from cookie sheet immediately.

Yield: 24 cookies

Exchange, 1 cookie: ⅓ bread
Each serving contains: Calories: 28, Carbohydrates: 4 g

Raspberry Chocolate Drops

1 c.	frozen or fresh raspberries	250 mL
1 T.	margarine	15 mL
2 T.	granulated sugar replacement	30 mL
1 T.	granulated fructose	15 mL
1 oz.	unsweetened premelted baking chocolate	28 g
1 T.	fat-free cream cheese	15 mL
½ t.	vanilla extract	2 mL
2	egg whites	2
1½ c.	all-purpose flour	375 mL
1 t.	baking powder	5 mL
½ t.	cream of tartar	2 mL
¼ t.	baking soda	1 mL

Place frozen raspberries in a microwave bowl. Cook in the microwave on High for 1½ minutes or until raspberries are thawed. Mash with a fork. Add margarine and return to microwave for 1 to 2 minutes or until margarine is melted and raspberries are warm. Allow to cool slightly. Beat in sugar replacement, fructose, baking chocolate, cream cheese, vanilla, and egg whites. Stir in flour, baking powder, cream of tartar, and baking soda. Spray cookie sheets lightly with a vegetable-oil spray. Drop cookie dough onto greased cookie sheets. Bake at 375°F (190°C) for 10 to 12 minutes. Remove from cookie sheets, and cool on racks.

Yield: 42 cookies

Exchange, 1 cookie: ¼ bread
Each serving contains: Calories: 21, Carbohydrates: 3 g

Vanilla Pillow Puffs

⅓ c.	unsweetened applesauce	90 mL
1	egg	1
1 t.	vanilla extract	5 mL
1 c.	all-purpose flour	250 mL
2 T.	granulated sugar replacement	30 mL
1 t.	baking powder	5 mL

Combine applesauce, egg, and vanilla in a medium-size bowl. Beat mixture with a fork until thoroughly blended. Thoroughly stir in flour, sugar replacement, and baking powder. Mixture will be sticky. Spray cookie sheet lightly with a vegetable-oil spray. Drop cookie dough onto the greased cookie sheet. Bake at 350°F (175°C) for 10 to 12 minutes. Cookies will be white; don't try to brown them. Remove from cookie sheet and cool.

Yield: 24 cookies

Exchange, 1 cookie: ⅓ bread
Each serving contains: Calories: 23, Carbohydrates: 4

Chocolate Pillow Puffs

⅓ c.	unsweetened applesauce	90 mL
1 oz.	unsweetened baking chocolate, melted	28 g
1	egg	1
1 t.	vanilla extract	5 mL
1 c.	all-purpose flour	250 mL
2 T.	granulated sugar replacement	30 mL
1 t.	baking powder	5 mL

Combine applesauce, melted baking chocolate, egg, and vanilla in a medium-size bowl. Beat with a fork until thoroughly blended, Thoroughly stir in flour, sugar replacement, and baking powder. Mixture will be sticky. Spray cookie sheet lightly with a vegetable-oil spray. Drop cookie dough onto the greased cookie sheet. Bake at 350°F (175°C) for 10 to 12 minutes. Remove from cookie sheet and cool.

Yield: 24 cookies

Exchange, 1 cookie: ⅓ bread, ¼ fat
Each serving contains: Calories: 29, Carbohydrates: 4 g

Chocolate Pecan Drops

1 T.	margarine, melted	15 L
1 oz.	unsweetened baking chocolate, melted	28 g
¼ c.	granulated fructose	60 mL
1	egg, slightly beaten	1
½ c.+ 2 T.	all-purpose flour	155 mL
½ t.	cream of tartar	2 mL
¼ t.	baking soda	1 mL
24	pecan halves	24

Stir melted margarine and chocolate until blended. Add fructose and egg. Stir until completely mixed. Add flour, cream of tartar, and baking soda. Stir until blended. Drop small balls of the cookie dough onto an ungreased cookie sheet. Bake at 350°F (175°C) for 5 minutes. Remove from oven, and press a pecan half into the top of each cookie. Continue baking for 5 minutes more. Remove from cookie sheet immediately.

Yield: 24 cookies

Exchange, 1 cookie: ¼ bread
Each serving contains: Calories: 22, Carbohydrates: 4 g

Apricot Snack Cookies

6 oz. jar	baby-food apricot purée	170 g jar
¼ c.	frozen orange juice concentrate	60 mL
1 T.	granulated fructose	15 mL
1	egg, slightly beaten	1
1 t.	vanilla extract	5 mL
1 c.	all-purpose flour	250 mL
1 t.	baking powder	5 mL

Combine apricot purée, orange juice concentrate, and fructose in a medium-size bowl. Stir to blend completely. Add egg and vanilla. Beat to mix. Add flour and baking powder. Stir until mixture is thoroughly blended (mixture will be soft). Spray cookie sheet with a vegetable-oil spray. Drop cookie dough onto the greased cookie sheet. Bake at 350°F (175°C) for 15 to 20 minutes. Move to cooling rack.

Yield: 24 cookies

Exchange, 1 cookie: ⅓ bread
Each serving contains: Calories: 26, Carbohydrates: 4 g

Banana Date Cookies

1 small	very ripe banana	1 small
½ c.	low-fat cottage cheese	125 mL
3 T.	granulated sugar replacement	45 mL
2 T.	granulated fructose	30 mL
1 t.	vanilla extract	5 mL
1	egg	1
1⅓ c.	biscuit mix	340 mL
⅓ c.	chopped dates	90 mL

Beat banana and cottage cheese until creamy. (This can be done in a food processor.) Add sugar replacement, fructose, and vanilla extract. Beat well. Beat in egg. Beat in biscuit mix, ⅓ c. (90 mL) at a time. (Beat well after each addition.) Fold in chopped dates. Allow cookie dough to rest 5 minutes before dropping onto cookie sheet. Adjust oven rack to upper half. Spray cookie sheet with a vegetable-oil spray. Drop cookie dough onto the greased cookie sheet. Bake at 375°F (190°C) for 12 to 15 minutes or until lightly browned. Move cookies to cooling rack immediately.

Yield: 36 cookies

Exchange, 1 cookie: ⅓ bread
Each serving contains: Calories: 29, Carbohydrates: 5 g

Bran Cookies

½ c.	100% bran cereal	125 mL
¼ c.	skim milk	60 mL
1 T.	margarine	15 mL
1	egg white	1
1 T.	granulated sugar replacement	15 mL
1 T.	granulated fructose	15 mL
1 t.	vanilla extract	5 mL
¾ c.	all-purpose flour	190 mL
1 t.	baking powder	5 mL

Combine bran cereal and skim milk in a medium-size microwave bowl. Cover with paper towels, and cook in the microwave on High for 1½ minutes. Stir in margarine until melted. Set aside to cool slightly. Add egg white, sugar replacement, fructose, and vanilla. Stir to blend thoroughly. Stir in flour and baking powder. Spray cookie sheet lightly with a vegetable-oil spray. Drop cookie dough onto the greased cookie sheet. Bake at 375°F (190°C) for 10 to 12 minutes. Remove from cookie sheet and cool on rack.

Yield: 24 cookies

Exchange, 1 cookie: ⅓ bread
Each serving contains: Calories: 29, Carbohydrates: 4 g

Raisin Bran Cookies

⅓ c.	raisins	90 mL
½ c.	water	125 mL
½ c.	100% bran cereal	125 mL
1 T.	margarine	15 mL
½ t.	brandy flavoring	2 mL
½ t.	vanilla extract	2 mL
1	egg white	1
2 T.	granulated sugar replacement	30 mL
1 c.	all-purpose flour	250 mL
1 t.	baking powder	5 mL
2 t.	aspartame sweetener	10 mL

Combine raisins and water in a medium-size microwave bowl. Cover with paper towels, and cook in the microwave on High for 5 minutes. Stir in bran cereal, margarine, brandy flavoring, and vanilla. Cover with paper towels, and set aside for 3 to 5 minutes, or until bran is soft. Place egg white in a small bowl or cup, and beat with a wire whisk until frothy. Add egg white and sugar replacement to cookie dough. Stir to thoroughly mix. Add flour and baking powder. Stir to blend completely. Spray cookie sheets lightly with a vegetable-oil spray. Drop cookie dough onto the greased cookie sheets. Flatten slightly, either with your fingers or the knife used for dropping the dough. Bake at 375°F (190°C) for 10 to 12 minutes. Remove from cookie sheets, and cool on racks. Sprinkle warm (not hot) cookies with aspartame sweetener.

Yield: 30 cookies

Exchange, 1 cookie: ⅓ bread
Each serving contains: Calories: 26, Carbohydrates: 4 g

Cranberry Walnut Bran Cookies

½ c.	100% bran cereal	125 mL
¼ c.	water	60 mL
1 T.	margarine	15 mL
1	egg white	1
2 T.	granulated sugar replacement	30 mL
1 T.	granulated fructose	15 mL
1 t.	vanilla extract	5 mL
¼ c.	chopped cranberries	60 mL
2 T.	chopped walnuts	30 mL
½ c. + 2 T.	all-purpose flour	155 mL
1 t.	baking powder	5 mL

Combine bran cereal and water in a medium-size microwave bowl. Cover with paper towels, and cook in the microwave on High for 1½ minutes. Stir in margarine until melted. Set aside to cool slightly. Add egg white, sugar replacement, fructose, and vanilla. Stir to blend thoroughly. Blend in cranberries and walnuts. Add flour and baking powder. Stir to blend completely. Spray cookie sheet lightly with a vegetable-oil spray. Drop cookie dough onto the greased cookie sheet. Bake at 375°F (190°C) for 10 to 12 minutes. Remove from cookie sheet, and cool on rack.

Yield: 24 cookies

Exchange, 1 cookie: ⅓ bread
Each serving contains: Calories: 22, Carbohydrates: 3 g

Pineapple Wheat Cookies

8 oz. can	crushed pineapple in juice	224 g can
½ c.	natural wheat and barley cereal (Grape-Nuts)	125 mL
1 T.	margarine	15 mL
1 t.	pineapple flavoring	5 mL
1	egg white	1
1 T.	granulated fructose	15 mL
1 T.	granulated sugar replacement	15 mL
1 c.	all-purpose flour	250 mL
1 t.	baking powder	5 mL

Combine crushed pineapple in juice with cereal in a medium-size microwave bowl. Cover with paper towels. Microwave on High for 2 to 3 minutes. Stir in margarine, re-cover, and allow to cool for 5 minutes. Add pineapple flavoring, egg white, fructose, and sugar replacement. Beat with a fork to blend completely. Stir in flour and baking powder thoroughly. Spray cookie sheets lightly with a vegetable-oil spray. Drop cookie dough onto the greased cookie sheets. Flatten slightly, either with your fingers or the knife used for dropping the dough. Bake at 375°F (190°C) for 12 to 15 minutes. Remove from cookie sheets, and cool on racks.

Yield: 30 cookies

Exchange, 1 cookie: ¼ bread
Each serving contains: Calories: 23, Carbohydrates: 3 g

Walnut Wheat Drops

⅓ c.	skim milk	90 mL
½ c.	natural wheat and barley cereal (Grape-Nuts)	125 mL
1 T.	margarine	15 mL
1 t.	vanilla extract	5 mL
1 t.	burnt-sugar flavoring	5 mL
1	egg white	1
1 T.	granulated fructose	15 mL
1 T.	granulated sugar replacement	15 mL
¼ c.	finely ground walnuts	60 mL
1 c.	all-purpose flour	250 mL
1 t.	baking powder	5 mL

Combine milk and cereal in a medium-size microwave bowl. Cover with paper towels. Microwave on High for 2 to 3 minutes. Stir in margarine, re-cover, and allow to cool for 5 minutes. Add vanilla, burnt-sugar flavoring, egg white, fructose, and sugar replacement. Beat with a fork to blend completely. Stir in walnuts, and allow to rest for 2 minutes. Thoroughly stir in flour and baking powder. Spray cookie sheets lightly with a vegetable-oil spray. Drop cookie dough onto the greased cookie sheets. Bake at 375°F (190°C) for 12 to 15 minutes. Remove from cookie sheets, and cool on racks.

Yield: 30 cookies

Exchange, 1 cookie: ⅓ bread
Each serving contains: Calories: 26, Carbohydrates: 4 g

Spicy Wheat Cookies

½ c.	water	125 mL
3 in.	cinnamon stick	7.5 cm
½ t.	allspice	2 mL
½ c.	natural wheat and barley cereal (Grape-Nuts)	125 mL
1 T.	margarine	15 mL
1	egg	1
2 T.	granulated sugar replacement	30 mL
½ c.	all-purpose flour	125 mL
½ t.	baking powder	2 mL

Combine water, cinnamon stick, and allspice in a small saucepan. Boil for 2 minutes. Stir in cereal. Cover and allow to rest 3 minutes. Remove cinnamon stick. Thoroughly stir in margarine, egg, and sugar replacement. Stir and completely work in flour and baking powder. Spray cookie sheet lightly with a vegetable-oil spray. Drop cookie dough onto the greased cookie sheet. If desired, flatten dough slightly, either with your fingers or the knife used for dropping the dough. Bake at 375°F (190°C) for 12 to 15 minutes. Remove from cookie sheet, and cool on rack.

Yield: 24 cookies

Exchange, 1 cookie: ¼ bread
Each serving contains: Calories: 20, Carbohydrates: 3 g

Triple-Juice Cookies

¼ c.	pineapple juice	60 mL
¼ c.	orange juice	60 mL
2 T.	lemon juice	30 mL
½ c.	natural wheat and barley cereal (Grape-Nuts)	125 mL
1 T.	margarine	15 mL
1 t.	vanilla extract	5 mL
2	egg whites	2
1 T.	granulated sugar replacement	15 mL
½ c.	all-purpose flour	125 mL
½ t.	baking powder	2 mL

Combine pineapple, orange, and lemon juice in a small saucepan. Bring to boil, and boil until liquid measures ⅓ c. (90 mL). Stir in cereal and margarine. Cover with paper towels, and allow to cool. Add vanilla, egg whites, and sugar replacement. Beat with a fork to blend completely. Thoroughly stir in flour and baking powder. Spray cookie sheet lightly with a vegetable-oil spray. Drop cookie dough onto the greased cookie sheet. Flatten dough slightly, either with your fingers or the knife used for dropping the dough. Bake at 375°F (190°C) for 12 to 15 minutes Remove from cookie sheet, and cool on rack.

Yield: 24 cookies

Exchange, 1 cookie: ¼ bread
Each serving contains: Calories: 23, Carbohydrates: 3 g

Easy Cranberry Cookies

8 oz. box	white cake mix, fructose-sweetened	226 g box
1	egg white	1
2 T.	water	30 mL
⅓ c.	chopped fresh cranberries	90 mL
½ t.	vanilla extract	2 mL

Combine cake mix, egg white, water, chopped cranberries, and vanilla extract in a medium-size bowl. Stir to blend completely. Drop on a cool, greased cookie sheet. Bake at 375°F (190°C) for 12 to 15 minutes or until golden brown. Move to cooling rack.

Yield: 24 cookies

Exchange, 1 cookie: ⅓ bread, ¼ fat
Each serving contains: Calories: 46, Carbohydrates: 4 g

Plum Spice Cookies

6 oz. jar	baby-food plum purée	170 g jar
¼ c.	frozen orange juice concentrate	60 mL
2 T.	granulated sugar replacement	30 mL
1	egg, slightly beaten	1
1 t.	vanilla extract	5 mL
¾ t.	allspice	3 mL
1 c.	all-purpose flour	250 mL
1 t.	baking powder	5 mL

Combine plum purée, orange juice concentrate, and sugar replacement in a medium-size bowl. Stir to blend completely. Add egg and vanilla. Beat to mix. Add allspice, flour, and baking powder. Stir until mixture is thoroughly blended (mixture will be soft). Spray cookie sheet with a vegetable-oil spray. Drop cookie dough onto the greased cookie sheet. Bake at 350°F (175°C) for 15 to 20 minutes. Move to cooling racks.

Yield: 30 cookies

Exchange, 1 cookie: ⅓ bread
Each serving contains: Calories: 20, Carbohydrates: 4 g

Apricot Raisin Cookies

6 oz. jar	baby-food apricot purée	170 g jar
¼ c.	frozen white grape juice concentrate	60 mL
1 T.	granulated fructose	15 mL
1	egg white	1
1 t.	vanilla extract	5 mL
1¼ c.	all-purpose flour	310 mL
1 t.	baking powder	5 mL
⅓ c.	raisins, chopped	90 mL

Combine apricot purée, grape juice concentrate, and fructose in a medium-size bowl. Stir to blend completely. Add egg white and vanilla. Beat to mix. Blend in flour and baking powder. Stir in chopped raisins. Spray cookie sheet with a vegetable-oil spray. Drop cookie dough onto the greased cookie sheet. Bake at 350°F (175°C) for 15 to 20 minutes. Move to cooling racks.

Yield: 30 cookies

Exchange, 1 cookie: ⅓ bread
Each serving contains: Calories: 27, Carbohydrates: 4 g

Brandy Pecan Cookies

8 oz. box	white cake mix, fructose-sweetened	227 g box
1	egg white	1
1 T.	brandy	15 mL
24	pecan halves	24

Combine cake mix, egg white, and brandy in a medium-size bowl. Stir to blend completely. Drop on a cool, greased cookie sheet. Press a pecan half into the top of each cookie. Bake at 375°F (190°C) for 12 to 15 minutes or until golden brown. Move to cooling rack.

Yield: 24 cookies

Exchange, 1 cookie: ⅓ bread, ¼ fat
Each serving contains: Calories: 50, Carbohydrates: 5 g

Toasted Almond Yogurt Drops

8 oz.	low-fat vanilla yogurt	224 g
2	egg whites	2
2 T.	granulated sugar replacement	30 mL
2 T.	granulated fructose	30 mL
1 t.	almond flavoring	5 mL
⅓ c.	toasted almonds, crushed*	90 mL
1¼ c.	all-purpose flour	310 mL
1 t.	baking powder	5 mL

Combine vanilla yogurt and egg whites in a mixing bowl. Beat until thoroughly blended, about 1 minute. Add sugar replacement, fructose, almond flavoring, toasted almonds, and ½ c. (125 mL) of the flour. Beat until smooth. Stir in remaining flour and baking powder. Spray cookie sheet with a vegetable-oil spray. Drop cookie dough onto the greased cookie sheet. Bake at 350 °F (175°C) for 12 to 15 minutes. Move to cooling racks.

Yield: 30 cookies

Exchange, 1 cookie: ⅓ bread, ¼ fat
Each serving contains: Calories: 34, Carbohydrates: 4 g

*To toast almonds: Sauté almond slices over low heat in a non-stick skillet until slices are lightly browned. Don't add any oil or shortening.

Caraway Yogurt Cookies

8 oz. box	yellow cake mix, fructose-sweetened	226 g box
⅓ c.	plain yogurt	90 mL
½ t.	ground nutmeg	2 mL
½ t.	caraway seeds	2 mL

Combine cake mix and yogurt in a medium-size bowl. Stir to blend completely. (Mix will seem sticky.) Stir in nutmeg and caraway seeds. Drop on a cool, greased cookie sheet. Bake at 375°F (190°C) for 12 to 15 minutes or until golden brown. Move to cooling rack.

Yield: 24 cookies

Exchange, 1 cookie: ⅔ bread
Each serving contains: Calories: 42, Carbohydrates: 7 g

Lemon Yogurt Drops

8 oz.	low-fat lemon yogurt	224 g
2	egg whites	2
2 T.	granulated sugar replacement	30 mL
2 T.	granulated fructose	30 mL
2 T.	freshly grated lemon rind	30 mL
1¼ c.	all-purpose flour	310 mL
1 t.	baking powder	5 mL

Combine lemon yogurt and egg whites in a mixing bowl. Beat until thoroughly blended, about 1 minute. Add sugar replacement, fructose, lemon rind, and ½ c. (125 mL) of the flour. Beat until smooth. Stir in remaining flour and baking powder. Spray cookie sheet with a vegetable-oil spray. Drop cookie dough onto the greased cookie sheet. Bake at 350°F (175°C) for 12 to 15 minutes. Move to cooling racks.

Yield: 30 cookies

Exchange, 1 cookie: ⅓ bread
Each serving contains: Calories: 27, Carbohydrates: 4 g

Rum Raisin Cookies

½ c.	raisins	125 mL
¼ c.	dark rum	60 mL
	water	
8 oz. box	yellow cake mix, fructose-sweetened	226 g box

Combine raisins and dark rum in a saucepan. Bring to a boil; then remove from heat and allow to cool. When cool, drain remaining rum liquid into a ⅓ c. (250 mL) measuring cup. Add enough water to make ⅓ c. (90 mL) of liquid. Combine cake mix and the ⅓ c. (90 mL) of rum liquid in a medium-size bowl. Stir to blend completely. (Mix will seem sticky.) Stir in raisins. Drop on a cool, greased cookie sheet. Bake at 375°F (190°C) for 12 to 15 minutes or until golden brown. Move to cooling rack.

Yield: 24 cookies

Exchange, 1 cookie: ¾ bread
Each serving contains: Calories: 54, Carbohydrates: 12 g

Swedish Classic Cookies

8 oz. box	yellow cake mix, fructose-sweetened	226 g box
⅓ c.	water	90 mL
2 t.	liquid fructose	10 mL
1 t.	ground coriander seeds	5 mL
½ t.	ground cinnamon	2 mL

Combine cake mix, water, and liquid fructose in a medium-size bowl. Stir to blend completely. (Mix will seem sticky.) Stir in coriander seeds and cinnamon. Drop on a cool, greased cookie sheet. Bake at 375°F (190°C) for 12 to 15 minutes or until golden brown. Move to cooling rack.

Yield: 24 cookies

Exchange, 1 cookie: ⅔ bread
Each serving contains: Calories: 43, Carbohydrates: 9 g

Whole Wheat Oatmeal Cookies

1½ c.	whole wheat flour	375 mL
1 t.	baking powder	5 mL
¼ t.	baking soda	1 mL
dash	salt	dash
1 c.	margarine	250 mL
⅔ c.	granulated sugar replacement	190 mL
⅓ c.	granulated fructose	90 mL
2	eggs	2
¼ c.	apple juice	60 mL
1 c.	quick-cooking oatmeal	250 mL

Combine whole wheat flour, baking powder, baking soda, and salt in a sifter. Sift together into a bowl. Set aside. Using an electric mixer, cream margarine. Gradually add granulated sugar replacement and fructose. Add eggs, one at a time, beating well after each addition. Add flour mixture alternately with apple juice. Beat until smooth. Stir in oatmeal. Drop onto ungreased cookie sheet. Bake at 350 °F (175°C) until edges are browned and top feels firm to the touch. Move to cooling rack.

Yield: 60 cookies

Exchange, 1 cookie: ⅓ bread, ½ fat
Each serving contains: Calories: 49, Carbohydrates: 5 g

Spice Whole Wheat Cookies

1½ c.	whole wheat flour	375 mL
1 t.	baking powder	5 mL
¼ t.	baking soda	1 mL
dash	salt	dash
2 t.	ground cinnamon	10 mL
1 t.	ground nutmeg	5 mL
¼ t.	ground cloves	1 mL
1 c.	margarine	250 mL
⅔ c.	granulated sugar replacement	190 mL
⅓ c.	granulated fructose	90 mL
2	eggs	2
¼ c.	white grape juice	60 mL

Combine whole wheat flour, baking powder, baking soda, salt, cinnamon, nutmeg, and cloves in a sifter. Sift together into a bowl. Set aside. Using an electric mixer, cream margarine. Gradually add granulated sugar replacement and fructose. Add eggs, one at a time, beating well after each addition. Add flour mixture alternately with grape juice. Beat until smooth. Drop onto ungreased cookie sheet. Bake at 350°F (175°C) until edges are brown and top feels firm. Move to wire racks.

Yield: 60 cookies

Exchange, 1 cookie: ⅓ bread, ½ fat
Each serving contains: Calories: 46, Carbohydrates: 4 g

Date Whole Wheat Cookies

1 c.	whole wheat flour	375 mL
1 t.	baking powder	5 mL
¼ t.	baking soda	1 mL
dash	salt	dash
1 c.	margarine	250 mL
⅔ c.	granulated sugar replacement	190 mL
⅓ c.	granulated fructose	90 mL
2	eggs	2
¼ c.	white grape juice	60 mL
⅓ c.	finely chopped dates	90 mL

Combine whole wheat flour, baking powder, baking soda, and salt in a sifter. Sift together into a bowl. Set aside. Using an electric mixer, cream margarine. Gradually add granulated sugar replacement and fructose. Add eggs, one at a time, beating well after each addition. Add flour mixture alternately with grape juice. Beat until smooth. Stir in finely chopped dates. Drop onto ungreased cookie sheet. Bake at 350°F (175°C) until edges are brown and top feels firm. Move to cooling racks.

Yield: 60 cookies

Exchange, 1 cookie: ½ bread, ½ fat
Each serving contains: Calories: 58, Carbohydrates: 7 g

Chocolate Chip Whole Wheat Cookies

1 c.	whole wheat flour	250 mL
1 t.	baking powder	5 mL
¼ t.	baking soda	1 mL
dash	salt	dash
1 c.	quick-cooking oatmeal	250 mL
1 c.	margarine	250 mL
⅔ c.	granulated sugar replacement	190 mL
⅓ c.	granulated fructose	90 mL
2	eggs	2
¼ c.	white grape juice	60 mL
½ c.	mini chocolate chips	125 mL

Combine whole wheat flour, baking powder, baking soda, and salt in a sifter. Sift together into a bowl. Stir in quick oatmeal. Set aside. Using an electric mixer, cream margarine. Gradually add granulated sugar replacement and fructose. Add eggs, one at a time, beating well after each addition. Add flour mixture alternately with grape juice. Beat until smooth. Stir in chocolate chips. Drop onto ungreased cookie sheet. Bake at 350°F (175°C) until edges are brown and top feels firm to the touch. Move to cooling racks.

Yield: 60 cookies

Exchange, 1 cookie: ⅓ bread, ⅓ fat
Each serving contains: Calories: 48, Carbohydrates: 4 g

Sweet Squash Cookies

⅓ c.	vegetable oil	90 mL
1	egg	1
1 c.	mashed acorn squash	250 mL
1½ c.	all-purpose flour	375 mL
1 t.	baking powder	5 mL
1 t.	allspice	5 mL
dash	cinnamon	dash

Combine oil, egg, and squash in a mixing bowl. Beat until thoroughly blended. Add flour, baking powder, and allspice. Beat well. Grease cookie sheet with a vegetable-oil spray. Drop cookie dough onto cookie sheet. If desired, sprinkle each cookie with a small amount of cinnamon. Bake at 350°F (175°C) for 10 to 12 minutes. Remove from oven, and cool on racks.

Yield: 36 cookies

Exchange, 1 cookie: ½ bread, ¼ fat
Each serving contains: Calories: 42, Carbohydrates: 7 g

Coconut Orange Cookies

1¾ c.	all-purpose flour	440 mL
¼ t.	baking soda	1 mL
¼ t.	salt	1 mL
½ c.	margarine	125 mL
⅔ c.	granulated sugar replacement	190 mL
2 T.	granulated fructose	30 mL
1	egg	1
½ t.	grated orange rind	2 mL
½ t.	grated lemon rind	2 mL
¼ c.	orange juice	60 mL
1 T.	lemon juice	15 mL
½ c.	unsweetened flaked coconut	125 mL

Sift together flour, baking soda, and salt. Set aside. Using an electric mixer, cream margarine, sugar replacement, and fructose. Beat in egg and grated orange and lemon rinds. Beat in dry ingredients alternately with juices. (Beat well after each addition.) Stir in coconut. Drop mixture onto greased cookie sheet. Bake at 350°F (175°C) for 12 to 14 minutes or until edges begin to lightly brown. Move cookies to cooling racks.

Yield: 48 cookies

Exchange, 1 cookie: ⅓ bread, ⅓ fat
Each serving contains: Calories: 41, Carbohydrates: 4 g

Lemon Yogurt Cake Cookies

8 oz. box	pound cake mix, fructose-sweetened	226 g box
⅓ c.	low-fat lemon yogurt	90 mL
2 t.	freshly grated lemon rind	10 mL

Combine cake mix, lemon yogurt, and lemon rind in a medium-size bowl. Stir to blend completely. (Mix will seem sticky.) Drop on a cool, greased cookie sheet. Bake at 375°F (190°C) for 12 to 15 minutes or until golden brown. Move to cooling rack.

Yield: 24 cookies

Exchange, 1 cookie: ⅔ bread
Each serving contains: Calories: 45, Carbohydrates: 8 g

Banana Cake Cookies

8 oz. box	pound cake mix, fructose-sweetened	226 g box
⅔ c.	mashed banana*	180 mL
1	egg white	1
½ c.	dietetic frosting mix	125 mL
2 T.	skim milk	30 mL
1 T.	margarine	15 mL

Combine cake mix, ⅓ c. (90 mL) of the mashed banana, and egg white in a medium-size bowl. Stir to blend completely. (Mix will seem sticky.) Drop on a cool, greased cookie sheet. Bake at 375°F (190°C) for 12 to 15 minutes or until golden brown. Move to cooling rack. Meanwhile, in a saucepan, combine the frosting mix, the remaining ⅓ c. (90 mL) mashed banana, and the skim milk. Stir to blend; then place saucepan over medium heat and continue stirring until mixture is very thick and paste like. Remove from heat, and stir in the margarine. Cool completely before frosting cookies.

Yield: 24 cookies

Exchange, 1 cookie. ½ bread, ⅓ fat
Each serving contains: Calories: 52, Carbohydrates: 8 g

*One large banana.

Brownie Espresso-Cream Cookies

1 T.	margarine	15 mL
1 oz.	unsweetened baking chocolate	28 g
1 t.	instant espresso granules or powder	5 mL
2 t.	granulated sugar replacement	30 mL
1 T.	granulated fructose	15 mL
2	egg whites	2
½ t.	vanilla extract	2 mL
1 c.	all-purpose flour	250 mL
1 t.	baking powder	5 mL
2 t.	sugar-free chocolate powdered-drink mix	10 mL

Combine margarine, baking chocolate, and espresso powder in a medium-size microwavable mixing bowl. Microwave on High for 1 minute, or until margarine and chocolate are melted. Stir to blend completely, and dissolve espresso powder. Set aside to cool slightly. Use a wire whisk to beat in sugar replacement, fructose, egg whites, and vanilla. Beat for 1 minute. Add flour and baking powder; stir until completely blended. Cover with plastic wrap, and refrigerate for at least 1 hour, or until needed. Form dough into small balls; then press balls into patties using the palm of your hand. Spray cookie sheet lightly with vegetable-oil spray. Place patties about 1 in. (2.5 cm) apart on the cookie sheet. Bake at 375°F (190°C) for 10 to 12 minutes. Remove from pan, and, while cookies are still hot, sprinkle with chocolate powdered-drink mix.

Yield: 24 cookies

Exchange, 1 cookie: ⅓ bread
Each serving contains: Calories: 24, Carbohydrates: 4 g

Chocolate Doodles

¼ c.	margarine	60 mL
3 oz.	semisweet baking chocolate	85 g
1¾ c.	all-purpose flour	440 mL
1½ t.	baking powder	7 mL
⅔ c.	granulated sugar replacement	190 mL
⅓ c.	granulated fructose	90 mL
3	eggs	3
2 t.	vanilla extract	10 mL

Combine margarine and baking chocolate in the top of a double boiler. Bring water to a boil, reduce heat to low, and heat until chocolate melts, stirring occasionally. Meanwhile, sift together the flour and baking powder. Remove double boiler from heat. Beat in the sugar replacement, fructose, and eggs. Add half of the flour mixture, and beat well. Remove the top half of the double boiler. Thoroughly stir in vanilla and remaining flour mixture. Cover and chill for at least 2 hours. Coat hands well with flour, and roll dough into 1 in. (2.5 cm) balls. Place balls on very lightly greased cookie sheet. Bake at 325°F (165°C) for 15 minutes. Move to cooling racks.

Yield: 60 cookies

Exchange, 1 cookie: ¼ bread, ¼ fat
Each serving contains: Calories: 32, Carbohydrates: 4 g

Cowboy Cookies

1 c.	all-purpose flour	250 mL
¾ t.	baking soda	3 mL
½ t.	baking powder	2 mL
½ c.	vegetable shortening	125 mL
⅔ c.	granulated sugar replacement	190 mL
⅓ c.	granulated fructose	90 mL
1	egg	1
½ t.	vanilla extract	2 mL
¾ c.	quick-cooking oatmeal	190 mL
¾ c.	toasted-rice cereal	190 mL

Sift together flour, baking soda, and baking powder; set aside. Using an electric mixer, beat shortening, sugar replacement, and fructose until fluffy. Beat in egg and vanilla extract. Gradually stir flour mixture into creamed mixture. Stir in oatmeal and rice cereal. Form into 1 in. (2.5 cm) balls. Place balls on a greased cookie sheet. Bake at 350°F (175°C) for 15 minutes. Move to cooling rack.

Yield: 36 cookies

Exchange, 1 cookie: ⅓ bread
Each serving contains: Calories: 28, Carbohydrates: 4 g

Brown Sugar Oatmeal Coconut Cookies

½ c.	all-purpose flour	125 mL
½ t.	baking soda	2 mL
dash	salt	dash
½ c.	vegetable shortening, melted	125 mL
¾ c.	granulated brown sugar replacement	190 mL
¼ c.	granulated fructose	60 mL
1	egg	1
½ t.	vanilla extract	2 mL
1 c.	quick-cooking oatmeal	250 mL
⅓ c.	unsweetened coconut	90 mL

Sift together flour, baking soda, and salt; set aside. Using an electric mixer, beat shortening, brown sugar replacement, and fructose on Medium until well blended. Add egg and beat well. Gradually stir flour mixture into creamed mixture. Stir in vanilla extract. Stir in oatmeal and coconut. Shape dough into balls, and place on greased cookie sheet. Bake at 325°F (165°C) for 12 to 15 minutes. Move to cooling racks.

Yield: 42 cookies

Exchange, 1 cookie: ¼ bread, ⅓ fat
Each serving contains: Calories: 40, Carbohydrates: 3 g

Pfeffernusse

2	eggs	2
1 c.	granulated brown sugar replacement	250 mL
½ c.	granulated fructose	125 mL
2 t.	fresh lemon juice	10 mL
2 c.	all-purpose flour	500 mL
2 t.	ground cinnamon	10 mL
½ t.	baking soda	2 mL
½ t.	ground cardamom	2 mL
½ t.	ground nutmeg	2 mL
½ t.	ground allspice	2 mL
½ t.	ground cloves	2 mL
¼ t.	salt	1 mL
¼ t.	ground black pepper	1 mL
¼ t.	ground blanched almonds	1 mL
	grated zest of one lemon	

Combine eggs, brown sugar replacement, and fructose in a mixing bowl. Beat to blend for 10 full minutes. Beat in lemon juice. In a bowl, combine flour, cinnamon, baking soda, cardamom, nutmeg, allspice, cloves, salt, and black pepper. Stir to mix. Gradually add flour mixture to egg mixture. Beat well after each addition. Add almonds and lemon zest. Stir to mix. Shape dough into balls, and place them on greased cookie sheets. Allow the balls to "ripen" overnight at room temperature. Bake at 350°F (175°C) for 15 minutes, or until cracks form in the tops. Move to cooling racks.

Yield: 70 balls

Exchange, 1 ball: ⅓ bread
Each serving contains: Calories: 21, Carbohydrates: 4 g

Old Fashioned Brown Sugar Cookies

2 c + 2 T.	all-purpose flour	530 mL
1 t.	baking soda	5 mL
1 t.	cream of tartar	5 mL
½ c.	margarine	125 mL
¾ c.	granulated brown sugar replacement	190 mL
¼ c.	granulated fructose	60 mL
2 t.	caramel flavoring	10 mL
2 small	eggs	2 small

Sift together flour, baking soda, and cream of tartar; set aside. Using an electric mixer, beat together margarine, brown sugar replacement, fructose, and caramel flavoring. Add eggs, one at a time, beating well after each addition. Stir flour mixture into creamed mixture, blending well. Shape dough into balls. Place balls on a greased cookie sheet. Dip a kitchen fork into flour, and flatten each cookie with the tines of the fork. Bake at 375°F (190°C) for 10 minutes. Move to cooling racks.

Yield: 42 cookies

Exchange, 1 cookie: ⅓ bread, ⅓ fat
Each serving contains: Calories: 42, Carbohydrates: 5 g

Date Delights

½ c.	margarine	125 mL
3 T.	granulated sugar replacement	45 mL
1 T.	granulated fructose	15 mL
1 t.	vanilla extract	5 mL
1 c.	all-purpose flour	250 mL
¼ c.	finely chopped dates	60 mL

Using an electric mixer, beat margarine, sugar replacement, and fructose until light and fluffy. Beat in vanilla. Stir in flour. Fold in dates until well blended. Shape dough into ½ in. (1.25 cm) balls. Place on lightly greased cookie sheets. Bake at 350°F (175°C) for 12 to 15 minutes. Cool on racks.

Yield: 42 balls

Exchange, 1 ball: ¼ bread, ¼ fat
Each serving contains: Calories: 30, Carbohydrates: 4 g

Whole Wheat Pineapple Cookies

½ c.	margarine	125 mL
⅔ c.	granulated sugar replacement	190 mL
¼ c.	granulated fructose	60 mL
1	egg	1
¼ c.	crushed pineapple in juice	60 mL
1 t.	pineapple flavoring	5 mL
2 c.	whole wheat flour	500 mL
1 t.	baking soda	5 mL

Using an electric mixer, beat margarine, sugar replacement, fructose, egg, crushed pineapple, and pineapple flavoring until well blended. In another bowl, mix flour and baking soda. Gradually beat about two-thirds of the whole wheat mixture into the creamed mixture. Stir in remaining flour until thoroughly mixed. Shape into small patties, and place on ungreased cookie sheets. Bake at 350°F (175°C) for 10 to 12 minutes. Move to cooling racks.

Yield: 54 cookies

Exchange, 1 cookie: ¼ bread
Each serving contains: Calories: 29, Carbohydrates: 4 g

Jellybean Tea Balls

½ c.	margarine	125 mL
3 T.	granulated sugar replacement	45 mL
1 T.	granulated fructose	15 mL
1 t.	vanilla extract	5 mL
1 c.	all-purpose flour	250 mL
2 T.	finely chopped dietetic jellybeans	30 mL

Using an electric mixer, beat margarine, sugar replacement, and fructose until light and fluffy. Beat in vanilla. Stir in flour until well blended. Fold in chopped jellybeans. Shape dough into ½ in. (1.25 cm) balls. Place on lightly greased cookie sheets. Bake at 350°F (175°C) for 12 to 15 minutes. Cool on racks.

Yield: 42 balls

Exchange, 1 ball: ¼ bread, ¼ fat
Each serving contains: Calories: 29, Carbohydrates: 3 g

Black Walnut Balls

¼ c.	margarine, melted	60 mL
2 T.	plain low-fat yogurt	30 mL
⅔ c.	granulated sugar replacement	190 mL
¼ c.	granulated fructose	60 mL
2	eggs	2
1 t.	vanilla extract	5 mL
½ c.	all-purpose flour	375 mL
1 t.	baking soda	5 mL
dash	salt	dash
⅓ c.	black walnuts, finely ground	90 mL

Combine melted margarine and the yogurt in a mixing bowl. Beat to blend. Beat in sugar replacement and fructose. Add eggs, one at a time beating well after each addition. Beat in vanilla. Stir in flour, baking soda, and salt. Fold in ground black walnuts. Cover and chill for at least 2 hours. Flour your hands, and shape dough into balls. Place on lightly greased cookie sheets. Bake at 350°F (175°C) for 8 to 9 minutes. Move to cooling racks.

Yield: 42 balls

Exchange, 1 ball: ¼ bread
Each serving contains: Calories: 19, Carbohydrates: 3 g

Cocoa Tea Balls

½ c.	margarine	125 mL
3 T.	granulated sugar replacement	45 mL
1 T.	granulated fructose	15 mL
1 t.	vanilla extract	5 mL
1 c.	all-purpose flour	250 mL
2 T.	baking cocoa	30 mL

Using an electric mixer, beat margarine, sugar replacement, and fructose until light and fluffy. Beat in vanilla. Stir in flour and cocoa until well blended. Shape dough into ½ in. (1.25 cm) balls. Place on lightly greased cookie sheets. Bake at 350°F (175°C) for 12 to 15 minutes. Cool on racks.

Yield: 42 balls

Exchange, 1 ball: ¼ bread, ¼ fat
Each serving contains: Calories: 25, Carbohydrates: 3 g

Deep Chocolate Cookies

½ c.	vegetable shortening	125 mL
3 oz.	unsweetened baking chocolate	85 g
1½ c.	granulated sugar replacement	375 mL
½ c.	granulated fructose	125 mL
4	eggs	4
2 t.	vanilla extract	10 mL
2 c.	all-purpose flour	500 mL
2 t.	baking soda	10 mL
¼ t.	salt	1 mL
42	pecan halves	42

Melt shortening and baking chocolate, either in the top of a double boiler, or in a microwavable cup. Pour into a mixing bowl. Beat in sugar replacement and fructose. (Mixture will look curdled.) Add eggs, one at a time, beating well after each addition. Beat in vanilla. Stir in flour, baking soda, and salt. Cover and chill at least 2 hours. Shape dough into balls. Place balls on lightly greased cookie sheets. Break each pecan half in half again. Place small pecan piece on top of dough. Then press pecan into dough, flattening dough slightly. Bake at 350°F (175°C) for 8 to 9 minutes. Move to cooling racks.

Yield: 84 cookies

Exchange, 1 cookie: ¼ bread, ¼ fat
Each serving contains: Calories: 33, Carbohydrates: 3 g

Deep Chocolate Coconut Balls

½ c.	vegetable shortening	125 mL
3 oz.	unsweetened baking chocolate	85 g
1½ c.	granulated sugar replacement	375 mL
½ c.	granulated fructose	125 mL
4	eggs	4
2 t.	vanilla extract	10 mL
2 c.	all-purpose flour	500 mL
2 t.	baking soda	10 mL
¼ t.	salt	1 mL
⅓ c.	unsweetened flaked coconut	90 mL

Melt shortening and baking chocolate, either in the top of a double boiler or in a microwavable cup. Pour into a mixing bowl. Beat in sugar replacement and fructose. (Mixture will look curdled.) Add eggs, one at a time, beating well after each addition. Beat in vanilla. Stir in flour, baking soda, and salt. Fold in coconut. Cover and chill at least 2 hours. Shape dough into balls. Place balls on lightly greased cookie sheets. Bake at 350°F (175°C) for 8 to 9 minutes. Move to cooling racks.

Yield: 84 balls

Exchange, 1 ball: ¼ bread, ¼ fat
Each serving contains: Calories: 33, Carbohydrates: 3 g

Chocolate Tuiles

2	egg whites, room temperature	2
⅓ c.	granulated sugar replacement	90 mL
2 T.	granulated fructose	30 mL
¼ c.	margarine	60 mL
1 oz.	semisweet baking chocolate	28 g
1 c.	all-purpose flour	250 mL
1 t.	chocolate flavoring	5 mL

Combine egg whites, sugar replacement, and fructose in a medium-size mixing bowl. Beat until foamy and well blended. Combine margarine and chocolate in a small cup; melt in microwave. Stir flour, melted margarine, chocolate mixture, and chocolate flavoring into egg mixture. Blend well. Drop onto a well-greased cookie sheet. Use a fork dipped in water to flatten dough wafer-thin. Bake at 350°F (175°C) for 8 minutes, or just until dough has lightly browned around edges. Use an oven mitt, and bend each wafer around a rolling pin. Press gently against the rolling pin for a few seconds. Slide wafer off pin, and place on cooling rack. Cool tuiles completely.

Yield: 30 tuiles

Exchange, 1 tuile: ¼ bread
Each serving contains: Calories: 21, Carbohydrates: 3 g

Vanilla Tuiles

2	egg whites, room temperature	2
⅓ c.	granulated sugar replacement	90 mL
2 T.	granulated fructose	30 mL
1 c.	all-purpose flour	250 mL
¼ c.	melted margarine	60 mL
1 t.	vanilla extract	5 mL

Combine egg whites, sugar replacement, and fructose in a medium-size mixing bowl. Beat until foamy and well blended. Stir in flour, melted margarine, and vanilla. Drop onto a well-greased cookie sheet. Use a fork dipped in water to flatten dough wafer-thin. Bake at 350°F (175°C) for 8 minutes, or just until lightly browned around edges. Use an oven mitt and bend each wafer around a rolling pin. Press gently against the rolling pin for a few seconds. Slide wafer off pin, and place on cooling rack. Cool tuiles completely.

Yield: 30 tuiles

Exchange, 1 tuile: ¼ bread
Each serving contains: Calories: 19, Carbohydrates: 3 g

Almond Tuiles

2	egg whites, room temperature	2
⅓ c.	granulated sugar replacement	90 mL
2 T.	granulated fructose	30 mL
¾ c.	all-purpose flour	190 mL
¼ c.	blanched almonds, finely ground	60 mL
¼ c.	melted margarine	60 mL
1 t.	almond extract	5 mL

Combine egg whites, sugar replacement, and fructose in a medium-size mixing bowl. Beat until foamy and well blended. Stir in flour, ground almonds, melted margarine, and almond extract. Mix well. Drop onto well-greased cookie sheet. Use a fork dipped in water to flatten dough wafer-thin. Bake at 350°F (175°C) for 8 minutes, or just until the dough has lightly browned around edges. Use an oven mitt, and bend each wafer around a rolling pin. Press gently against the rolling pin for a few seconds. Slide wafer off pin, and place on cooling rack. Cool tuiles completely.

Yield: 30 tuiles

Exchange, 1 tuile: ¼ bread
Each serving contains: Calories: 20, Carbohydrates: 3 g

Currant Clusters

¼ c.	margarine, melted	60 mL
2 T.	plain low-fat yogurt	30 mL
¾ c.	granulated sugar replacement	190 mL
¼ c.	granulated fructose	60 mL
2	eggs	2
1 t.	vanilla extract	5 mL
1½ c.	all-purpose flour	375 mL
1 t.	baking soda	5 mL
dash	salt	dash
⅓ c.	currants	90 mL

Combine melted margarine and the yogurt in a mixing bowl. Beat to blend. Beat in sugar replacement and fructose. Add eggs, one at a time, beating well after each addition. Beat in vanilla. Stir in flour, baking soda, and salt. Fold in currants. Cover and chill at least 2 hours. Flour your hands, and shape dough into balls; then flatten balls slightly in the palm of your hand. Place on lightly greased cookie sheets. Bake at 350°F (175°C) for 8 to 9 minutes. Move to cooling racks.

Yield: 42 cookies

Exchange, 1 cookie: ¼ bread
Each serving contains: Calories: 20, Carbohydrates: 4 g

Vanilla-Cream Cookies

¼ c.	margarine, melted	60 mL
2 T.	plain low-fat yogurt	30 mL
¾ c.	granulated sugar replacement	190 mL
¼ c.	granulated fructose	60 mL
2	eggs	2
1 t.	vanilla extract	5 mL
1½ c.	all-purpose flour	375 mL
1 t.	baking soda	5 mL
dash	salt	dash

Combine melted margarine and the yogurt in a mixing bowl. Beat to blend. Beat in sugar replacement and fructose. Add eggs, one at a time, beating well after each addition, Beat in vanilla. Stir in flour, baking soda, and salt. Cover and chill at least 2 hours. Flour your hands, and shape dough into balls; then flatten balls slightly in the palm of your hand, Place on lightly greased cookie sheets. Using a table fork, press tines gently around the edge of each cookie. Bake at 350°F (175°C) for 8 to S minutes. Move to cooling racks.

Yield: 42 cookies

Exchange, 1 cookie: ⅓ bread
Each serving contains: Calories: 19, Carbohydrates: 3 g

Chocolate Rounds

2 oz.	semisweet baking chocolate, melted and cooled	57 g
½ c.	margarine	125 mL
⅓ c. + 2 T.	granulated sugar replacement	120 mL
¼ c.	granulated fructose	60 mL
3	egg yolks	3
1 t.	vanilla extract	5 mL
1½ c.	all-purpose flour	375 mL
½ t.	baking powder	2 mL
dash	salt	dash

Beat chocolate and margarine until light and fluffy. Add sugar replacement and fructose; beat at least 2 minutes. Beat in egg yolks and vanilla. Gradually stir in flour, baking powder, and salt. Shape dough into small balls; then flatten balls into 1 in. (2.5 cm) rounds. Place on a very lightly greased cookie sheet. Bake at 375°F (190°C) for 10 minutes, or until lightly browned. Move to cooling rack.

Yield: 36 cookies

Exchange, 1 cookie: ⅓ bread
Each serving contains: Calories: 28, Carbohydrates: 4 g

Hazelnut Puffs

½ c.	margarine	125 mL
⅓ c.	granulated sugar replacement	90 mL
⅓ c.	granulated fructose	90 mL
3	egg yolks	3
1 t.	vanilla extract	5 mL
1½ c.	all-purpose flour	375 mL
½ t.	baking powder	2 mL
dash	salt	dash
⅓ c.	hazelnuts, finely chopped	90 mL

Beat margarine until light and fluffy. Add sugar replacement and fructose; beat at least 2 minutes. Beat in egg yolks and vanilla. Gradually stir in flour, baking powder, and salt. Then stir in hazelnuts. Shape dough into balls. Place on a very lightly greased cookie sheet. Bake at 375°F (190°C) for 10 minutes, or until lightly browned. Move to cooling rack.

Yield: 36 cookies

Exchange, 1 cookie: ⅓ bread, ¼ fat
Each serving contains: Calories: 29, Carbohydrates: 4 g

Old Fashioned Ice-Box Cookies

½ c.	margarine	125 mL
⅓ c.	granulated sugar replacement	90 mL
¼ c.	granulated fructose	60 mL
2 T.	skim milk	30 mL
1	egg	1
1 t.	vanilla extract	5 mL
1¾ c.	all-purpose flour	440 mL
dash	salt	dash
¼ c.	pecans, finely chopped	60 mL

Using an electric mixer, thoroughly cream together margarine, sugar replacement, and fructose. Beat in skim milk, egg, and vanilla. Gradually add flour and salt. Stir to completely blend. Divide dough in half. Shape each half into a 6 in. (15 cm) roll. Roll dough in the chopped pecans. Wrap each roll in wax paper. Chill dough in refrigerator overnight. Cut each roll into 18 slices. Place slices on a greased cookie sheet. Bake at 350°F (175°C) for 10 to 12 minutes. Remove from cookie sheet, and cool on rack.

Yield: 36 cookies

Exchange, 1 cookie: ⅓ bread, ½ fat
Each serving contains: Calories: 42, Carbohydrates: 4 g

Thin Lemon Refrigerator Cookies

2 c.	all-purpose flour	500 mL
½ t.	baking powder	2 mL
1 c.	margarine	250 mL
½ c.	granulated sugar replacement	125 mL
1	egg	1
1 T.	lemon juice	15 mL
½ t.	lemon peel, freshly grated	2 mL

Sift together flour and baking powder; set aside. Using an electric mixer on Medium, beat the margarine and sugar replacement until well blended. Add egg, lemon juice, and lemon peel. Beat well. Gradually stir dry ingredients into creamed mixture, mixing well. Divide dough in half. Shape each half into a 6 in. (15 cm) roll. Wrap each roll in plastic wrap. Chill in refrigerator overnight. Cut each roll into 30 thin slices. Place slices on ungreased cookie sheets. Bake at 375°F (190°C) for about 8 to 10 minutes, or until golden brown. Remove from cookie sheets, and place on racks.

Yield: 60 cookies

Exchange, 1 cookie: ⅓ bread, ⅓ fat
Each serving contains: Calories: 32, Carbohydrates: 4 g

Cinnamon Almond Refrigerator Cookies

2¼ c.	all-purpose flour	560 mL
2 t.	ground cinnamon	10 mL
¼ t.	salt	1 mL
1 c.	margarine	250 mL
⅔ c.	granulated sugar replacement	180 mL
⅓ c.	granulated fructose	90 mL
1	egg	1
½ c.	chopped toasted almonds	125 mL

Sift together flour, cinnamon, and salt; set aside. Using an electric mixer on Medium, beat the margarine, sugar replacement, and fructose until well blended. Add egg and beat well. Gradually stir dry ingredients into creamed mixture, mixing well. Stir in almonds. Divide dough in half. Shape dough into two 6 in. (15 cm) rolls. Wrap each roll in plastic wrap. Chill dough in refrigerator overnight. Cut each roll into 24 slices. Place slices on greased cookie sheets. Bake at 350°F (175°C) for about 8 to 10 minutes, or until golden brown. Remove from cookie sheets, and place on racks.

Yield: 48 cookies

Exchange, 1 cookie: ⅓ bread, ⅓ fat
Each serving contains: Calories: 33, Carbohydrates: 4 g

Sunflower Cookies

1½ c.	quick-cooking oatmeal	375 mL
¾ c.	whole wheat flour	190 mL
¼ c.	wheat germ	60 mL
½ t.	baking soda	2 mL
dash	salt	dash
½ c.	margarine	125 mL
⅔ c.	granulated sugar replacement	180 mL
⅓ c.	granulated fructose	90 mL
1	egg	1
1 t.	brandy flavoring	5 mL
½ t.	vanilla extract	2 mL
½ c.	dry-roasted sunflower seeds	125 mL
	aspartame sweetener	

Combine oatmeal, whole wheat flour, wheat germ, baking soda, and salt in a bowl; set aside. Using an electric mixer on Medium, beat the margarine, sugar replacement, and fructose until well blended. Add egg and beat well. Beat in brandy flavoring and vanilla. Stir dry ingredients into creamed mixture, mixing well. Stir in sunflower seeds. Divide dough in half. Shape each half into an 8 in. (20 cm) roll. Wrap each roll in plastic wrap. Chill in refrigerator overnight. Cut each roll into 24 slices. Place slices on ungreased cookie sheets. Bake at 375°F (190°C) for about 10 to 12 minutes, or until golden brown. Remove from cookie sheets, and place on racks. While warm, sprinkle with aspartame sweetener.

Yield: 48 cookies

Exchange, 1 cookie: ⅓ bread, ¼ fat
Each serving contains: Calories: 29, Carbohydrates: 3 g

Walnut Butterscotch Cookies

2 c.	all-purpose flour	500 mL
½ t.	baking soda	2 mL
½ t.	cream of tartar	2 mL
¾ c.	margarine	190 mL
¾ c.	granulated brown sugar replacement	190 mL
¼ c.	granulated fructose	60 mL
1	egg	1
1 t.	vanilla extract	5 mL
½ c.	chopped walnuts	125 mL

Sift together flour, baking soda, and cream of tartar; set aside. Using an electric mixer on Medium, beat the margarine, brown sugar replacement, and fructose until well blended. Add egg and beat well. Beat in vanilla. Gradually stir dry ingredients into creamed mixture, mixing well. Stir in walnuts. Shape dough into one 13 in. (33 cm) roll. Wrap dough in wax paper, and refrigerate at least 4 hours, or overnight. Cut roll into 54 slices. Place slices on greased cookie sheets. Bake at 400°F (200°C) for about 10 to 12 minutes, or until golden brown. Remove from cookie sheets and place on racks.

Yield: 54 cookies

Exchange, 1 cookie: ⅓ bread, ⅓ fat
Each serving contains: Calories: 30, Carbohydrates: 4 g

Papaya Sugar Slices

1¾ c.	all-purpose flour	440 mL
½ t.	baking soda	2 mL
½ c.	margarine	125 mL
⅔ c.	granulated sugar replacement	180 mL
¼ c.	granulated fructose	60 mL
2	eggs	2
2 t.	vanilla extract	10 mL
2 T.	all-purpose flour	30 mL
2.5 oz.	unsweetened dried papaya, cubed	71 g

Sift together the 1¾ c. (440 mL) of flour and the baking soda; set aside. Using an electric mixer on Medium, beat the margarine, sugar replacement, and fructose until well blended. Add eggs, one at a time, beating well after each addition. Stir in vanilla. Gradually stir flour mixture into creamed mixture, mixing well. Combine the 2 T. (30 mL) of flour and cubed papaya in a blender. Process on Low or Medium until papaya is powdered. Stir into cookie dough. Shape dough into a 12 in. (30 cm) roll. Wrap in plastic wrap, and refrigerate overnight. Cut roll into 48 slices. Place slices on greased cookie sheets. Bake at 400°F (200°C) for about 5 minutes, or until golden brown. Remove from cookie sheets, and place on racks.

Yield: 48 cookies

Exchange, 1 cookie: ⅓ bread
Each serving contains: Calories: 28, Carbohydrates: 5 g

Pumpkin Pinwheels

1½ c.	all-purpose flour	375 mL
1 c.	quick-cooking oatmeal	250 mL
¼ t.	baking soda	1 mL
1 c.	granulated sugar replacement	250 mL
¼ c. + 2 T.	granulated fructose	60 mL + 30 mL
½ c.	margarine	125 mL
2	egg whites	2
1 c.	canned pumpkin	250 mL
1 t.	pumpkin-pie spices	5 mL

Combine flour, oatmeal, and baking soda in a small bowl; stir to mix. Set aside. Using an electric mixer, beat ¾ c. (190 mL) of the granulated sugar replacement and ¼ c. (60 mL) of the fructose with the margarine until fluffy. Beat in egg whites. Stir in flour mixture. Turn dough out onto a large piece of wax paper. Press dough into a 16 × 12 in. (40 × 30 cm) rectangle. In another bowl, combine pumpkin, pumpkin-pie spices, the remaining ¼ c. (60 mL) of sugar replacement, and the remaining 2 T. (30 mL) of fructose. Blend thoroughly. Spread pumpkin mixture over flattened dough. Roll dough, beginning at the narrow end. Wrap in wax paper; freeze overnight or until firm. Cut frozen dough into 48 slices. Place slices on greased cookie sheets. Bake at 400°F (200°C) for 8 to 9 minutes, or until golden brown. Move to cookie racks, and cool completely.

Yield: 48 cookies

Exchange, 1 cookie: ⅓ bread
Each serving contains: Calories: 38, Carbohydrates: 6 g

Black-Walnut Chocolate Cookies

2½ c.	all-purpose flour	625 mL
2 t.	baking powder	10 mL
½ t.	salt	2 mL
½ c.	margarine	125 mL
¾ c.	granulated sugar replacement	190 mL
½ c.	granulated fructose	125 mL
1	egg	1
1 t.	vanilla extract	5 mL
½ t.	black-walnut flavoring	2 mL
2 oz.	unsweetened baking chocolate, melted and cooled	57 g
¼ c.	skim milk	60 mL
½ c.	black walnuts, chopped	125 mL

Sift together flour, baking powder, and salt; set aside. Using an electric mixer on Medium, beat the margarine, sugar replacement, and fructose until well blended. Add egg and beat well. Beat in vanilla, black-walnut flavoring, and baking chocolate. Add dry ingredients alternately with milk to creamed mixture, mixing well. Stir in black walnuts. Divide dough in half. Shape each half into an 8 in. (20 cm) roll. Wrap in wax paper, and refrigerate at least 4 hours or overnight. Cut each roll into 30 slices. Place slices on greased cookie sheets. Bake at 350°F (175°C) for about 10 to 12 minutes. Remove from cookie sheets, and place on racks.

Yield: 60 cookies

Exchange, 1 cookie: ⅓ bread, ½ fat
Each serving contains: Calories: 50, Carbohydrates: 5 g

Cardamom Maple Spritz Cookies

1 c.	vegetable shortening	250 mL
½ c.	granulated sugar replacement	125 mL
¼ c.	granulated fructose	60 mL
1	egg	1
1 t.	vanilla extract	5 mL
1 t.	maple flavoring	5 mL
2½ c.	all-purpose flour	625 mL
2 t.	ground cardamom	10 mL
½ t.	baking powder	2 mL
dash	salt	dash

Using an electric mixer, beat shortening until light. Combine sugar replacement and fructose in a bowl; stir to mix. Gradually beat sugar-replacement mixture into creamed shortening. Beat in egg, vanilla, and maple flavoring. Combine flour, cardamom, baking powder, and salt in a mixing bowl; stir to mix. Gradually stir flour mixture into creamed mixture. Press dough from a cookie press (use thin setting or small tip) onto ungreased cookie sheets, following press manufacturer's directions. Bake at 375°F (190°C) for 8 to 10 minutes, or until edges of cookies are delicately browned. Move to cooling racks.

Yield: 75 cookies

Exchange, 1 cookie: ¼ bread
Each serving contains: Calories: 19, Carbohydrates: 3 g

Basic Spritz Cookies

1 c.	vegetable shortening	250 mL
½ c.	granulated sugar replacement	125 mL
¼ c.	granulated fructose	60 mL
1	egg	1
1 t.	vanilla or almond extract	5 mL
2¼ c.	all-purpose flour	560 mL
½ t.	baking powder	2 mL
dash	salt	dash

Using an electric mixer, beat shortening until light. Combine sugar replacement and fructose in a bowl; stir to mix. Gradually beat sugar-replacement mixture into creamed shortening. Beat in egg and vanilla. Combine flour, baking powder, and salt in a mixing bowl; stir to mix. Gradually stir flour mixture into creamed mixture. Press dough from a cookie press (use thin setting or small tip) onto ungreased cookie sheets, following press manufacturer's directions. Bake cookies at 375°F (190°C) for 8 to 10 minutes, or until edges of cookies are delicately browned. Move to cooling racks.

Yield: 70 cookies

Exchange, 1 cookie: ⅓ bread
Each serving contains: Calories: 23, Carbohydrates: 2 g

Spice Spritz Cookies

2¼ c.	all-purpose flour	560 mL
¼ t.	baking soda	1 mL
1 t.	ground cinnamon	5 mL
½ t.	ground ginger	2 mL
½ t.	ground allspice	2 mL
½ t.	ground nutmeg	2 mL
¼ t.	ground cloves	1 mL
¼ t.	salt	1 mL
½ c.	margarine	125 mL
⅓ c.	granulated sugar replacement	90 mL
3 T.	granulated fructose	45 mL
1	egg	1
¼ c.	liquid fructose	60 mL

Sift together flour, baking soda, cinnamon, ginger, allspice, nutmeg, cloves, and salt; set aside. Using an electric mixer, beat margarine until light. Add granulated sugar replacement and granulated fructose. Beat until fluffy. Beat in egg and liquid fructose. Gradually beat flour mixture into creamed mixture. Press dough from a cookie press onto ungreased cookie sheets, following press manufacturer's directions. Bake at 350°F (175°C) for 8 to 10 minutes, or until cookies are lightly browned. Move to cooling racks.

Yield: 75 cookies

Exchange, 1 cookie: ⅓ bread
Each serving contains: Calories: 21, Carbohydrates: 2 g

Butter-Flavored Spritz Cookies

2½ c.	all-purpose flour	625 mL
½ t.	baking powder	2 mL
¼ t.	salt	1 mL
1 c.	margarine	250 mL
½ c.	granulated sugar replacement	125 mL
¼ c.	granulated fructose	60 mL
1	egg	1
1½ t.	butter flavoring	7 mL

Sift together flour, baking powder, and salt; set aside. Using an electric mixer, beat margarine until light. Combine sugar replacement and fructose in a bowl; stir to mix. Gradually beat sugar-replacement mixture into creamed margarine. Beat in egg and butter flavoring. Gradually stir flour mixture into creamed mixture. Press dough from a cookie press (use thin setting or small tip) onto ungreased cookie sheets, following press manufacturer's directions. Bake cookies at 375°F (190°C) for 8 to 10 minutes, or until edges of cookies are delicately browned. Move to cooling racks.

Yield: 80 cookies

Exchange, 1 cookie: ⅓ bread
Each serving contains: Calories: 22, Carbohydrates: 3 g

Wheat Germ Cookies

2¼ c.	all-purpose flour	560 mL
3 t.	baking powder	15 mL
½ t.	salt	2 mL
¼ c.	wheat germ	60 mL
½ c.	margarine	125 mL
¼ c.	granulated sugar replacement	190 mL
¼ c.	granulated fructose	60 mL
2	eggs	2
1 t.	vanilla extract	5 mL

Sift together flour, baking powder, and salt. Stir in wheat germ; set aside. Beat margarine, sugar replacement, and fructose until light and fluffy. Add eggs, one at a time, beating well after each addition. Beat in vanilla. Gradually stir flour mixture into creamed mixture. Mix well. Cover and chill dough for at least 1 hour. Divide dough in half. Roll out each half of the dough on floured surface to scant ¼ in. (8 mm) thickness. Cut dough with a floured 1½ in. (3.7 cm) cookie cutter. Place cookies on a greased cookie sheet. Bake at 400°F (200°C) for 8 minutes, or until golden brown. Move to cooling rack.

Yield: 30 cookies

Exchange, 1 cookie: ½ bread
Each serving contains: Calories: 42, Carbohydrates: 9 g

Holiday Star Cookies

2 c.	all-purpose flour	500 mL
⅛ t.	ground nutmeg	0.5 mL
⅛ t.	ground cinnamon	0.5 mL
½ c.	margarine	125 mL
¾ c.	granulated sugar replacement	190 mL
¼ c.	granulated fructose	60 mL
2	eggs	2

Sift together flour, nutmeg, and cinnamon; set aside. Using an electric mixer, beat together margarine, sugar replacement, and fructose until light and fluffy. Add eggs, one at a time, beating well after each addition. Gradually stir flour into creamed mixture. Cover and chill overnight. Divide dough in half; then roll out each half on lightly floured surface to ⅛ in. (4 mm) thickness. Cut with a small star cookie cutter. Place onto greased cookie sheets. Bake at 350°F (175°C) for 10 to 12 minutes. Move to cooling racks.

Yield: 96 cookies

Exchange, 1 cookie: ¼ bread
Each serving contains: Calories: 17, Carbohydrates: 2 g

Brown Sugar Press Cookies

1 c.	margarine	250 mL
⅔ c.	granulated brown sugar replacement	190 mL
1	egg yolk	1
1 t.	vanilla extract	5 mL
½ t.	caramel flavoring	2 mL
¼ t.	salt	1 mL
2 c.	all-purpose flour	500 mL

Using an electric mixer, beat margarine in a large mixing bowl. Gradually add brown sugar replacement, beating until light and fluffy. Beat in egg yolk, vanilla, caramel flavoring, and salt. Stir in flour. Chill for at least 2 hours. Press dough from cookie press onto ungreased cookie sheets, following press manufacturer's directions. Bake at 350°F (175°C) for 8 to 10 minutes. Move to cooling racks.

Yield: 60 cookies

Exchange, 1 cookie: ⅓ bread
Each serving contains: Calories: 23, Carbohydrates: 3 g

Caraway Diamonds

1½ c.	all-purpose flour	375 mL
2 T.	vegetable shortening	30 mL
2 T.	margarine	30 mL
¼ c.	granulated sugar replacement	60 mL
1	egg	1
½ t.	vanilla extract	2 mL
½ t.	crushed caraway seeds	2 mL

Sift flour, and set aside. Using an electric mixer, beat together shortening, margarine, and sugar replacement until light and fluffy. Beat in egg and vanilla. Gradually add flour to creamed mixture. Stir in caraway seeds. Roll out dough on lightly floured surface to ⅛ in. (4 mm) thickness. Cut into 2 in. (5 cm) diamonds. Place dough on greased cookie sheets. Bake at 325°F (165°C) for 10 to 12 minutes. Move to cooling racks.

Yield: 40 cookies

Exchange, 1 cookie: ¼ bread
Each serving contains: Calories: 21, Carbohydrates: 3 g

Langues de Chat

My grandmother served these with coffee on her sunporch on summer afternoons. I've changed the recipe, but the wonderful rich character remains.

2 T.	butter or margarine	30 mL
2 T.	fat-free cream cheese	30 mL
3 pkgs.	acesulfame-K sugar substitute	3 pkgs.
3 T.	sugar	45 mL
1 large	egg or equivalent egg substitute, lightly beaten	1 large
1 t.	vanilla extract	5 mL
¼ t.	butter extract	2 mL
½ c.	flour, sifted	125 mL

In a medium bowl, beat the butter, cream cheese, acesulfame-K, and sugar until light and fluffy. Slowly beat in the egg and the two extracts. Fold in the flour to make a soft dough. Spoon the dough carefully into a pastry bag fitted with a ⅜ in. (1 cm) plain tip. Squeeze out 3 in. (7.5 cm) lengths onto greased baking sheets that have been lined with parchment or waxed paper. Cut off the dough with a sharp knife in between the cookies. Bake in a preheated 425°F (220°C) oven for 8–10 minutes, until the edges are lightly browned. Cool the sheets on a wire rack before removing the cookies.

Yield: 30 cookies

Exchange: free
Each serving contains: Calories: 23, Total fat: 1 g, Carbohydrates: 3 g, Protein: 1 g, Sodium: 14 mg, Cholesterol: 9 mg

Ground Almond Cookies

1¾ c.	all-purpose flour	440 mL
½ t.	salt	2 mL
1 c.	margarine	250 mL
⅓ c.	granulated sugar replacement	90 mL
¾ t.	almond extract	4 mL
1 c.	blanched almonds, ground or very finely chopped	250 mL
¼ c.	Powdered Sugar Replacement	60 mL

Measure flour onto waxed paper. Add salt and stir to blend. Cream thoroughly the margarine, granulated sugar replacement, and almond extract. Add blended dry ingredients and almonds to creamed mixture. Mix well. Shape dough into 1 in. (2.5 cm) balls or crescents. Place on ungreased baking sheets. Bake at 375°F (190°C) for 10 to 12 minutes until lightly browned. Remove from baking sheets. Cool slightly on rack. Roll in powdered sugar replacement. Cool.

Yield: 4 dozen cookies

Exchange, 1 cookie: ⅓ bread, 1 fat
Each serving contains: Calories: 60, Carbohydrates: 7 g

Cheesecakes

An entire chapter on cheesecakes! Why? Because the new nonfat dairy products make it easy to make cheesecakes that fit into diabetic meal plans. These products also add calcium and protein. Here are a few hints about using these new nonfat products.

Nonfat ricotta cheese

Check the dates on the label before you buy; use the cheese while it's still fresh. Nonfat ricotta is used not only in cooking, it also makes a nice (and fat-free) spread for toast and other foods; try it with a little added nutmeg and aspartame.

Nonfat cottage cheese

Process in a food processor or blender for a full two to three minutes to eliminate the curds before using in cooking.

Nonfat cream cheese

Microwave for 30 seconds to soften before adding it to a recipe.

Yogurt

Don't be misled by clever labels. Be sure the yogurt is 100% nonfat. It should also be free of sugar and other caloric sweeteners such as fruit purées. Some yogurts are sweetened with only aspartame or NutraSweet.

Skim milk

Skim milk does not create rich, creamy desserts the way cream does, although it's fairly innocuous. So add a little cornstarch dissolved in water to thicken dishes made with skim milk. Opinions vary on the use of canned evaporated skim milk. Some people like it when it is disguised by tasty ingredients—others avoid it like the plague.

Egg substitutes

These are a popular way to avoid cholesterol and are more convenient to use in cooking than whole eggs. Egg substitutes can be found in supermarkets either chilled near the eggs or frozen in the freezer section. Some egg substitutes are totally non-fat, others have a very small amount of fat. We had more success cooking with a defrosted egg substitute that has a tiny amount of corn oil than with the totally fat-free versions.

Egg substitutes and egg whites, which is basically what egg substitutes are, have a tendency to become rubbery, especially if exposed to too much heat. To minimize this problem, cook cheesecakes in a hot-water bath, the traditional way to bake custards. In a hot-water bath, food cooks in a smaller pan or pans set inside a larger pan of hot water.

Here's an easy way to manage: Preheat the oven, open the oven door, and slide the lower oven rack partway out. Set the larger pan on this rack. Put the smaller pan(s) of uncooked food in the center of the larger pan. Take a teakettle of boiling water and very carefully pour boiling water into the larger pan. Be sure you do not spill or splatter any water inside the smaller pan. Also, if you're using a springform pan, which is great for cheesecake, be sure the rim is tightly attached to the bottom rim.

Gelatin in cheesecake

Opinions vary on this subject. Some people declare vehemently that "real" cheesecake does not have gelatin. Others like gelatin-based desserts. We give you lots of choice; you decide which you prefer.

Crust

As far as crusts are concerned, you can decide for yourself. Some people like a graham cracker crust, which is described in the chapter on pies. To save calories, many cheesecake recipes suggest you simply sprinkle a few tablespoons of graham cracker crumbs on the base of the pan. Of course, you can make a cheesecake with no crust or bottom layer.

Granola Cheesecake

A super combination—creamy cheesecake with a crunch.

Crust

¼ c.	margarine or butter, melted	60 mL
1 T.	water	15 mL
3 pkts	concentrated acesulfame-K	3 pkts.
1 c.	Granola Topping	250 mL

Filling

8 oz.	nonfat cream cheese, softened	250 mL
1 c.	nonfat cottage cheese, drained	250 mL
½ c.	egg substitute or 2 eggs	125 mL
3 pkts.	concentrated acesulfame-K	3 pkts.
1 t.	vanilla extract	5 mL
1 T.	flour	15 mL

Topping

⅓ c.	Granola Topping	90 mL

Stir the crust ingredients together and press the mixture into the bottom of a 9 in. (23 cm) springform pan. Set aside. Beat the filling ingredients together until smooth. Spoon this carefully over the crust. Sprinkle the top with granola topping. Bake in a 375°F (190°C) oven for 40 minutes or until set. Cool before removing cake from the pan.

Yield: 10 servings

Exchange, 1 serving: 1 meat
Each serving contains: Calories: 88, Carbohydrates: 11 g, Fiber: trace, Sodium: 186 mg, Cholesterol: 5.2 mg

Healthy Cheesecake

This is a healthy version of the old fashioned cheesecake everyone loves. We don't think you'll miss the fat!

¼ c.	graham cracker crumbs	60 mL
2 c.	yogurt cheese*	500 mL
2 t.	vanilla extract	10 mL
½ c.	egg substitute	125 mL
2 T.	cornstarch	30 mL
6 pkts.	concentrated acesulfame-K	6 pkts.

Topping

½ c.	nonfat sour cream	125 mL
2 t.	sugar	10 mL
2 t.	concentrated acesulfame-K	2 t.
1 t.	vanilla extract	5 mL

Spray a 9 in. (23 cm) springform (or other) pie pan with non-stick cooking spray. Sprinkle it evenly with graham cracker crumbs. Set aside.

Use an electric mixer to combine the next five ingredients. Beat until creamy. Pour the mixture onto the crumbs. Bake in a preheated 325°F (160°C) oven for 35 minutes. Remove from the oven and let cool. Refrigerate. Combine the topping ingredients and pour the mixture over the baked, chilled cheesecake. Return it to the oven for 10 minutes. Chill. Run a knife around the edge of the pan to loosen the cheesecake.

Yield: 12 servings

Exchange, 1 serving: ½ bread
Each serving contains: Calories: 49, Carbohydrates: 8 g, Fiber: trace, Sodium: 68 mg, Cholesterol: 2 mg

*Yogurt cheese is made by letting yogurt drip through cheesecloth overnight in the refrigerator.

Apple Cheesecake

This cheesecake is fabulous. Some people like to pour the batter into a prebaked graham cracker crust.

1 lb.	nonfat cottage cheese	450 g
⅔ c.	nonfat sour cream	180 mL
4 t.	fructose	20 mL
2	eggs	2
1 T.	all-purpose flour	15 mL
½ t.	nutmeg	5 mL
pinch	cinnamon	pinch
1	juice of one lemon	1
4	small apples, peeled, cored, and sliced into half moons	4
	Graham Cracker Crust (optional)	

Beat the cottage cheese, sour cream, fructose, eggs, flour, nutmeg, and cinnamon until smooth. Stir in the lemon juice. Spread half the apples in the bottom, over a crust if you like. Pour the cottage cheese mixture over the apples. Top with the remaining apples. Bake in a preheated oven at 375°F (190°C) or until set. Cool completely.

Yield: 10 servings

Exchange, 1 serving: 1 bread
Each serving contains: Calories: 101, Carbohydrates: 10 g Fiber: 1.1 g, Sodium: 36 mg, Cholesterol: 61 mg

Cheesecake with Jelly Glaze

This looks more like a pie than a cheesecake, but it tastes like a cheesecake. The top looks lovely with slices of kiwi and raspberry or strawberry halves.

8 oz. pkg.	nonfat cream cheese	250 mL pkg.
1 c.	nonfat yogurt sweetened with aspartame	250 mL
1 pkg.	unsweetened gelatin	1 pkg.
⅓ c.	water	90 mL
1 T.	measures–like–sugar aspartame	15 mL
1 c.	fresh fruit cut into pieces, or canned, no sugar added	250 mL
3 T.	jelly, made with saccharin	45 mL

Combine the cream cheese and yogurt and beat until smooth. In a small saucepan, sprinkle the gelatin into the water; let soften for 2 minutes. Over low heat, stir to dissolve the gelatin. Remove from the heat and add to cream cheese mixture. Add the aspartame. With an electric mixer, beat until smooth. Pour into a crust of your choice (A graham cracker crust is traditional.) Arrange the fruit on top. Microwave the jelly for 30 seconds or heat in a saucepan over low heat. When jelly is liquefied, use a pastry brush to glaze the top of the pie.

Yield: 8 servings

Exchange, 1 serving: 1 milk
Each serving contains: Calories: 60, Carbohydrates: 13 g Fiber: 0.5 g, Sodium: 164 mg, Cholesterol: 4 mg

Pumpkin Cheesecake

This is a wonderful cheesecake, creamy and smooth, with a hint of your favorite pumpkin-pie taste.

1 lb.	nonfat cream cheese	450 g
12 t.	fructose	60 mL
¼ c.	egg substitute	60 mL
1 (16 oz.) can	pumpkin	1 (488 mL) can
1½ t.	cinnamon	7.5 mL
1 t.	allspice	5 mL
¼ t.	ginger	1.25 mL
¼ t.	mace	1.25 mL
1	unbaked crust, preferably graham (optional)	1

Spray an 8 in. (20 cm) springform pan with non-stick vegetable cooking spray. Line the bottom of the sprayed pan with crust, if desired. Beat the cream cheese, fructose, and egg substitute until smooth. Beat the pumpkin and spices into the cheese mixture. Spoon the filling into the crust, if used. Bake in a preheated 350°F (180°C) oven for 45 minutes or until set. Cool the cake completely before removing it from the pan.

Yield: 10 servings

Exchange, 1 serving: 1 milk
Each serving contains: Calories: 82, Carbohydrates: 28 g, Fiber: 2 g, Sodium: 244 mg, Cholesterol: 6.4 mg

Ricotta Pie

This is a traditional Italian Easter dessert. You'll like it at any time of the year.

2 lb.	fat-free ricotta	900 g
6	eggs	6
⅓ c.	sugar	90 mL
⅓ c.	measures-like-sugar saccharin	90 mL
2 t.	vanilla extract	10 mL
2 t.	butter-flavored extract	10 mL
1 t.	cinnamon	5 mL

With an electric mixer, beat all the ingredients except the cinnamon until smooth. Pour the batter into a 10 in. (25 cm) pie crust of your choice. Sprinkle with cinnamon. Bake at 350°F (180°C) for 50 to 60 minutes until a knife inserted comes out clean. Cool. Refrigerate.

Yield: 8 servings

Exchange, 1 serving: 1½ milk + 1 meat
Each serving contains: Calories: 159, Carbohydrates: 28 g, Fiber: 1 g, Sodium: 178 mg, Cholesterol: 10 mg

No-Bake Orange Cheesecake

Make this a day or two ahead of time. Keep it covered and refrigerated until serving time. Garnish with the oranges just before serving.

Crust

1 c.	finely crushed graham cracker crumbs	250 mL
3 T.	melted margarine or butter	45 mL

Cheesecake Filling

¼ c.	cold water	60 mL
1 env.	unflavored gelatin	1 env.
16 oz.	nonfat cream cheese, at room temperature	450 g
¼ c.	sugar	60 mL
6 pkts.	concentrated acesulfame-K	6 pkts.
1 c.	nonfat sour cream	250 mL
¾ c.	freshly squeezed orange juice	180 mL
1 t.	freshly grated orange peel	5 mL
2 t.	orange flavoring	10 mL

Topping

3	navel oranges, peeled, tbitter parts removed	3

To make the crust: Mix the graham cracker crumbs and margarine. Spread this over the bottom and a little up the sides of a 9 in. (23 cm) springform pan. Freeze the crust while mixing the filling.

To make the filling: Put the water in a small saucepan and sprinkle the gelatin on top. After 1 minute turn the heat on low and, stirring constantly, heat for 2–3 minutes until the gelatin is dissolved. Remove from heat.

With an electric mixer, beat the cream cheese, sugar, and acesulfarne-K in a large bowl. When the mixture is fluffy, add the sour cream and beat well. Mix in the orange juice, gelatin, peel, and flavoring. Pour into a chilled crust. Refrigerate for 4–6 hours until firm.

Before serving, run a thin knife around the edge of the cake to loosen it. Remove the springform from the outside. Top the cake with sliced oranges.

Yield: 12 servings

Exchange, 1 serving: 1 bread + ½ fat + ½ milk
Each serving contains: Calories: 164, Carbohydrates: 18 g, Fiber: 1.2 g, Sodium: 265 mg, Cholesterol: 9.1 mg

Creamy Amaretto Cheesecake

2 (8 oz.) pkgs.	nonfat cream cheese	2 (244 g) pkgs.	
2 T.	cornstarch	30 mL	
2 t.	concentrated acesulfame-K	10 mL	
2 T.	sugar	30 mL	
¼ c.	Amaretto	60 mL	
1 t.	vanilla extract	5 mL	
½ c.	egg substitute	125 mL	
1	graham cracker crust (optional)	1	
	fresh fruit (optional)		

Cream the first six ingredients together. Pour in the egg substitute and beat with an electric mixer until creamy. Pour the batter into an 8 in. (20 cm) graham cracker crust, if desired. Bake in a preheated 325°F (160°C) oven for 35 minutes. Chill. Before serving, top with fruit, if desired.

Yield: 8 servings

Exchange, 1 serving: 1 milk
Each serving (without crust) contains: Calories: 108, Carbohydrates: 34 g, Fiber: 0, Sodium: 303 mg, Cholesterol: 8 mg

Strawberry Cream Cheese Tarts

These are very light and fluffy and have a wonderful, rich flavor. No one will guess they aren't loaded with fat and calories.

6 oz.	nonfat cream cheese	200 g	
¾ c.	nonfat cottage cheese	190 mL	
⅔ c.	nonfat sour cream	180 mL	
3	eggs separated	3	
7 t.	fructose	35 mL	
1	graham cracker crust recipe pressed into 18 tart pans	1	
	Strawberry Topping		

To prepare the filling, beat the cream cheese, cottage cheese, sour cream, egg yolks, and fructose in a large bowl until smooth. In another bowl, beat the egg whites until soft peaks form; fold them into the cheese mixture. Spoon the filling into the prepared crusts. Chill until set. Garnish with Strawberry Topping.

Yield: 18 tarts

Exchange, 1 serving: ½ milk
Each serving contains: Calories: 44, Carbohydrates: 14 g, Fiber: 0, Sodium: 63 mg, Cholesterol: 49 mg

Marble Cheesecake

This is a spectacular-looking dessert. We made it with 2 T. (30 mL) sugar and remade it with fructose. Although the sugar version won out in the taste and texture contest, the fructose version was quite good too.

2 c.	nonfat ricotta cheese	500 mL
8 oz.	nonfat cream cheese	250 g
¼ c.	egg substitute	60 mL
3	egg whites	3
2 T.	sugar	30 mL
12 pkts.	concentrated acesulfame-K	12 pkts.
1 T.	vanilla extract	15 mL
1½ t.	lemon juice	7.5 mL
3 T.	cocoa	45 mL
3 T.	water	45 mL
2 pkts.	concentrated acesulfame-K	2 pkts.
3 T.	crumbs made from 2 chocolate cookies sweetened with fructose	45 mL

Put the ricotta cheese in a food processor or blender and process for a full minute. Soften the cream cheese in a microwave oven for 30 seconds. Add it to the food processor with the egg substitute, egg whites, sugar, acesulfame-K, vanilla extract, and lemon juice. Process to combine. In a medium bowl, whisk together the cocoa, water, and acesulfame-K.

Pour approximately 1 c. (250 mL) cheese batter from the food processor into the cocoa. Whisk to combine. Set aside this "chocolate" batter. Then take a 9 in. (23 cm) springform baking pan that has been sprayed with non-stick vegetable cooking spray. Pour most of the white batter into this prepared pan. Pour all the chocolate batter in the center on top of the white batter. There will be a white ring all around the edge of the pan. Carefully pour the rest of the white batter into the center of the chocolate batter. Use a knife to marble the batters by making an "S" curve through the batter. Do not mix completely.

Place the springform pan in the center of a baking pan. Slowly and carefully pour boiling water into the outer baking pan, smoothing the batter in the springform pan. (This hot-water bath will help the cheesecake bake like a custard.) Bake in a preheated 325°F (160°C) oven for 50 minutes or until it starts to shrink away from the sides of the pan. Remove the cake from the hot-water bath and chill it completely overnight. Press chocolate cookie crumbs onto the sides of the cake.

Yield: 16 servings

Exchange, 1 serving: ½ milk
Each serving contains: Calories: 57, Carbohydrates: 10 g, Fiber: trace, Sodium: 112 mg, Cholesterol: 4.5 mg

Cheese Flan

You'll love serving this elegant dessert. It rivals the desserts in fancy restaurants, yet it's so easy to make and virtually foolproof!

4	eggs or equivalent egg substitute	4
½ c.	nonfat sour cream	125 mL
8 oz.	nonfat cream cheese	250 g
¼ c.	lemon juice	125 mL
2 t.	vanilla extract	10 mL
1 pkt.	concentrated acesulfame-K	1 pkt.
dash	nutmeg	dash
4 T.	chopped walnuts	60 mL
2 T.	measures-like-sugar aspartame	30 mL
1	unbaked crust (optional)	1

Spread the crust on the bottom of a flan pan or quiche dish. Put the next seven ingredients into a blender. Pour the blender contents onto a graham cracker or other crust, if desired. Bake at 375°F (190°C) for 25 minutes. Mix together the walnuts and aspartame. Sprinkle over the flan. Cool. Store the flan in the refrigerator.

Yield: 16 servings

Exchange, 1 serving: ½ milk
Each serving contains: Calories: 41, Carbohydrates: 8 g, Fiber: trace, Sodium: 111 mg, Cholesterol: 3 mg

Lemon Cheesecake

Crust

1 c.	saltine-cracker crumbs	250 mL
1 T.	soft margarine	15 mL
1 t.	grated lemon peel	5 mL

Filling

1 pkg.	sugar-free lemon gelatin	1 pkg.
2 c.	hot water	500 mL
2 T.	finely grated lemon peel	30 mL
8 oz. pkg.	light cream cheese	227 g pkg.
1 c.	prepared nondairy whipped topping	250 mL

Crust: Mix together the saltine-cracker crumbs, margarine, and 1 t. (5 L) of the lemon peel. Press into the bottom and slightly up the sides of an 8 in. (20 cm) pie pan. Refrigerate until ready to use.

Filling: Dissolve the lemon gelatin in the hot water. Stir in the 2 remaining (30 mL) of lemon peel, and allow to cool until mixture is a thick syrup. Whip cream cheese until light and fluffy. Gradually add lemon-gelatin mixture. Fold in nondairy whipped topping. Transfer to saltine-cracker crust. Refrigerate at least 2 to 3 hours or until firm.

Yield: 8 servings

Exchange, 1 serving: 1 bread, ¾ low-fat milk, 1 fat
Each serving contains: Calories: 224, Carbohydrates: 23 g

Fresh Strawberry Cheesecake

Crust

1½ c.	graham cracker crumbs	375 mL
1 T.	soft margarine	15 mL
1/2 t.	ground nutmeg	2 mL
1 T.	water	5 mL

Filling

8 oz.	low-fat cottage cheese	227 g
8 oz. pkg.	light cream cheese	227 g pkg.
⅔ c.	granulated sugar replacement	180 mL
1½ t.	vanilla extract	7 mL
2 env.	unflavored gelatin	2 env.
½ c.	cold water	125 mL
2 c.	prepared nondairy whipped topping	500 mL
3	egg whites, beaten stiff	3
2 c.	halved strawberries	500 mL

Crust: Mix the graham cracker crumbs, margarine, and nutmeg together. Stir in the water until mixture is moist. Press into the bottom and slightly up the sides of a 10 in. (25 cm) springform pan. Refrigerate until ready to use.

Filling: Combine cottage cheese and cream cheese in a food processor or large bowl. Process or beat until cheeses are blended and creamy. Beat in sugar replacement and vanilla. Sprinkle and soften the gelatin in the cold water in a microwave-proof cup or bowl. Heat in the microwave for 1 to 2 minutes. Stir to dissolve the gelatin. Then completely fold the gelatin into the cheese mixture. Fold 1 c. (250 mL) of the prepared whipped topping and the three stiffly beaten egg whites into the cheese mixture. Transfer mixture to prepared crust. Chill thoroughly.

To serve: Remove sides of pan. Place cheesecake on decorative serving plate. Spread remaining 1 c. (250 mL) of nondairy whipped topping over top of cheesecake. Arrange the halved strawberries in the whipped topping.

Yield: 20 servings

Exchange, 1 serving: ¾ whole milk
Each serving contains: Calories: 140, Carbohydrates: 9 g

Cherry Cheesecake

Crust

1½ c.	cornflake crumbs	375 mL
1 T.	soft margarine	15 mL
1 T.	granulated sugar replacement	15 mL
2 t.	water	5 mL

Filling

8 oz. pkg.	light cream cheese	227 g pkg.
½ c.	granulated sugar replacement	125 mL
2	eggs, separated	2
1½ T.	all-purpose flour	21 mL
⅛ t.	salt	½ mL
½ t.	vanilla extract	2 mL
½ c.	evaporated milk, chilled	125 mL
1½ T.	lemon juice	1 mL

Topping

½ c.	fresh tart red cherries	375 mL
½ c.	water	125 mL
½ c.	granulated sugar replacement	125 mL
1 env.	unflavored gelatin	1 env.
2 T.	cold water	30 mL
	red food coloring	

Crust: Mix together cornflake crumbs, margarine, and the 1 T. (15 mL) of granulated sugar replacement. Add the 1 t. (5 mL) of water and thoroughly blend. Press into bottom and slightly up sides of a 9 in. (23 cm) springform pan. Refrigerate until ready to use.

Filling: Whip the cream cheese until soft and fluffy. Beat in ½ c. (125 mL) of granulated sugar replacement and egg yolks (one at a time). Beat in the flour, salt, and vanilla extract. Whip the evaporated milk until thick, add the lemon juice, and continue beating until stiff. Gently fold into cream mixture. Beat the egg whites until stiff. Fold into the cream mixture. Transfer to prepared cornflake crust. Bake at 325°F (165°C) for 1 hour. Turn off heat and allow cheesecake to cool in oven.

Topping: Combine tart cherries, the ½ c. (125 mL) of water, and the ½ c. (125 mL) of granulated sugar replacement in a saucepan. Mix well and bring to a boil. Reduce heat and simmer for 8 minutes. Dissolve the gelatin in 2 T. (30 mL) of cold water. Stir into cherry mixture. Cook until gelatin is dissolved. Remove from heat. Add a few drops of red food coloring. Cool until thickened. At serving time, spread cherry mixture over cheesecake.

Yield: 20 servings

Exchange, 1 serving: 1 bread, 1 fat
Each serving contains: Calories: 125, Carbohydrates: 15 g

Cinnamon Apple Cheesecake

Crust

1 c.	graham cracker crumbs	250 mL
1 T.	soft margarine	5 mL
1 t.	ground cinnamon	5 mL

Filling

2 c.	cinnamon apple juice	500 mL
1 env.	unflavored gelatin	1 env.
1 pkg.	sugar-free vanilla pudding mix (to cook)	1 pkg.
3 in.	cinnamon stick	7.5 cm
8 oz. pkg.	light cream cheese	227 g pkg.

Crust: Mix together the graham cracker crumbs, margarine, and cinnamon. Press into the bottom and slightly up the sides of an 8 in. (20 cm) pie pan. Refrigerate until ready to use.

Filling: Pour cinnamon apple juice in a saucepan. Sprinkle gelatin over top and allow to soften for 3 to 4 minutes. Stir in pudding mix. Add cinnamon stick. Cook and stir over medium heat until mixture is smooth and thickened. Remove from heat and allow to cool to room temperature. Remove cinnamon after mixture is cooled. Whip cream cheese until light and fluffy. Slowly add cooled cinnamon-apple mixture. Beat thoroughly. Pour into 8 in. (20 cm) graham cracker crust. Refrigerate at least 2 to 3 hours or until firm.

Yield: 8 servings

Exchange, 1 serving: 1 bread, 1 low-fat milk, 1 fat
Each serving contains: Calories: 240, Carbohydrates: 26 g

Prize Chocolate Cheesecake

Crust

32	graham crackers, crumbed	32
¼ c.	margarine, melted	60 mL
2 t.	granulated sugar replacement	10 mL
½ c.	semisweet chocolate chips	125 mL

Filling

8 oz. pkg.	cream cheese	226 g pkg.
2 T.	lemon juice	30 mL
1	egg, separated	1
2 T.	granulated sugar replacement	30 mL
⅔ c.	skim milk	180 mL
½ t.	lemon rind, freshly grated	2 mL
1 env.	unflavored gelatin	1 env.
2 T.	boiling water	30 mL

Decorative Topping

¼ c.	semisweet chocolate chips, chopped	60 mL

To make the crust, mix graham cracker crumbs, margarine and sugar replacement together. Press into bottom and sides of a 9 in. (23 cm) springform pan. Chill until firm. Melt chocolate chips and spread on top of crust. Refrigerate.

For the filling, beat cream cheese with lemon juice until smooth. Place egg yolk, sugar replacement and milk in saucepan. Heat gently until thick enough to coat the back of a spoon, but *do not boil.* Remove from heat. Gradually stir in the cream cheese mixture and grated lemon rind. Dissolve gelatin in boiling water. Stir into mixture and blend thoroughly. Beat egg white until stiff and fold into the filling. Pour the filling over chocolate-layered crust. Refrigerate to completely set. Decorate top with chopped chocolate chips. Refrigerate until serving time.

Yield: 20 servings

Exchange, 1 serving: 1 bread, 2 fat
Each serving contains: Calories: 149, Carbohydrates: 22 g

Fruit Desserts and Cobblers

Many people with diabetes save a fruit to have as their dessert. You don't need a cookbook for this. In this chapter we offer fancier desserts that are basically fruits. Taking a fruit exchange and turning it into an attractive healthy dessert makes sense for everyone in the family.

Sweet and Sour Strawberries

Surprisingly flavorful and so easy! Serve in fancy glasses.

2 c.	fresh or frozen strawberries with no sugar added	500 mL
3 pkts.	concentrated acesulfame-K	3 pkts.
2 T.	balsamic vinegar	30 mL

Slice the strawberries in half. Sprinkle them with acesulfame-K and vinegar. Stir to combine. This is best served chilled.

Yield: 4 servings

Exchange: free
Each serving contains: Calories: 24, Carbohydrates: 5 g, Fiber: 2 g, Sodium: trace, Cholesterol: 0 mg

Zesty Strawberries

Adding black pepper to strawberries is unusual but very tasty. Try it! You'll like it.

2 c.	fresh strawberries, sliced	500 mL
1½ t.	concentrated aspartame	7 mL
½ t.	cracked black pepper	2 mL
½ t.	brandy extract	2 mL
2 T.	diet cream soda	30 mL

Stir all the ingredients together and chill before serving. Zesty Strawberries can be served plain or over a frozen ice cream substitute.

Yield: 8 servings

Exchange: free
Each serving contains: Calories: 11, Carbohydrates: 3 g, Fiber: trace, Sodium: trace, Cholesterol: 0 mg

Cool Strawberry Fluff

A light, frothy dessert, Cool Strawberry Fluff will melt in your mouth. Serve it after a heavy meal for the best effect.

10 oz. (1¼ c.)	fresh or frozen strawberries, sliced, no sugar added	300 g (310 mL)
2 env. (2 T.)	unflavored gelatin	2 env. (30 mL)
1 c.	coarsely crushed ice	250 mL

Put ½ c. (125 mL) strawberries into a blender and blend them for about 5 seconds. Pour them into a small saucepan and heat over low heat until they begin to boil, then transfer them back into the blender. Sprinkle the gelatin over the hot strawberries, cover, and blend for about 30 seconds more. Add the crushed ice and blend at the lowest speed for 20 seconds. Put the remaining strawberries in a bowl, add the puréed mixture, and mix together for about 30 seconds. Pour into individual dishes or a serving bowl. Chill.

Yield: 4 servings

Exchange: free
Each serving contains: Calories: 26, Carbohydrates: 4 g, Fiber: trace, Sodium: 3 mg, Cholesterol: 0 mg

Fresh Strawberry-Melon Medley

This is a favorite among dinner guests. They love the festive way it looks and tastes and can't believe how simple it is to prepare!

10 oz.	defrosted sliced strawberries, no sugar added	300 g
1½ c.	water	375 mL
½	stick cinnamon	½
3 T.	cornstarch	45 mL
¼ c.	cold water	60 mL
3 pkts.	concentrated acesulfame-K	3 pkts.
2 c.	fresh strawberries, quartered	500 mL
2 c.	honeydew melon balls (fresh or frozen)	500 mL

In a saucepan combine the thawed strawberries, 1½ c. (375 mL) water, and cinnamon; bring to a boil, then simmer for five minutes. Purée in a blender or food processor. In another bowl, blend the cornstarch, ¼ c. (60 mL) cold water, and acesulfame-K. Stir into the purée. Bring to a boil, stirring constantly, then simmer for one minute. Pour into a bowl; place a piece of wax paper on the surface; let cool, then refrigerate.

Before serving, remove the wax paper. Beat the purée until fluffy. Fold in the fresh strawberries and melon balls, reserving a few of each for the garnish. Spoon into parfait glasses; top with the reserved strawberries and melon balls.

Yield: 6 servings

Exchange, 1 serving: 1½ fruit
Each serving contains: Calories: 104, Carbohydrates: 18 g, Fiber: 3 g, Sodium: 18 mg, Cholesterol: 0 mg

Double Melon Dessert

If you don't have a melon ball scoop, dice 3 c. melon or use frozen melon. This is perfect for an afternoon snack on a summer day or as a sorbet after a fancy meal.

2	cantaloupes (or 1 large honeydew melon)	2
2 pkgs.	sugar-free orange-flavored gelatin	2 pkgs.
1	orange	1

Scoop out enough melon balls to equal 3 c. (750 mL). Chill. Using a spoon, scrape out the remainder of the melon. Purée. Measure the puréed melon. Add water, if needed, to make 4 c. Pour into a saucepan. Heat until steaming. Remove from the heat, add gelatin, and stir until the gelatin is dissolved. Pour into six custard cups and chill until firm. Garnish each serving with ½ c. (125 mL) of melon balls and orange slices.

Yield: 6 servings

Exchange, 1 serving: 1 bread
Each serving contains: Calories: 88, Carbohydrates: 12 g, Fiber: 2 g, Sodium: 83 mg, Cholesterol: 0 mg

Applesauce

Unsweetened applesauce in a glass jar is about as convenient as a diabetic dessert can be. A diabetic friend suggested putting applesauce in the cookbook because he always likes it dressed up with aspartame and cinnamon. I didn't think that just adding aspartame and cinnamon to commercial applesauce was actually a recipe! But maybe the advice on sweet sprinkles will give you some good ideas.

Sweet Sprinkles

Mix an artificial sweetener of your choice with other spices. Put the mixture into a clean salt shaker or other small shaker container. Here are some combinations our tasters liked: equal parts of aspartame and cinnamon; aspartame and cardamom; aspartame and pumpkin pie spice.

Baked Apples

Baked apples are easy to make, and the apple juice makes them especially moist. Just put them in the oven before you start the rest of your dinner preparations. The smell coming from the oven will tantalize you.

4 med.	baking apples	4 med.
1 t.	fructose	5 mL
⅓ c.	canned crushed pineapple packed in juice, drained	90 mL
2 T.	raisins (optional)	30 mL
¼ t.	cinnamon	1 mL
2–4 c.	unsweetened apple juice	500 mL

Peel the top of each apple. Use a sharp knife to remove the core, but leave the bottom intact so the hollow can be filled. Cut a thin slice from the bottom, if necessary, so the apple stands upright. In a small bowl, combine the fructose, pineapple, raisins, and cinnamon. Spoon the mixture equally into each apple hollow. Place the apples in a shallow baking dish. Surround the apples with apple juice to a depth of about ½ inch (1.25 cm). Bake in a preheated 350°F (180°C) oven for about an hour. The apples should be tender, but not mushy. Serve warm, at room temperature, or chilled and garnish with sugar-free nonfat whipped topping just before serving.

Yield: 4 servings

Exchange, 1 serving: 2 fruits
Each serving contains: Calories: 110, Carbohydrates: 77 g, Fiber: 4 g, Sodium: 8, Cholesterol: 0 mg

Apple Crisp

An apple crisp baking fills a home with the most wonderful aroma.

4 c.	apples, sliced	1 L
¼ c.	water	60 mL
1 T.	molasses	15 mL
3 pkts.	concentrated acesulfame-K	3 pkts.
1 T.	lemon juice	15 mL
1 t.	cinnamon	5 mL
¼ t.	cloves	1 mL
¾ c.	oatmeal	190 mL
2 t.	margarine or butter	10 mL
2 pkts.	concentrated acesulfame-K	2 pkts.

Combine the apples, water, molasses, acesulfame-K, lemon juice, cinnamon, and cloves. Mix well. Arrange the apple mixture in an 8 in. (20 cm) square baking dish coated with non-stick cooking spray. Combine the remaining ingredients and sprinkle the mixture over the apples. Bake at 375°F (190°C) for 30 minutes or until the apples are tender and the topping is lightly browned.

Yield: 8 servings

Exchange, 1 serving: 1 bread
Each serving contains: Calories: 84, Carbohydrates: 22 g, Fiber: 2 g, Sodium: 12 mg, Cholesterol: 0 mg

Apple Betty

Apple Betty is a casserole of apples and bread crumbs. It's rich and delicious.

1½ c.	fresh bread crumbs	375 mL
¼ c.	melted margarine or butter	60 mL
4 pkts.	concentrated acesulfame-K	4 pkts.
¼ t.	nutmeg	1 mL
¼ t.	cinnamon	1 mL
3 med.	apples, pared, cored, and sliced thin	3 med.
1½ t.	lemon juice	7 mL
3 T.	water	45 mL
1 pkt.	concentrated acesulfame-K	1 pkt.

Toss the bread crumbs and margarine. In a small bowl, combine the four packets of acesulfame-K and the nutmeg and cinnamon. In a 1-qt. (1 L) casserole arrange one-third of the crumbs. On top of the crumbs arrange one-third of the apples. Sprinkle the apples with one-third of the cinnamon mixture. Add another layer of crumbs, and apples. Do this again. Top with the remaining crumbs. Mix together the lemon juice, water, and one packet of acesulfame-K. Drizzle over the top layer of crumbs. Cover and bake in a preheated 350°F (180°C) oven for 15 minutes, then uncover and bake 30 minutes longer. Serve warm or cold.

Yield: 8 servings

Exchange, 1 serving: 1 fat + ½ bread + ½ fruit
Each serving contains: Calories: 117, Carbohydrates: 22 g, Fiber: 2 g, Sodium: 83 mg, Cholesterol: 0 mg

Apple Dessert

This recipe is wonderful because it's fast and easy to make with ingredients that are usually on hand. Shake on a little nutmeg and cinnamon if you like.

1 c.	unsweetened applesauce	250 mL
½ T.	lemon juice	7 mL
½ t.	vanilla extract	2 mL
1 env.	gelatin	1 env.
¼ c.	cold water	60 mL
¼ c.	hot water	60 mL

Mix together the applesauce, lemon juice, and vanilla extract. Soften the gelatin in cold water for five minutes. Add the hot water and stir until it is dissolved. Then add the water and gelatin to the applesauce mixture. Refrigerate the mixture. When it begins to stiffen, beat it until light.

Yield: 6 servings

Exchange: free
Each serving contains: Calories: 22, Carbohydrates: 5 g, Fiber: trace, Sodium: 2 mg, Cholesterol: 0 mg

Nectarine Crisp

Nectarines are available fresh most of the year and are great to cook with.

1 c.	rolled oats	250 mL
¼ c.	apple juice concentrate	60 mL
1 t.	cornstarch	5 mL
4	nectarines, peeled and sliced thin	4
3 T.	flour	45 mL
1½ t.	cinnamon	7 mL
¼ t.	nutmeg	1 mL
3 pkts.	acesulfame-K	3 pkts.
2 T.	diet pancake syrup, sugar-free	30 mL
2 T.	nonfat sour cream	30 mL

Spread the rolled oats flat in a large pan. Bake in a preheated 325°F (160°C) oven for 10 minutes. Remove from the oven and set aside. Meanwhile, in a saucepan stir together the apple juice concentrate and cornstarch and cook over medium heat until thickened, stirring constantly. Spread the nectarine slices evenly over the bottom of a small ovenproof dish that has been coated with non-stick cooking spray. Pour the apple juice-cornstarch mixture over the slices. Then combine the flour, cinnamon, nutmeg, and acesulfame-K with the oatmeal. Add the pancake syrup and sour cream to the flour-oatmeal and stir to combine. Crumble this mixture over the nectarines. Bake in a preheated 325°F (160°C) oven for 45 minutes.

Yield: 6 servings

Exchange, 1 serving: 1 bread + ½ fruit
Each serving contains: Calories: 140, Carbohydrates: 32 g, Fiber: 3 g, Sodium: 16 mg, Cholesterol: trace

Nectarine Purée

Use fresh, sweet nectarines in season for the best result.

3	nectarines	3
2 t.	lemon juice	10 mL
2 t.	concentrated aspartame	10 mL

Drop the nectarines into a large pan of boiling water. Shut off the heat. Let stand for one minute to loosen the skins. Drain the hot water; then pour cold water over the fruit and slip off their skins. Place the nectarines in a food processor or blender with the lemon juice and aspartame. The amount of aspartame will vary, depending on the tartness of the fruit. Purée. Spoon into glass dessert dishes.

Yield: 3 servings

Exchange, 1 serving: 1 fruit
Each serving contains: Calories: 68, Carbohydrates: 16 g, Fiber: 3 g, Sodium: trace, Cholesterol: 0 mg

Elegant Blueberry Dessert

A very fancy way to serve a dessert that is basically just fruit.

½ c.	nonfat milk	125 mL
2 t.	cornstarch	10 mL
2 T.	orange liqueur (optional)	30 mL
2 pkts.	concentrated acesulfame-K	2 pkts.
2 t.	vanilla extract	10 mL
1 t.	concentrated aspartame-K	5 mL
1	egg white	1
pinch	cream of tartar	pinch
2 c.	blueberries (fresh or frozen without sugar and defrosted)	500 mL

Stir together the milk, cornstarch, liqueur if desired, and acesulfame-K in a medium saucepan. Use a wire whisk to be sure the cornstarch is dissolved. Bring to a boil and reduce the heat to a simmer, stirring constantly. Turn off the heat and stir in the vanilla extract and aspartame.

In a separate bowl, beat the egg white until it holds its peaks, add the cream of tartar, and continue beating until the white is stiff. Fold it into the milk-cornstarch mixture. Then stir in the blueberries. Pour the mixture into four fancy glasses, such as wine glasses. Chill.

Yield: 4 servings

Exchange, 1 serving: 1 bread
Each serving contains: Calories: 60, Carbohydrates: 12 g, Fiber: 2 g, Sodium: 33 mg, Cholesterol: trace

Watermelon Pudding

This is a great way to serve the watermelon left over after a picnic.

3 c.	puréed watermelon	750 mL
1 T.	lemon juice	15 mL
1 env.	unflavored gelatin	1 env.
1 pkg.	strawberry-flavored gelatin dessert	1 pkg.
¾ lb.	nonfat cottage cheese	340 g

In a saucepan, combine the watermelon purée, lemon juice, and unflavored gelatin. Let it stand for five minutes or so to soften. Heat gently until the gelatin dissolves. Remove from the heat and stir in the strawberry-flavored gelatin. Stir until the mixture is smooth and the gelatin is dissolved. Pour half the mixture into six custard cups coated with non-stick cooking spray. Chill until set. Pour the remainder into a blender or food processor. Add the cottage cheese and blend. Pour the blended cheese on top of the first mixture. Chill until firm.

Serve in cups or unmold onto dessert plates. (To unmold custard cups, run a hot knife around the inside of each cup, dip the knife into a pan of hot water for a few seconds. Put a plate over the top of the cup. Invert, shake onto the plate.)

Yield: 6 servings

Exchange, 1 serving: 1 fruit
Each serving contains: Calories: 85, Carbohydrates: 8 g, Fiber: 1.6 g, Sodium: 7 mg, Cholesterol: 0 mg

Poached Pears and Raspberries

When you find out how easy this fabulous recipe is, you'll stop being so impressed with poached pear desserts at the most chic restaurants.

6 med	pears	6 med
1 pkt.	concentrated acesulfame-K, or 1 T. (15 mL) sugar	1 pkt.
¼ c.	water	60 mL
1 in.	vanilla bean, slit	2.5 cm
2 c.	raspberries, fresh or frozen, unsweetened	500 mL
2 T.	fruit-only jam (seedless raspberry is a good choice	30 mL

Peel, core, and halve the pears. Combine the acesulfame-K or sugar and water in a saucepan and bring to a boil. Reduce the heat to low and add the vanilla bean and pear halves. Cover. Simmer for 5 minutes or so, until the pears are fork-tender. Cool. Drain. In a small bowl, gently toss the raspberries and jelly. Put two pear halves on each serving plate. Mound the raspberries on top of the pears.

Yield: 6 servings

Exchange, 1 serving: 2 fruits
Each serving contains: Calories: 168, Carbohydrates: 35 g, Fiber: 7 g, Sodium: 0, Cholesterol: 0 mg

Pears à la Crème

When you see pears in the grocery store, think of this recipe and the fabulous dessert it makes.

2 large	firm pears, peeled, cored	2 large
1 pkt.	concentrated acesulfame-K, or 1 T. (15 mL) sugar	1 pkt.
¼ c.	unsweetened pineapple juice	60 mL
1 c.	sugar-free whipped topping	250 mL
4 pkts.	concentrated aspartame	4 pkts.

Cut the pears into large chunks. Combine the pears, acesulfame-K, and pineapple juice. Bring to a boil, stirring constantly until the sugar dissolves. Cover, reduce heat, and cook until the fruit is fork-tender. The time will vary depending on the hardness of the fruit. This step may be very short. Uncover, increase the heat, and cook until the juices thicken. Cool until serving time. Fold in the topping and aspartame just before serving.

Yield: 6 servings

Exchange, 1 serving: 1 fruit
Each serving contains: Calories: 52, Carbohydrates: 23 g, Fiber: 1.6 g, Sodium: 7 mg, Cholesterol: 0 mg

Ambrosia

When oranges are sweet and juicy, ambrosia can be as delectable as any elaborate dessert.

2	oranges, peeled with any bitter white skin removed	2
2 t.	measures-like-sugar aspartame	10 mL
2	bananas, peeled	2
¼ c.	shredded coconut (optional)	125 mL

Slice the oranges and bananas thin. Place a layer of orange slices in the bottom of a serving bowl. Sprinkle with some of the aspartame. Place a layer of bananas over the oranges, then a layer of coconut. Make many layers of fruit, ending with a layer of coconut. Cover with plastic wrap; refrigerate for at least an hour before serving.

Yield: 4 servings

Exchange, 1 serving: 1½ fruit
Each serving contains: Calories: 84, Carbohydrates: 26 g, Fiber: 3 g, Sodium: trace, Cholesterol: 0 mg

Grapefruit Meringue

Grapefruit isn't just for breakfast anymore! Baked with a crown of meringue, the grapefruit becomes sweet and dramatic.

2 med.	grapefruit	2 med.
3	egg whites	3
3 pkts.	concentrated acesulfame-K	3 pkts.

Cut the grapefruit in half; snip the center core from each half, then cut around all sections, and arrange the halves in a shallow baking dish lined with aluminum foil. Beat the egg whites until they are stiff enough to hold their shape; gradually add the acesulfame-K, beating until they are stiff. Pile some of meringue mixture on top of each grapefruit half. Bake for 15 minutes in a 375°F (190°C) oven.

Yield: 4 servings

Exchange, 1 serving: 1 fruit
Each serving contains: Calories: 50, Carbohydrates: 10 g, Fiber: trace, Sodium: 38 mg, Cholesterol: 0 mg

Mixed Berry Smoothie

Many grocery stores sell unsweetened fruits in collections. The combination of raspberries, strawberries, and blueberries is a natural for easy desserts.

12 oz. can	evaporated nonfat milk	354 mL can
1 T.	cornstarch	15 mL
3 pkts.	concentrated acesulfame-K	3 pkts.
1 t.	almond extract	5 mL
1 t.	concentrated aspartame	5 mL
12 oz. bag	frozen mixed berries	340 g bag
2 c.	nonfat yogurt, no sugar added (plain or vanilla)	500 mL

Combine the first three ingredients and stir them together in a saucepan. Heat just to the boil, then reduce the heat and simmer for 5 minutes or until the sauce thickens. Stir constantly with a wire whisk. Turn off the heat; stir in the almond extract, aspartame, and berries. Let cool and then fold in the yogurt.

Yield: 8 servings

Exchange, 1 serving: 1 milk
Each serving contains: Calories: 99, Carbohydrates: 22 g, Fiber: 1 g, Sodium: 93 mg, Cholesterol: 0 mg

Elegant Fruit with Almonds

This really is an elegant dessert that you can put together with cans from your shelf. Leave the almonds out if you don't need the fat.

20 oz.	pineapple chunks, packed in juice (reserve the juice)	600 g
16 oz.	sliced peaches, fresh or canned, unsweetened	480 g
1 T.	safflower oil	15 mL
4 T.	slivered almonds	60 mL
1 T.	lemon juice	15 mL
5 T.	unsweetened pineapple juice (from the can of pineapple)	75 mL

Drain the canned fruits and save the juice. Drop the fruit into a serving bowl and refrigerate. Heat the oil in a small frying pan; add the almonds and cook gently, stirring until they are lightly browned. Remove from the heat and let cool. Add the lemon juice and pineapple juice to the almonds and stir; toss over fruit. Refrigerate until serving time. This is best served chilled.

Yield: 6 servings

Exchange, 1 serving: 1 fruit + 1 fat + ½ bread
Each serving contains: Calories: 153, Carbohydrates: 23 g, Fiber: 2 g, Sodium: 6 mg, Cholesterol: 0 mg

Four Fruit Compote

Oranges, cantaloupe, grapes, and pears are the four fruits we used in this compote. They blend together very well to make an attractive and succulent dessert.

1	large orange	1
1	small cantaloupe	1
½ lb.	seedless grapes	225 g
3	ripe pears	3
½ c.	water	125 mL
3 T.	lemon juice	45 mL
3 pkts.	concentrated acesulfame-K	3 pkts.
¼ t.	mace	1 mL
2 T.	rum (optional)	30 mL

Cut the orange into segments, remove the membrane, and put the segments into a large bowl. Cut the cantaloupe into wedges about 2 inches (5 cm) wide. Remove the seeds and skin. Cut the wedges into large cubes. Add the cubes and the stemmed grapes to the oranges. Cut the pears into quarters, remove the cores, then cut the pears into large cubes. Sprinkle them with lemon juice and add them to the fruit mixture.

Mix together the water, lemon juice, acesulfame-K, and mace. Add the rum, if desired. Cover; refrigerate for an hour or more before serving.

Yield: 8 servings

Exchange, 1 serving: 1 fruit
Each serving contains: Calories: 76, Carbohydrates: 19 g, Fiber: 3 g, Sodium: 8 mg, Cholesterol: 0 mg

Peaches and Black Cherries

Take advantage of succulent, fresh, ripe peaches when they are in season and make this dramatic combination.

6	peaches	6
1 T.	sugar or 1 pkt. concentrated acesulfame-K	15 mL
⅓ c.	water	60 mL
12	black cherries	12
¾ c.	sugar-free soda (black cherry or raspberry is a good choice)	190 mL

Dip the peaches one at a time in a pan of boiling water. Plunge them into cold water and slip off the skins. Discard the water. Mix the sugar or acesulfame-K and ⅓ c. water in a saucepan large enough to hold all six peaches. Bring the sugar and water to boiling point. Cook gently and add the peaches. Continue to cook gently for 5 more minutes or so. Cool the peaches and their liquid. Before serving, drain the peaches, saving the liquid. Slice the peaches into dessert glasses. Add the cherries. Mix the soda and peach juice together and pour it over the fruit.

Yield: 6 servings

Exchange, 1 serving: ½ fruit
Each serving contains: Calories: 43, Carbohydrates: 15 g, Fiber: 1 g, Sodium: 5 mg, Cholesterol: 0 mg

Spiced Purple Plums

4	firm purple plums	4
½ c.	water	125 mL
1	clove, whole	1
1	bay leaf	1
1	cinnamon stick	1
1 T.	granulated sugar replacement	15 mL

Peel, pit and quarter plums. Combine water, clove, bay leaf, cinnamon, and sugar replacement in saucepan. Bring just to boiling; add plums. Bring back to boiling, reduce heat and cook 5 minutes. With a slotted spoon, remove plums to heated serving dish.

Yield: 2 servings

Exchange, 1 serving: 1 fruit
Each serving contains: Calories: 51, Carbohydrates: 23 g

Poached Figs

1 c.	water	250 mL
¼ c.	wine vinegar	60 mL
3 T.	granulated sugar replacement	45 mL
2	cinnamon sticks	2
15	dried figs	15

Combine water, vinegar, sugar replacement and cinnamon sticks in saucepan, and bring to a boil. Add figs, reduce heat, cover, and simmer for 15 minutes. Add extra water if needed. Remove figs with slotted spoon. Chill thoroughly.

Yield: 15 servings

Exchange, 1 serving: 1 fruit
Each serving contains: Calories: 60, Carbohydrates: 15 g

Strawberries Romanoff

2 c.	fresh strawberries, hulled	500 mL
1 c.	French Vanilla Ice Cream, softened	250 mL
1 T.	Orange Marmalade	15 mL
2 t.	rum extract	10 mL
½ c.	low-calorie whipped topping, prepared	125 mL

Divide strawberries evenly between 4 serving dishes and chill thoroughly. At serving time, fold together ice cream, orange marmalade, rum extract, and topping. Spoon over cold strawberries. Serve immediately.

Yield: 4 servings

Exchange, 1 serving: ½ fruit, ½ medium-fat meat, 1 fat
Each serving contains: Calories: 75, Carbohydrates: 18 g

Berries with Cream

1½ c.	creamed cottage cheese	375 mL
¼ c.	buttermilk	60 mL
2 c.	fresh blueberries	500 mL
2 c.	fresh raspberries	500 mL

Place cottage cheese in strainer over bowl. Drain thoroughly for at least 1 hour in refrigerator. Add buttermilk to cottage cheese liquid; stir to blend. Cover and refrigerate dry cottage cheese mixture. Gently combine blueberries with half of milk mixture, and the raspberries with the remaining half. Cover both and refrigerate. Shortly before serving, mold one-sixth of the cottage cheese into the center of each of the 6 chilled dessert plates. Arrange one-sixth of the blueberries opposite one-sixth of the raspberries in a crescent pattern around each mound of cottage cheese. Serve immediately.

Yield: 6 servings

Exchange, 1 serving: 1 fruit, 1 lean meat
Each serving contains: Calories: 94, Carbohydrates: 14 g

Fruit Flower

¼ c.	buttermilk	60 mL
2 t.	granulated sugar replacement	10 mL
2 t.	cornstarch	10 mL
3 T.	hazelnuts, skinned	45 mL
1	firm peach	1
1	firm purple plum	1
1	firm red plum	1
	lemon juice	
6	sour cherries	6

Combine buttermilk, sugar replacement, and cornstarch in small saucepan. Cook and stir over low heat until thickened. Toast hazelnuts and process them in blender or food processor until they are fine crumbs; reserve.

Peel, pit and slice peach and plums. Dip in lemon juice. Pit cherries. Arrange sliced fruit alternately in circle on two small serving plates. Spoon thickened milk in center and top with cherries. Sprinkle toasted hazelnut crumbs over fruit plate. Serve immediately.

Yield: 2 servings

Exchange, 1 serving: 1 bread, 1 fat
Each serving contains: Calories: 124, Carbohydrates: 31 g

Christmas Pear

1	pear	1
½ c.	water	125 mL
2 T.	granulated sugar replacement	30 mL
4 drops	red food color	4 drops
1 in.	cinnamon stick	2.5 cm

Peel and core pear. Cut in half or into slices. Combine water, sugar replacement, food color, and cinnamon stick in saucepan. Bring to a boil, add the pear, reduce heat and simmer for 3 minutes. Turn pear several times to completely color. Remove with slotted spoon. Serve hot or cold.

Yield: 1 serving

Exchange, 1 serving: 1 fruit
Each serving contains: Calories: 60, Carbohydrates: 50 g

Apricot-Banana Sauté

4	apricots	4
1	banana	1
2 t.	margarine	10 mL
1 T.	low-calorie maple syrup	15 mL
1 t.	almond extract	5 mL
½ t.	vanilla extract	2 mL

Peel, pit and quarter apricots. Peel and slice bananas into 1 in. (2.5 cm) slices. Melt margarine in skillet, add maple syrup and extracts, and stir just to blend. Add fruit and sauté, turning once, for 2 minutes. Spoon into heated serving dishes.

Yield: 2 servings

Exchange, 1 serving: 2 fruit, ⅓ bread
Each serving contains: Calories: 126, Carbohydrates: 25 g

Orange Marmalade

1	orange	1
1 c.	water	250 mL
1 T.	low-calorie pectin	15 mL
1 t.	granulated sugar replacement	5 mL

With a vegetable peeler, remove peel from orange. Combine orange peel and water in saucepan, bring to boil, and boil for 3 minutes. Cut off membrane from fruit. Place fruit, orange water (with peel), and pectin in blender or food processor. Work until completely blended. Pour into saucepan, bring to boil, and boil for 1 minute. Allow to cool slightly. Stir in sugar replacement. Pour into serving dish or jelly jar. Chill.

Microwave: Follow directions using at least 1 qt. (1 L) microwave dish. Cook on High.

Yield: 1¼ c. (310 mL)

Exchange, 2 T. (30 mL): ¼ fruit
Each serving contains: Calories: 10, Carbohydrates: 3 g

Red Fruit Compote

1 lb. can	tart cherries	460 g can
10 oz. pkg.	unsweetened frozen raspberries, thawed	280 g pkg.
10 oz. pkg.	unsweetened frozen strawberries, thawed	280 g pkg.
2 T.	granulated sugar replacement	30 mL
2 T.	cornstarch	30 mL
1 T.	lemon juice	15 mL

Drain fruit; reserve liquids. Add enough water to reserved fruit liquid to make 2½ c. (625 mL). Blend liquid, sugar replacement and cornstarch in saucepan; cook and stir over medium heat until clear and thickened. Remove from heat; stir in lemon juice. Fold in cherries, raspberries, and strawberries. Chill thoroughly.

Yield: 8 servings

Exchange, 1 serving: 1 fruit
Each serving contains: Calories: 42, Carbohydrates: 23 g

Frozen Fruit

¼ c.	fresh grapefruit sections	60 mL
¼ c.	fresh orange sections	60 mL
¼ c.	fresh tart cherries	60 mL
¼ c.	banana slices	60 mL
1 t.	lemon juice	5 mL
1 t.	unflavored gelatin	5 mL
2 T.	cold water	15 mL
1 t.	liquid sugar replacement	5 mL
1 c.	low-calorie whipped topping (prepared)	250 mL

Combine fruits and lemon juice in bowl; toss to coat. Cover and refrigerate. Sprinkle gelatin over cold water, and allow it to rest 5 minutes to soften. Heat just until gelatin is completely dissolved. Add gelatin and sugar replacement to fruit; toss to coat. Fold topping into fruit mixture. Spoon into mold, freezer tray or individual dishes. Freeze until firm.

Yield: 8 servings

Exchange, 1 serving: ½ fruit, ⅓ fat
Each serving contains: Calories: 29, Carbohydrates: 7 g

Cranberries and Peaches

6	fresh peach halves, peeled	6
	lemon juice	
1¼ c.	unsweetened cranberry juice	310 mL
1 T.	cornstarch	15 mL
2 T.	granulated sugar replacement	30 mL
½ t.	orange peel, grated	2 mL
¼ t.	salt	1 mL
1	cinnamon stick	1
5	whole cloves	5

Dip peach halves in lemon juice to preserve color; place in serving dish. Combine cranberry juice, cornstarch, sugar replacement, orange peel, salt, cinnamon stick, and cloves in saucepan. Cook and stir over medium heat until mixture boils and is clear. Remove from heat. Remove cinnamon stick and cloves, and pour hot liquid over peaches. Serve hot or cold.

Yield: 6 servings

Exchange, 1 serving: ½ fruit
Each serving contains: Calories: 22, Carbohydrates: 20 g

Melon and Grapes

½	cantaloupe melon	½	
1 c.	green grapes	250 mL	
¼ c.	buttermilk	60 mL	
1 t.	liquid sugar replacement	5 mL	
1 t.	water	5 mL	

Peel and cube melon into the size of the grapes and place in bowl. Peel grapes and add to melon. Combine buttermilk, sugar replacement, and water in cup, stirring to blend. Pour over fruit mixture. Fold in gently to coat the fruit. Cover and refrigerate at least 1 hour. Drain thoroughly and divide between 2 cold serving dishes. Serve immediately.

Yield: 2 servings

Exchange, 1 serving: 1 fruit
Each serving contains: Calories: 72, Carbohydrates: 26 g

Apple Fritters

⅓ c.	flour	90 mL	
½ t.	baking powder	2 mL	
dash	salt	dash	
2 T.	milk	30 mL	
1	apple, peeled and sliced	1	

Combine flour, baking powder, salt, and milk in small bowl, beating until smooth. If batter is too stiff, add a little water. Dip apple slices into batter and fry until golden brown.

Yield: 2 servings

Exchange, 1 serving: 1 bread
Each serving contains: Calories: 105

Plum Whip

½ lb.	fresh plums	250 g	
1 t.	lemon juice	5 mL	
1	egg white	1	
1 T.	granulated sugar replacement	15 mL	

Pit and quarter plums. Purée plums and lemon juice in blender or food processor. Beat egg white and sugar replacement into stiff peaks. Gradually, beat plum purée into egg-white mixture. Spoon into dessert glasses.

Yield: 4 servings

Exchange, 1 serving: 1 fruit
Each serving contains: Calories: 38

Nectarine with Pistachio Cream

1 T.	pistachio-flavored sugar-free instant pudding mix	15 mL
⅔ c.	skim milk	180 mL
2	nectarines	2
4 t.	nonfat strawberry yogurt	20 mL

Combine pistachio pudding mix and milk in a small mixing bowl. Beat with a fork or whipping whisk for 1 to 2 minutes or until well blended. Set aside for 5 to 8 minutes to allow to thicken. (Mixture should be a light-syrup consistency) Divide and spread pistachio mixture on the bottom of four small dessert plates. Cut nectarines in half. Cut each half into ten very thin slices. Arrange slices in a fan fashion on one side of the plate on top of the pistachio mixture. Place a 1 t. (5 mL) "dot" of strawberry yogurt at the base of the nectarine fan. Chill or serve immediately

Yield: 4 servings

Exchange, 1 serving: ½ fruit, ¼ skim milk
Each serving contains: Calories: 50, Carbohydrates: 12 g

Nectarine with Rum Cream

1	nectarine	1
½ c.	nonfat plain yogurt	125 mL
1 env.	aspartame low-calorie sweetener	1 env.
¼ t.	rum extract	2 mL

Divide nectarine in half and remove seed. Slice each half into eight slices and arrange each half on a plate in a daisy petal-type design. Combine yogurt, sweetener, and rum extract in a small bowl. Stir to completely blend. Divide mixture evenly between the two plates, spooning it into the middle of the two daisy forms.

Yield: 2 servings

Exchange, 1 serving: ½ fruit, ¼ skim milk
Each serving contains: Calories: 52, Carbohydrates: 11 g

Nectarine with Strawberry Sauce

1	nectarine, cubed	1
4 t.	all-natural strawberry preserves	20 mL
1 T.	prepared nondairy whipped topping	15 mL

Divide the nectarine cubes evenly and place them in two dishes. Spoon strawberry preserves into a small microwave or heat-proof dish. Heat until melted. Pour warmed preserves over nectarine cubes. Top with nondairy whipped topping. Serve immediately.

Yield: 2 servings

Exchange, 1 serving: ¾ fruit
Each serving contains: Calories: 45, Carbohydrates: 11 g

Kiwi and Pineapple with Raspberry Dip

1	kiwi, peeled and sliced	1	
1	pineapple ring	1	
2 T.	low-fat raspberry yogurt	30 mL	

Arrange kiwi slices on one side edge of a dessert plate. Place pineapple ring slightly over the inside edge of the kiwi slices. (Pineapple ring should be approximately in middle of plate.) Spoon raspberry yogurt into the hole of the pineapple ring. Cover and chill or serve immediately.

Yield: 2 servings

Exchange, 1 serving: 1 fruit
Each serving contains: Calories: 56, Carbohydrates: 12 g

Melon with Blueberry Glaze

¼	cantaloupe, peeled	¼	
½ c.	fresh blueberries, washed	125 mL	
2 T.	all-natural blueberry preserves	30 mL	

Cut cantaloupe into four slices; then arrange in a double circle on a serving plate. Place blueberries in the middle of the circle. Melt blueberry preserves in a small bowl in the microwave or small saucepan. Pour liquid preserves lightly over the melon and blueberries.

Yield: 1 serving

Exchange, 1 serving: 2 fruit
Each serving contains: Calories: 128, Carbohydrates: 28 g

Berries with Lemon Custard

3 c.	strawberries, hulled and quartered lengthwise	750 mL	
2 env.	aspartame low-calorie sweetener	2 env.	
1 t.	grated lemon peel	5 mL	
1 recipe	Lemon Custard	1 recipe	

Mix strawberries, aspartame sweetener, and lemon peel in a bowl. Refrigerate 3 to 4 hours or overnight. Spoon ¼ c. (60 mL) of the Lemon Custard into the middle of a dessert plate. Drain berries and spoon over custard. Top with remaining custard.

Yield: 6 servings

Exchange, 1 serving: ⅔ low-fat milk, ⅓ fruit
Each serving contains: Calories: 87, Carbohydrates: 7 g

White Chocolate-Dipped Strawberries

| ½ c. | dietetic white chocolate chips | 125 mL |
| 24 | large strawberries with stems | 24 |

Line a cookie sheet with wax paper. Melt white chocolate in double boiler over very low heat, stirring until smooth. Remove from heat. Holding one strawberry at a time from the stem, dip halfway into chocolate, tipping pan if necessary. Shake excess chocolate back into pan. Place on prepared cookie sheet. Refrigerate until chocolate sets, about 30 minutes.

Yield: 24 strawberries or 8 servings

Exchange, 1 serving: ⅓, fruit, ¼ fat
Each serving contains: Calories: 25, Carbohydrates: 3 g

Double Chocolate with Raspberries

For Dark Chocolate Sauce

| ¼ c. | semisweet chocolate chips | 60 mL |
| 3 T. + 1 t. | low-fat milk | 50 mL |

For White Chocolate Sauce

| ¼ c. | white chocolate chips | 60 mL |
| 3 T. + 1t. | low-fat milk | 50 mL |

Berries

| 90 | fresh raspberries | 90 |

Fill a small saucepan with about ¾ in. of water. Bring water to a simmer. Place chocolate chips in a custard cup. Place custard cup in the simmering water. When the chips just begin to melt, add 1T (15 mL) of the milk. Cook and stir until mixture is smooth and creamy. Continue stirring and slowly add remaining milk. Remove custard cup from water and set aside.

Proceed as for Dark Chocolate Sauce.

To serve: Measure 2 t. (10 mL) of each chocolate sauce onto a small dessert plate or saucer, with dark chocolate on one side of plate and white chocolate on the other. Gently pull the tips of a fork through both sauces to give a spiral appearance. Decorate each plate of the swirled chocolate sauces with 15 raspberries. Serve immediately.

Yield: 6 servings

Exchange, 1 serving: 1⅓ fruit, 1 fat
Each serving contains: Calories: 92, Carbohydrates: 5 g

Peach Clafouti

Clafouti is like a cobbler. It's just one dish, easy with fruit and pastry.

1 lb.	peaches, sliced	450 g
1 c.	skim milk	250 mL
2 whole	eggs or equivalent egg substitute	2 whole
2 T.	peach-flavored brandy (optional)	30 mL
2 T.	sugar	30 mL
2 pkgs.	acesulfame-K	2 pkgs.
½ c.	flour	125 mL
¼ t.	nutmeg	2 mL

Coat a 1 qt. (1 L) shallow baking dish with non-stick vegetable cooking spray. Arrange peach slices evenly on the bottom of it.

Put the milk, eggs, brandy (if you are using it), sugar, and acesulfame-K in a blender or food processor. Use a 1 T. (15 mL) measure and remove 1 T. (15 mL) flour from the half-cup (125 mL) measure and mix in the nutmeg. Set aside. Add the ½ cup minus 1 T. (125 mL minus 5 mL) flour to the mixture in the blender or food processor and process until smooth. Pour over the peaches.

Sprinkle with the flour-nutmeg mixture. Bake in a preheated 350°F (180°C) oven for 30–35 minutes. The topping will be golden and puffed.

Yield: 6 servings

Exchange, 1 serving: 1½ starch/bread
Each serving contains: Calories: 126, Total fat: 2 g, Carbohydrates: 23 g, Protein: 5 g, Sodium: 248 mg, Cholesterol: 72 mg

Peach Crème Fraîche

20 oz.	peach slices in juice	550 g
1 c.	frozen low-fat non-dairy whipped topping	250 mL
1 t.	almond extract	5 mL
1 env.	plain gelatin	1 env.
3 T.	water	45 mL

Drain the peaches. Reserve four slices for garnish. Discard the juice or reserve it for another use. Put the peaches, whipped topping, and almond extract in a blender or food processor. Blend until smooth. In a small saucepan, mix together the gelatin and water. Let stand five minutes. Heat over low flame, stirring constantly until the gelatin is dissolved. Add to the peach mixture. Blend another few seconds. Spoon into four dessert dishes. Refrigerate until serving time. Garnish with the reserved peach slices and additional whipped topping, if desired.

Yield: 4 servings

Exchange, 1 serving: 1 starch/bread; ½ fruit
Each serving contains: Calories: 114, Total fat: 2 g, Carbohydrates: 22 g, Protein: 2 g, Sodium: 1 mg, Cholesterol: 0 mg

Fried Spiced Apples

This is a wonderfully satisfying dessert for a winter evening.

4 large	cooking apples, peeled and cored	4 large
1 t.	sugar	5 mL
¼ t.	ginger	2 mL
¼ t.	cinnamon	2 mL
2 T.	butter or margarine	30 mL
1 c.	frozen low-fat nondairy whipped topping	250 mL

Cut the apples into ¼ in. (6 mm) thick slices. On a dinner plate, mix together the sugar, ginger, and cinnamon. In a large, heavy-bottomed frying pan, melt the butter or margarine. Dip the apple slices in the sugar and cinnamon mixture. Fry 3–5 minutes on each side or until lightly browned. Remove slices to a serving dish. Serve immediately with whipped topping.

Yield: 4 servings

Exchange, 1 serving: 2 fruit; 1½ fat
Each serving contains: Calories: 176, Total fat: 8 g, Carbohydrates: 26 g, Protein: 0.3 g, Sodium: 58 mg, Cholesterol: 15 mg

Marinated Blueberries

Delicious when blueberries are fresh and plentiful.

2 c.	fresh blueberries	500 mL
1 t.	grated orange rind	5 mL
2 T.	Triple Sec or other orange-flavored liqueur	30 mL
2 t.	sugar	10 mL
½ c.	frozen low-fat nondairy whipped topping	125 mL

In a shallow mixing bowl, combine the blueberries, orange rind, Triple Sec, and sugar. Toss to coat the berries. Cover loosely and refrigerate for an hour or more. Before serving, mix a few times. Serve with whipped topping.

Yield: 4 servings

Exchange, 1 serving: 1 starch/bread
Each serving contains: Calories: 69, Total fat: 1 g, Carbohydrates: 14 g, Protein: 1 g, Sodium: 4 mg, Cholesterol: 0 mg

Oranges and Grapes

Make a glamorous-looking fresh dessert with fresh winter fruits.

4	oranges, peeled	4
1 c.	grapes, halved and seeded, if necessary	250 mL
¼ c.	water	60 mL
1 t.	rum flavoring	5 mL
2 pkgs.	sugar substitute	2 pkgs.

Slice the oranges into layers. Arrange with grape halves in a glass serving dish. Mix together the water, flavoring, and sugar substitute.

Pour the mixture over the fruit. Cover the bowl and refrigerate for at least an hour before serving.

Yield: 4 servings

Exchange, 1 serving: 1 starch/bread; ½ fruit
Each serving contains: Calories: 90, Total fat: 0.3 g, Carbohydrates: 23 g, Protein: 2 g, Sodium: 3 mg, Cholesterol: 0 mg

Piña Colada Sherbet

You don't make this sherbet and freeze it, you freeze the pineapple ahead of time.

20 oz	pineapple chunks in juice, no sugar added	550 g
2 t.	coconut extract	10 mL
1 c.	frozen low-fat nondairy whipped topping	250 mL

Drain and freeze the pineapple chunks. Put them into a food processor. If the pineapple sticks to the container, run water on the outside. Add the coconut extract and blend until mushy. Transfer to a medium mixing bowl. Fold in the whipped topping. Serve immediately.

Yield: 4 servings

Exchange, 1 serving: 2 fruit; ½ fat
Each serving contains: Calories: 127, Total fat: 2 g, Carbohydrates: 26 g, Protein: 0.6 g, Sodium: 1 mg, Cholesterol: 0 mg

Fruit Platter with Mango Sauce

2 large	mangos, pitted	2 large
⅓ c.	unsweetened pineapple juice	90 mL
2 T.	fresh lime juice	0 mL
1 T.	granulated fructose	15 mL
2	papayas, peeled, seeded, and cut into 12 slices	2
1	pineapple, peeled, cored, and cut into 12 slices	1
1	honeydew melon, peeled and cut into 12 wedges	1
1 T.	grated lime peel	30 mL

Cut away mango flesh from skin. Combine mango, pineapple juice, lime juice, and fructose in a blender. Process to a purée. Cover and refrigerate. Arrange papaya slices, pineapple slices, and honeydew wedges on a large platter. Pour mango sauce over fruit. Sprinkle with lime peel.

Yield: 12 servings

Exchange, 1 serving: 2 fruit
Each serving contains: Calories: 126, Carbohydrates: 26 g

Fruit Chutney

1 c.	raspberry vinegar	250 mL
½ c.	red wine vinegar	125 mL
2 c.	dry white wine	500 mL
½ c.	frozen orange juice concentrate	125 mL
1 c.	crushed pineapple in juice	250 mL
1 c.	diced apple	250 mL
⅔ c.	diced papaya	180 mL
⅔ c.	diced mango	180 mL
½ c.	thinly sliced green bell pepper	
½ c.	thinly sliced red bell pepper	125 mL
½ c.	thinly sliced yellow bell pepper	125 mL
¼ c.	granulated sugar replacement	60 mL
6 whole	peppercorns	6 whole
1	bay leaf	1
2 T.	minced fresh mint	30 mL

Combine vinegars in a large saucepan. Bring to a boil, reduce heat, and simmer to reduce liquid to about ½ c. (125 mL). Add wine, orange juice concentrate, fruit, bell peppers, sugar replacement, peppercorns, and bay leaf. Cook until fruit is soft. Transfer fruit and bell peppers to a bowl. Simmer liquid for about 5 minutes. Return fruit and bell peppers to saucepan. Cook over low heat, stirring occasionally, and reduce mixture to about 2½ c. Remove from heat. Remove peppercorns and bay leaf. Stir in mint. Cover and chill.

Yield: 20 servings

Exchange, 1 serving: negligible
Each serving contains: Calories: negligible, Carbohydrates: negligible

Glazed Apricots

½ c.	water	125 mL
2 T.	all-natural orange marmalade	30 mL
16	moist dried apricots	16

Combine water and marmalade in a small nonstick saucepan. Heat and stir over medium heat until marmalade is melted. Add apricots. Reduce heat; then cover and simmer until apricots are tender and syrup is reduced and coats apricots (about 20 to 25 minutes). Cool apricots in syrup. Remove apricots from syrup. Drain to remove excess syrup.

Yield: 8 servings

Exchange, 1 serving: ½ fruit
Each serving contains: Calories: 24, Carbohydrates: 6 g

Cranberry and Raspberry Fool

1½ c.	fresh cranberries	375 mL
1½ c.	fresh raspberries	375 mL
¼ c.	granulated fructose	60 mL
¼ c.	raspberry juice	60 mL
2 c.	prepared nondairy whipped topping	500 mL

Combine cranberries, raspberries, and fructose in a food processor or blender. Process into a purée. Transfer to a nonstick saucepan. Stir in raspberry juice. Cook and stir over medium heat until mixture is a thick purée. If desired, press through a sieve to remove seeds. Transfer mixture to a large bowl. Cover and chill mixture thoroughly. To serve: Swirl nondairy whipped topping into cranberry-raspberry mixture. Do not mix thoroughly. Divide evenly among six decorative glasses. Serve immediately.

Yield: 6 servings

Exchange, 1 serving: ⅓ fruit, 1 fat
Each serving contains: Calories: 69, Carbohydrates: 4 g

Strawberries with Cinnamon Sauce

⅔ c.	water	180 mL
1 t.	ground cinnamon	5 mL
6 in.	cinnamon stick, broken in pieces	9 cm
1 T.	cold water	15 mL
1 t.	cornstarch	5 mL
3 env.	aspartame sweetener	3 env.
2 c.	frozen, unsweetened strawberries*	500 mL
2 T.	prepared nondairy whipped topping	30 mL

Combine the ⅔ c. (180 mL) of water and the ground cinnamon and broken cinnamon pieces in a saucepan. Bring to a boil, reduce heat, and simmer until liquid is about ½ c. (125 mL). Remove cinnamon pieces. Dissolve the cornstarch in the 1 T. (15 mL) of cold water. Pour into cinnamon water. Cook and stir until mixture becomes the consistency of a thin syrup. Remove from heat. Allow to cool until pan is cool enough to comfortably put on your hand. Stir in the aspartame sweetener. Place frozen strawberries in a narrow bowl. Pour warm cinnamon mixture over the strawberries. Cover and refrigerate until strawberries are thawed and liquid is chilled. To serve: Divide berries and juice evenly between two decorative glasses. Top each glass with 1 T. (15 mL) of nondairy whipped topping.

Yield: 2 servings

Exchange, 1 serving: 1 fruit
Each serving contains: Calories: 55, Carbohydrates: 13 g

*This recipe can be made with fresh strawberries, but there will be less juice.

Ginger Pear Crumble

30	gingersnaps	30
30 oz.	pear halves, in juice can	855 g can
1 T.	lemon juice	15 mL
½ t.	ground cinnamon	2 mL
¼ t.	salt	1 mL
¼ t.	ground nutmeg	1 mL

Using a food processor or blender, grind the gingersnaps into crumbs. Arrange half of the gingersnap crumbs on the bottom of a 1½ qt. (1½ L) baking dish that has been sprayed with vegetable oil. Drain pears, reserving ¼ c. (60 mL) of the liquid. Place pears on the crumbs. Add lemon juice to the reserved pear liquid and sprinkle over pears. Mix cinnamon, salt, and nutmeg together. Sprinkle on top of pears. Top with remaining gingersnap crumbs. Bake at 350°F (175°C) for about 25 minutes.

Yield: 6 servings

Exchange, 1 serving: ½ bread, ⅓ fruit
Each serving contains: Calories: 160, Carbohydrates: 21 g

Blueberry Crisp

1 qt.	frozen or fresh blueberries	1 L
2 T.	granulated fructose	30 mL
2 T.	lemon juice	30 mL
2 T.	water	30 mL

Topping

1 c.	quick-cooking oatmeal	250 mL
¼ c.	all-purpose flour	60 mL
¼ c.	chopped walnuts	60 mL
3 T.	granulated fructose	45 mL
⅓ c.	firm margarine	90 mL

Place the blueberries in a shallow 1½ qt. (1½ L) baking dish. Sprinkle with 2 T. (30 mL) of the fructose, lemon juice, and water. Stir to mix evenly. Combine oatmeal, flour, walnuts, and 3 T. (45 mL) of the fructose in a small bowl. Cut margarine into mixture or rub with the fingers until mixture becomes coarse crumbs. Sprinkle evenly over the top of the blueberry mixture. Bake at 350°F (175°C) uncovered for 30 to 40 minutes or until topping is browned and berries are tender. Serve hot or cold.

Yield: 8 servings

Exchange, 1 serving: 1 fruit, ⅓ bread, 2 fat
Each serving contains: Calories: 187, Carbohydrates: 21 g

Pear and Mandarin Orange Crisp

1 lb. can	pear halves in juice	454 g can
15 oz. can	mandarin orange sections in water	425 g can
2 t.	granulated fructose	10 mL
1 t.	cornstarch	5 mL

Topping

6	graham cracker squares	6
⅓ c.	all-purpose flour	90 mL
1 t.	granulated fructose	5 mL
1 t.	vanilla extract	5 mL
3 T.	firm margarine	45 mL

Drain ½ c. (125 mL) of the pear juice from the can into a measuring cup; reserve. Drain the pears, and arrange pear halves in the bottom of a 1 qt. (1 L) well-greased baking dish. Drain the mandarin oranges, and pour orange sections over the pear halves. Add the 2 t. (10 mL) of fructose and the cornstarch to the reserved pear juice; stir to dissolve. Pour over fruit in baking dish. Crush graham crackers. Combine graham cracker crumbs, flour, 1 t. (5 mL) of the fructose, and vanilla in a small bowl. Cut the margarine into the flour mixture or rub with the fingers until the mixture becomes coarse crumbs. Sprinkle evenly over the fruit. Bake at 350°F (175°C) for 30 to 35 minutes or until topping is browned. Serve hot or cold.

Yield: 8 servings

Exchange, 1 serving: ⅔ fruit, ½ bread, 1 fat
Each serving contains: Calories: 119, Carbohydrates: 18 g

Royal Anne Cherry Coconut Crisp

16 oz. can	Royal Anne cherries in water	454 g can
1 t.	lemon juice	5 mL
2 t.	water	10 mL
1 T.	granulated fructose	15 mL
1 t.	ground nutmeg	5mL

Topping

½ c.	quick-cooking oatmeal	125 mL
2 T.	all-purpose flour	30 mL
¼ c.	unsweetened coconut	60 mL
2 T.	granulated fructose	30 mL
¼ c.	firm margarine	60 mL

Drain cherries. Divide evenly between four oven-proof serving dishes. Sprinkle with lemon juice and water. Combine 1 T. (15 mL) of the fructose and the nutmeg; sprinkle evenly over the four servings. Combine oatmeal, flour, coconut, and 2 T. (30 mL) of the fructose in a bowl. Cut margarine into mixture, forming coarse crumbs. Sprinkle evenly over the top of cherries. Bake at 350°F (175°C) for 20 to 30 minutes or until topping is browned. Serve hot or cold.

Yield: 4 servings

Exchange, 1 serving: 1 fruit, 1 fat
Each serving contains: Calories: 120, Carbohydrates: 18 g

Banana Crisp on a Stick

1 pkg.	sugar-free orange gelatin	1 pkg.
¼ c.	corn flakes	60 mL
1 t.	granulated fructose	5 mL
1	large banana	1

Prepare gelatin as directed on package. Allow to cool until thick but not set. Crush corn flakes and spread on a small plate. Sprinkle with fructose. Peel banana and cut in half horizontally. Place each half on the end of a wooden popsicle or lollipop stick. Dip banana halves into thickened gelatin. Then roll each banana half in the corn-flake crumbs. Press crumbs lightly into sides of banana. Cool or eat immediately (You will not use all of the gelatin.) Children love 'em.

Yield: 2 servings

Exchange, 1 serving: 1 fruit, ¼ bread
Each serving contains: Calories: 76, Carbohydrates: 20 g

Apple Cranberry Shortcake

Shortcake

3 c.	biscuit mix	750 mL
3 T.	firm shortening	45 mL
1	egg	1
⅓ c.	skim milk	180 mL
1 T.	margarine, melted	15 ml

Sauce

1 qt.	apples, peeled and thinly sliced	1 L
1 c.	cranberries	250 mL
¼ c.	water	60 mL
⅓ c.	granulated brown sugar replacement	90 mL
¼ c.	granulated fructose	60 mL
1 t.	caramel flavoring	5 mL
dash	salt	dash

Combine biscuit mix and shortening in a medium-sized bowl. Cut shortening into mix to form coarse crumbs. Combine egg and skim milk in a bowl. Beat slightly to blend. Pour into biscuit mix. Stir to moisten dry ingredients. Divide dough in half. Pat half of the dough on the bottom of a 9 in. (23 cm) layer cake pan. Brush with the melted margarine. Roll out remaining dough and place on top of dough in cake pan. Bake at 425°F (220°C) for 20 to 25 minutes. Meanwhile, combine ingredients for sauce in a heavy nonstick saucepan. Bring to a boil and boil until apple slices are tender. Turn shortcake out onto serving tray. Remove top layer of cake. Fill bottom layer with half of the apple cranberry sauce. Return top to cake, and spoon remaining sauce over top. To serve: Cut cake into nine wedges.

Yield: 9 servings

Exchange, 1 serving: 1⅓ bread, 1 fruit, 1½ fat
Each serving contains: Calories: 314, Carbohydrates: 36 g

Fruit Cobblers

1 tube (10 count)	ready-to-bake biscuits	1 tube (10 count)	Prepare any of the fruit fillings below. Pour filling into an 8 in. (20 cm) round baking pan. Lay biscuits on top of filling. Bake at 400°F (200°C) for 20 to 25 minutes. Serve warm or chilled.

Tart Cherry Filling

1 lb. 4 oz. can	pitted tart cherries (water packed)	545 g can	Do not drain the cherries. Combine ingredients in a saucepan. Cook and stir until boiling and slightly thickened.
¼ c.	granulated fructose	60 mL	
1 T.	quick-cooking tapioca	15 mL	**Yield: 10 servings**
	red food coloring (optional)		*Exchange, 1 serving: 1 bread, ⅓ fruit* *Each serving contains: Calories: 90, Carbohydrates: 20 g*

Fresh Peach Filling

1½ T.	cornstarch	23 mL	Combine cornstarch, sugar replacement, nutmeg, and water in a saucepan. Cook and stir until thickened. Add sliced peaches and lemon juice. Cook 5 minutes longer.
¼ c.	granulated sugar replacement	60 mL	
¼ t.	ground nutmeg	1 mL	
½ c.	water	125 mL	
1 qt.	peaches, peeled and sliced	1 L	**Yield: 10 servings**
1 T.	lemon juice	15 mL	*Exchange, 1 serving: 1 bread, ½ fruit* *Each serving contains: Calories: 103, Carbohydrates: 25 g*

Apple Filling

1 lb. 4 oz. can	Musselman's sliced apples	567 g can	Combine all ingredients in a saucepan. Stir to mix. Cook and stir until hot.
¼ c.	water	60 mL	
1½ T.	cornstarch	23 mL	**Yield: 10 servings**
2 T.	granulated fructose	30 mL	*Exchange, 1 serving: 1 bread, ⅓ fruit*
½ t.	ground cinnamon	2 mL	*Each serving contains: Calories: 92, Carbohydrates: 21 g*
¼ t.	ground nutmeg	1 mL	

Rhubarb Cobbler

1 lb.	fresh or frozen rhubarb cut in 1 in. (2.5 cm) pieces	500 g
½ c.	granulated fructose	125 mL
¼ c.	water	60 mL
⅔ c.	all-purpose flour	180 mL
⅓ c.	whole wheat pastry	90 mL
1½ t.	baking powder	7 mL
dash	salt	dash
2 T.	firm margarine	30 mL
½ c.	skim milk	125 mL

Place rhubarb in a bowl. Sprinkle with fructose and water. Toss to completely coat. Place in a 1½ qt. (1½ L) well-greased baking dish. Combine all-purpose flour, wheat flour, baking powder, and salt in a bowl. Cut the firm margarine into the flour mixture until mixture becomes coarse crumbs. Stir in the skim milk. Drop the cobbler batter in eight equal spoonfuls on top of rhubarb. Bake at 375°F (190°C) for 25 to 30 minutes or until batter is golden brown and rhubarb is tender.

Yield: 8 servings

Exchange, 1 serving: 1 bread, ½ fat
Each serving contains: Calories: 107, Carbohydrates: 18 g

Strawberries Chantilly

Don't forget to let the strawberries stand. That's the secret of getting them juicy.

2 c.	fresh strawberries or frozen (no sugar), thawed	500 mL
1 T.	sugar	15 mL
1 T.	Kirsch or cherry liqueur (optional)	15 mL
1 c.	frozen low-fat nondairy whipped topping, thawed	250 mL
⅓	angel food cake	⅓

Cut the strawberries in half. In a mixing bowl, combine the strawberries, sugar, and liqueur, if you are using it. Let stand ½ hour to 1 hour. Just before serving fold together the strawberries and the whipped topping. Put one slice of angel food cake on each of four dessert plates. Spoon the strawberry mixture on top.

Yield: 4 servings

Exchange, 1 serving: 1 starch/bread; 2 fruit
Each serving contains: Calories: 202, Total fat: 2 g, Carbohydrates: 41 g, Protein: 3 g, Sodium: 254 mg, Cholesterol: 0 mg

Spicy Orange Slices

2 large	oranges	2 large
2 T.	all-purpose flour	30 mL
½ c.	graham cracker crumbs	125 mL
½	allspice	2 mL
	vegetable spray	

Cut oranges (with peel on) into slices about ¼ in. (8 mm) thick, removing the seeds. Combine flour, graham cracker crumbs, and allspice in a bowl. Stir to mix. Dip orange slices into mixture, making sure to coat well. Place oranges coated with mixture into skillet oiled with vegetable spray. Do not crowd pan. Brown orange slices on both sides. Re-spray pan if necessary.

Yield: 8 servings

Exchange, 1 serving: ½ starch/bread
Each serving contains: Calories: 40, Carbohydrates: 7 g

Strawberry Dream

1 qt.	strawberries	1 L
¼ c.	granulated fructose	60 mL
½ c.	quick-cooking tapioca	125 mL
¼ t.	salt	1 mL
2 c.	boiling water	500 mL
2 c.	prepared nondairy whipped topping	500 mL

Reserve five strawberries for garnish. Crush remaining strawberries and mix them with fructose. Allow to stand at least an hour. Mix tapioca with salt and boiling water. Cook over low heat, stirring constantly, until tapioca is clear. Drain juice from berries into a measuring cup. Add enough water to berry juice to make 2 c. (500 mL) of liquid. Stir in crushed strawberries. Stir into tapioca mixture and cook 6 minutes longer. Cool completely. Divide half of the tapioca mixture among 10 dessert dishes. Fold the nondairy whipped topping into the remaining tapioca mixture; then divide it evenly among the dessert dishes. Now cut the reserved strawberries in half, and use them to garnish the top of each dish. Chill thoroughly before serving.

Yield: 10 servings

Exchange, 1 serving: ½ starch/bread, ½ fruit
Each serving contains: Calories: 72, Carbohydrates: 14 g

Peach Slump

6 c.	sliced peaches, peeled	1500 mL
⅓ c.	granulated fructose	90 mL
1½ t.	cinnamon	7 mL
½ c.	water	125 mL
12	unbaked biscuits	12
12 T.	prepared nondairy whipped topping	180 mL

Combine peaches, fructose, cinnamon, and water in a nonstick skillet. Bring to a simmer. Top with biscuits. Cover and simmer for 25 to 30 minutes. Top each serving with 1 T. (15 mL) of nondairy whipped topping.

Yield: 12 servings

Exchange, 1 serving: 1 starch/bread, 1 fruit
Each serving contains: Calories: 112, Carbohydrates: 19 g

Brandied Apples

6	tart apples	6
1 T.	lemon juice	15 mL
¼ c.	brandy	60 mL
⅛ t.	cinnamon	½ mL
12 T.	prepared nondairy whipped topping	180 mL

Core apples and then cut them into quarters. Place quarters in a bowl. Sprinkle with lemon juice, tossing to coat. Drain off any excess lemon juice. Pour brandy and cinnamon over apple quarters, tossing to coat. Cover tightly and marinate for several hours or overnight. Toss several times during marinating. For each of the 12 servings, place two quarters in a small dessert dish and top with 1 T. (15 mL) nondairy whipped topping.

Yield: 12 servings

Exchange, 1 serving: 1 fruit
Each serving contains: Calories: 57, Carbohydrates: 13 g

Hidden Apple

1	cored apple	1
2 T.	orange juice	30 mL
dash each	nutmeg, cinnamon, sugar replacement	dash each
	uncooked dough for 1 biscuit	

Prick the inside of the apple cavity with a fork or toothpick. Sprinkle with orange juice, spices, and sugar replacement. Place the biscuit dough on a lightly floured surface. Flatten the dough into a square that is large enough to wrap completely around the apple. Place the apple in the middle of the dough. Bring the corners of the dough up to the top of the apple. Secure with a toothpick or press the edges together firmly. Place in a baking dish. Then bake at 375°F (190°C) for 20 to 25 minutes or until done.

Yield: 1 serving

Exchange, 1 serving: 1 fruit, 1 starch/bread
Each serving contains: Calories: 135, Carbohydrates: 29 g

Date Nut Dish

2	eggs	2
1 T.	granulated sugar replacement	15 mL
⅔ c.	all-purpose flour	180 mL
1 t.	baking powder	5 mL
½ c.	coarsely chopped walnuts	125 mL
1 c.	chopped dates	250 mL

Beat eggs until thick and lemon-colored. Stir in sugar replacement. Combine flour and baking powder in sifter; then sift into egg mixture. Beat until well blended. Fold in walnuts and dates. Transfer to a well greased 9 in. (23 cm) layer cake pan, Bake at 350°F (175°C) for 20 to 30 minutes or until golden brown on top. Serve warm.

Yield: 10 servings

Exchange, 1 serving: 1 fruit, ½ starch/bread, ½ fat
Each serving contains: Calories: 131, Carbohydrates: 22 g

Apple-Go-Round

1	firm apple	1	
¼ c.	orange juice	60 mL	
1 t.	lemon juice	5 mL	
1 T.	raisins	15 mL	
1 T.	celery, diced	15 mL	
2 T.	applesauce	30 mL	
	lettuce leaf		

Slice off top of apple; remove core. Prick outside with sharp fork. Place apple in tall narrow bowl. Combine orange and lemon juice; pour over apple. (Add extra water if apple is not covered.) Marinate in refrigerator 4 to 5 hours. Combine raisins, celery, and applesauce. Allow to mellow at room temperature 2 hours. Chill thoroughly. Drain apple. Cut apple into 8 sections, slicing almost to the bottom. Fill with applesauce mixture. Place on crisp lettuce leaf.

Yield: 1 serving

Exchange, 1 serving: 2 fruit
Each serving contains: Calories: 54, Carbohydrates: 68 g

Peach Melba

½ c.	raspberries	125 mL	
½ t.	sugar replacement	5 mL	
½ c.	dietetic vanilla ice cream	125 ml	
½	peach, sliced	½	

Slightly mash raspberries and sugar replacement. Allow to rest 5 minutes. Place ice cream in dish. Top with peach slices and raspberries.

Yield: 1 serving

Exchange, 1 serving: 1 bread, 1 fruit
Each serving contains: Calories: 120, Carbohydrates: 32 g

Baked Apple Dumpling

1 t.	raisins	5 mL	
2 T.	orange juice	30 mL	
½ t.	sugar replacement	3 mL	
1 small	apple	1 small	
	dough for 1 biscuit		

Combine raisins and orange juice in saucepan. Heat to a boil. Add sugar replacement. Cover. Allow to rest while preparing remaining ingredients. Core apple; with a fork or toothpick, prick inside the apple cavity. On floured board, roll biscuit dough very thin and large enough to wrap around apple. Place apple in center of dough. Fill apple cavity with raisin mixture. Wrap dough around apple and secure at top. Place in baking dish. Bake at 375°F (190°C) for 25 to 30 minutes.

Yield: 1 serving

Exchange, 1 serving: 1 bread, 1 fruit
Each serving contains: Calories: 142, Carbohydrates: 68 g

Wheat and Oat Fruit Cobbler

16 oz. can	pitted tart cherries	480 g can
¼ c.	granulated sugar replacement	60 mL
2 T.	cornstarch	30 mL
5 drops	red food coloring (optional)	5 drops
2 c.	fresh or frozen blueberries, rinsed and drained	500 mL
½ t.	almond extract	2 mL
1 c.	graham flour	250 mL
3 T.	granulated sugar replacement	45 mL
1½ t.	baking powder	7 mL
½ t.	salt	2 mL
¼ c.	margarine	60 mL
½ c.	quick-cooking or old fashioned oatmeal	125 mL
⅓ c.	skim milk	90 mL
1	egg, lightly beaten	1

Drain cherries and save the liquid. Add enough water to make 1 c. (250 mL). Combine ¼ c. (60 mL) sugar replacement and cornstarch in a medium saucepan. Add cherry liquid, cherries, and food coloring, if using. Stir to blend. Cook over medium heat until mixture comes to a boil. Reduce heat. Cook 1 minute, stirring constantly, until mixture thickens and is clear. Remove from heat. Add blueberries and almond extract. Pour mixture into 2 qt. (2 L) casserole. Set aside while preparing topping.

Measure flour into a bowl. Add 3 T. (45 mL) sugar replacement, baking powder and salt to flour. Stir well to blend. Cut in the margarine until mixture looks like coarse meal. Stir in oats. Add milk and egg. Stir just to moisten dry ingredients. Drop dough by spoonfuls onto warm fruit. Spread carefully to cover top. Bake at 400°F (200°C) for 25 to 30 minutes. Serve warm.

Yield: 8 servings

Exchange, 1 serving: 1 bread, 2 fruit, 1½ fat
Each serving contains: Calories: 173, Carbohydrates: 44 g

Prune Casserole

A sweet ending to any meal.

4 c.	whole wheat bread cubes, toasted	1 L
2 c.	prunes, cooked, pitted and sliced	500 mL
1 c.	apples, chopped	250 mL
½ c.	prune juice	125 mL
1¼ c.	water	310 mL
½ t.	salt	2 mL
½ t.	ground cinnamon	2 mL
2 T.	margarine	10 mL

Place half of the toasted bread cubes in a well-greased 1½ qt. (1½ L) casserole. Spread the prunes in a layer over the bread cubes. Arrange the apples in a layer over the prunes, then layer the remaining bread cubes. Combine prune juice, water, salt, cinnamon, and margarine in a saucepan. Bring to a boil; cook for 3 minutes. Pour over prume casserole. Cover. Bake at 375°F (190°C) for 1 hour.

Yield: 8 servings

Exchange, 1 serving: ¾ bread, 2 fruit
Each serving contains: Calories: 137, Carbohydrates: 77 g

Flaming Peaches

A fast but exotic dessert.

6	canned peach halves in their own juice	6
¼ c.	Raspberry Preserves	60 mL
¼ c.	brandy	60 mL

Drain peach halves. Arrange in 6 shallow baking dishes. Melt preserves, stirring constantly. Brush peaches with preserves. Drizzle brandy over peaches; ignite. Serve immediately.

Yield: 6 servings

Exchange, 1 serving: 1 fruit
Each serving contains: Calories: 30, Carbohydrates: 16 g

Frosty Pineapple Dessert

20 oz. can	Featherweight water-packed pineapple chunks, drained	600 g can
3½ c.	chopped ice	875 mL
½ t.	vanilla extract	2 mL
dash	mint extract	dash
6	mint sprigs	6

Combine all ingredients except the mint sprigs in a blender. Blend at high speed until finely crushed. Serve immediately in chilled dessert dishes with mint sprigs on top.

Yield: 6 servings

Exchange, 1 serving: 1 fruit
Each serving contains: Calories: 50, Carbohydrates: 14 g

Based on a recipe from Featherweight Brand Foods.

Tarts

Chocolate Almond Tart

Crust

¼ c.	flour, sifted	190 mL
2 t.	granulated sugar replacement	10 mL
5 T.	margarine	75 mL
½ t.	vanilla extract	2 mL
2–3 T.	water	30–45 mL

Filling

1	egg	1
1 T.	flour	15 mL
¼ c.	skim milk	60 mL
¼ c.	heavy cream	60 mL
⅓ c.	granulated sugar replacement	90 mL
1 oz.	baking chocolate, melted	30 g
½ c.	almonds, slivered	125 mL
2 t.	brandy flavoring	10 mL
dash	salt	dash

In a bowl or food processor, combine flour, sugar replacement, and margarine. With a steel blade or knife work into a mixture like cornmeal. Add vanilla extract and enough water to make a soft dough. Press dough evenly into a 9 in. (23 cm) false-bottom tart pan. Chill in refrigerator for 45 minutes. Cover the chilled dough with aluminum foil and fill with dried beans or pie weights. Bake in the lower part of a 400°F (200°C) oven for 8 minutes. Remove foil and beans and bake the crust for 5 minutes longer. Remove from oven. Combine filling ingredients and beat well. Pour into partially baked shell. Set on the middle rack of the oven and bake for 20 to 30 minutes, until filling is set and a knife inserted in center comes out clean. Cool before serving.

Yield: 14 servings

Exchange, 1 serving: ½ bread, 2 fat
Each serving contains: Calories: 120, Carbohydrates: 7 g

Lemon Tarts

10	prepared tart shells	10
½ c.	granulated fructose	125 mL
2 T.	low-calorie margarine	30 mL
1 t.	butter flavoring	5 mL
¼ c.	lemon juice	60 mL
1 t.	grated lemon zest	5 mL
1	egg, beaten	1

Combine fructose, margarine, butter flavoring, lemon juice, lemon zest, and egg in top of double boiler. Stir to mix. Cook and stir over hot water until mixture thickens. Pour into the 10 tart shells. Chill until firm.

Yield: 10 servings

Exchange, 1 serving (without crust): ½ fruit
Each serving contains: Calories: 31, Carbohydrates: 5 g

Apricot Tarts

12	prepared tart shells	12	
1 c.	fresh apricots, cut in eighths	375 mL	
2 t.	lemon juice	10 mL	
2 drops	almond extract	2 drops	
12 T.	prepared nondairy whipped topping	180 mL	

Combine apricots, lemon juice, and almond extract in a bowl. Toss to mix. Fold apricots into nondairy whipped topping. Divide mixture evenly between the 12 tart shells. Chill thoroughly before serving.

Yield: 12 servings

Exchange, 1 serving (without crust): ⅓ fruit
Each serving contains: Calories: 25, Carbohydrates: 8 g

Tart-Cherry Tarts

4	baked tart shells	4	
2 c.	frozen tart cherries	500 mL	
⅔ c.	sorbitol	180 mL	
¼ t.	lavender leaves	1 mL	
2	cardamom pods	2	
1 T.	cornstarch	15 mL	

Allow cherries to thaw. Drain liquid into a 1 c. (250 mL) measuring cup, pressing cherries with back of spoon to extract juice. Add extra water, if juice does not measure 1 c. (250 mL). Reserve cherries. Pour juice into a saucepan; then add sorbitol. Stir to mix. Either in the palm of your hand or in a mortar, crush lavender leaves and cardamom seeds from pod. Add to juice with cornstarch. Stir to dissolve cornstarch. Cook and stir over medium heat until mixture becomes clear and thick. Allow to cool for 3 minutes. Pour two-thirds of the liquid over the cherries; then fold to blend. Divide cherry mixture evenly between the four tart shells. Pour remaining liquid over cherry mixture in tart shells. Chill until firm.

Yield: 4 servings

Exchange, 1 serving (without crust): 1 fruit
Each serving contains: Calories: 57, Carbohydrates: 15 g

Strawberry Tarts

6	prepared tart shells	6
3 c.	fresh strawberries	750 mL
½ c.	apple juice	125 mL
2 t.	unflavored gelatin	10 mL
½ c.	prepared nondairy whipped topping	125 mL

Clean the strawberries and then slice them in half lengthwise. Combine apple juice and gelatin in saucepan. Allow gelatin to soften for 5 minutes. Bring to a boil. Remove from heat and allow mixture to cool and thicken. Divide the strawberries evenly between the six tart shells. Pour gelatin over the top. Chill until firm. Divide the nondairy whipped topping evenly among the strawberry tarts.

Yield: 6 servings

Exchange, 1 serving (without crust): ¾ fruit
Each serving contains: Calories: 42, Carbohydrates: 12 g

Dried Apricot and Prune Tarts

10	unbaked tart shells	10
1 c.	dried prunes	250 mL
1 c.	dried apricots	250 mL
dash	salt	dash
1 t.	cinnamon	5 mL
¾ c.	prune liquid	190 mL

Place prunes in saucepan. Cover with water and boil for about 15 minutes. Drain, reserving liquid. Remove pits from prunes; then cut them in half and place them back in saucepan. Rinse apricots (do not cook). Cut apricots in half and add to prunes. Next, add salt, cinnamon, and ¼ c. (190 mL) of the reserved prune liquid. If the liquid drained from the prunes does not measure ¾ c. (190 mL), add water to liquid. Bring to a boil; then reduce heat and cook until mixture thickens. Divide mixture evenly between the 10 tart shells. Bake at 425°F (220°C) for 15 minutes.

Yield: 10 servings

Exchange, 1 serving (without crust): 1 fruit
Each serving contains: Calories: 56, Carbohydrates: 15 g

Currant Tartlets

18	unbaked tartlets	18
⅓ c.	dried currants	90 mL
1 t.	low-calorie margarine	5 mL
⅓ c.	granulated brown sugar replacement	90 mL
1	egg white, slightly beaten	1
¼ t.	vanilla extract	1 mL

Wash currants and then cover with boiling water. Allow to soften for 5 minutes and then drain. While still hot, stir in margarine, brown sugar replacement, egg white, and vanilla. Divide mixture evenly among the 18 tartlets. Cover tartlets loosely with aluminum foil. Bake at 350°F (175°C) for 15 minutes; then remove aluminum foil, reduce heat to 300°F (150°C), and cook for 10 more minutes.

Yield: 18 tartlets

Exchange, 2 tartlets (without crust): ⅓ fruit
Each serving contains: Calories: 17, Carbohydrates: 4 g

Raspberry Cranberry Tarts

10	unbaked tart shells	10
10 oz. pkg.	frozen unsweetened raspberries	289 g pkg.
3 c.	fresh cranberries	750 mL
1 c.	granulated sugar replacement	250 mL
3 T.	cornstarch	45 mL
dash	salt	dash
3 T.	cold water	45 mL

Allow raspberries to thaw. Drain juice from raspberries by lightly pressing them with the back of a spoon into a 1 c. (250 mL) measuring cup. If juice does not measure 1 c. (250 mL), add water. Set raspberries aside. Combine the 1 c. (250 mL) of raspberry juice and the cranberries in a saucepan. Cook and stir over medium heat until cranberries begin to "pop." Remove from heat. Combine sugar replacement, cornstarch, and salt in a small mixing bowl. Stir in cold water to dissolve cornstarch; then add to cranberry mixture. Return to heat and cook until thickened. Remove from heat, and allow to cool for 5 minutes. Now stir in raspberries. Divide mixture evenly among the 10 tart shells. Bake at 400°F (200°C) for 10 to 15 minutes.

Yield: 10 servings

Exchange, 1 serving (without crust): ⅔ fruit
Each serving contains: Calories: 40, Carbohydrates: 9 g

Date Tarts

8	prepared tart shells	8
2 c.	pitted dates	500 mL
1 c.	water	250 mL
2 T.	orange juice	30 mL

Combine dates and water in a saucepan; then cook to a thick paste. Remove from heat, and add orange juice. Allow mixture to cool. Divide mixture evenly among the eight tart shells.

Yield: 8 servings

Exchange, 1 serving (without crust): 1 fruit
Each serving contains: Calories: 62, Carbohydrates: 16 g

Strawberry Chiffon Tarts

12	prepared tart shells	12
2 c.	strawberries	500 mL
1 env.★	low-calorie strawberry-flavored gelatin	1 env.★
¼ c.	cold water	60 mL
½ c.	boiling water	125 mL
dash	salt	dash
1 c.	prepared nondairy whipped topping	250 mL
2	egg whites, stiffly beaten	2
12	whole strawberries	12 whole

Crush the 2 c. (500 mL) of strawberries. Set aside. Soften strawberry gelatin in cold water for 5 minutes. Add boiling water and then stir to dissolve gelatin. Stir in salt. Allow to cool to room temperature, but do not allow to set. Fold in the crushed strawberries. Cool until mixture is soft but no longer runny. Fold nondairy whipped topping and beaten egg whites into strawberry gelatin. (If mixture is too soft, chill until it holds a soft shape.) Divide mixture evenly among the 12 tart shells. Chill thoroughly. Just before serving, top each tart with a whole strawberry.

Yield: 12 servings

Exchange, 1 serving (without crust): ⅓ fruit
Each serving contains: Calories: 20, Carbohydrates: 5 g

★four-servings size

Strawberry Cheese Tarts

10	prepared tart shells	10
3 oz.	cream cheese	90 g
¼ c.	half-and-half	60 mL
3 T.	granulated sugar replacement	45 mL
2 c.	sliced fresh strawberries	500 mL
10 T.	prepared nondairy whipped topping	150 mL

Beat cream cheese and half-and-half together until stiff and smooth. With the back of a spoon or a small knife, line the tart shell with the cream cheese mixture. Combine sugar replacement and strawberries in a bowl. Toss to mix. Divide the strawberries evenly among the 10 tart shells. Top each tart with 1 T. (15 mL) of nondairy whipped topping.

Yield: 10 servings

Exchange, 1 serving (without crust): ¼ fruit, ⅔ fat
Each serving contains: Calories: 51, Carbohydrates: 3 g

Pumpkin Chiffon Tarts

12	prepared tart shells	12
1 env.	unflavored gelatin	1 env.
⅔ c.	granulated brown sugar replacement	180 mL
1 t.	pumpkin pie spice	5 mL
3	egg yolks, slightly beaten	3
⅔ c.	skim milk	180 mL
1 c.	canned pumpkin	250 mL
3	egg whites, stiffly beaten	3

Combine gelatin, brown sugar replacement, and pie spice in a saucepan. Combine egg yolks and milk, mixing to blend. Pour into the saucepan. Stir to blend mixture. Allow gelatin to soften for 5 minutes. Bring mixture to boiling; then remove from heat and stir in canned pumpkin. Allow to cool until mixture holds a soft shape (do not allow to set). Fold in stiffly beaten egg whites. Divide mixture evenly among the 12 tart shells. Chill thoroughly before serving.

Yield: 10 servings

Exchange, 1 serving (without crust): ⅓ fruit
Each serving contains: Calories: 19, Carbohydrates: 3 g

Pineapple Tarts

	unbaked double crust	
2 c.	canned crushed pineapple, in its own juice, but drained	500 mL
2 T.	juice from crushed pineapple	30 mL
¼ c.	fresh sweet cherries	60 mL
¼ t.	grated lemon rind	1 mL

Roll out dough into a square. Cut into eight 5 in. (12 cm) squares. Arrange dough squares in muffin pans. Combine remaining ingredients in a bowl. Divide mixture evenly among the dough squares. Draw the corners of the squares together over the filling; then pinch the edges together. Bake at 425°F (220°C) for 20 to 25 minutes or until golden brown.

Yield: 8 servings

Exchange, 1 serving (without crust): ½ fruit
Each serving contains: Calories: 27, Carbohydrates: 7 g

Raisin Nut Tarts

8	unbaked tart shells	8
⅓ c.	low-calorie margarine	90 mL
½ c.	granulated sugar replacement	125 mL
3	egg yolks, beaten	3
1	egg white, stiffly beaten	1
1 c.	chopped raisins	250 mL
1 c.	chopped walnuts	250 mL
1 t.	vanilla extract	5 mL

Cream margarine and sugar replacement together. Beat in egg yolks. Fold in stiffly beaten egg white. Next, add raisins, walnuts, and vanilla. Divide evenly between the eight tart shells. Bake at 350°F (175°C) for 10 to 15 minutes or until tops become slightly browned.

Yield: 8 servings

Exchange, 1 serving (without crust): 1 fruit, 1⅓ fat
Each serving contains: Calories: 199, Carbohydrates: 14 g

Pistachio Pineapple Tart

A real treat for the eyes and taste buds.

1	phyllo dough tart shell for 12 in. (30 cm) tart, baked	1
1 pkg.	sugar-free pistachio no-cook pudding mix	1 pkg.
1¾ c.	skim milk	435 mL
20 oz.	pineapple slices, packed in juice, drained	565 g
8 t.	fresh cherries, pitted	40 mL

Prepare the phyllo tart shell. Put the phyllo shell on a dessert plate. Put the pudding mix into a medium mixing bowl. Add the milk and combine according to the directions on the package. Spoon into the tart shell. Dry the drained pineapple slices on paper towels. Arrange them on the pistachio pudding. Put the cherries in the center.

Yield: 10 servings

Exchange, 1 serving: 1 starch/bread; ½ fruit
Each serving contains: Calories: 105, Total fat: 0.6 g, Carbohydrates: 24 g, Protein: 2 g, Sodium: 85 mg, Cholesterol: 1 mg

Chocolate Tart Filling

You might want to use this plain, as an alternative to the chocolate-fruit combination.

¼ c.	sugar	60 mL
3 pkgs.	acesulfame-K or saccharin	3 pkgs.
2 T.	cocoa powder, unsweetened	30 mL
3 T.	cornstarch	45 mL
1¾ c.	skim milk	435 mL
1 t.	vanilla extract	5 mL
1 t.	crème de cacao liqueur (optional)	5 mL

Combine the sugar, sugar substitute, cocoa powder, and cornstarch in a medium saucepan. Add a small amount of the milk. Stir with a wire whisk until the mixture is evenly moistened. Add the remainder of the milk, the vanilla extract, and the crème de cacao, if desired. Cook, stirring constantly until filling is thick and you can see whisk marks as you stir. Cool before pouring into tart shell. Makes 2 cups (500 mL).

Yield: 10 servings

Exchange, 1 serving: ⅔ starch/bread
Each serving contains: Calories: 56, Total fat: 0.3 g, Carbohydrates: 1 g, Protein: 2 g, Sodium: 54 mg, Cholesterol: 1 mg

Vanilla Tart Filling

This has the taste and consistency of a bakery tart filling. It's easy to prepare.

1¾ c.	skim milk	435 mL
2 T.	butter or margarine	30 mL
3 T.	cornstarch	45 mL
2 T.	sugar	30 mL
3 pkgs.	acesulfame-K	3 pkgs.
1 large	egg or equivalent egg substitute	1 large
1 T.	vanilla extract	15 mL

Heat the milk and butter over simmering water in the top of a double boiler. In a bowl, mix together the cornstarch, sugar, and acesulfame-K. Add the egg and then the vanilla, blending well after each addition. Pour the cornstarch mixture into the warm milk. Mix with a wire whisk over simmering water until the mixture is thick. When the whisk leaves patterns, the pudding is finished cooking. Cool before using. Makes 2 cups (500 mL).

Yield: 10 servings

Exchange, 1 serving: ½ starch/bread; ½ fat
Each serving contains: Calories: 63, Total fat: 3 g, Carbohydrates: 7 g, Protein: 2 g, Sodium: 52 mg, Cholesterol: 28 mg

Chocolate Pear Tart

Since this uses canned pears, you can make it anytime.

1	phyllo dough tart shell for 12 in. (30 cm)	1
2 c.	Chocolate Tart Filling	500 mL
15 oz	pear halves in water, no added sugar, drained	430 g

Prepare the phyllo tart shell. Spoon the chocolate filling into the tart shell. Slice the pears thin (if this has not been done by the processor.) Put the slices onto paper towels to dry. Arrange the pears on the chocolate filling starting at the outside edge. Make a floral pattern in the center. This may be refrigerated for an hour before serving.

Yield: 10 servings

Exchange, 1 serving: 1 starch/bread
Each serving contains: Calories: 85, Total fat: 0.7 g, Carbohydrates: 17 g, Protein: 2 g, Sodium: 82 mg, Cholesterol: 1 mg

Chocolate Raspberry Tart

Chocolate and raspberry are a wonderful combination. You can make this all year round since the fresh raspberries are optional.

1	phyllo dough tart shell for 12 in. (30 cm)	1
¼ c.	seedless raspberry preserves, fruit only (no sugar added)	60 mL
2 c.	Chocolate Tart Filling (optional: add 2 T. (30 mL) crème de cacao)	500 mL
½ c.	frozen lo-fat nondairy whipped topping, thawed (optional)	125 mL
¼ c.	fresh seedless raspberries (optional)	60 mL

Prepare the phyllo tart shell. Smooth the raspberry preserves on the bottom of the inside of the tart shell. Spoon the chocolate filling on top of the preserves. Garnish with whipped topping and raspberries, if desired. May be refrigerated an hour or two before serving.

Yield: 10 servings

Exchange, 1 serving: 1 starch/bread
Each serving contains: Calories: 87, Total fat: 0.7 g, Carbohydrates: 18 g, Protein: 2 g, Sodium: 82 mg, Cholesterol: 1 mg

Banana Walnut Tart

A great solution for those ripe bananas.

1	phyllo dough tart shell for 12 in. (30 cm)	1
¼ c.	finely chopped walnuts	60 mL
2 c.	Vanilla Tart Filling	500 mL
2 large	large ripe bananas	2 large
1 t.	lemon juice	5 mL
3	mint leaves (optional)	3

Prepare the phyllo tart shell. Mix the walnuts into the Vanilla Tart Filling before spooning it into the tart shell. Slice the bananas into a bowl. Add the lemon juice and, using a fork, toss gently to coat. Arrange the bananas in a spiral pattern on top of the filling. When you come around to the starting slice, move in one and repeat. A few mint leaves strategically placed in the center make a nice touch. May be refrigerated an hour or two before serving.

Yield: 10 servings

Exchange, 1 serving: 1 starch/bread, 1 fat
Each serving contains: Calories: 120, Total fat: 5 g, Carbohydrates: 16 g, Protein: 3 g, Sodium: 80 mg, Cholesterol: 28 mg

Tangerine Tart

A nice winter treat when tangerines are at their sweetest and cheapest!

1	phyllo dough tart shell for 12 in. (30 cm)	1
2 c.	Vanilla Tart Filling, except use 1 t. (5 mL) orange extract and 1 t. (5 mL) vanilla extract instead of 1 T. (15 mL) vanilla extract	500 mL
5	tangerines, peeled	5
5	cherries, pitted	5
2 T.	shredded coconut meat (optional)	30 mL

Prepare the phyllo tart shell. Spoon the Vanilla Tart Filling into the prepared shell. Remove any white strings or rind from the tangerine segments and separate the segments. Slice the inner skin carefully and slip out any seeds. Arrange the tangerine segments as spokes of wheels with a cherry in the center of each group on top of the tart filling. Sprinkle coconut over the top of the tangerine-and-cherry pattern. May be refrigerated an hour or two before serving.

Yield: 10 servings

Exchange, 1 serving: 1 starch/bread; ½ fat
Each serving contains: Calories: 99, Total fat: 3 g, Carbohydrates: 15 g, Protein: 2 g, Sodium: 80 mg, Cholesterol: 28 mg

Peach and Raspberry Tart

This is easy to create but looks fabulous. Try it when raspberries are in season.

1	phyllo dough tart shell for 12 in. (30 cm)	1
2 c.	Vanilla Tart Filling (optional: use Triple Sec instead of vanilla extract)	500 mL
15 oz. can	sliced peaches, packed without sugar in fruit juice	420 g can
1 c.	fresh raspberries	250 mL

Prepare the phyllo tart shell. Spoon the Vanilla Tart Filling into the tart shell. Drain the peaches and dry them on paper towels. Lay the peach slices on them flat-side-down, making a swirling pattern on the outside of the tart. Make a circle of raspberries inside. Then make a flower of peach slices and raspberries in the center. May be refrigerated for an hour before serving.

Yield: 10 servings

Exchange, 1 serving: 1 starch/bread; ½ fat
Each serving contains: Calories: 88, Total fat: 3 g, Carbohydrates: 13 g, Protein: 2 g, Sodium: 54 mg, Cholesterol: 28 mg

Strawberry-Kiwi Tart

1	phyllo dough tart shell for 12 in. (30 cm)	1
2 c.	Vanilla Tart Filling	500 mL
3 large	ripe kiwis, peeled and sliced	3 large
1 c.	strawberries, hulled	250 mL

Prepare the phyllo tart shell. Spoon the Vanilla Tart Filling into the prepared tart shell. Arrange the kiwi slices around the edge of the tart. Stand a circle of strawberries inside the kiwi circle. Arrange the remaining fruit on the inside of the tart. Serve immediately. This may be refrigerated for an hour or two.

Yield: 10 servings

Exchange, 1 serving: 1 starch/bread; ½ fat
Each serving contains: Calories: 98, Total fat: 4 g, Carbohydrates: 14 g, Protein: 2 g, Sodium: 81 mg, Cholesterol: 28 mg

Orange Tart

If you use Triple Sec, it's very elegant.

1	phyllo dough tart shell for 12 in. (30 cm)	1
2 c.	Vanilla Tart Filling, except use 1 t. (5 mL) or 2 t. (10 mL) Triple Sec in place of the vanilla extract	500 mL
2	sweet oranges, peeled	2

Prepare the phyllo tart shell. Spoon the tart filling into the tart shell. Pull any white strings off the oranges. With a sharp knife cut away any white areas. These will be bitter, so cut them away ruthlessly. Cut the orange crosswise into thin slices. Lay the slices in an overlapping pattern covering the entire surface of the tart. May be refrigerated for an hour or two before serving.

Yield: 10 servings

Exchange, 1 serving: 1 starch/bread; ½ fat
Each serving contains: Calories: 90, Total fat: 3 g, Carbohydrates: 14 g, Protein: 2 g, Sodium: 80 mg, Cholesterol: 28 mg

July 4th Tart

The red, white, and blue pattern is very patriotic. Sometimes we try to arrange the fruit in a flag design.

1	phyllo dough tart shell for 12 in. (30 cm)	1
2 c.	Vanilla Tart Filling	500 mL
1 c.	fresh blueberries	250 mL
1 c.	fresh whole strawberries, hulled	250 mL

Prepare the phyllo tart shell. Spoon the Vanilla Tart Filling into the prepared shell. Arrange the blueberries in a circle around the edge. Put the strawberries in a line across diagonally. Do this again to divide the tart into four sections. Arrange any remaining fruit in patterns in the open areas. May be refrigerated for an hour or two.

Yield: 10 servings

Exchange, 1 serving: 1 starch/bread; ½ fat
Each serving contains: Calories: 92, Total fat: 3 g, Carbohydrates: 13 g, Protein: 2 g, Sodium: 81 mg, Cholesterol: 28 mg

Fresh Apple Tarts

	Margarine Pastry	
3 large	tart apples, peeled, cored, paper-thinly sliced	3 large
3 T.	Mazola regular or unsalted margarine, melted	45 mL
1 T.	brown sugar	15 mL
¼ t.	ground cinnamon	1 mL
2 T.	confectioners' sugar	30 mL

Divide Margarine Pastry into eight sections. Between 2 sheets waxed paper, roll each pastry section into a 5½ in. (14 cm) circle. Place oil cookie sheets. Slightly flute edge. Top each pastry round with apple slices in overlapping rows. Stir together next 3 ingredients. With pastry brush coat apple slices with margarine mixture. Bake at 425°F (220°C) for 10 to 12 minutes or until golden brown. Sift confectioners' sugar over top. Broil 6 in. (15 cm) from heat for 1 minute or until bubbly. Serve warm.

Yield: 8 tarts

Exchange, 1 tart: 2 bread, 1 fat
Each serving contains: Calories: 158, Carbohydrates: 33 g

Pies

issing from most discussions of pie is an honest acknowledgment of how high the fat content is. One small slice of a traditional two-crust pie has more than three fat exchanges, and that's just the crust. These numbers assume that a standard nine-inch pie is cut into eight slices. If you eat one-sixth of a two-crust pie, you get four fat exchanges, again for just the crust portion.

What to do about this depressing pie crust news? It's up to you to decide how many calories and fat exchanges you are willing to spend on pie crust—to follow, there are a range of fat levels and calories. The current standard practice is that one serving is one-eighth of a nine-inch pie.

Many of the following recipes separate crusts from the recipes for fillings. You decide which crust you wish to pair with which filling. Be sure to combine the calories, exchanges, etc., for the total.

For meringue pie crust, the crust portion of one slice is only 30 calories. There is no fat or cholesterol, and there are no exchanges. The trade-off is that with a meringue pie crust, you have to plan ahead and give it time to cook and cool, although it is very easy to do. Another trade-off is that a meringue pie crust can be unexciting.

Next best, in terms of fat and calorie scores, is the cottage cheese-based pie crust. One slice of this crust has only 52 calories and 2.8 grams of fat, for half a fat exchange.

After that, the next best is a graham cracker crust. One slice is only 86 calories and 2.2 grams of fat, also half a fat exchange.

Next comes a flour-based pie crust which uses half margarine and half nonfat cream cheese. One slice of a pie with a bottom crust only has 97 calories and 4.3 grams of fat. It looks beautiful, but it is not as flaky as a traditional lard and flour pie crust.

When you use all margarine for a flour-based pie crust, one slice of bottom-crust-only pie has 140 calories and 8.5 grams of fat. A slice from a pie with a top and bottom crust has 241 calories and 15.5 grams of fat. All these figures are for the crust portion only.

Some other crust suggestions: You can use phyllo dough to make a nice top crust; the cost per slice is low in calories. It is not recommended to use phyllo dough for a bottom crust; the dough dissolves into an unattractive goo. The idea of putting a fruit filling into an empty pie pan and then covering it with phyllo dough may seem strange when you first hear about it, but it works quite well and is low in calories.

Creamy Prune Pie Filling

The combination of prunes, lemon flavor, and cardamom makes a special "European" dish.

10 pkts.	concentrated acesulfame-K	10 pkts.
⅓ c.	flour	90 mL
pinch	salt (optional)	pinch
2 c.	skim milk	500 mL
⅓ c.	egg substitute	90 mL
1 c.	nonfat sour cream	250 mL
1 t.	vanilla extract	5 mL
2 t.	grated lemon peel	10 mL
1 t.	lemon juice	5 mL
½ c.	pitted prunes, cut into small pieces	125 mL

Topping

3	egg whites	3
¼ t.	cream of tartar	1.25 mL
2 t.	sugar	10 mL
3 pkts.	concentrated acesulfame-K	3 pkts.
½ t.	cardamom	2.5 mL

Combine the 10 packets of acesulfame-K, flour, and salt in a saucepan. Add the milk and stir to combine. Bring to a boil and cook for 1–2 minutes, stirring with a wire whisk. Turn off the heat. In a separate container, add a small amount of the hot milk and the egg substitute. Return this to the saucepan and cook for several minutes over low heat, stirring with a wire whisk. Let cool for a few minutes. Add the sour cream, vanilla extract, lemon peel, lemon juice, and prune pieces. Whisk together. Pour into a prepared pie shell or into an empty 9 in. (23 cm) pan if you wish to reduce calories.

Then prepare the topping. Beat the egg whites with an electric mixer, add in the cream of tartar near the end. Then beat in the sugar, acesulfame-K, and cardamom. Spread the meringue over the top of the pie. Use a rubber spatula to be sure the topping goes all the way to the edges. Bake in a preheated 350°F (180°C) oven for 13 minutes. Cool in the refrigerator.

Yield: 8 servings

Exchange, 1 serving: 1 milk
Each serving contains: Calories: 97, Carbohydrates: 16 g, Fiber: trace, Sodium: 110 mg, Cholesterol: 5 mg

Not-Quite-American Apple (or Cherry) Pie

This is an example of how to combine a dough or crust recipe with a filling recipe.

4 pieces	phyllo dough	4 pieces	
4 c.	apple or cherry filling (from this book)	1 L	

First make the fruit filling. Turn the filling into a 9 in. (23 cm) pie pan that has been coated with non-stick vegetable cooking spray. Set aside. Following the general instructions for using phyllo dough, spread one sheet of dough onto a work surface and coat it with cooking spray. Spread the second sheet of dough over the first. Spray. Repeat until there are four layers on top of one another. Lift these four layers together and center them over the fruit-filled pie pan. Use a pair of clean scissors to trim away all but one in. (2.5 cm) around the edge of the dough. Use your fingers to crimp together the edge to reassemble a traditional pie crust. Bake in a preheated 375°F (190°C) oven for 15 minutes or until the top is nicely browned. Watch carefully that it does not overcook.

Yield: 8 servings

Each serving contains: Carbohydrates: 65 g

Apple Pie Filling for Pie or Tarts

The sweetness of the filling depends on the type of apple you choose.

4 c.	apple, peeled, sliced thin	1 L
1 T.	cinnamon	15 mL
1 t.	nutmeg	5 mL
1 T.	vanilla extract	15 mL
2 T.	lemon juice	30 mL
6 pkts.	concentrated acesulfame-K	6 pkts.
1 t.	grated lemon peel	5 mL

Put the apple slices into a large non-stick pan that has been coated with non-stick cooking spray. Cover and cook for about 10 minutes. Stir occasionally. When the apple slices are soft, add the remaining ingredients and stir to mix.

This recipe makes enough for one 9 in. (23 cm) pie or 12 tarts.

Yield: 8 servings

Exchange, 1 serving: 1½ fruit
Each serving contains: Calories: 89, Carbohydrates: 15 g, Fiber: 4 g, Sodium: 1 mg, Cholesterol: 0 mg

Cherry Pie Filling

Be sure to buy cherries packed in water or juice with no sugar.

2 (14.5 oz) cans	cherries, in water	2 (411 g) cans
3 T.	quick-cooking tapioca	45 mL
5 pkts.	concentrated acesulfame-K	5 pkts.
¼ t.	almond extract	1 mL
5 drops	red food coloring	5 drops
1 t.	lemon peel	5 mL

Drain the cherries, reserving ⅓ c. (90 mL) of the liquid. Whisk together all the remaining ingredients, then let the mixture thicken for 15 minutes. Use a two-crust pastry recipe for the crust or use the phyllo recipe below.

To make a cherry pie with a phyllo dough crust, follow the general instructions for phyllo dough. Spread out one layer and coat it with non-stick cooking spray. Top it with a second layer, and spray. Repeat until there are four layers on top of one another. Lift the dough onto the fruit in the pie pan. Coat with non-stick cooking spray. Use scissors to trim away all but one in. (2.5 cm) around the edge. Use your fingers to crimp it in to form an edge. Bake in a preheated 375°F (190°C) oven for 15 minutes.

Yield: 8 servings

Exchange, 1 serving: 1 fruit
Each serving contains: Calories: 55, Carbohydrates: 12 g, Fiber: trace, Sodium: 1.3 mg, Cholesterol: 0 mg

Lemon Chiffon Pie Filling

If you like a light, tart lemon chiffon pie, this easy recipe is for you. It's perfect on a hot summer evening. Our friend Marge thinks it's wonderful after a lobster dinner.

1 env.	unflavored gelatin	1 env.
6 pkts.	concentrated acesulfame-K	6 pkts.
4	eggs, separated	4
½ c.	lemon juice (fresh is best)	125 mL
¼ c.	water	60 mL

Thoroughly mix the gelatin and three packets of acesulfame-K in the top of a double boiler. Beat together the egg yolks, lemon juice, and water; add this to the gelatin.

Cook the mixture over boiling water, stirring constantly until the gelatin is dissolved, about 5 minutes. Remove from the heat. Chill, stirring occasionally until the mixture mounds slightly when dropped from a spoon. Beat the egg whites until stiff. Beat in the remaining acesulfame-K. Fold the gelatin mixture into the stiffly beaten egg whites. Turn into a baked pie shell, if desired. Chill until firm.

Yield: 8 servings

Exchange, 1 serving: ½ meat
Each serving contains: Calories: 46, Carbohydrates: 0 g, Fiber: trace, Sodium: 38 mg, Cholesterol: 137 mg

Frozen Raspberry Pie Filling

This is another of Marion's recipes, modified for diabetic use. It tastes very rich and creamy.

½ c.	sugar-free, reduced-fat vanilla ice cream	375 mL
½ c.	raspberries	125 mL
1	prepared pie crust	1

Allow the ice cream to soften at room temperature for approximately an hour; add the raspberries and process until smooth in a food processor. Pour into a pie crust shell. Freeze. Allow the pie to soften for a few minutes at room temperature before serving.

Yield: 8 servings

Exchange, 1 serving: ½ bread
Each serving contains: Calories: 41, Carbohydrates: 17 g, Fiber: trace, Sodium: 17 mg, Cholesterol: 6 mg

Blueberry Pie Filling

Everyone we know likes blueberry pie. If you can afford the calories and fat exchanges, put this filling between a bottom and top pie crust. If you want a lighter version, put just the filling in an empty pie pan and top it with a phyllo crust. This filling is great in a turnover made from phyllo dough.

12 oz. bag	frozen blueberries	356 g bag
3 pkts.	concentrated acesulfame-K	3 pkts.
1½ T.	cornstarch dissolved in 2 T. (30 mL) water	22 mL
½ t.	vanilla extract	2 mL
½ T.	lemon juice	7 mL
¼ t.	cinnamon	1 mL

Partially defrost the blueberries at room temperature or in a microwave oven for 60 seconds. Combine all the other ingredients in a saucepan, add the blueberries, and heat over medium heat, stirring constantly until the mixture thickens.

Yield: 8 servings

Exchange, 1 serving: ½ fruit
Each serving contains: Calories: 23, Carbohydrates: 7 g, Fiber: trace, Sodium: 2 mg, Cholesterol: 0 mg

Pistachio Pineapple Pie Filling

This is very quick to put together and sets up quickly too. It's the type of recipe that makes non-cooks feel successful.

2 pkg.	sugar-free pistachio pudding mix	2 pkg.
2¼ c.	nonfat milk	560 mL
1 t.	almond extract	5 mL
8 oz. can	crushed pineapple (in unsweetened juice)	250 mL can
1	prepared pie shell	1

Combine the pudding, milk, and almond extract and beat with an electric mixer for one minute. Add the pineapple and its juice and beat for an additional minute. Pour into a prepared pie shell.

Yield: 8 servings

Exchange, 1 serving: 1 bread
Each serving contains: Calories: 71, Fiber: trace, Sodium: 366 mg, Cholesterol: 1.1 mg

Sheer Delight Pie Filling

This dessert is rich and delicious, a special-occasion treat. It's great in a baked graham cracker crust.

1 pkg.	sugar-free, fat-free instant pudding	1 pkg.
1½ c.	nonfat sour cream	310 mL
1 T.	rum extract	15 mL
2 T.	measures-like-sugar aspartame	30 mL
2 T.	nonfat milk	30 mL
8 oz. can	crushed unsweetened pineapple in juice, drained	1 pkg.
½ c.	flaked coconut	125 mL
1	prepared pie shell	1
	banana slices (optional)	
	whipped topping (optional)	

Combine instant pudding, sour cream, rum extract, aspartame, and milk in a medium bowl. Beat the mixture with a wire whisk until blended and smooth, about a minute, then fold in the pineapple and coconut. Spoon everything into a pie shell. Chill for three hours. Before serving, garnish with sliced bananas or your favorite topping (optional).

Yield: 8 servings

Exchange, 1 serving: 1 bread + 1 fat + 1 fruit
Each serving contains: Calories: 181, Fiber: 2 g, Sodium: 227 mg, Cholesterol: 6 mg

Tutti-Frutti Pie

Count the calories and exchanges for the pie crust separately from the filling, depending on which crust you choose. If you choose no crust, just pour the mixture into a pie pan and chill it; you save yourself the trouble of making a crust, and you save calories. This filling is really good and it's quick and easy.

1 env.	plain gelatin	1 env.
2 T.	cold water	30 mL
¾ c.	nonfat cottage cheese	190 mL
⅓ c.	boiling water	90 mL
¼ c.	skim milk	60 mL
2 t.	vanilla extract	10 mL
½ t.	almond extract	2.5 mL
1 t.	concentrated aspartame	10 mL
1 lb.	light mixed fruit chunks, drained	450 g

Sprinkle the gelatin over the cold water. Set aside to soften for a few minutes. Meanwhile, put the cottage cheese into a food processor or blender and process for a full 2 minutes to make it very creamy. Add the boiling water to the softened gelatin. Stir until the gelatin is completely dissolved. Add this mixture, milk, extracts, and aspartame to the blender. Blend until the mixture is smooth. Put the canned fruit into the food processor or blender and blend for a few seconds. Pour into a pie crust or into a plain pie pan. Chill until set.

Yield: 8 servings

Exchange, 1 serving: ½ bread
Each serving contains: Calories: 52, Fiber: trace, Sodium: 7 mg, Cholesterol: 2 mg

Luscious Strawberry Pie Filling

If you can find sugar-free, nonfat frozen yogurt, use it as a base for other flavors. By itself it's a little unexciting, but strawberries bring their own special taste.

2 c.	frozen whole strawberries with no sugar added	500 mL
1 t.	sugar	5 mL
1 t.	concentrated aspartame	5 mL
1 t.	lemon juice	5 mL
1 c.	boiling water	250 mL
1 pkg. (.3 oz.)	triple berry sugar-free gelatin	1 pkg. (8.5 g)
2 t.	strawberry extract	10 mL
1 pint	sugar-free vanilla nonfat yogurt	475 mL
1	prepared pie shell	1

Mix the strawberries in a bowl with the sugar, aspartame, and lemon juice. Set aside for approximately an hour. Combine the boiling water and gelatin and stir until completely dissolved. Add the strawberry extract and stir to combine. Add the frozen yogurt and stir until it melts and the mixture is smooth. Freeze for 10 minutes, until the gelatin starts to set. Add the strawberries. Pour into a pie shell of your choice. Refrigerate. Serve when set.

Yield: 8 servings

Exchange, 1 serving: 1 fruit
Each serving contains: Calories: 58, Fiber: trace, Sodium: 63 mg, Cholesterol: 0 mg

Quick Banana Cream Pie Filling

This would be a good project for a cook-in-training. You just can't go wrong. Banana cream pie is traditionally served in a flour-based bottom crust.

1	banana, ripe, sliced thin	1
3 c.	skim milk	750 mL
2 pkgs.	sugar-free fat-free vanilla pudding	2 pkgs.

Place the banana slices in the bottom of the pie shell of your choice. Using an electric mixer, combine the milk and pudding. Pour the mixture over the banana slices. Chill until serving time. Add additional thin slices of banana or whipped topping just before serving, if desired.

Yield: 8 servings

Exchange, 1 serving: 1 bread
Each serving contains: Calories: 70, Fiber: trace, Sodium: 377 mg, Cholesterol: 1.5 mg

Golden Treasure Pie Filling

This is a sugar-free version of an old family favorite. Karin served this on New Year's Day, and no one guessed it was sugar-free.

2 T.	cornstarch	30 mL
2 T.	water	30 mL
3 pkts.	concentrated saccharin	3 pkts.
3 pkts.	concentrated acesulfame-K	3 pkts.
1 T.	margarine	15 mL
2 T.	sifted flour	30 mL
½ c.	nonfat cottage cheese	125 mL
1 t.	vanilla extract	5 mL
1	egg white or egg	1
¾ c.	nonfat milk	190 mL
2 (8½ oz.) cans	crushed pineapple, packed in juice, undrained	2 (256 g) cans

Combine the cornstarch and water in a small saucepan. Bring to a boil, then cook one minute, stirring constantly. Cool. Stir in the saccharin. In a mixing bowl, blend the acesulfame-K and margarine. Add the flour, cottage cheese, and vanilla. Beat until smooth. Slowly add the egg, and then the milk, to the cheese mixture, beating constantly. Pour the pineapple into a 10-in. (25 cm) crust, if desired, spreading the mixture evenly. Gently pour the cottage cheese over the pineapple, being careful not to disturb the first layer. Bake at 450°F (230°C) for 15 minutes, then reduce the heat to 325°F (160°C) and bake for 45 minutes longer.

Yield: 10 servings

Exchange, 1 serving: 1 bread
Each serving contains: Calories: 68, Carbohydrates: 24 g, Fiber: trace, Sodium: 36 mg, Cholesterol: 1.3 mg

Boston Cream Pie

No one will ever guess this is a diabetic dessert. Your guests will be impressed.

2 c.	cake flour	500 mL
1 T.	baking powder	15 mL
¼ t.	salt (optional)	1 mL
1 c.	egg substitute	250 mL
⅓ c.	sugar	90 mL
6 pkts.	concentrated saccharin	6 pkts.
1½ t.	vanilla extract	7 mL
½ t.	butter-flavored extract	2 mL
⅓ c.	canola oil	90 mL
1 c.	egg whites at room temperature	250 mL
½ t.	cream of tartar	2 mL

Cream Filling

1½ c.	skim milk	375 mL
1 pkg.	fat-free, sugar-free vanilla instant pudding	1 pkg.

Sift together the flour, baking powder, and salt. Set aside. In a separate bowl, beat the egg substitute until light and fluffy. Add the sugar, saccharin, vanilla and butter extracts. Add the oil. Add the flour mixture. In another bowl, beat the egg whites until thick. Add the cream of tartar and continue beating until stiff. Stir about one-third of the stiff egg whites into the flour mixture to tighten. Then fold in the remaining egg whites. Pour into 2 8 in. (20 cm) cake pans that have been coated with non-stick cooking spray. Bake in a preheated 350°F (180°C) oven for 25 minutes or until done.

To make the cream filling: Mix together the milk and pudding mix until thick. Spread half the cream filling between the layers.

Boston Cream Pie (continued)

Chocolate Topping

½	Cream Filling	½
1 T.	cocoa	15 mL

To make the chocolate topping: Combine the other half of the cream topping with cocoa. Spread on top of the cream pie.

Yield: 12 servings

Exchange, 1 serving: 1 bread, 1 milk
Each serving contains: Calories: 172, Carbohydrates: 44 g, Fiber: 0.5 g, Sodium: 63 mg, Cholesterol: 0.5 mg

Chocolate Cream Pie

2½ c.	skim milk	625 mL
2 oz.	baking chocolate	60 g
2 T.	flour	30 mL
3 T.	cornstarch	45 L
¼ c.	granulated sugar replacement	60 mL
½ t.	salt	2 mL
4	egg yolks, beaten	4
1 T.	butter	15 mL
1½ t.	vanilla extract	7 mL
10 in.	Basic Pie Shell, baked	25 cm
1c.	low-calorie whipped topping	250 mL

Combine 2 c. (500 mL) of the milk with baking chocolate in top of double boiler. Cook and stir over simmering water until chocolate has melted and mixture is smooth. Sift together twice the flour, cornstarch, sugar replacement and salt. Mix flour mixture with remaining ½ c. (125 mL) milk. Add to chocolate mixture, stirring constantly, until thickened. Cook 10 minutes longer. Remove from heat, gradually add some of the chocolate mixture to the beaten egg yolks, then stir into the pan and return to heat. Cook 2 minutes longer; remove from heat, add butter and vanilla. Pour into baked pie shell. Chill in refrigerator until cool and set. Decorate with whipped topping.

Yield: 8 servings

Exchange, 1 serving: ¾ bread, 2 fat plus pie crust exchange
Each serving contains: Calories: 147 plus pie crust calories, Carbohydrates: 35 g

Angel Pie

Crust

4	egg whites	4
¼ t.	cream of tartar	1 mL
3 T.	granulated sugar replacement	45 mL

Filling

4	egg yolks	4
3 T.	granulated sugar replacement	45 mL
1 oz.	baking chocolate, melted	30 g
dash	salt	dash
1c.	low-calorie whipped topping	250 mL

Beat egg whites until frothy; add cream of tartar and sugar replacement. Beat until stiff. Line a 9 in. (23 cm) pie pan with meringue mixture. Bake at 275°F (135°C) for 45 minutes.

Beat egg yolks in top of double boiler; add sugar replacement, baking chocolate and salt. Cook and stir until thick, about 10 minutes. Cool. Fold in whipped topping. Pour mixture into angel shell.

Yield: 8 servings

Exchange, 1 serving: ½ bread, 1 fat plus pie crust exchange
Each serving contains: Calories: 70 plus pie crust calories, Carbohydrates: 14 g

South Seas Pie

¼ c.	unsweetened coconut, shredded	60 mL
9 in.	Basic Pie Shell, unbaked	23 cm
1 c.	water	250 mL
2 T.	cornstarch	30 mL
⅓ c.	mini chocolate chips	90 mL
4	eggs, slightly beaten	4
2 T.	granulated sugar replacement	30 mL
¼ t.	salt	1 mL
1½ t.	vanilla extract	7 mL
1 c.	unsalted macadamia nuts, finely chopped	250 mL

Press unsweetened coconut into bottom and sides of unbaked pie shell. Set aside. Combine water and corn-starch in saucepan, cook and stir over medium heat until mixture is thick and clear. Remove from heat and stir in mini chocolate chips. Cool to room temperature. Add eggs, sugar replacement, salt and vanilla extract. Beat with electric mixer until fluffy; fold in macadamia nuts. Pour into pie shell. Bake 325°F (165°C) for 40 to 45 minutes or until filling is set. Cool.

Yield: 8 servings

Exchange, 1 serving: ¾ bread, 3 fat plus pie crust exchange
Each serving contains: Calories: 186 plus pie crust calories, Carbo-hydrates: 49 g

Creamy Custard Pie

2 c.	skim milk	500 mL
¼ c.	flour	60 mL
¼ c.	cocoa	60 mL
⅛ t.	salt	.5 mL
3 T.	granulated sugar replacement	45 mL
3	egg yolks	3
1 T.	butter	15 mL
1 T.	vanilla extract	15 mL
8 in.	Basic Pie Shell, baked	20 cm

Scald 1 c. (250 mL) of the milk. Mix dry ingredients with remaining milk. Add to hot milk and cook until custard coats the spoon, about 15 minutes. Add butter and vanilla. Stir to blend. Remove from heat. When partially cooled, pour into baked pie shell. Chill thoroughly before serving.

Yield: 8 servings

Exchange, 1 serving: ½ bread, 1 fat plus pie crust exchange
Each serving contains: Calories: 81 plus pie crust calories, Carbo-hydrates: 42 g

Banana Chocolate Pie

⅓ c.	flour	90 mL
3 T.	granulated sugar replacement	45 mL
⅛ t.	salt	.5 mL
2 c.	skim milk, scalded	500 mL
3	egg yolks, beaten	3
1 T.	butter	15 mL
1 t.	vanilla extract	5 mL
2	bananas, sliced	2
¼ c.	mini chocolate chips	60 mL
9 in.	Basic Pie Shell, baked	23 cm

Combine flour, sugar replacement, and salt in top of double boiler. Blend in milk slowly. Cook until thickened. Add beaten egg yolks and cook 2 minutes longer, stirring constantly. Remove from heat, add butter and vanilla extract. Cool. Add sliced bananas and chocolate chips. Fold to completely blend. Turn into baked pie shell. Chill for at least 2 hours before serving.

Yield: 8 servings

Exchange, 1 serving: ¾ lean meat, ½ fruit plus pie crust exchange
Each serving contains: Calories: 129 plus pie crust calories, Carbo-hydrates: 34 g

Maple-Nut Chocolate Pie

A New England turnabout.

1 env.	unflavored gelatin	1 env.
2 T.	cold water	30 mL
½ c.	skim milk	125 mL
⅓ c.	low-calorie maple syrup	90 mL
¼ c.	semisweet mini chocolate chips	60 mL
⅛ t.	salt	.5 mL
2	egg yolks	2
1 c.	low-calorie whipped topping	250 mL
2	egg whites, beaten stiff	2
¼ c.	walnuts, chopped	60 mL
9 in.	Basic Pie Shell, baked	23 cm

Soften gelatin in water. Combine milk, syrup, chocolate chips, salt, and egg yolks in top of double boiler. Cook and stir until mixture is thickened. Add gelatin and stir to dissolve completely. Allow to cool. Fold whipped topping into mixture. Fold egg whites into mixture. Fold in nuts and pour mixture into baked pie shell. Refrigerate until set.

Yield: 8 servings

Exchange, 1 serving: 1 bread, 1 fat plus pie crust exchanges
Each serving contains: Calories: 106 plus pie crust calories, Carbohydrates: 21 g

Coconut Chocolate Pie

3 T.	cocoa	45 mL
2 T.	granulated sugar replacement	30 mL
3	eggs, well beaten	3
⅛ t.	salt	½ mL
1 t.	vanilla extract	5 mL
¼ c.	unsweetened coconut, chopped	60 mL
2 c.	skim milk, scalded	500 mL
9 in.	Basic Pie Shell, unbaked	23 cm

Blend cocoa, sugar replacement, eggs, salt, vanilla, and coconut. Add scalded milk slowly. Pour into unbaked pie shell. Bake at 425°F (220°C) for 40 minutes or until set.

Yield: 8 servings

Exchange, 1 serving: ⅓ bread, ½ fat plus pie crust exchange
Each serving contains: Calories: 64 plus pie crust calories, Carbohydrates: 32 g

Coffee Chiffon Pie

The coffee is what makes it GOOD.

1 c.	skim evaporated milk	250 mL
½ c.	very strong coffee	125 mL
1 env.	unflavored gelatin	1 env.
¼ c.	cold water	60 mL
3	eggs separated	3
3 T.	granulated sugar replacement	45 mL
3 T.	cocoa	45 mL
⅛ t.	salt	½ mL
¼ t.	nutmeg	1 mL
½ t.	vanilla extract	2 mL
2 T.	chocolate sprinkles or jimmies	30 mL
9 in.	Basic Pie Shell, baked	23 cm

Scald milk and coffee. Sprinkle gelatin on cold water, allow to soften. Beat egg yolks, sugar replacement, cocoa, salt, and nutmeg. Slowly add hot milk and coffee mixture. Add vanilla and softened gelatin. Chill until partially set. When mixture is partially set, beat well. Beat egg whites until stiff. Fold into cooled chocolate-coffee mixture. Pour into baked pie shell. Sprinkle top with chocolate sprinkles. Chill 2 to 3 hours or until firm.

Yield: 8 servings

Exchange, 1 serving: ¼ bread, ½ fat plus pie crust exchange
Each serving contains: Calories: 55 plus pie crust calories, Carbohydrates: 22 g

Peanut Butter Pie

1¼ c.	hot water	60 mL
¼ c.	creamy peanut butter	60 mL
1 oz.	baking chocolate	30 g
¼ c.	sorbitol	60 mL
2 T.	granulated sugar replacement	30 mL
1¼ c.	skim evaporated milk	310 mL
3 T.	flour	45 mL
3 T.	cornstarch	45 mL
2	egg yolks, slightly beaten	2
1 t.	vanilla extract	5 mL
9 in.	Basic Pie Shell, baked	23 cm

Combine water, peanut butter and baking chocolate in top of double boiler. Cook and stir over simmering water until peanut butter and chocolate are melted. Stir in sorbitol and granulated sugar replacement. In a bowl, blend milk, flour and cornstarch together until smooth; gradually pour into chocolate mixture. Cook and stir until thickened. Pour small amount of chocolate mixture into beaten egg yolks and stir. Add egg mixture to pan. Cook and stir 2 minutes longer. Remove from heat; stir in vanilla. Cool slightly. Pour into baked pie shell. Chill in refrigerator until set, at least 2 hours.

Yield: 8 servings

Exchange, 1 serving: 1 high-fat meat, 1 fat, ½ fruit plus pie crust exchange
Each serving contains: Calories: 138 plus pie crust calories, Carbohydrates: 8 g

White Raisin Pie

Thank you, Mrs. Danalo.

¼ c.	water	190 mL
¼ c.	semisweet chocolate chips	60 mL
1 c.	white raisins (sultanas)	250 mL
½ c.	skim evaporated milk	125 mL
1 t.	vanilla extract	5 mL
1 T.	granulated sugar replacement	15 mL
¼ c.	cornstarch	60 mL
⅛ t.	salt	½ mL
⅛ t.	cinnamon	½ mL
2	eggs	2
9 in.	Basic Pie Shell, unbaked	23 cm

Place water in heavy saucepan and bring to boil. Add chocolate chips and white raisins. Remove from heat, cover and allow to rest 15 minutes. Return to heat and add milk; warm slightly. Remove from heat and stir in vanilla extract. Mix together sugar replacement, cornstarch, salt and cinnamon. Stir into chocolate mixture. Beat eggs with electric mixer until frothy; stir into chocolate mixture. Pour into unbaked pie shell. Bake at 375°F (190°C) for 40 to 45 minutes or until set. Cool.

Yield: 8 servings

Exchange, 1 serving: 1½ bread, ½ fat plus pie crust exchange
Each serving contains: Calories: 121 plus pie crust calories, Carbohydrates: 34 g

Triple Decker Pie

Pretty and different—nice to serve.

9 in.	Chocolate Crust, unbaked	23 cm
Layer 1		
2	eggs	2
¼ c.	milk chocolate chips, melted	60 mL
dash	salt	dash
1 t.	vanilla extract	5 mL
1 c.	skim milk	250 mL
Layer 2		
1 c.	skim milk	250 mL
2 T.	flour	30 mL
1.5 oz.	baking chocolate	45 g
2 T.	sugar replacement	30 mL
2	egg yolks, slightly beaten	2
1 t.	vanilla extract	5 mL

Layer 1: Have the unbaked pie crust ready. Beat eggs in medium bowl until well blended. Add melted chocolate, salt, and vanilla extract. Beat one more minute. Stir in milk. Pour into pie shell. Bake at 300°F (150°C) for 50 minutes or until a knife inserted in center comes out clean. Cool.

Layer 2: Combine milk, flour, baking chocolate and sugar replacement in top of double boiler; cook and stir over medium heat until mixture thickens. Pour a small amount of chocolate mixture into egg yolks, then add to the large amount in the pan. Cook and stir until mixture is thick. Remove from heat and cover with waxed paper. When almost cool, remove paper and spread onto baked custard layer. Cool completely.

Triple Decker Pie *(continued)*

Layer 3

2 env.	unflavored gelatin	2 env.
¾ c.	water	190 mL
3 T.	sorbitol	45 mL
or		
2 T.	granulated sugar replacement	30 mL
2 t.	white vanilla extract	10 mL
2	egg whites	2

Layer 3: In a saucepan, sprinkle gelatin over water, allow to soften for 5 minutes. Place pan over medium heat and bring to a boil. Cook until gelatin is dissolved. Remove from heat, add sorbitol and white vanilla. Stir to blend completely. Allow to cool until mixture is consistency of thick syrup. Beat egg whites into soft peaks. With a slow stream, add gelatin mixture, beating constantly into stiff peaks. Spread over entire surface of pie. Chill until firm.

Yield: 8 servings

Exchange, 1 serving: 1 high-fat meat , 1 fruit, ½ fat plus pie crust exchange
Each serving contains: Calories: 125 plus pie crust calories, Carbohydrates: 66 g

Pecan Chocolate Chip Pie

½ c.	butter, softened	125 mL
2 T.	granulated sugar replacement	30 mL
3	eggs	3
1 t.	vanilla extract	5 mL
1 T.	flour	15 mL
⅓ c.	semisweet chocolate chips	90 mL
¼ c.	pecans, chopped	60 mL
10 in.	Basic Pie Shell, unbaked	25 cm

Cream butter and sugar replacement in large bowl until fluffy. Beat in eggs and vanilla extract. Add flour and blend until smooth; fold in chocolate chips and pecans. Pour mixture into unbaked pie shell. Bake at 325°F (165°C) for about 50 minutes or until center is set and top is golden.

Yield: 8 servings

Exchange, 1 serving: 1 high-fat meat, 3 fat, ½ fruit plus pie crust exchange
Each serving contains: Calories: 220 plus pie crust calories

Perfection Pie

3 T.	chocolate chips	45 mL
⅓ c.	water, boiling	90 mL
3	eggs	3
1 T.	cornstarch	15 mL
3 T.	granulated sugar replacement	45 mL
2 T.	vegetable shortening, melted	30 mL
8 in.	Basic Pie Shell, unbaked	20 cm

Melt chocolate chips in boiling water; set aside to cool. Beat eggs; blend in cornstarch and sugar replacement. Continue beating and add the shortening and, gradually, the chocolate mixture. Pour into pie shell. Bake at 400°F (200°C) for about 35 minutes or until custard is set.

Yield: 8 servings

Exchange, 1 serving: ⅓ bread, 1 fat plus pie crust exchange
Each serving contains: Calories: 86 plus pie crust calories, Carbohydrates: 19 g

Gooseberry Pie

	unbaked double crust	
3 c.	gooseberries	750 mL
¾ c.	granulated fructose	190 mL
3½ T.	quick-cooking tapioca	52 mL
1 T.	low-calorie margarine	15 mL

Slightly crush the gooseberries. Stir in fructose and tapioca. Transfer to 9 in. (23 cm) pastry-lined pie pan. Dot with margarine. Adjust top crust, flute or pinch edges, and cut slits in top to allow steam to escape. Bake at 425°F (220°C) for 40 to 45 minutes or until lightly browned.

Yield: 8 servings

Exchange, 1 serving (without crust): 2 fruit
Each serving contains: Calories: 122, Carbohydrates: 28 g

Wild Blueberry Pie

9 in.	baked pie shell	23 cm
5 T.	granulated fructose	75 mL
3 T.	cornstarch	45 mL
dash	salt	dash
¼ c.	water	60 mL
1 qt.	wild blueberries*	1 L
1 T.	low-calorie margarine	15 mL

Combine fructose, cornstarch, and salt in heavy nonstick saucepan. Add water and 1½ c. (375 mL) of the blueberries. Cook over medium heat until mixture thickens. Remove from heat and stir in margarine. Pour remaining 2½ c. (625 mL) of the blueberries into bottom of baked shell. Top with blueberry glaze. Chill thoroughly.

Yield: 8 servings

Exchange, 1 serving (without crust): 1 fruit, ⅓ fat
Each serving contains: Calories: 75, Carbohydrates: 16 g

*Fresh cultivated blueberries can be substituted for wild blueberries.

Summer Mulberry Pie

	unbaked double crust	
5 T.	granulated fructose	75 mL
¼ c.	all-purpose flour	60 mL
2 T.	cornstarch	30 mL
dash	salt	dash
1 qt.	mulberries, cleaned	1 L
2 T.	low-calorie margarine	30 mL

Combine fructose, flour, cornstarch, and salt in a bowl. Toss to mix. Sprinkle half of mixture into bottom of 9 in. (23 cm) pastry-lined pie pan. Fill with mulberries. Sprinkle remaining mixture over top. Dot with margarine. Adjust top crust, flute or pinch edges, and cut slits in top to allow steam to escape. Bake at 425°F (220°C) for 40 to 50 minutes or until lightly browned.

Yield: 8 servings

Exchange, 1 serving (without crust): 1 fruit, ½ fat
Each serving contains: Calories: 91, Carbohydrates: 17 g

Fresh Elderberry Pie

	unbaked double crust	
4 c.	elderberries, cleaned	1000 mL
1 T.	cider vinegar	15 mL
½ c.	granulated sugar replacement	125 mL
⅓ c.	all-purpose flour	90 mL
2 t.	cornstarch	10 mL
dash	salt	dash

Place elderberries into bottom of 9 in. (23 cm) pastry-lined pie pan. Sprinkle with vinegar. Combine sugar replacement, flour, cornstarch, and salt in medium-size bowl. Stir to blend. Sprinkle mixture over berries. Adjust top crust, flute or pinch edges, and cut slits in top to allow steam to escape. Bake at 400°F (200°C) for 35 to 45 minutes or until lightly browned.

Yield: 8 servings

Exchange, 1 serving (without crust): 1 fruit
Each serving contains: Calories: 69, Carbohydrates: 15 g

Purple Plum Pie

9 in.	unbaked pie shell	23 cm
1 qt.	sliced purple plums	1 L
⅓ c.	granulated sugar replacement	90 mL
¼ c.	all-purpose flour	60 mL
2 t.	cider vinegar	10 mL

Combine plums, sugar replacement, flour, and cider vinegar in a large bowl. Toss to mix. Transfer to pie shell. Place pie in a baking bag, and fasten bag securely. Bake at 425°F (220°C) for 50 to 60 minutes. Remove bag from oven. Allow pie to cool inside the bag until lukewarm. Remove pie from bag to cooling rack.

Yield: 8 servings

Exchange, 1 serving (without crust): 1 fruit
Each serving contains: Calories: 58, Carbohydrates: 15 g

Fresh Raspberry Pie

	baked pie shell	
1 qt.	fresh raspberries	1 L
1 c.	cold water	250 mL
½ c.	granulated fructose	125 mL
3 T.	cornstarch	45 mL
1 t.	fresh lemon juice	5 mL

Wash and thoroughly drain raspberries. Combine 1 c. (250 mL) of the raspberries, water, fructose, and cornstarch in nonstick saucepan. Stir to blend. Cook and stir over medium heat until thickened. Remove from heat and add lemon juice. Cool to lukewarm. Pour the remaining 3 c. (750 mL) of drained raspberries into bottom of baked pie shell. Top with raspberry glaze. Chill until firm.

Yield: 8 servings

Exchange, 1 serving (without crust): 1 fruit
Each serving contains: Calories: 68, Carbohydrates: 16 g

Fresh Tart-Cherry Pie

	unbaked double crust	
½ c.	granulated fructose	125 mL
⅓ c.	all-purpose flour	90 mL
¼ c.	granulated sugar replacement	60 mL
1 qt.	pitted tart cherries	1 L
2 or 3 drops	almond extract	2 or 3 drops
2 T.	low-calorie margarine	30 mL

Combine fructose, flour, and sugar replacement in a large bowl. Add cherries and almond extract. Toss to coat. Transfer cherry mixture to bottom of 9 in. (23 cm) pastry-lined pie pan. Dot with margarine. Adjust top crust, flute or pinch edges, and cut slits in top to allow steam to escape. Bake at 425°F (220°C) for 40 to 50 minutes or until lightly browned.

Yield: 8 servings

Exchange, 1 serving (without crust): 1 fruit, ⅓ bread
Each serving contains: Calories: 106, Carbohydrates: 22 g

Fresh Sweet Cherry Pie

9 in.	baked pie shell	23 cm
1 qt.	pitted sweet cherries	1 L
½ c.	granulated sugar replacement	125 mL
3 T.	cornstarch	45 mL
dash	salt	dash
1 t.	lemon juice	5 mL

Place sweet cherries in medium-size bowl. With the back of a spoon, push to extract the juice. Drain juice into medium-size saucepan. Reserve cherries. Add sugar replacement, cornstarch, and salt to cherry juice in saucepan. Stir to blend. Cook and stir over medium heat until clear and thickened. Remove from heat, and stir in lemon juice. Cool to lukewarm. Fold cherries into cooled glaze. Chill to re-thicken. Transfer to baked pie shell. Chill until firm.

Yield: 8 servings

Exchange, 1 serving (without crust): 1 fruit
Each serving contains: Calories: 64, Carbohydrates: 15 g

Peach Pie

	unbaked double crust	
2 (1 lb.) cans	sliced peaches, in their own juice	2 (489 g) cans
2 T.	granulated fructose	30 mL
3 T.	cornstarch	45 mL
½ t.	nutmeg	2 mL
dash	salt	dash
⅛ t.	almond extract	½ mL

Drain juice from peaches into a saucepan by pushing down lightly on peaches in can. Transfer peaches from can to strainer, allowing any excess juice to run off. Add fructose, cornstarch, nutmeg, salt, and almond extract to juice in saucepan. Cook and stir over medium heat until clear and thickened. Arrange peaches in the bottom of a 9 in. (23 cm) pastry-lined pie pan. Pour juice mixture over peaches. Adjust top crust, and pinch or flute edges; then cut in vents to allow steam to escape. Bake at 400°F (200°C) for 40 to 45 minutes.

Yield: 8 servings

Exchange, 1 serving (without crust): 1 fruit
Each serving contains: Calories: 66, Carbohydrates: 16 g

Apple 'n' Cheese Pie

	unbaked double crust	
6 c.	sliced apples (peeled)	1500 mL
1 T.	apple juice	15 mL
⅓ c.	granulated fructose	90 mL
2 T.	all-purpose flour	30 mL
¾ t.	apple pie spice	4 mL
¼ lb.	grated sharp cheddar cheese	120 g

Combine apples and apple juice in bowl, and toss to mix. Combine fructose, flour, and apple pie spice in another bowl. Stir to mix. Sprinkle a third of the fructose mixture on bottom of 8 in. (20 cm) pastry-lined deep-dish pie pan. Transfer apple and juice to pie pan. Sprinkle with remaining fructose mixture. Top with grated cheese. Adjust top crust, and flute or pinch edges. Then score top to allow steam to escape. Bake at 400°F (200°C) for 50 to 60 minutes or until top becomes lightly browned.

Yield: 8 servings

Exchange, 1 serving (without crust): 1½ fruit, ⅓ whole milk
Each serving contains: Calories: 162, Carbohydrates: 27 g

Nectarine Pie

	unbaked double crust	
5 c.	sliced nectarines (peeled)	1250 mL
1 t.	lemon juice	5 mL
½ c.	granulated fructose	125 mL
⅓ c.	all-purpose flour	90 mL
¼ t.	nutmeg	1 mL
1 T.	low-calorie margarine	15 mL

Combine nectarines, lemon juice, fructose, flour, and nutmeg in a large bowl. Toss to mix. Transfer to 9 in. (23 cm) pastry-lined pie pan. Dot with margarine. Adjust top crust, and pinch or flute edges; then cut in vents to allow steam to escape. Bake at 425°F (220°C) for 40 to 50 minutes.

Yield: 8 servings

Exchange, 1 serving (without crust): 1⅔ fruit
Each serving contains: Calories: 104, Carbohydrates: 24 g

Fresh Pineapple Pie

	unbaked double crust	
3½ c.	fresh pineapple chunks	875 mL
2	eggs, slightly beaten	2
¾ c.	granulated sugar replacement	190 mL
2½ T.	all-purpose flour	37 mL
1 T.	grated lemon zest	15 mL
1 t.	lemon juice	5 mL
dash	salt	dash

Put pineapple chunks in bottom of 9 in. (23 cm) pastry-fined pie pan. Combine eggs, sugar replacement, flour, lemon zest, lemon juice, and salt in bowl. Beat to blend. Pour over pineapple chunks. Adjust top crust, and pinch or flute edges; then cut in vents to allow steam to escape. Bake at 425°F (220°C) for 40 to 50 minutes.

Yield: 8 servings

Exchange, 1 serving (without crust): 1 fruit
Each serving contains: Calories: 63, Carbohydrates: 10 g

Strawberry and Rhubarb Pie

	unbaked double crust	
⅔ c.	sorbitol	180 mL
⅓ c.	all-purpose flour	90 mL
½ t.	grated fresh orange zest	2 mL
2 c.	fresh strawberries	500 mL
2 c.	cubed fresh rhubarb	500 mL
2 T.	low-calorie margarine	30 mL

Combine sorbitol, flour, and orange zest in a bowl. Stir to mix. Place half of the strawberries and half of the rhubarb in the bottom of a 9 in. (23 cm) pastry-lined pie pan. Sprinkle with half of the sorbitol-flour mixture. Arrange the remaining fruit in the pie pan. Sprinkle with remaining sorbitol-flour mixture. Dot with margarine. Adjust top crust, and pinch or flute edges, then cut in vents to allow steam to escape. Bake at 425°F (220°C) for 40 to 50 minutes.

Yield: 8 servings

Exchange, 1 serving (without crust): ½ fruit
Each serving contains: Calories: 25, Carbohydrates: 7 g

Dried-Fruit Pie

	unbaked double crust	
½ c.	dried apricots	125 mL
½ c.	dried prunes	125 mL
⅓ c.	raisins	90 mL
¼ c.	orange juice	60 mL
⅛ t.	mace	½ mL

Pour boiling water over apricots and prunes, and allow to sit for 3 minutes. Drain and cover with a bath of cold water. Allow to soften for 3 hours. Then drain the liquid into a saucepan. Cut fruit into quarters, and put in saucepan with liquid. Cook and stir until fruit is completely softened and liquid is reduced to about ⅓ c. (90 mL). Remove from heat, and stir in raisins, orange juice, and mace. Transfer to 8 or 9 in. (20 or 23 cm) pastry-lined pie pan. Adjust top crust, and pinch or flute edges; then cut in vents to allow steam to escape. Bake at 400°F (200°C) for 30 to 35 minutes.

Yield: 8 servings

Exchange, 1 serving (without crust): 1 fruit
Each serving contains: Calories: 60, Carbohydrates: 15 g

Cream Pie

8 in.	baked pie shell	20 cm
⅓ c.	granulated sugar replacement	90 mL
3 T.	cornstarch	45 mL
dash	salt	dash
½ c.	cold skim milk	125 mL
1½ c.	scalded skim milk	375 mL
3	egg yolks, beaten	3
2 t.	vanilla extract	10 mL
1 recipe	meringue topping	1 recipe

Combine sugar replacement, cornstarch, and salt in the top of a double boiler. Stir in cold milk to dissolve cornstarch. Slowly add scalded milk. Place over hot water. Cook and stir until mixture thickens. Pour small amount of thickened mixture into beaten egg yolks, stirring to mix. Return to pan. Cook 4 to 5 minutes longer. Stir in vanilla. Remove from heat and allow to cool. Transfer to baked pie shell. Top with meringue, sealing edges. Bake at 350°F (175°C) for 7 to 10 minutes or until peaks are browned.

Yield: 8 servings

Exchange, 1 serving (no crust): 1 low-fat milk
Each serving contains: Calories: 58, Carbohydrates: 6 g

Apricot Cream Pie

8 in.	baked pie shell	20 cm
¼ c.	granulated sugar replacement	60 mL
3 T.	cornstarch	45 mL
dash	salt	dash
½ c.	cold skim milk	125 mL
1½ c.	scalded skim milk	375 mL
3	egg yolks, beaten	3
1 c.	apricot purée	250 mL
½ t.	vanilla extract	2 mL
2 c.	prepared nondairy whipped topping	500 mL

Combine sugar replacement, cornstarch, and salt in the top of a double boiler. Stir in cold milk to dissolve cornstarch. Slowly add scalded milk. Place over hot water. Cook and stir until mixture thickens. Pour small amount of thickened mixture into beaten egg yolks, stirring to mix. Return to pan. Cook 4 to 5 minutes longer. Stir in apricot purée and vanilla. Cook for 2 minutes. Remove from heat and allow to cool. Transfer to baked pie shell. Cool thoroughly. Top with nondairy whipped topping.

Yield: 8 servings

Exchange, 1 serving (without crust): ¾ fruit, low-fat milk
Each serving contains: Calories: 103, Carbohydrates: 18 g

Fresh-Peach Cream Pie

8 in.	baked pie shell	20 cm
4	fresh peaches	4
2 t.	lemon juice	10 mL
¼ c.	granulated fructose	60 mL
3 T.	cornstarch	45 mL
dash	salt	dash
½ c.	cold skim milk	125 mL
1½ c.	scalded skim milk	375 mL
3	egg yolks, beaten	3
1 t.	almond extract	5 mL

Pour boiling water over peaches. Peel, remove the pits, and cut into thin slices. Place sliced peaches into a bowl of ice water; then add lemon juice and stir. Combine fructose, cornstarch, and salt in the top of a double boiler. Stir in cold milk to dissolve cornstarch. Slowly add scalded milk. Place over hot water. Cook and stir until mixture thickens. Pour small amount of thickened mixture into beaten egg yolks, stirring to mix. Return to pan. Cook 4 to 5 minutes longer. Stir in almond extract. Remove from heat and allow to cool. Transfer to baked pie shell. Chill until top becomes firm. Thoroughly drain peach slices and then pat them dry. Arrange peach slices on top of pie.

Yield: 8 servings

Exchange, 1 serving (without crust): ⅓ fruit, ½ low-fat milk
Each serving contains: Calories: 78, Carbohydrates: 11 g

Pineapple Cream Pie

9 in.	baked pie shell	23 cm
1½ c.	crushed pineapple, in its own juice	375 mL
2 t.	cornstarch	10 mL
⅓ c.	granulated sugar replacement	90 mL
3 T.	cornstarch	45 mL
dash	salt	dash
½ c.	cold skim milk	125 mL
1½ c.	scalded skim milk	375 mL
3	egg yolks, beaten	3
1 t.	vanilla extract	5 mL
2 T.	grated semisweet chocolate	30 mL

Combine pineapple with juice and the 2 t. (10 mL) cornstarch in a saucepan. Stir to blend. Cook and stir over medium heat until mixture thickens. Set aside. Combine sugar replacement, the 3 T. (45 mL) cornstarch, and salt in the top of a double boiler. Stir in cold milk to dissolve cornstarch. Slowly add scalded milk. Place over hot water. Cook and stir until mixture thickens. Pour small amount of thickened mixture into beaten egg yolks, stirring to mix. Return to pan. Cook 4 to 5 minutes longer. Stir in vanilla. Remove from heat and allow to slightly cool. Pour just enough of the cream filling into pie shell to cover bottom. Spread pineapple filling on top. Allow to cool. Top with remaining cream filling. Then garnish with grated semisweet chocolate.

Yield: 8 servings

Exchange, 1 serving (without crust): ⅓ fruit, ½ low-fat milk
Each serving contains: Calories: 76, Carbohydrates: 6 g

Banana Cream Pie

8 in.	baked pie shell	20 cm
⅓ c.	granulated fructose	90 mL
3 T.	cornstarch	45 mL
dash	salt	dash
½ c.	cold skim milk	125 mL
1½ c.	scalded skim milk	375 mL
3	egg yolks, beaten	3
2 t.	vanilla extract	10 mL
3	sliced ripe bananas	3
1 recipe	meringue topping	1 recipe

Combine fructose, cornstarch, and salt in the top of a double boiler. Stir in cold milk to dissolve cornstarch. Slowly add scalded milk. Place over hot water. Cook and stir until mixture thickens. Pour small amount of thickened mixture into beaten egg yolks, stirring to mix. Return to pan. Cook 4 to 5 minutes longer. Stir in vanilla. Remove from heat and allow to cool completely. Alternate layers of sliced bananas and cream filling in pie shell, ending with bananas. Top with meringue, sealing edges. Bake at 350°F (175°C) for 5 to 7 minutes or until peaks become slightly browned.

Yield: 8 servings

Exchange, 1 serving (without crust): ¼ fruit, low-fat milk
Each serving contains: Calories: 95, Carbohydrates: 16 g

Raspberry Cream Pie

9 in.	baked pie shell	23 cm
1½ c.	skim milk	375 mL
¼ c.	granulated sugar replacement	60 mL
¼ t.	salt	1 mL
3 T.	all-purpose flour	45 mL
1	egg yolk, beaten	1
1 T.	low-calorie margarine	15 mL
½ t.	vanilla extract	2 mL
1 c.	fresh raspberries	250 mL
2 c.	prepared nondairy whipped topping	500 mL

Combine skim milk, sugar replacement, salt, and flour in a heavy saucepan. Cook and stir until mixture thickens. Stir small amount of mixture into beaten egg yolk; then return to saucepan. Cook and stir 1 or 2 minutes longer. Stir in margarine and vanilla. Remove from heat and allow to cool. Fold in fresh raspberries. Transfer to baked pie shell. Top with nondairy whipped topping. Chill.

Yield: 8 servings

Exchange, 1 serving (without crust): ¼ fruit
Each serving contains: Calories: 47, Carbohydrates: 11 g

Blackberry Cream Pie

8 in.	baked pie shell	20 cm
1½ c.	evaporated skim milk	375 mL
½ c.	granulated sugar replacement	125 mL
2 T.	cornstarch	30 mL
1 t.	lemon juice	5 mL
1½ c.	fresh blackberries	375 mL

Combine evaporated milk, sugar replacement, cornstarch, and lemon juice in the top of a double boiler. Stir to dissolve cornstarch. Place over simmering water; then cook and stir until mixture thickens. Allow to cool slightly; then fold in blackberries. Transfer to baked pie shell. Allow to cool.

Yield: 8 servings

Exchange, 1 serving (without crust): ¾ fruit
Each serving contains: Calories: 45, Carbohydrates: 9 g

Old-Fashioned Pumpkin Pie

9 in.	unbaked pie shell	23 cm
1¼ c.	canned pumpkin	310 mL
⅓ c.	granulated fructose	90 mL
1 c.	evaporated skim milk	250 mL
2	eggs	2
1 T.	cornstarch	15 mL
2 T.	cold water	30 mL
1 t.	cinnamon	5 mL
½ t.	nutmeg	2 mL
¼ t.	salt	1 mL
¼ t.	ginger	1 mL

Combine pumpkin, fructose, evaporated milk, and eggs in a large bowl. Beat to blend. Blend cornstarch in cold water. Beat into pumpkin mixture. Beat in cinnamon, nutmeg, salt, and ginger. Pour into unbaked pie shell. Bake at 400°F (200°C) for 45 to 50 minutes or until knife inserted in center comes out clean.

Yield: 8 servings

Exchange, 1 serving (without crust): 1¼ fruit
Each serving contains: Calories: 80, Carbohydrates: 18 g

Pecan Pumpkin Pie

9 in.	unbaked pie shell	23 cm
1 lb. can	canned pumpkin	458 g can
2	eggs	2
½ c.	granulated sugar replacement	125 mL
½ t.	salt	2 mL
1 t.	cinnamon	5 mL
½ t.	ginger	2 mL
¼ t.	cloves	1 mL
1½ c.	half-and-half	375 mL
1 recipe	Pecan Topping	1 recipe
3 1	dietetic maple syrup	45 mL

Combine pumpkin, eggs, sugar replacement, salt, cinnamon, ginger, cloves, and half-and-half in a large bowl. Beat to blend thoroughly. Pour into unbaked pie shell. Bake at 400°F (200°C) for 45 to 50 minutes or until knife inserted in center comes out clean. Sprinkle with Pecan Topping and dietetic maple syrup.

Yield: 8 servings

Exchange, 1 serving (without crust): ¾ low-fat milk, 1⅔ fat
Each serving contains: Calories: 167, Carbohydrates: 9 g

Pumpkin Meringue Pie

9 in.	unbaked pie shell	23 cm
1½ c.	canned pumpkin	375 mL
1½ c.	skim milk	375 mL
3	eggs	3
⅔ c.	granulated brown sugar replacement	180 mL
1¼ t.	cinnamon	6 mL
½ t. each	salt, ginger, nutmeg	2 mL each
1 recipe	meringue topping	1 recipe

Combine pumpkin, skim milk, eggs, brown sugar replacement, and spices in a large bowl. Beat to blend. Pour into unbaked pie shell. Bake at 400°F (200°C) for 45 to 50 minutes or until knife inserted in center comes out clean. Cool slightly. Spread meringue over pie, sealing edges. Bake at 350°F (175°C) for 10 to 12 minutes or until the peaks begin to brown.

Yield: 8 servings

Exchange, 1 serving (without crust): ½ low-fat milk
Each serving contains: Calories: 63, Carbohydrates: 7 g

Sweet Potato Pie

9 in.	unbaked pie shell	23 cm
2 c.	sweet potato purée	500 mL
2	eggs	2
½ c.	granulated sugar replacement	125 mL
2 T.	dietetic maple syrup	30 mL
1 t.	vanilla extract	5 mL
½ t. each	cinnamon, nutmeg, salt	2 mL each
1½ c.	skim milk	375 mL
1 recipe	meringue topping	1 recipe

Combine sweet potato purée, eggs, sugar replacement, maple syrup, vanilla, spices, and skim milk in a large bowl. Beat to blend. Pour into unbaked pie shell. Bake at 400°F (200°C) for 45 to 50 minutes or until knife inserted in center comes out clean. Cool slightly. Spread meringue over pie, sealing edges. Bake at 350°F (175°C) for 10 to 12 minutes or until the peaks begin to brown.

Yield: 8 servings

Exchange, 1 serving (without crust): 1 fruit
Each serving contains: Calories: 55, Carbohydrates: 12 g

Sliced Yam Pie

	unbaked double crust	
1 lb.	yams	500 g
2 med	apples	2 med
1 t.	lemon juice	5 mL
½ c.	granulated brown sugar replacement	125 mL
3 T.	granulated fructose	45 mL
½ t.	cinnamon	2 mL
½ t.	ginger	2 mL
dash	salt	dash
⅛ t.	cloves	½ mL
3 T.	low-calorie margarine	45 mL
½ c.	skim milk	125 mL

Boil yams until half-cooked; then cool with cold running water. Peel and slice. Peel, core, and slice apples. Combine yam and apple slices in a bowl. Sprinkle with lemon juice. Combine brown sugar replacement, fructose, cinnamon, ginger, salt, and cloves in a bowl. Stir to mix. Layer a third of the yam-and-apple slices mixture in the bottom of a 8 or 9 in. (20 or 23 cm) pastry-lined pie pan. Sprinkle with a third of the sugar replacement mixture; then dot with 1 T. (15 mL) of the margarine. Repeat these layers two more times. Pour skim milk over entire surface. Adjust top crust and seal edges securely. Bake at 425°F (220°C) for 35 to 45 minutes or until yams become soft.

Yield: 8 servings

Exchange, 1 serving (without crust): ½ starch/bread, ½ fruit
Each serving contains: Calories: 73, Carbohydrates: 15 g

Slip Custard Pie

9 in.	baked pie shell	23 cm
4	eggs, slightly beaten	4
2½ c.	warm skim milk	625 mL
¼ c.	granulated fructose	60 mL
1 t.	vanilla extract	5 mL
dash	salt	dash
½ t.	nutmeg	2 mL

Combine eggs, skim milk, fructose, vanilla, and salt in a bowl. Beat to blend. Pour mixture into a 9 in. (23 cm) pie pan. Sprinkle with nutmeg. Place the filled pie pan into another pan containing water. (Water should reach halfway up sides of pie pan.) Bake at 350°F (175°C) for 30 to 35 minutes or until knife inserted in center comes out clean. Cool to room temperature. Carefully loosen around the edge of the custard with a sharp knife or thin spatula. Gently shake pie pan to further loosen custard. Then slip custard from pie pan into baked pie shell.

Yield: 8 servings

Exchange, 1 serving (without crust): ½ medium-fat meat, ½ skim milk
Each serving contains: Calories: 89, Carbohydrates: 8 g

Coconut Custard Pie

9 in.	unbaked pie shell	23 cm
4	eggs, slightly beaten	4
2 c.	warm skim milk	500 mL
½ c.	granulated sugar replacement	125 mL
1 t.	vanilla extract	5 mL
⅓ c.	flaked coconut	180 mL

Combine eggs, skim milk, sugar replacement, and vanilla in a bowl. Beat to blend. Sprinkle ⅓ c. (90 mL) of the coconut on the bottom of the unbaked pie shell. Pour custard mixture over coconut. Top with remaining coconut. Bake at 350°F (175°C) for 30 to 35 minutes or until knife inserted in center comes out clean. Cool to room temperature.

Yield: 8 servings

Exchange, 1 serving (without crust): ½ medium-fat meat, 1 fat
Each serving contains: Calories: 82, Carbohydrates: 4 g

Vanilla Pie

9 in.	baked pie shell, chilled	23 cm
¾ c.	granulated sugar replacement	190 mL
5 T.	cornstarch	75 mL
1½ c.	boiling water	375 mL
3	egg whites	3
dash	salt	dash
1 T.	vanilla extract	15 mL
1 c.	prepared nondairy whipped topping	250 mL

Combine sugar replacement and cornstarch in a heavy saucepan. Slowly add boiling water, stirring constantly. Cook and stir until clear and thickened. Combine egg whites and salt in a large mixing bowl. Beat until stiff. Then beat in vanilla. Continue beating until whites are creamy. Slowly pour cornstarch mixture over egg whites, beating continually. Cool slightly. Transfer to baked pie shell. Cool completely. Top with whipped topping.

Yield: 8 servings

Exchange, 1 serving (without crust): ½ starch/bread
Each serving contains: Calories: 31, Carbohydrates: 6 g

Lemon Meringue Pie I

9 in.	baked pie shell	23 cm
¾ c.	granulated fructose	190 mL
1½ c.	water	375 mL
¼ t.	salt	1 mL
½ c.	cornstarch	125 mL
¼ c.	cold water	60 mL
4	egg yolks, slightly beaten	4
½ c.	freshly squeezed lemon juice	125 mL
3 T.	low-calorie margarine	45 mL
1½ t.	grated fresh lemon peel	7 mL
4	egg whites	4
dash	salt	dash
¼ c.	granulated sugar replacement	60 mL

Combine fructose, the 1½ c. (375 mL) water, and salt in a medium-size, heavy saucepan. Heat to boiling. Combine cornstarch and the ¼ c. (60 mL) cold water, stirring to blend thoroughly. Add to boiling mixture, stirring constantly. Cook and stir until mixture is clear and thickened. Remove from heat. Beat egg yolks and lemon juice together. Slowly stir into hot mixture. Return to heat and cook until mixture begins to boil. Stir in margarine and lemon peel. Cover and cool to room temperature. Beat egg whites and salt together until soft peaks form. Gradually add sugar replacement. Beat just until peaks are stiff. Pour lemon mixture into pie shell. Top with egg whites, sealing edges. Bake at 350°F (175°C) until peaks begin to brown.

Yield: 8 servings

Exchange, 1 serving (without crust): ½ medium-fat meat, ⅓ fruit
Each serving contains: Calories: 88, Carbohydrates: 6 g

Lemon Meringue Pie II

9 in.	baked pie shell	23 cm
1¼ c.	granulated sugar replacement	310 mL
7 T.	cornstarch	105 mL
¼ t.	salt	1 mL
1½ c.	water	375 mL
3	egg yolks, beaten	3
1 T.	low-calorie margarine	15 mL
1 t.	grated lemon peel	5 mL
½ c.	lemon juice	125 mL
1 recipe	Basic Meringue	1 recipe

Combine sugar replacement, cornstarch, salt, and water in a heavy saucepan. Stir to blend. Cook and stir over medium heat until mixture is clear and thickened. Remove from heat. Stir small amount of hot mixture into egg yolks; then return to saucepan. Cook and stir 2 to 3 minutes longer. Remove from heat and stir in margarine, lemon peel, and lemon juice. Cool slightly. Transfer to baked pie shell. Top with Basic Meringue, sealing edges. Bake at 350°F (175°C) for 7 to 10 minutes or until peaks begin to brown.

Yield: 8 servings

Exchange, 1 serving (without crust): ¾ medium-fat meat
Each serving contains: Calories: 42, Carbohydrates: 3 g

Lime Pie

9 in.	baked pie shell	23 cm
1 c.	sorbitol	250 mL
⅓ c.	cornstarch	90 mL
¼ t.	salt	1 mL
1½ c.	water	375 mL
3	egg yolks, beaten	3
¼ c.	freshly squeezed lime juice	60 mL
1 T.	grated fresh lime zest	15 mL
	green food coloring (optional)	
1 recipe	Basic Meringue	1 recipe

Combine sorbitol, cornstarch, and salt in heavy saucepan. Stir to mix. Slowly stir water into mixture. Cook and stir over medium heat until mixture is clear and thickened. Remove from heat. Pour small amount of hot mixture into egg yolks; then return to saucepan. Bring to boil and cook for 1 minute. Remove from heat. Stir in lime juice and lime zest. Add green food coloring, if desired. Transfer immediately to baked pie shell. Top with Basic Meringue, sealing edges. Bake at 350°F (175°C) for 7 to 10 minutes or until peaks begin to brown.

Yield: 8 servings

Exchange, 1 serving (without crust): ½ medium-fat meat, 1 fruit
Each serving contains: Calories: 103, Carbohydrates: 13 g

Open-Faced Green-Apple Pie

	baked pie shell	
6 c.	sliced green apples, peeled	1500 mL
½ c.	apple juice	125 mL
3 T.	all-purpose four	45 mL
8 T.	prepared nondairy whipped topping	120 mL

Combine apples, apple juice, and flour in a nonstick saucepan. Cook and stir until thickened. Transfer to baked pie shell. Chill or serve warm with 1 T. (15 mL) of the nondairy whipped topping on each slice.

Yield: 8 servings

Exchange, 1 serving (without crust): 1⅓ fruit
Each serving contains: Calories: 98, Carbohydrates: 22 g

Hot-Fudge Pie

9 in.	unbaked pie shell, chilled	23 cm
3 sq. (1 oz. each)	semisweet chocolate	3 sq. (30 g each)
⅓ c.	low-calorie margarine	90 mL
1 env.	butter-flavoring dry mix	1 env.
3	eggs, beaten	3
1 c.	sorbitol	250 mL
¼ c.	all-purpose flour	60 mL
2 t.	skim milk	10 mL
1 t.	vanilla extract	5 mL
dash	salt	dash

Combine chocolate and margarine in top of double boiler. Cook over boiling water until chocolate melts. Remove from heat and allow to cool to room temperature. Combine chocolate mixture, butter-flavoring mix, and eggs in large mixing bowl. Beat 10 to 15 minutes or until slightly thickened. Beat in sorbitol, flour, skim milk, vanilla, and salt. Transfer to unbaked pie shell. Bake at 375°F (190°C) for 35 to 40 minutes or until knife inserted in center comes out clean. Serve warm.

Yield: 8 servings

Exchange, 1 serving (without crust): ¾ fruit, ⅓ medium-fat meat, 1 fat
Each serving contains: Calories: 189, Carbohydrates: 12 g

Chocolate Chip Pie

9 in.	unbaked pie shell	23 cm
¼ c.	low-calorie margarine	60 mL
3	eggs, beaten	3
½ c.	liquid fructose	125 mL
¼ t.	salt	1 mL
1 t.	vanilla extract	5 mL
½ c.	chocolate chips	125 mL
¼ c.	chopped pecans	60 mL
2 T.	water	30 mL
2 t.	bourbon flavoring	10 mL

Cream margarine until light and fluffy. Beat in eggs, liquid fructose, salt, and vanilla. Continue beating 3 more minutes. Stir in chocolate chips, pecans, water, and bourbon flavoring. Transfer to unbaked pie shell. Bake at 375°F (190°C) for 35 to 40 minutes or until knife inserted in center comes out clean. Allow to cool.

Yield: 8 servings

Exchange, 1 serving (without crust): ½ fruit, ⅓ medium-fat meat, 1 fat

Each serving contains: Calories: 162, Carbohydrates: 6 g

Cocoa Pie

9 in.	unbaked pie shell	23 cm
¾ c.	granulated fructose	190 mL
¼ c.	cocoa powder	60 mL
dash	salt	dash
2	eggs	2
¼ c.	low-calorie margarine	60 mL
15 oz. can	evaporated skim milk	427 g can
2 t.	vanilla extract	10 mL

Combine fructose, cocoa, and salt in a bowl, stirring to mix thoroughly. Combine eggs, margarine, evaporated milk, and vanilla in a mixing bowl; then beat to blend. Add cocoa mixture in small amounts, beating well after each addition. Transfer to unbaked pie shell. Bake at 350°F (175°C) for 45 to 50 minutes or until knife inserted in center comes out clean. Cool before serving.

Yield: 8 servings

Exchange, 1 serving (without crust): ¾ fruit, ¼ medium-fat meat, ½ fat

Each serving contains: Calories: 162, Carbohydrates: 13 g

Mincemeat Pie

9 in.	unbaked Basic Pie Shell	23 cm
½ lb.	beef stew meat	250 g
2 med	apples	2 med
1	orange with rind	1
½	lemon with rind	½
¼ lb.	suet	125 g
½ c.	raisins	125 mL
½ c.	currants	125 mL
3 T.	granulated sugar replacement	45 mL
½ c.	orange juice	125 mL
½ t.	salt	2 mL
¼ t.	nutmeg	1 mL
dash	cinnamon	dash
dash	mace	dash

Prepare, but do not bake, pie shell. Place stew meat in covered saucepan; cover meat with water. Place over medium heat and cook about 1 hour, or until very tender. Drain thoroughly. Core apples and slice; cut orange and lemon into small pieces. Combine beef, suet, apples, orange, and lemon in food processor or food chopper, chopping into coarse-meal consistency. Pour back into saucepan, add remaining ingredients, cover and simmer over low heat for 1 hour. Pour into unbaked pie shell. Bake at 400°F (200°C) for 25 minutes.

Yield: 8 servings

Exchange, 1 serving: 1 bread, 1 high-fat meat, 2 fat, plus pie shell exchange
Each serving contains: Calories: 284 plus pie shell calories, Carbohydrates: 35 g

Raisin Pecan Pie

9 in.	unbaked Basic Pie Shell	23 cm
1½ c.	evaporated skimmed milk	375 mL
¼ c.	granulated sugar replacement	60 mL
1 T.	butter	15 mL
4	eggs	4
2 t.	cornstarch	10 mL
¼ t.	salt	1 mL
1 c.	pecans, chopped	250 mL
1 t.	vanilla extract	5 mL
⅓ c.	raisins	90 mL

Prepare, but do not bake, pie shell. Combine milk, sugar replacement, butter, eggs, cornstarch and salt in heavy saucepan. Cook and stir over medium-low heat until well blended and slightly thickened. Remove from heat, stir in pecans and vanilla and allow filling to rest 10 minutes. Sprinkle raisins on bottom of unbaked pie shell and pour pecan mixture over them. Bake at 375°F (190°C) for 45 to 50 minutes, or until knife inserted in center comes out clean.

Yield: 8 servings

Exchange, 1 serving: 1 full-fat milk, 1 fat, plus pie shell exchange
Each serving contains: Calories: 199 plus pie shell calories, Carbohydrates: 49 g

Chocolate Rum Pie

9 in.	baked Basic Pie Shell	23 cm
1 env.	unflavored gelatin	1 env.
1 c.	skim milk	250 mL
2	egg yolks	2
2 T.	granulated sugar replacement	30 mL
dash	salt	dash
¼ c.	cocoa	60 mL
2 t.	rum flavoring	10 mL
2	egg whites	2
1 T.	liquid sugar replacement	15 mL
2 c.	low-calorie whipped topping (prepared)	500 mL

Prepare and bake pie shell. Combine gelatin, milk, egg yolks, granulated sugar replacement, salt, and cocoa in heavy saucepan. Cook and stir over low heat until completely blended and slightly thickened. Remove from heat. Stir in rum flavoring and chill until partially set. Beat egg whites and liquid sugar replacement into stiff peaks and fold into cooled chocolate mixture. Layer chocolate mixture and topping into baked pie shell, ending with topping. Chill until firm.

Yield: 8 servings

Exchange, 1 serving: ½ high-fat meat, ⅓ fruit, plus pie shell exchange
Each serving contains: Calories: 74 plus pie shell calories, Carbo-hydrates: 8 g

Tart Rhubarb Soufflé Pie

9 in.	unbaked Basic Pie Shell	23 cm
1 qt.	rhubarb, cut into 1 in. (2.5 cm) pieces	1 L
⅓ c.	water	90 mL
1 env.	unsweetened strawberry drink mix	1 env.
2 T.	cornstarch	30 mL
¼ c.	granulated sugar replacement	60 mL
2	egg whites	2

Prepare, but do not bake, pie shell. Combine rhubarb and water in saucepan, and cook over medium heat until rhubarb is tender. Pour into blender or food processor, add strawberry drink mix, cornstarch and sugar replacement, and purée. Refrigerate to chill completely. Beat egg whites until stiff; beat rhubarb mixture to loosen. Blend egg whites into rhubarb mixture and pour into pie shell, spreading evenly. Attach a 2 in. (5 cm) collar of flour-dusted waxed paper. Preheat oven to 400°F (200°C); reduce heat to 375°F (190°C). Place pie in lower third of oven. Bake for 30 or 35 minutes. Insert wire cake tester in center; soufflé is done if tester comes out clean. (Place waxed paper over collar to keep top from getting too brown.)

Yield: 8 servings

Exchange, 1 serving: negligible plus pie shell exchange
Each serving contains: Calories: 12 plus pie shell calories, Carbo-hydrates: 26 g

Pumpkin Cheese Pie

9 in.	unbaked Basic Pie Shell	23 cm
Cheese Layer		
8 oz. pkg.	cream cheese (softened)	220 g pkg.
2 T.	granulated sugar replacement	30 mL
1 t.	vanilla extract	5 mL
1	egg	1
Pie Layer		
1½ c.	cooked pumpkin (unsweetened)	375 mL
1 c.	evaporated skimmed milk	250 mL
2	eggs	2
2 T.	granulated sugar replacement	30 mL
1 t.	cinnamon	5 mL
¼ t.	ginger	1 mL
¼ t.	nutmeg	1 mL

Prepare, but do not bake, pie shell. Combine cream cheese, sugar replacement, vanilla, and 1 egg in mixing bowl; stir to mix well. Spread in bottom of unbaked pie shell. Combine pumpkin, milk, 2 eggs, sugar replacement and spices in a mixing bowl or food processor, beating to blend thoroughly. Carefully pour over cheese layer. Bake at 350°F (175°C) for 65 to 70 minutes, or until knife inserted in center comes out clean.

Microwave: Cook on Medium for 20 to 25 minutes, or until edges are set and center is soft but not runny. Allow to rest 15 to 20 minutes before serving.

Yield: 8 servings

Exchange, 1 serving: 1 high-fat meat, 1 fat, ½ fruit, plus pie shell exchange
Each serving contains: Calories: 173 plus pie shell calories, Carbohydrates: 18 g

Black Bottom Lemon Cream Pie

	baked pastry shell	
2 pkgs.	sugar-free lemon gelatin	2 pkgs.
2 t.	grated lemon rind	10 mL
½ c.	sugarless carob drops	125 mL
1 c.	prepared nondairy whipped topping	250 mL

In a large bowl, prepare lemon gelatin as directed on package with the addition of the lemon rind. Set completely. Melt carob drops over hot water. Spread evenly over bottom of pastry shell. With an electric mixer, beat the set gelatin until fluffy. Beat in the nondairy whipped topping. Pile gelatin mixture into pastry shell. Chill thoroughly.

Yield: 8 servings

Exchange, 1 serving (without pastry shell): ½ bread
Each serving contains: Calories: 48, Carbohydrates: 8 g

Black Raspberry and Strawberry Layered Pie

	baked pastry shell	

Strawberry Layer

16 oz. bag	Flavorland frozen strawberries	453 g bag
⅔ c.	water	180 mL
2 T.	cornstarch	30 mL
2 T.	granulated fructose	30 mL
1 t.	strawberry flavoring	5 mL

Black Raspberry Layer

12 oz. bag	Flavorland frozen black raspberries	340 g bag
½ c.	water	125 mL
2 T.	cornstarch	30 mL
2 T.	granulated fructose	30 mL
1 t.	vanilla flavoring or extract	5 mL
½ t.	grated orange peel	2 mL

For strawberry layer: Remove four large frozen strawberries from bag. Set aside reserved strawberries and allow remaining strawberries to partially thaw. Combine water, cornstarch, fructose, and strawberry flavoring in a saucepan. Cook and stir over medium heat until mixture is a very thick paste. Mixture will not be clear. Fold partially frozen strawberries into paste mixture until all berries are coated and mixture is clear. (If not clear, return to stove and heat slightly. Cool completely.) Set aside.

For black raspberry layer: Partially thaw black raspberries. Combine water, cornstarch, fructose, vanilla, and orange peel in a saucepan. Cook and stir over medium heat until mixture is a very thick paste. Fold partially frozen black raspberries into paste mixture until all berries are coated and mixture is clear. (If not clear, return to stove and heat slightly. Cool completely before continuing.)

To complete pie: Transfer strawberry mixture to bottom of baked pastry shell. Arrange evenly. Top with black raspberry mixture. Cut the four reserved strawberries in half lengthwise, and decorate with the eight halves around the top of the pie. Chill thoroughly.

Yield: 8 servings

Exchange, 1 serving (without pastry shell): 1¼ fruit
Each serving contains: Calories: 72, Carbohydrates: 18 g

Lime Fluff Pie

	pastry shell, baked	
1 pkg.	sugar-free lime gelatin	1 pkg.
1 pkg.	vanilla-flavored sugar-free pudding mix	1 pkg.
2 c.	skim milk	500 mL

Prepare lime gelatin as directed on package. Pour into a medium-sized narrow bowl to chill. Refrigerate until completely set. Meanwhile, combine vanilla pudding mix and milk in a saucepan. Cook and stir over medium heat until mixture comes to a full boil. Cover and allow to cool. With an electric mixer, beat the set gelatin until frothy. Then beat the cooled pudding into the gelatin. Transfer mixture to prepared pie shell. Refrigerate until thoroughly set.

Yield: 8 servings

Exchange, 1 serving (without pastry shell): ⅓ bread
Each serving contains: Calories: 38, Carbohydrates: 6 g

Sweet Cherry Coconut Pie

	baked pastry shell	
2 bags (16 oz.)	Flavorland frozen dark sweet cherries	2 bags (453 g)
¾ c.	water	190 mL
3 T.	cornstarch	45 mL
2 T.	granulated fructose	30 mL
1 t.	lemon juice	5 mL
3 oz. pkg.	cream cheese, room temperature	86 g pkg.
⅓ c.	unsweetened grated or shredded coconut, toasted	90 mL

Partially thaw cherries. Combine water, cornstarch, fructose, and lemon juice in a saucepan. Cook and stir over medium heat until mixture is a very thick paste. Remove from heat and fold in cherries until all cherries are coated and mixture is clear. Set aside to cool. Spread softened cream cheese on the bottom of the baked pastry shell. Sprinkle with the toasted coconut. Press the coconut slightly into the cheese. Transfer sweet cherry mixture to the shell and arrange evenly. If desired, decorate with pastry cutouts. Chill thoroughly.

Yield: 8 servings

Exchange, 1 serving (without pastry shell): 1½ fruit, 1¼ fat
Each serving contains: Calories: 133, Carbohydrates: 22 g

Red Raspberry Pie

	baked pastry shell	
1 qt.	frozen unsweetened red raspberries	1 L
1 c.	water	250 mL
3 T.	cornstarch	45 mL
⅓ c.	granulated fructose	90 mL
2 t.	lemon juice	10 mL
3 oz. pkg.	cream cheese, room temperature	86 g pkg.
1 T.	skim milk	15 mL

Partially thaw red raspberries. Combine water, cornstarch, fructose, and lemon juice in a saucepan. Cook and stir over medium heat until mixture is very thick. Fold partially frozen raspberries into mixture until all berries are coated and mixture is evenly distributed throughout the berries. Set aside to cool. Combine cream cheese and milk, and beat to blend. Spread cream cheese mixture over bottom of baked pastry shell. Spread cooled berry mixture over cream cheese mixture. Chill until firm. If desired, serve with a dot of nondairy whipped topping on each piece of pie.

Yield: 8 servings

Exchange, 1 serving (without pastry shell): 1¾ fruit, ¼ fat
Each serving contains: Calories: 96, Carbohydrates: 11 g

Chocolate Raspberry Pie

	pastry shell, baked★	
2 pkgs.	chocolate-flavored sugar-free pudding mix	2 pkgs.
1 qt.	skim milk	1 L
2 c.	fresh raspberries	500 mL

Combine chocolate pudding mix and milk in a saucepan. Cook and stir over medium heat until mixture comes to a full boil. Allow to cool for 5 to 10 minutes or until pan can comfortably be held. Fold in raspberries. Transfer to pastry shell. Chill until thoroughly set and ready to serve.

Yield: 8 servings

Exchange, 1 serving (without pastry shell): ¾ skim milk, ¼ fruit
Each serving contains: Calories: 93, Carbohydrates: 16 g

*★This pie is good with a cracker crumb crust.

Peach Blueberry Pie

	pastry shell, baked★	
1 pkg.	vanilla-flavored sugar-free pudding mix	1 pkg.
1 t.	almond flavoring	5 mL
2 c.	sliced fresh peaches	500 mL
	juice of 1 lemon	
2 c.	fresh blueberries, cleaned	500 mL

Prepare vanilla pudding mix as directed on package for pie, adding the almond flavoring. Allow to cool for 5 to 10 minutes. Pour filling into prepared pastry shell. Chill until set. Just before serving, sprinkle peaches with lemon juice. Arrange peaches and blueberries on pie. Chill until serving time.

Yield: 8 servings

Exchange, 1 serving (without pastry shell): 1 fruit
Each serving contains: Calories: 54, Carbohydrates: 13 g

*★This pie is good with a graham cracker or meringue crust.

Chocolate Chip Mint Cream Pie

	pastry shell, baked	
2 pkgs.	vanilla-flavored sugar-free pudding mix	2 pkgs.
1 qt.	skim milk	1 L
1½ t.	peppermint flavoring	7 mL
4 drops	green food coloring	4 drops
¼ c.	minichocolate chips	60 mL
1 c.	prepared nondairy whipped topping	250 mL

Combine vanilla pudding mix, milk, flavoring, and food coloring in a saucepan. Stir to dissolve pudding mix. Cook and stir over medium heat until mixture comes to a full boil. Set aside and allow to cool. Fold in chocolate chips. Transfer to prepared pastry shell. Refrigerate until set. Decorate with nondairy whipped topping. Refrigerate until ready to serve.

Yield: 8 servings

Exchange, 1 serving (without pastry shell): 1 skim milk, ¾ fat
Each serving contains: Calories: 124, Carbohydrates: 17 g

Plain Custard Pie

	unbaked pastry shell	
4	eggs, slightly beaten	4
¼ t.	salt	1 mL
¼ c.	granulated fructose	60 mL
3 c.	skim milk	750 mL
1 t.	vanilla flavoring or extract	5 mL
	ground nutmeg	

Combine eggs, salt, and fructose in a mixing bowl. Beat with a wire whisk or fork until thoroughly blended. Beat in skim milk and vanilla flavoring. Pour into unbaked pastry shell. Sprinkle with nutmeg. Bake at 425 °F (220 °C) for 10 minutes. Reduce heat to 300 °F (150 °C) and continue baking for 30 to 40 more minutes or until knife inserted in middle comes out clean.

Yield: 8 servings

Exchange, 1 serving (without pastry shell): ⅔ skim milk, 1 fat
Each serving contains: Calories: 86, Carbohydrates: 8 g

Cool Strawberry Pie

	pastry shell, baked	
1 pkg.	sugar-free strawberry gelatin	1 pkg.
1 qt.	fresh strawberries, rinsed and hulled	1 L

Prepare gelatin as directed on package. Cool until gelatin resembles a thick syrup. Arrange strawberries in the pastry shell. Spoon thickened gelatin over the top. Refrigerate until thoroughly set.

Yield: 8 servings

Exchange, 1 serving (without pastry shell): ⅓ fruit
Each serving contains: Calories: 22, Carbohydrates: 5 g

Ginger Banana Pie

9 in.	baked pie shell	23 cm
6	gingersnaps	6
1 env.	unflavored gelatin	1 env.
⅔ c.	granulated sugar replacement	180 mL
¾ c.	water	190 mL
3	bananas	3
3 T.	fresh lemon juice	45 mL
1 t.	grated lemon peel	5 mL
2	egg whites	2
	lemon juice	

Powder gingersnaps in a food processor or blender. Set aside. Combine gelatin, sugar replacement, and water in a small saucepan or microwave-safe bowl. Stir to mix. Heat until gelatin is completely dissolved. Remove from heat. Meanwhile, mash two of the bananas. Stir the 3 T. (45 mL) of lemon juice and the lemon peel into the mashed bananas. Stir banana mixture into gelatin; then allow to cool until mixture is the consistency of thick cream. Add egg whites. Beat with a rotary beater until mixture begins to hold its shape. Chill if necessary. Spoon mixture into the baked pie shell. Chill thoroughly. At serving time, slice remaining banana and dip each slice in lemon juice. Garnish top of pie with banana slices; then sprinkle with powdered gingersnaps.

Yield: 8 servings

Exchange, 1 serving: 1 bread, ½ fat, ⅔ fruit
Each serving contains: Calories: 159, Carbohydrates: 23 g

Orange Juice Angel Pie

1 recipe	Meringue Pie Shell	1 recipe
4	egg yolks	4
1	egg	1
½ c.	granulated sugar replacement	125 mL
or		
2 T.	granulated fructose	30 mL
¼ c.	frozen orange juice concentrate, undiluted	60 mL
1 T.	fresh lemon juice	15 mL
2 c.	prepared nondairy whipped topping	60 mL

Beat egg yolks and egg until thick and lemon-colored. Beat in sweetener of your choice, orange juice concentrate, and lemon juice. Pour into a saucepan. Cook and stir until mixture is very thick. Chill thoroughly. Stir slightly to loosen mixture. Fold nondairy whipped topping into cold orange mixture. Transfer to pie shell. Chill thoroughly.

Yield: 8 servings, with granulated sugar replacement

Exchange, 1 serving: ⅓ fruit, 1½ fat
Each serving contains: Calories: 94, Carbohydrates: 4 g

Buttermilk Raisin Crustless Pie

1 env.	unflavored gelatin	1 env.
¼ c.	cold water	60 mL
2 c.	buttermilk	500 mL
1 c.	raisins	250 mL
3 T.	all-purpose flour	45 mL
¼ c.	sugar-free maple-flavored syrup	60 mL
½ t.	ground cinnamon	2 mL
¼ t.	ground nutmeg	1 mL

Lightly grease the bottom and sides of a 9 in. (23 cm) pie pan. Sprinkle unflavored gelatin over cold water. Stir slightly; then allow to soften for 1 minute. Meanwhile, combine buttermilk, raisins, and flour in a saucepan. Whisk until flour is completely blended and mixture is smooth. Cook over medium-low heat until mixture is warm. Pour in softened gelatin, and continue cooking until gelatin is completely dissolved. Remove from heat. Cover and allow to cool for at least ½ hour to plump the raisins. Add maple syrup, cinnamon, and nutmeg. Pour into prepared pie pan. Bake at 350°F (175°C) for 45 minutes. Cool to room temperature; then chill.

Yield: 8 servings

Exchange, 1 serving: 1 fruit, ¼ low-fat milk
Each serving contains: Calories: 77, Carbohydrates: 18 g

Blueberries-in-Milk Crustless Pie

2 c.	unsweetened, frozen blueberries	500 mL
3 T.	granulated fructose	45 mL
¾ c.	buttermilk	190 mL
¼ c.	low-fat milk	60 mL
3 T.	all-purpose flour	45 mL

Lightly grease the bottom and sides of a 9 in. (23 cm) pie pan. Place blueberries in pie pan and level. Sprinkle 1 T. (15 mL) of the granulated fructose over the top of the blueberries. Bake at 375°F (190°C) for 15 minutes. Meanwhile, combine remaining fructose, buttermilk, milk, and flour in a bowl. Beat or whisk until flour is completely blended and mixture is smooth. Pour buttermilk mixture over blueberries. Return to oven and continue baking for 30 minutes more or until middle of pie is just set. Cool to room temperature; then chill.

Yield: 8 servings

Exchange, 1 serving: ½ fruit, ¼ low-fat milk
Each serving contains: Calories: 53, Carbohydrates: 10 g

Raspberry Ribbon Pie

The ribbon in the title refers to the red and white layers.

1 pkg.	sugar-free raspberry gelatin mix	1 pkg.
1¼ c.	boiling water	310 mL
10 oz.	frozen whole red raspberries	300 g
1 T.	lemon juice	15 mL
3 oz.	fat-free cream cheese	80 g
2 t.	aspartame sweetener	10 mL
1 t.	vanilla extract	5 mL
1 c.	frozen low-fat nondairy whipped topping, thawed	250 mL
1	frozen pie crust, baked	1

To prepare the red layers: Put the raspberry gelatin mix into a mixing bowl. Add the boiling water. Add the frozen raspberries and lemon juice. Stir until the raspberries are defrosted. Refrigerate 1–2 hours until partially set.

To prepare the white layers: In a mixing bowl, combine the cream cheese, aspartame, and vanilla. Add a spoonful of the whipped topping. Fold to mix. Continue adding the topping spoonful by spoonful, folding in each addition. Refrigerate until the white layer is partially set.

Spread half the white mixture on the bottom of the pie shell. Cover with half the red gelatin mixture. Repeat with white and red layers, ending with the white mixture. Chill until set, 3 hours or more.

Yield: 8 servings

Exchange, 1 serving: 1 starch/bread, 1 fat
Each serving contains: Calories: 132, Total fat: 6 g, Carbohydrates: 16 g, Protein: 2 g, Sodium: 182 mg, Cholesterol: 2 mg

Hawaiian Pineapple Pie

I don't think I was ever served this in Hawaii, but the spirit of the islands is here.

20 oz.	crushed pineapple in juice	570 g
1 pkg.	sugar-free vanilla pudding	1 pkg.
½ c.	water	125 mL
1 t.	butter or margarine	5 mL
1	frozen pie crust, baked	1
½ c.	frozen low-fat nondairy whipped topping	125 mL
2 T.	coconut flakes (optional)	30 mL

Drain the can of pineapple pieces, saving the juice. In a saucepan, combine the pudding mix, water, and reserved pineapple juice. Cook over medium heat. Stir constantly. When mixture comes to a full boil, add the pineapple chunks and butter. Stir well. Pour into the pie crust. Cool. Just before serving, top with the non-dairy topping and sprinkle with coconut flakes, if desired.

Yield: 8 servings

Exchange, 1 serving: 1 starch/bread, 1 fat
Each serving contains: Calories: 140, Total fat: 6 g, Carbohydrates: 21 g, Protein: 1 g, Sodium: 136 mg, Cholesterol: 1 mg

Peach Cream Cheese Pie

This pie is not very sweet. It's perfect after dinner on a hot summer evening.

½ c.	orange juice	125 mL
2 envs.	plain gelatin	2 envs.
2 t.	orange extract	10 mL
1 c.	fat-free cream cheese	250 mL
1 c.	frozen low-fat nondairy whipped topping, thawed	250 mL
16 oz.	"lite" peach slices in juice, drained and chopped	450 g
1	frozen pie crust, baked	1

In a small saucepan, heat the orange juice until simmering. Pour into a blender or food processor. Add the gelatin and orange extract. Blend for 30 seconds or so before adding the cream cheese, topping, and peaches. Blend until smooth, another 20 seconds or more. Pour quickly into the pie crust. Refrigerate 3 hours or so before serving.

Yield: 8 servings

Exchange, 1 serving: 1 starch/bread, ½ fruit, 1 fat
Each serving contains: Calories: 170, Total fat: 6 g, Carbohydrates: 22 g, Protein: 4 g, Sodium: 245 mg, Cholesterol: 5 mg

Strawberry Ice Cream Pie

Let the ice cream soften before beginning the rest of the recipe.

1 pkg.	sugar-free strawberry gelatin powder	1 pkg.
⅔ c.	boiling water	165 mL
2 c.	sugar-free low-fat strawberry ice cream, softened	500 mL
1 c.	frozen low-fat nondairy whipped topping, thawed	250 mL
1	frozen pie crust, baked	1
1 c.	fresh or frozen (no sugar added) strawberries (optional)	250 mL

Put the gelatin powder into a large mixing bowl. Add the boiling water. Stir until gelatin is dissolved. Add the ice cream slowly. Stir until the mixture is smooth (except for the strawberry pieces, of course). Stir in the whipped topping by spoonfuls. Beat after each addition. A whisk works well. Spoon the mixture into the prepared pie crust. Freeze a few hours until firm. For easiest cutting, run a sharp knife under hot running water between each cut. Garnish with strawberries and whipped topping, if desired.

Yield: 8 servings

Exchange, 1 serving: 1 starch/bread, 1 fat
Each serving contains: Calories: 128, Total fat: 6 g, Carbohydrates: 17 g, Protein: 0.9 g, Sodium: 148 mg, Cholesterol: 0 mg

Strawberry Meringue Pie

A baked Alaska-style pie with strawberries. Dessert lovers will be delighted with the ice cream-meringue combination.

4 c.	sugar-free, low-fat vanilla ice cream, softened	1 L
1	frozen pie crust, baked	1
3 c.	fresh strawberries or frozen, unsweetened, thawed	750 mL
2 large	egg whites	2 large
¼ t.	cream of tartar	2 mL
1½ t.	aspartame sweetener	8 mL

Spread the ice cream into the pie shell, pushing it to the edges. Freeze all day or overnight. Just before serving, spread the strawberries on top of the ice cream and preheat the oven to 500°F (250°C). Put the egg whites, cream of tartar, and aspartame into an electric mixing bowl. Beat at high speed until the whites are stiff and form peaks but are not dry. Spoon this meringue on top of the strawberries using the spoon to make decorative peaks. Be sure all the surface is covered right up to the crust. Put the pie on a wooden bread board and place it in the oven. Bake for 5 minutes or so in the hot oven until meringue is lightly browned. Serve at once.

Yield: 8 servings

Exchange, 1 serving: 1 starch/bread, ½ fruit, 1 fat
Each serving contains: Calories: 150, Total fat: 5 g, Carbohydrates: 24 g, Protein: 1 g, Sodium: 138 mg, Cholesterol: 0 mg

Cocoa Chiffon Pie

This needs at least eight hours to chill. Prepare it the night before you plan to serve it or in the morning if you want to serve it in the evening. It's worth planning ahead.

1 env.	unflavored gelatin	1 env.
3 T.	unsweetened cocoa powder	45 mL
1¾ c.	skim milk	435 mL
1 t.	vanilla extract	5 mL
1½ c.	frozen low-fat nondairy whipped topping, thawed	375 mL
1½ t.	aspartame sweetener	8 mL
1	frozen pie crust, baked	1

In a medium saucepan, mix together the gelatin, cocoa powder, and skim milk. Let stand for 5 minutes or so. Place over low heat. Stir with a wire whisk until the gelatin is dissolved, about 5 minutes. Remove from heat and stir in the vanilla. Refrigerate the mixture while preparing the rest of the pie. Put the whipped topping and aspartame in a mixing bowl. Mix to combine. Add the cocoa mixture. Mix at the lowest speed until blended. Turn into prepared pie crust. Refrigerate 8 hours or overnight before serving.

Yield: 8 servings

Exchange, 1 serving: 1 starch/bread, 1½ fat
Each serving contains: Calories: 145, Total fat: 7 g, Carbohydrates: 16 g, Protein: 3 g, Sodium: 133 mg, Cholesterol: 1 mg

Squash Pie

This tastes like coconut custard. If the top is brown but the center isn't cooked, cover the pie with aluminum foil and bake for a few minutes more.

2 c.	yellow squash, freshly grated, peeled	500 mL
¼ c.	sugar	60 mL
6 pkgs.	saccharin or acesulfame-K sugar substitute	6 pkgs.
1 t.	cornstarch	5 mL
1 t.	vanilla	5 mL
2 t.	coconut extract	10 mL
1 T.	flour	15 mL
3 large	eggs or equivalent egg substitute, slightly beaten	3 large
¼ c.	butter or margarine, melted	60 mL
1	Deep Dish Pie Shell, unbaked	1

In a large mixing bowl, combine all the ingredients except the pie shell, and mix well. Pour into the unbaked pie shell. Put the pie into a preheated 400°F (200°C) oven for 10–15 minutes. Reduce the temperature to 350°F (180°C) for 40–50 minutes until the top is golden brown.

Yield: 8 slices

Exchange, 1 serving: 2 starch/bread, 1 fruit, 1 fat
Each slice contains: Calories: 280, Total fat: 4 g, Carbohydrates: 46 g, Protein: 6 g, Sodium: 93 mg, Cholesterol: 95 mg

Blueberry Sour Cream Pie

I have used both fresh and frozen blueberries and they work equally well in this pie.

2 c.	fresh or frozen blueberries	500 mL
1	frozen pie crust, unbaked, or Deep Dish Pie Shell, unbaked	1
1 c.	fat-free sour cream	250 mL
2 T.	sugar	30 mL
3 pkgs.	saccharin or acesulfame-K sugar substitute	3 pkgs.
1 large	egg yolk, lightly beaten	1 large
1 t.	vanilla	1 t.

Put the blueberries in the crust. Mix all the other ingredients in a mixing bowl. Pour this mixture over the blueberries. Bake in a preheated 375°F (190°C) oven for 45 minutes. The pie top will be lightly browned. Cool and chill before serving.

Yield: 8 servings

Exchange, 1 serving: 1 starch/bread, 1 fat
Each serving contains: Calories: 143, Total fat: 6 g, Carbohydrates: 19 g, Protein: 2 g, Sodium: 132 mg, Cholesterol: 27 mg

Strawberry Cream Pie

9 in.	baked pie shell	23 cm
1 pkg.	low-calorie vanilla pudding	1 pkg.
1½ c.	Strawberry Topping	375 mL
¼ c.	fresh strawberries (halved)	60 mL
1 pkg.	low-calorie whipped topping (prepared)	1 pkg.

Prepare pudding as directed on package; cool slightly. Pour into baked pie shell. Cover with waxed paper; chill until set. Combine Strawberry Topping with fresh strawberries. Spread evenly on top of pudding. Top with prepared whipped topping.

Yield: 8 servings

Exchange, 1 serving: 1½ fruit, ½ milk, plus pie shell exchange
Each serving contains: Calories: 75, plus pie shell calories, Carbohydrates: 18 g

Strawberry Topping

2 c.	fresh or frozen strawberries (unsweetened)	500 mL
1½ t.	cornstarch	7 mL
¼ c.	cold water	60 mL
2 t.	sugar replacement	10 mL

Place strawberries in top of double boiler. Cook over boiling water until soft and juicy. Blend cornstarch and cold water. Add to strawberries. Cook until clear and slightly thickened. Remove from heat; add sugar replacement. Cool. Topping can also be made with blueberries or raspberries.

Yield: 1½ c. (375 mL)

Exchange, ½c. (125 mL): 1 fruit
Each serving contains: Calories: 40

Lemon Cake Pie

9 in.	unbaked pie shell	23 cm
½ c.	sugar replacement	125 mL
2 T.	flour	30 mL
2 T.	soft margarine	30 mL
1 T.	lemon rind	15 mL
3 T.	lemon juice	45 mL
1 c.	skim milk	250 mL
2	eggs, separated	2

Combine sugar replacement, flour, margarine, lemon rind and juice, skim milk, and egg yolks. Beat vigorously. Fold in egg whites (well beaten). Pour into unbaked pie shell. Bake at 325°F (165°C) for 1 hour, or until set.

Yield: 8 servings

Exchange, 1 serving: 1 milk, plus pie shell exchange
Each serving contains: Calories: 40, plus pie shell calories, Carbohydrates: 43 g

Fresh Rhubarb Pie

9 in.	unbaked pie shell	23 cm
1 qt.	1 in. (2.5 cm) pieces rhubarb	1 L
4 T.	flour	60 mL
½ c.	sugar replacement	125 mL
2	eggs (beaten)	2

Mix rhubarb, flour, sugar replacement, and eggs. Pour into unbaked pie shell. Bake at 350°F (175°C) for 40 to 50 minutes, or until set.

Yield: 8 servings

Exchange, 1 serving: ½ fruit, plus pie shell exchange
Each serving contains: Calories: 68, plus pie shell calories

CRUSTS

Basic Pie Shell

⅓ c.	shortening	90 mL
1 c.	flour, sifted	250 mL
¼ t.	salt	1 mL
2 to 4 T.	ice water	30 to 60 mL

Chill shortening. Cut shortening into flour and salt until mixture forms crumbs. Add ice water, 1 T. (15 mL) at a time, and flip mixture around in bowl until a ball forms. Wrap ball in plastic wrap and chill at least 1 hour. Roll to fit 9 in. (23 cm) pie pan. Fill with pie filling or prick with fork. Bake at 425°F (220°C) for 10 to 12 minutes or until firm, or leave unbaked.

Yield: 8 servings

Exchange, 1 serving: 1 bread, 1 fat
Each serving contains: Calories: 120, Carbohydrates: 10 g

Cocoa-Flavored Crisp Cereal Crust

2 c.	cocoa-flavored cereal	500 mL
1½ T.	water	21 mL

In a food processor, blend the dry cereal on high until it becomes a medium-fine grain. Add water and then process for another minute. Press mixture into an ungreased 8 or 9 in. (20 or 23 cm) pie pan.

Yield: 8 servings or single pie crust

Exchange, 1 serving: ⅓ starch/bread
Each serving contains: Calories: 25, Carbohydrates: 4 g

Graham Cracker Crust

20	2 in. (5 cm) square graham crackers	20
2 T.	water	30 mL
½ t.	cinnamon	2 mL

Using food processor, crush crackers to make a cup of fine crumbs. Add water and cinnamon. Blend until sticky. Press mixture into an ungreased 8 or 9 in. (20 or 23 cm) pie pan.

Yield: 8 servings or single pie crust

Exchange, 1 serving: ¾ starch/bread
Each serving contains: Calories: 68, Carbohydrates: 12 g

Cocoa-Flavored Puffed Cereal Crust

2½ c.	cocoa-flavored cereal	625 mL
1½ T.	water	21 mL

Blend dry cereal on high in a food processor. Add water and then blend for another minute. Press mixture into ungreased 8 or 9 in. (20 or 23 cm) pie pan.

Yield: 8 servings or single pie crust

Exchange, 1 serving: ⅓ starch/bread
Each serving contains: Calories: 27, Carbohydrates: 5 g

Ginger Cookie Crust #1

| 20 | 2 in. (5 cm) ginger cookies | 20 |
| 1 T. | water | 15 mL |

Blend cookies on high in a food processor. Add water and blend until moist. Press crust into ungreased 8 or 9 in. (20 or 23 cm) pan.

Yield: 8 servings or single pie crust

Exchange, 1 serving: ¾ starch/bread
Each serving contains: Calories: 56, Carbohydrates: 13 g

Ginger Cookie Crust #2

| 20 | 2 in. (5 cm) ginger cookies | 20 |
| 2 T. | skim milk | 30 mL |

Crush cookies in food processor on high. Process until crumbs become very fine. Add milk and process until dough forms a ball. Press into ungreased 8 or 9 in. (20 or 23 cm) pie pan or torte pan, or chill and roll dough.

Yield: 8 servings or single pie crust

Exchange, 1 serving: ¾ starch/bread
Each serving contains: Calories: 56, Carbohydrates: 13 g

Corn Cereal Crust

| 3 c. | cornflake cereal | 750 mL |
| 1½ T. | water | 21 mL |

Crush cornflakes in food processor on high to make 1¼ c. (310 mL) of fine crumbs. Add water and blend until moist. Press crust into ungreased 8 or 9 in. (20 or 23 cm) pie pan.

Yield: 8 servings or single pie crust

Exchange, 1 serving: ½ starch/bread
Each serving contains: Calories: 35, Carbohydrates: 8 g

Bran Cereal-with-Raisins Crust

| 2 c. | raisin bran cereal | 500 mL |
| 2 t. | rum flavoring | 10 mL |

Using a blender, chop cereal thoroughly, one cup at a time. Make sure to stir cereal from underneath blender's blades when blender is turned off. Transfer to food processor and add rum flavoring. Process until sticky. Press mixture into ungreased 8 or 9 in. (20 or 23 cm) pie pan.

Yield: 8 servings or single pie crust

Exchange, 1 serving: ½ starch/bread
Each serving contains: Calories: 35, Carbohydrates: 8 g

Cinnamon Crunch Cereal Crust

| 3 c. | cinnamon cereal | 750 mL |
| 1½ T. | water | 21 mL |

Crush cereal on high in food processor until crumbs become fine. Add water and blend to moisten. Press crumbs into ungreased 8 or 9 in. (20 or 23 cm) pie pan.

Yield: 8 servings or single pie crust

Exchange, 1 serving: ⅔ starch/bread
Each serving contains: Calories: 50, Carbohydrates: 12 g

Meringue Crust

3	egg whites, at room temperature	3
¼ t.	cream of tartar	1 mL
dash	salt	dash
¼ c.	granulated sugar replacement	60 mL

Combine egg whites, cream of tartar, and salt in a mixing bowl. Beat until soft peaks form. Gradually add sugar replacement. Beat to stiff peaks. Spread over bottom and sides of 8 or 9 in. (20 or 23 cm) pie pan. Bake at 275°F (135°C) for an hour or until lightly browned and crisp. Cool before filling.

Yield: 8 servings

Exchange, 1 serving: negligible
Each serving contains: Calories: negligible, Carbohydrates: negligible

Flavored-Meringue Crust

3	egg whites, at room temperature	3
¼ t.	cream of tartar	1 mL
dash	salt	dash
1 t.	one of the following: vanilla extract, ground cardamom, nutmeg, cinnamon, lavender leaves, pumpkin-pie spice, mace, lemon juice	5 mL

Combine egg whites, cream of tartar, and salt in a mixing bowl. Beat until soft peaks form. Add flavoring of your choice. Beat to stiff peaks. Spread over bottom and sides of 8 or 9 in. (20 or 23 cm) pie pan. Bake at 275°F (135°C) for an hour or until lightly browned and crisp. Cool before filling.

Yield: 8 servings

Exchange, 1 serving: negligible
Each serving contains: Calories: negligible, Carbohydrates: negligible

Orange Crust

3 c.	all-purpose flour	750 mL	
1 c.	solid shortening	250 mL	
1 t.	granulated sugar replacement	5 mL	
2 t.	grated orange peel	10 mL	
7 T.	orange juice	105 mL	

Combine flour, shortening, sugar replacement, and orange peel in a bowl or food processor. Cut until mixture is the consistency of cornmeal. Make a well in the middle of the mixture; then add orange juice. Toss until mixture is moist enough to hold a shape. If needed, add a small amount of water, 1 t. (5 mL) at a time. Form into a ball, wrap in plastic wrap, and chill for at least 2 hours. Then divide dough in half. Roll out both halves on a lightly floured surface. Arrange bottom crust in pie pan. Add filling. Adjust top crust, scoring or cutting slits to allow steam to escape. Seal edges. Bake as directed in your pie recipe.

Yield: 8 servings or double pie crust

Exchange, 1 serving: 2 starch/bread, 3 fat
Each serving contains: Calories: 310, Carbohydrates: 30 g

Puff Pastry Crust

1 c.	unsalted butter	250 mL	
2 c.	sifted cake flour	500 mL	
½ c.	ice water	125 mL	

Cut ½ c. (90 mL) of butter into the cake flour. Allow the remaining butter to become soft but not runny. Add ice water to flour mixture, 1 T. (15 mL) at a time, until a soft dough forms. Chill for an hour. Then roll out dough on a lightly floured surface. Brush with one-fourth of the softened butter. Fold in half, brush with 2 T. (30 mL) of the softened butter, and fold in half again. Place in plastic wrap and chill for an hour. Then roll out and repeat brushing with half of the remaining softened butter. Repeat process a third time with the remaining butter. This can be baked immediately as directed in your pie recipe, refrigerated for up to 2 days, or frozen.

Yield: 16 servings

Exchange, 1 serving: 1 starch/bread, 2½ fat
Each serving contains: Calories: 140, Carbohydrates: 16 g

Cottage Cheese Crust

⅓ c.	butter-flavored shortening	90 mL
1 c.	sifted all-purpose flour	250 mL
½ c.	low-calorie cottage cheese	125 mL

Cut shortening into flour; then add cottage cheese and mix into a smooth dough. Wrap dough in plastic wrap and chill for at least an hour. Roll to desired shape.

Yield: 8 servings or single pie crust

Exchange, 1 serving: ⅔ starch/bread, 1½ fat
Each serving contains: Calories: 156, Carbohydrates: 12 g

Cheddar Cheese Crust

1½ c.	all-purpose flour	375 mL
dash	salt	dash
¾ c.	grated sharp cheddar cheese	190 mL
½ c.	solid shortening	125 mL
5 to 6 T.	ice water	75 to 90 mL

Combine flour, salt, cheese, and shortening in a food processor with a steel blade. Process on High with alternate on/off switch until mixture turns into coarse crumbs. On Low, add water through the feeder tube, 1 T. (15 mL) at a time, until dough starts to ball. Form dough into a ball with your hands. Wrap in plastic wrap and chill for 2 hours. Then divide dough in half and roll out both halves on lightly floured surface. Arrange bottom crust in pie pan. Add filling. Adjust top crust, scoring or cutting slits to allow steam to escape. Seal edges. Bake as directed in your pie recipe.

Yield: 8 servings or double pie crust

Exchange, 1 serving: 1 starch/bread, 2½ fat
Each serving contains: Calories: 200, Carbohydrates: 15 g

Egg Yolk Crust

1 c.	sifted all-purpose flour	250 mL
dash	salt	dash
1 T.	granulated sugar replacement	15 mL
¼ c.	butter-flavored shortening	60 mL
1	egg yolk, slightly beaten	1

Combine flour, salt, and sugar replacement in food processor or bowl. Cut in shortening, using on/off switch or short cuts. Add egg yolk and mix thoroughly. Press dough into bottom of 8 or 9 in. (20 or 23 cm) pie pan, springform pan, or tart pans. Add filling as directed in your pie recipe or fill with pie weights. Bake at 425°F (220°C) for 10 minutes or until crust is slightly brown.

Yield: 8 servings or single pie crust

Exchange, 1 serving: ⅔ starch/bread, 1 fat
Each serving contains: Calories: 115, Carbohydrates: 12 g

Pastry Crust

2 c.	sifted all-purpose flour	500 mL
dash	salt	dash
1 c.	butter-flavored shortening	250 mL
⅓ c.	ice water	90 mL

Combine flour and salt in bowl or food processor. Cut in shortening until mixture is in fine crumbs. Add water and mix to a dough. Chill for an hour. Divide dough in half. Roll out half on lightly floured surface. Line pan, fill, and then roll out top crust. Slit top crust to allow steam to escape. Place on top of filling and seal edges. Bake as directed in your pie recipe.

Yield: 8 servings or double pie crust

Exchange, 1 serving: 1⅓ starch/bread, 5 fat
Each serving contains: Calories: 326, Carbohydrates: 21 g

Chocolate Crust

¾ c.	flour	190 mL
3 T.	cocoa	45 mL
⅓ c.	vegetable shortening, softened	90 mL
1 t.	liquid fructose	5 mL
or		
1	granulated sugar replacement	15 mL
2 to 3 T.	cold water	30 to 45 mL

In a food processor or bowl, combine flour, cocoa, shortening and fructose; work into crumbs. Add enough water to make a soft ball. Roll up or press into sides and bottom on pie pan. Use as directed in recipe.

Yield: 8 servings

Exchange, 1 serving: ¾ bread, 2 fat
Each serving contains: Calories: 129

Nut Meringue Pie Shell

3	egg whites	3
½ t.	vanilla extract	2 mL
¼ t.	cream of tartar	1 mL
dash	salt	dash
½ c.	granulated sugar replacement	125 mL
¼ c.	chopped nuts	60 mL

Combine egg whites, vanilla, cream of tartar, and salt in a bowl. Beat to soft peaks. Gradually beat in sugar replacement. Beat to stiff peaks. Spread on the bottom and sides of a 9 in. (23 cm) pie pan. Sprinkle with chopped nuts. Bake at 275°F (135°C) for 1 hour. Cool completely before using.

Yield: 8 servings

Exchange, 1 serving: ½ fat
Each serving contains: Calories: 23, Carbohydrates: negligible

Deep Dish Pie Shell

2 c.	flour	500 mL
11 T.	fat-free butter and oil replacement product	165 mL
3–4 T.	ice water	45–60 mL

Put the flour into a bowl. Using two knives or a pastry blender, cut in the butter and oil replacement until the mixture resembles coarse meal. Add about two tablespoons (30 mL) of water and work it in gently with a fork. Gradually add the ice water a little at a time, using fingers or a fork to work the dough into a ball. Don't let the ball become sticky, the result of too much water. Chill the dough for 30 minutes. On a lightly floured surface, flatten the dough into a circle with roundish edges or rectangular edges, depending on your deep dish pie pan.

With a rolling pin, roll the dough slightly larger than the pan, rolling from the center outward, the thinner the better. Fold the dough in half and gently lift it onto a pie pan coated with non-stick vegetable spray, being careful not to stretch it. Unfold the dough and pat it gently into the pan. Using a kitchen knife, cut away any dough that extends more than ¾ in. (3 cm) beyond the edge of the pan. Fold the outside dough over to make a double thickness around the rim of the pan. Press the edge down with a fork, or use your fingers to make a fluted edge. If the crust will be baked without any filling, prick the crust all over with a fork. Bake in 425°F (220°C) oven for approximately 12 to 15 minutes or until it looks as brown as you would like, or follow the directions of the recipe contained with the filling recipe.

Yield: 1 Deep Dish Pie Shell, or 8 servings

Exchange, 1 serving: 1 starch/bread, 1 fruit
Each serving contains: Calories: 162, Total fat: 0.2 g, Carbohydrates: 36 g, Protein: 3 g, Sodium: 8 mg, Cholesterol: 0 mg

Cakes

Making "diabetic" cakes is a challenge; we offer you some tips here. Because sugar is needed to add lightness and a tender texture, it cannot be eliminated completely. We use a bare minimum of sugar and then bolster the sweet taste with artificial sweeteners. We substitute some new no-fat products, such as nonfat sour cream, yogurt, buttermilk, mayonnaise, cream cheese, etc. We offer a few other hints on making "diabetic" cakes.

- Watch cakes carefully near the end of the baking time. Low-sugar, low-fat cakes can easily overcook. Set your timer for the minimum time, then test for doneness. With most cakes, a toothpick inserted in the middle should come out clean.
- Use lots of beaten egg whites to add a light touch; using a minimum amount of sugar and fat can lead to a dense texture. You may want to save the unwanted egg yolks as "pet" food; animals don't suffer from cholesterol problems as some humans do.
- It often works well to use cake flour rather than regular flour. This too lightens a low-sugar, low-fat product.
- Bake cakes in fairly small containers to minimize the amount of time needed for baking. In larger pans cakes with only egg whites can become rubbery. Cupcake pans work well, as do small loaf pans.

- Slice leftover cake and freeze the individual slices well wrapped. That way you can defrost just the right amount. Do not expect low-sugar, low-fat cakes to remain fresh for a long time. Freezing works well. Take a few strawberries or raspberries out of a freezer bag and serve them with a defrosted cake slice.
- A person with a sweet tooth may want a little extra sweetness. As soon as a cake is out of the oven, poke a few holes in the top with a fork and drizzle in aspartame dissolved in an equal amount of water. Cupcakes can be rolled in the dissolved aspartame.

Making frosting is another real challenge since traditional frostings are basically mixtures of sugar and fat. The challenge is to make something that tastes good. A combination of artificial sweetener, cornstarch, and nonfat dry milk may look like frosting but the taste is disappointing. Our frosting recipes, based on ingredients such as nonfat cream cheese, are quite tasty. But to be honest, plan to serve the cake within a few hours of frosting it. These frostings do not have the staying power of sugary, fatty frostings. You can eliminate frosting by serving a slice of cake with a small amount of unsweetened applesauce; try adding a little cinnamon and aspartame. Or try our other toppings from the "Frostings and Toppings" section.

Gingerbread

This cake looks ordinary, but the taste is quite special. If you want to add something on top, try our Lemon Sauce or an appropriate whipped topping.

1 c.	flour	250 mL
¾ t.	baking soda	4 mL
1 t.	cinnamon	5 mL
½ t.	dry mustard	2.5 mL
1 t.	ginger	5 mL
dash	salt (optional)	dash
2 T.	nonfat yogurt	30 mL
2 T.	melted margarine or butter	30 mL
¼ c.	molasses	40 mL
6 pkts.	concentrated acesulfame-K	6 pkts.
2 T.	Prune Purée	30 mL
3	egg whites	3

Glaze ingredients

2 T.	hot water	30 mL
2 t.	measures-like-sugar aspartame	10 mL
½ t.	lemon extract	2.5 mL

Sift together the flour, baking soda, cinnamon, mustard, ginger, and salt. Set aside. In a separate bowl, whisk together the yogurt, margarine, molasses, acesulfame-K, and prune purée. Add the flour-and-spice mixture to the wet mixture and stir together. In a separate bowl, beat the egg whites until stiff. Gradually beat the beaten egg whites into the batter. Pour the batter into an 8 inch (20 cm) round pan that has been sprayed with non-stick vegetable cooking spray. Bake in a preheated 325°F (160°C) oven for 20–25 minutes or until a toothpick comes out clean. As soon as the gingerbread is out of the oven, combine the glaze ingredients. Use a toothpick to poke holes in the top of the gingerbread. Then use a pastry brush to brush the glaze over the top.

Yield: 10 servings

Exchange, 1 serving: 1 bread
Each serving contains: Calories: 89, Carbohydrates: 17 g, Fiber: 0.4 g, Sodium: 130 mg, Cholesterol: 0 mg

Angel Food Cake I

Did you know that you should "break" angel food cake apart instead of using a knife to slice it? With a knife you compress the cake. Instead, use a special slicer or take two forks (one in each hand), and starting with the inside hole, jab the tines into the cake, keeping the forks very close together. Then work a line across to the outside by tearing the cake as you gently separate the forks.

1 c.	flour	250 mL
¼ c.	sugar	60 mL
3 pkts.	concentrated acesulfame-K	3 pkts.
1½ c.	egg whites (12)	375 mL
1½ t.	cream of tartar	7 mL
¼ t.	salt	60 mL
¼ c.	sugar	60 mL
4 pkts.	concentrated acesulfame-K	4 pkts.
1½ t.	vanilla extract	7 mL
½ t.	almond extract	2 mL

Sift together the flour, first amount of sugar, and first amount of acesulfame-K. Set aside. In a large mixing bowl, combine the egg whites, cream of tartar, and salt. With an electric mixer, beat until foamy. Mix together the second amount of sugar and the second acesulfame-K. Gradually add this mixture, 1 T. (15 mL) at a time, to the egg whites. Continue beating until stiff peaks form. Fold in the vanilla and almond extracts. Sprinkle the flour mixture over the beaten egg whites. Fold gently just until the flour disappears. Fold the batter into an ungreased 10 × 4 in. (25 × 10 cm) tube pan.

Bake in a 375°F (190°C) oven for 30–35 minutes, until no imprint remains after finger lightly touches the top of the cake. The top should be golden brown. To cool, turn the baked cake over. For best results stand the tube pan on a custard cup or put a bottle in the center hole to hold the top away from the counter so circulation will occur. Remove the cake from the pan only after it is thoroughly cool. Drizzle with bittersweet topping, fruit topping, or sliced fresh fruit.

Yield: 24 slices

Exchange, 1 serving: ½ bread
Each serving contains: Calories: 42, Carbohydrates: 7 g, Fiber: 1 g, Sodium: 178 mg, Cholesterol: 0.7 mg

Angel Food Cake II

During a recent insulin reaction, Edith's friend Bob wondered aloud why he had low blood sugar and thought it was because he had eaten some of this angel cake. Edith reminded him that the cake was only egg whites, flour and almost no sugar. The cake tastes so sweet, Bob had been fooled. And he hates artificial sweeteners.

¼ c.	sugar	60 mL
½ c.	measures-like-sugar saccharin	125 mL
6 pkts.	concentrated acesulfame-K	6 pkts.
1¼ c.	cake flour	310 mL
12	egg whites	12
1½ t.	cream of tartar	7 mL
pinch	salt (optional)	pinch
1 t.	vanilla extract	5 mL
1 t.	almond extract	5 mL

Stir together the sugar, measures-like-sugar saccharin, and acesulfame-K. Divide approximately in half. Set aside one half. Put the other half of the sugar substitute/acesulfame-K mixture in a sifter with all the cake flour. Sift twice and set aside. Using an electric mixer, beat the egg whites with the cream of tartar, salt, and vanilla and almond extracts. Gradually add the reserved sugar-substitute/acesulfame-K mixture to the beaten egg whites. They should hold stiff peaks. Fold in the flour-sugar mixture, a small amount at a time, until it is all folded in.

Pour the batter into an angel cake pan that has been sprayed very lightly with non-stick cooking spray. Bake in a preheated 375°F (190°C) oven for 40 minutes or until the top is lightly browned, or until a toothpick inserted comes out clean. As soon as it is out of the oven, invert the pan on a rack and let cool completely before removing from the pan.

Yield: 24 servings

Exchange, 1 serving: ½ bread
Each serving contains: Calories: 45, Carbohydrates: 10 g, Fiber: 0, Sodium: 26 mg, Cholesterol: 0 mg

Lemony Angel Food

The perfect solution for leftover angel food cake that is getting stale. The topping revives the cake.

½	angel food cake, cut into 6 pieces	½
1 pkg.	sugar-free lemon pudding mix (prepared according to package directions)	1 pkg.
1¼ c.	water or skim milk	310 mL
1 t.	lemon juice	5 mL
1 recipe	Lemon Sauce	1 recipe
½ c.	frozen low-fat nondairy whipped topping (optional)	125 mL

Cut each of the six pieces of cake into chunks and arrange them in six serving dishes. Mix the lemon pudding, made with water or skim milk, with the lemon juice and spoon over the angel food cake. Drizzle Lemon Sauce over the mixture. Top with a dollop of white topping, if desired.

Yield: 6 servings

Exchange, 1 serving: 1 starch/bread; 1½ fruit
Each serving contains: Calories: 149, Total fat: 1 g, Carbohydrates: 35 g, Protein: 4 g, Sodium: 304 mg, Cholesterol: 35 mg

Lemon Sauce

This lemon sauce is best when used in a day or two. Keep it refrigerated.

⅓ c.	fresh lemon juice	80 mL
6 pkgs.	saccharin or acesulfame-K sugar substitute	6 pkgs.
1 large	egg or equivalent egg substitute	1 large
1 T.	cornstarch	15 mL
1 T.	water	15 mL
1 t.	vanilla extract	5 mL
1 t.	aspartame sweetener	5 mL

Combine the lemon juice and saccharin or acesulfame-K in a saucepan over medium heat. Bring to a simmer. In a medium mixing bowl, beat the egg. Using a fork, blend together the cornstarch and water in a cup. Add this to the egg. Add a small amount of the lemon juice mixture to the egg mixture. Now put this into the saucepan with the remaining lemon mixture. Cook over medium heat, stirring constantly until thickened. Remove from heat. Cool. Stir in the vanilla and aspartame.

Yield: ⅔ c., or 6 servings

Exchange: free
Each serving contains: Calories: 27, Total fat: 0.8 g, Carbohydrates: 4 g, Protein: 1 g, Sodium: 15 mg, Cholesterol: 35 mg

Chocolate Mayonnaise Cake

This would have been loaded with fat before fat-free mayonnaise. It's a moist, rich chocolate cake.

2 c.	sifted flour	500 mL
¼ c.	sugar	0 mL
6 pkgs.	saccharin or acesulfame-K sugar substitute	6 pkgs.
1½ t.	baking soda	8 mL
4 T.	unsweetened cocoa powder	60 mL
1 c.	cold water	250 mL
1 c.	fat-free mayonnaise	250 mL

Mix together the dry ingredients in a large mixing bowl. In another bowl, beat together the cold water and mayonnaise. Add the water mixture to the dry ingredients. Mix well to combine. Prepare an 8 × 12 in. (20 × 30 cm) sheet cake pan, coating it with non-stick cooking spray. Pour the batter into the pan and bake it in a preheated 350°F (180°C) oven for 45 minutes or until a tester comes out clean. Cut into eight sections.

Yield: 8 pieces

Exchange, 1 serving: 1 starch/bread; 1 fruit
Each piece contains: Calories: 147, Total fat: 0.7 g, Carbohydrates: 32 g, Protein: 4 g, Sodium: 241 mg, Cholesterol: 0 mg

Cherry Cheese Suzette

Rich and sweet. A brunch favorite.

Batter

¼ c.	fat-free butter and oil replacement product	60 mL
2 large	eggs or equivalent egg substitute	2 large
1¼ c.	flour	310 mL
1 t.	baking powder	5 mL
¾ c.	skim milk	185 mL

Filling

2 c.	fat-free cottage cheese	500 mL
1 t.	butter extract	5 mL
1 pkg.	saccharin or acesulfame-K sugar substitute	1 pkg.
½ c.	fruit-only cherry preserves	125 mL

Put the butter replacement in the mixing bowl of an electric mixer. Add the eggs and beat until smooth. In another bowl, combine the flour and baking powder. With mixer running at low speed, add the flour mixture to the egg mixture alternately with the milk. Blend for two minutes at low speed. Coat an 8 in. (20 cm) pan with non-stick cooking spray. Spoon half the batter into the pan. In a mixing bowl, combine the cottage cheese, butter extract, and sugar substitute. Pour the filling over the batter. Spread so the filling is evenly distributed. Dot with cherry filling. Carefully pour the remaining batter on top. Bake in a preheated 350°F (180°C) oven for 50–60 minutes. The top will be lightly browned.

Yield: 9 servings

Exchange, 1 serving: 2 starch/bread
Each serving contains: Calories: 164, Total fat: 1 g, Carbohydrates: 29 g, Protein: 10 g, Sodium: 201 mg, Cholesterol: 52 mg

Carrot Cake with Cream Cheese Icing

I made this carrot cake to taste as much as possible like those served at the old Commissary Restaurant in Philadelphia, my absolute favorite carrot cake.

2 c.	flour	500 mL
2 t.	cinnamon	10 mL
1 t.	baking powder	5 mL
⅓ c.	fat-free butter and oil replacement product	80 mL
4 T.	sugar	60 mL
6 pkgs.	saccharin or acesulfame-K sugar substitute	6 pkgs.
3 large	eggs or egg substitute	3 large
3 med	carrots, grated	3 med
½ c.	finely chopped walnuts (optional)	125 mL
1 recipe	cream cheese icing	1 recipe

In a medium mixing bowl, blend together the flour, cinnamon, and baking powder. In another bowl, beat together the butter replacement, sugar, and sugar substitute. Beat in the eggs, one at a time, alternating with the flour mixture. Stir in the carrots and walnuts, if you are using them. Pour the batter into a 9 in. (14 cm) cake pan coated with non-stick vegetable spray. Bake in a 350°F (180°C) oven for 40 minutes. Cool the cake on a wire rack for 10 minutes before removing it from the pan. Ice with cream cheese frosting.

Yield: 8 servings

Exchange, 1 serving: 2 starch/bread 1 vegetable, 1 fruit
Each serving contains: Calories: 250, Total fat: 2 g, Carbohydrates: 47 g, Protein: 8 g, Sodium: 223 mg, Cholesterol: 85 mg

Yield: 10 servings

Exchange, 1 serving: 2 starch/bread, ½ fruit
Each serving contains: Calories: 200, Total fat: 2 g, Carbohydrates: 38 g, Protein: 6 g, Sodium: 179 mg, Cholesterol: 68 mg

Snowball Cake

Impressive! Prepare this any time you want to show off. It looks fabulous on a buffet table.

1 pkg.	sugar-free strawberry gelatin mix	1 pkg.
1 c.	hot water	250 mL
1 c.	cold water	250 mL
1 c.	frozen low-fat nondairy whipped topping, thawed	250 mL
2 c.	fresh strawberries or frozen, sugar-free, defrosted	500 mL
1	angel food cake, cut into 1 in. (2.5 cm) cubes	1

Prepare the gelatin by putting the powder into a mixing bowl. Add the hot water and stir until the powder is dissolved. Add the cold water and stir to combine. Refrigerate an hour or so until partially set. In another bowl, fold together the whipped topping and the strawberries. Fold into the partially set gelatin. Return to the refrigerator.

Line a deep mixing bowl with long pieces of waxed paper. The pieces should extend over the edge, travel down the inside of the bowl and up the other side, extending past the rims. Use several overlapping strips so the inside of the bowl is totally covered. Alternate layers of the gelatin mixture with cake cubes in the bowl. Refrigerate 8 hours or overnight. Before serving, put a cake plate upside down on top of the bowl. Turn the whole thing over. Peel off the waxed paper carefully.

Yield: 16 servings

Exchange, 1 serving: 1 starch/bread, ½ fruit
Each serving contains: Calories: 112, Total fat: 0.7 g, Carbohydrates: 25 g, Protein: 3 g, Sodium: 204 mg, Cholesterol: 0 mg

Gourmet Strawberries and Mint

Not your run-of-the-mill strawberry shortcake. This is a nice treat at a luncheon.

4 c.	fresh strawberries, sliced	1 L
2 T.	powdered sugar	30 mL
1 T.	fresh mint leaves, finely chopped	15 mL
1 c.	fat-free sugar-free lemon yogurt	250 mL
¼ c.	fat-free sour cream	60 mL
1	angel food cake, cut in 16 slices	1

Mix the strawberries, powdered sugar, and mint together in a mixing bowl. Set aside for an hour at room temperature. This will cause the strawberries to let out their juice. When you are ready to serve, mix the yogurt and sour cream together in a small bowl. Put one slice of cake on each of 8 dessert plates. Put a spoonful of strawberries on top and then the second slice of cake. Top with the rest of the strawberries and distribute the yogurt-sour cream mixture.

Yield: 8 servings

Exchange, 1 serving: 1 starch/bread, 1½ fruit
Each serving contains: Calories: 161, Total fat: 0.3 g, Carbohydrates: 36 g, Protein: 3 g, Sodium: 272 mg, Cholesterol: 0 mg

Strawberry Charlotte

This charlotte is layered angel food cake filled with pudding and strawberry preserves. If the preserves are too rigid to spread, add a little hot water and mix well, to soften them up.

1	angel food cake	1
⅓ c.	fruit-only strawberry preserves	80 mL
1 recipe	Vanilla Tart Filling, or sugar-free low-fat strawberry pudding made with skim milk according to package directions	1 recipe

Slice the angel food cake crosswise into three sections. Lay the bottom part, cut-side-up, on a serving plate. Spread with one-third of the jam, Prepare the tart filling and then spoon one- third of the vanilla filling or pudding evenly on top of the jam layer. Spread jam on top of the next layer of angel food cake and place it on top of the pudding layer. Repeat, ending with pudding on top. Refrigerate until serving.

Yield: 12 servings

Exchange, 1 serving: 1½ starch/bread, 1 fruit
Each serving contains: Calories: 196, Total fat: 3 g, Carbohydrates: 39 g, Protein: 5 g, Sodium: 296 mg, Cholesterol: 23 mg

Peach Charlotte

A taste of Georgia. Use fresh peaches instead of canned, if you have them, for the most authentic charlotte of all.

1	angel food cake	1
⅓ c.	fruit-only peach preserves	80 mL
1 recipe	Vanilla Tart Filling or sugar-free low-fat vanilla pudding, made with skim milk according to package directions	1 recipe
15 oz.	canned peaches, sliced, packed in juice without sugar, drained and chopped	425 g

Slice the angel food cake crosswise into three sections. Place the bottom part, cut-side-up, onto a serving plate. Prepare the tart filling. Spread the cut side of the cake on the plate with one-third of the jam. Mix the vanilla filling with the drained, chopped peaches. Spoon one-third of this mixture onto the first layer of the cake. Spread jam on top of the next layer of the cake and repeat, ending with pudding. Refrigerate until serving time.

Yield: 12 servings

Exchange, 1 serving: 2 starch/bread, 1 fruit, ½ fat
Each serving contains: Calories: 211, Total fat: 3 g, Carbohydrates: 43 g, Protein: 5 g, Sodium: 296 mg, Cholesterol: 23 mg

Chocolate Charlotte

I've made this several different ways. In a pinch I use the pudding mix and whichever fruit preserves I have enough of. The raspberry-chocolate combination is the one you'd expect in an expensive restaurant.

1	angel food cake	1	
⅓ c.	fruit-only cherry preserves or seedless raspberry fruit-only preserves	80 mL	
1 recipe	Chocolate Tart Filling, or sugar-free low-fat chocolate pudding, made with skim milk according to package directions	1 recipe	

Follow the directions for Strawberry Charlotte.

Yield: 12 servings

Exchange, 1 serving: ½ milk, 2 fruit
Each serving contains: Calories: 190, Total fat: 0.4 g, Carbohydrates: 43 g, Protein: 5 g, Sodium: 298 mg, Cholesterol: 1 mg

Shortcake

People who like genuine shortcake with their strawberries or peaches will love this! Of course, others enjoy angel cake as a base for sweetened fruit.

Those who wish to cut back on calories or exchanges can spoon fruit over half a shortcake.

1¾ c.	flour	340 mL
1 t.	sugar	5 mL
3 pkts.	concentrated acesulfame-K	3 pkts.
2 t.	baking powder	10 mL
½ t.	baking soda	1 mL
dash	salt (optional)	dash
3 T.	margarine or butter	45 mL
⅝ c.	nonfat milk or nonfat buttermilk	150 mL

Combine the flour, sugar, acesulfame-K, baking powder, baking soda, and salt. Cut in the margarine. Using a food processor makes this very quick and easy. Then add the milk and process, or use your hands to gather the dough into a ball.

Put the dough on a lightly floured surface. Work it briefly into a ball and then flatten it. Use a rolling pin to flatten it out; the dough should be about ¾ in. (1.75 cm) thick. Use a round biscuit cutter to cut out 10 circles. Place the biscuits on a baking sheet. Bake in a preheated 450°F (230°C) oven for 8–9 minutes, until lightly brown.

To serve, halve each biscuit and serve with fruit and whipped topping, if desired.

Yield: 10 servings

Exchange, 1 serving: 1 bread + ½ fat
Each serving contains: Calories: 111, Carbohydrates: 17 g, Fiber: trace, Sodium: 103 mg, Cholesterol: trace

Hot-Milk Sponge Cake

1 c.	sifted cake flour	250 mL
1 t.	baking powder	5 mL
3	eggs	3
¼ c.	sugar	60 mL
3 pkts.	concentrated acesulfame-K	3 pkts.
¼ c.	hot milk	60 mL
1 t.	vanilla extract	5 mL
	fruit (optional)	
	whipped topping (optional)	

Grease two 8 in. (30 cm) round layer-cake pans. Dust lightly with flour and baking powder mixed together. Using an electric mixer at high speed, beat the eggs in a small, deep bowl until they are light and fluffy; slowly beat in the sugar and acesulfame-K until the mixture is almost double in volume and is very thick. Turn the speed to low; beat in the hot milk and vanilla. Fold in the flour mixture, a third at a time, until just blended. Pour into the prepared pan.

Bake in a 350°F (180°C) oven for 15–20 minutes or until the centers spring back when lightly pressed with a fingertip. Cool in the pans on wire racks for 10 minutes. Then loosen cakes carefully around the edges with a knife, turn out onto the wire racks, and cool completely. To serve, put fresh fruit (or well-drained canned fruit packed in its own unsweetened juice) and your favorite whipped topping between the two layers and on top of the cake.

Yield: 8 servings

Exchange, 1 serving: 1 bread
Each serving contains: Calories: 108, Carbohydrates: 14 g, Fiber: 0, Sodium: 79 mg, Cholesterol: 103 mg

Oat Bran Cake

Oat bran is recommended especially for diabetics because it can help stabilize blood sugar. Here's a delicious way to serve it. Use the whole batter to make four large oat bran pancakes, about the size of a small cake. To turn this into a cake, assemble them in a stack with fillings in between. We like this combination.

1	pancake	1
¼ c.	raspberry or strawberry purée	60 mL
1	pancake	1
¼ c.	Lemon Curd	60 mL
1	pancake	1
¼ c.	raspberry or strawberry purée	60 mL
1	pancake	1
¼ c.	whipped topping	60 mL

Layer ingredients in order shown. Cut and serve like a cake.

Yield: 8 servings

Each serving contains: Carbohydrates: 17 g

Rich Chocolate Cake

Don't let the long list of ingredients intimidate you; this cake is worth the effort!

1⅓ c.	cake flour	340 mL
⅓ c.	unsweetened cocoa powder	90 mL
¼ t.	baking powder	1 mL
¼ t.	baking soda	1 mL
pinch	salt (optional)	pinch
½ c.	egg substitute	125 mL
1 t.	vanilla extract	5 mL
1 T.	raspberry liqueur	45 mL
½ c.	nonfat buttermilk	125 mL
4 T.	margarine or butter	90 mL
2 T.	prune purée	30 mL
15 pkts.	concentrated acesulfame-K	15 pkts.
3 T.	sugar	45 mL
6	egg whites	6
¼ t.	cream of tartar	1 mL
½ c.	frozen raspberries	125 mL
½ t.	concentrated aspartame	2 mL

Sift the first five ingredients together twice; set aside. Combine the egg substitute and vanilla extract, raspberry liqueur, and buttermilk. Using an electric mixer, cream the margarine or butter and the prune purée. Add acesulfame-K and sugar and beat well. Gradually add the egg substitute alternately with the flour mixture. Beat until well combined. Beat the egg whites until stiff. Add the cream of tartar and continue beating. Add a small amount of egg whites to the batter to lighten it. With a rubber spatula, fold in the remaining beaten whites. Pour into two 8 in. (20 cm) round cake pans that have been coated with non-stick cooking spray. Bake in a preheated 350°F (180°C) oven for 30–35 minutes. Cool, then invert onto a plate. Combine the raspberries and aspartame in a food processor to make raspberry purée.

Spread raspberry purée over the top of one layer. Put the other layer on top and cover with raspberry purée.

Decorate top with whole raspberries if desired.

Yield: 10 servings

Exchange, 1 serving: 2 bread + 1½ fat
Each serving contains: Calories: 189, Carbohydrates: 39 g, Fiber: 1.74 g, Sodium: 90 mg, Cholesterol: 0 mg

Chocolate Eclair Cake

Karin made this for her mother's 75th-birthday party. It was easy to make, looked impressive, and tasted delicious. Everyone gave it rave reviews.

Dough

1 c.	water	250 mL
½ c.	canola oil	125 mL
1 c.	flour	250 mL
4	eggs	4
1 t.	butter-flavored extract	5 mL

Filling

2 (8 oz.) pkg.	sugar-free vanilla pudding	2 (244 g) pkg.
2½ c.	skim milk	625 mL
¾ c.	prepared sugar-free, low-fat whipped topping from mix	190 mL

Topping

6 T.	unsweetened cocoa powder	90 mL
2 T.	canola oil	30 mL
2 T.	skim milk	30 mL
¾ c.	aspartame	190 mL
1 t.	vanilla extract	5 mL
	extra milk, if needed	
1 t.	butter-flavored extract	5 mL

To make the dough: Heat the water and oil to a rolling boil. Stir in the flour over low heat until the mixture forms a ball. Remove from the heat. Using an electric mixer, beat in the eggs thoroughly, one at a time. Put in the butter extract. Spoon onto an ungreased cookie sheet in the shape of a ring or wreath. Bake until golden brown and dry at 400°F (200°C) for 35 to 40 minutes. Cool away from drafts. Slice in half horizontally. Just before serving add the filling by removing the top half, adding the filling, and replacing the top. Add the topping.

To make the filling: Whisk the pudding and milk until the mixture thickens. Fold in the whipped topping.

To make the topping: Melt the cocoa powder with the oil and milk. Cool. Add the aspartame and vanilla and beat until the mixture is the desired consistency. Add a little extra milk if necessary, one teaspoon at a time. Drizzle on top of the cake.

Yield: 24 servings

Exchange, 1 serving: 1 bread, 1 fat
Each serving contains: Calories: 100, Carbohydrates: 21 g, Fiber: trace, Sodium: 156 mg, Cholesterol: trace

Applesauce Carrot Cake

Carrot cakes tend to be very high in fat because of the large amount of oil used. This recipe gets its moist good taste from pineapple, applesauce, and nonfat sour cream. It has a wonderful texture and tastes very rich.

2 c.	flour	500 mL
2 t.	baking powder	10 mL
2 t.	baking soda	10 mL
1 T.	cinnamon	15 mL
1 t.	allspice	5 mL
1 t.	nutmeg	5 mL
½ c.	pineapple, canned, crushed	125 mL
¼ c.	raisins	60 mL
½ c.	walnuts, chopped	125 mL
¼ c.	sugar	60 mL
3 pkts.	concentrated acesulfame-K	3 pkts.
¾ c.	egg substitute or 3 eggs	190 mL
½ c.	measures-like-sugar saccharin	125 mL
½ c.	nonfat sour cream	125 mL
½ c.	unsweetened applesauce	125 mL
2 t.	vanilla extract	10 mL
2 c.	shredded carrots	500 mL
⅔ c.	shredded coconut (optional)	180 mL

Sift together the flour, baking powder, baking soda, and spices. In a blender or food processor, blend the pineapple, raisins, nuts, and sugar. Do not liquefy. Mix together the acesulfame-K, eggs, saccharin, sour cream, applesauce, vanilla, and the blender mixture. Beat well. Add the flour mixture. Mix well. Add the carrots and coconut. Stir gently. Pour into a 10 in. (25 cm) cake pan coated with non-stick cooking spray. Bake at 350°F (180°C) for 50–60 minutes or until a cake tester inserted into the center comes out clean. Cool in the pan on a cooling rack. Remove from the pan and cut horizontally to make a two-layer cake. Frost between the layers and on top with Applesauce-Carrot Cake Frosting (recipe below).

Yield: 12 servings

Exchange, 1 serving: 2 breads
Each serving contains: Calories: 165, Carbohydrates: 37 g, Fiber: 1.6 g, Sodium: 304 mg, Cholesterol: 1.3 mg

Applesauce-Carrot Cake Frosting

Although this is a variation of the classic carrot cake frosting, you might want to try it on other flavorful cakes as well.

8 oz.	nonfat cream cheese, softened	250 mL
½ c.	bulk aspartame	125 mL
1 t.	lemon extract	5 mL
1 t.	butter-flavored extract	5 mL

Beat all ingredients together until smooth.

Yield: 12 T.

Exchange: free
Each serving contains: Calories: 17, Fiber: 0, Sodium: 90 mg, Cholesterol: 2.7 mg

Holiday Cranberry Cake

It's worth keeping cranberries in the freezer so you can make this cake year round. Buy cranberries around Thanksgiving, when stores are well stocked with them.

2 c.	cake flour	500 mL
1 t.	baking powder	5 mL
½ t.	baking soda	2 mL
pinch	salt (optional)	pinch
2 T.	orange peel granules	30 mL
4 T.	margarine or butter	60 mL
¼ c.	sugar	30 mL
12 pkts.	concentrated acesulfame-K	12 pkts.
2 c.	cranberries (fresh or frozen)	500 mL
½ c.	egg substitute	125 mL
¾ c.	nonfat sugar-free plain yogurt	190 mL
¼ c.	Triple Sec	60 mL
1 t.	vanilla extract	5 mL

Glaze

2 oz.	nonfat cream cheese	60 mL
1 t.	concentrated aspartame	5 mL
2 T.	skim milk	30 mL
½ t.	clear vanilla extract	2 mL

Sift together the first four ingredients, add the orange peel, and set aside. With an electric mixer, soften the margarine. Add the sugar and acesulfame-K and beat for a few minutes. Add the egg substitute slowly and beat. Alternately add the flour mixture and the yogurt, liqueur, and vanilla extract. Beat for a few minutes, then fold in the cranberries. Pour the batter into a tube pan that has been coated with non-stick cooking spray. Bake in a preheated 350°F (180°C) oven for 45 minutes. Cool and then remove from the pan. Prepare the glaze and drizzle it over the top of the cake.

To make the glaze, soften the cream cheese by microwaving it for about 20 seconds or by heating it in a saucepan over very low heat. Set aside. Use a wire whisk to combine the other ingredients; then whisk in the softened cream cheese for a few minutes until it is creamy. Use large spoon to drizzle glaze over top of the cake.

Yield: 12 servings

Exchange, 1 serving: 1 fruit + 1 bread
Each serving contains: Calories: 164, Carbohydrates: 28 g, Fiber: 1 g,
*   Sodium: 178 mg, Cholesterol: 0.7 mg*

French Pastry Cake

The word for this cake is "Wow!" It would have been out of this world in fat and calories before the new nonfat ingredients, but once the cake is made, no one can tell.

½ c.	margarine or butter	125 mL
½ c.	nonfat cream cheese	125 mL
¼ c.	sugar	60 mL
½ c.	measures-like-sugar saccharin	125 mL
2	eggs or equivalent egg substitute	2
1 c.	nonfat sour cream	250 mL
1 c.	nonfat mayonnaise	250 mL
1 T.	vanilla extract	15 mL
2 c.	flour	500 mL
1 t.	baking powder	5 mL
1 t.	baking soda	5 mL

Cinnamon Mixture

1 T.	cinnamon	15 mL
2 pkts.	concentrated acesulfame-K	2 pkts.
½ c.	chopped almonds	125 mL

Cream margarine or butter and cream cheese with sugar and saccharin. Add the eggs, sour cream, mayonnaise, and vanilla extract; beat well. Mix the flour, baking powder, and baking soda and add to the batter. Put half the batter into a tube pan or bundt pan coated with non-stick cooking spray. Mix together the cinnamon, acesulfame-K, and chopped almonds. Sprinkle half the cinnamon mixture on top of the batter in the pan, then add the rest of the batter. Sprinkle the rest of the cinnamon mixture on top of the batter. Bake at 350°F (180°C) 60–75 minutes or until the top is light brown and the cake pulls away from the pan.

Yield: 20 servings

Exchange, 1 serving: 1 fat + 1 bread
Each serving contains: Calories: 155, Carbohydrates: 17 g, Fiber: 0.6 g, Sodium: 274 mg, Cholesterol: 30 mg

Banana Cake

Egg whites lighten this cake. You'll be proud to serve it.

2 c.	flour	500 mL
1 T.	baking powder	15 mL
2 T.	fructose	30 mL
¼ c.	fat-free mayonnaise	60 mL
½ c.	egg substitute	125 mL
1½ c.	mashed banana	375 mL
½ t.	vanilla extract	2 mL
1 t.	banana extract	5 mL
3	egg whites	3
¼ t.	cream of tartar	1 mL

Sift together the flour, baking powder, and fructose. In a bowl, mix the mayonnaise, egg substitute, banana, and flavorings. Beat until smooth. Gradually add the flour mixture and beat to combine.

In a separate bowl, beat the egg whites until foamy. Add cream of tartar and beat until stiff. Add approximately a third of the whites to the flour mixture to lighten it. Gently fold in the rest.

Pour into two 8 in. (20 cm) cake pans that have been coated with nonstick cooking spray. Bake in a 350°F (180°C) oven for 20 minutes. Frost with Applesauce-Carrot Cake Frosting, Creamy Frosting, or your favorite whipped topping and sliced ripe bananas.

Yield: 12 servings

Exchange, 1 serving: 1½ bread
Each serving contains: Calories: 121, Carbohydrates: 18 g, Fiber: 1 g, Sodium: 183 mg, Cholesterol: 0 mg

Spragg Cake

Dedicated to W. Spragg, a diligent helper in the diabetes work being done in Iowa. This is yours, Mr. Spragg.

¼ c.	almonds, toasted and ground	60 mL
½ c.	semisweet chocolate chips	125 mL
2 T.	butter	30 mL
¼ c.	skim milk	60 mL
5	egg yolks	5
5 T.	cornstarch	75 mL
4 T.	granulated sugar replacement	60 mL
1 T.	almond extract	15 mL
1 t.	instant coffee	5 mL
1 T.	flour	15 mL
5	egg whites	5

Combine ground almonds, chocolate chips, butter, and milk in saucepan. Cook and stir over low heat until chocolate is melted; cool. Beat egg yolks with an electric mixer on high speed until pale yellow, gradually adding 3 T. (45 mL) of the cornstarch and 2 T. (30 mL) of the sugar replacement. Add egg yolk mixture to cooled chocolate mixture. Fold in almond extract, coffee and flour. In another bowl, with clean beaters beat egg whites until stiff. Gradually add remaining 2 T. (30 mL) cornstarch and 2 T. (30 mL) sugar replacement. Gently fold a large spoonful of whites into chocolate mixture to lighten, then fold remaining whites into chocolate mixture. Pour batter into well greased 10 in. (25 cm) springform pan. Bake at top of 350°F (175°C) oven for 40 to 50 minutes or until cake springs back when lightly touched.

Yield: 20 servings

Exchange, 1 serving: ½ bread, 1 fat
Each serving contains: Calories: 69, Carbohydrates: 7 g

Rum Roll

An extra-special cake with few calories.

¾ c.	cake flour	190 mL
1 t.	baking powder	5 mL
½ t.	baking soda	2 mL
dash	salt	dash
3	egg whites	3
1 T.	white vinegar	15 mL
1 T.	water	15 mL
¼ c.	semisweet chocolate chips	60 mL
3 T.	sorbitol	45 mL
3 T.	granulated sugar replacement	45 mL
⅓ c.	water, boiling	90 mL
3	egg yolks	3
2 T.	rum flavoring	30 mL
1 t.	vanilla extract	5 mL
1 recipe	Chocolate Whipped Topping	1 recipe

Sift together 3 times the cake flour, baking powder, baking soda, and salt. Whip egg whites until soft peaks form; gradually, add vinegar and water and continue whipping into stiff peaks. In a bowl combine chocolate chips, sorbitol, and sugar replacement. Add boiling water and stir until chocolate is melted. Add egg yolks, rum and vanilla extract. Beat until smooth and slightly fluffy. Fold in dry flour mixture. Fold in egg whites. Do not over mix; some streaks of egg white may remain. Gently, spread mixture into papered, well greased and floured jelly roll pan. Bake at 325°F (165°C) for 13 to 15 minutes or until cake tests done. Invert cake onto a lightly floured pastry towel or cloth. Peel off paper. Gently roll up cake and towel. Place on cooling rack and allow to cool. Unroll cake, spread with the chocolate whipped topping. Roll up without squeezing whipped topping from cake. Chill in refrigerator or freeze.

Yield: 24 servings

Exchange, 1 serving: ½ bread
Each serving contains: Calories: 29, Carbohydrates: 9 g

Fudge Cupcakes

½ c.	butter	125 mL
3 oz.	baking chocolate	90 g
½ c.	granulated sugar replacement	125 mL
2 c.	flour	500 mL
dash	salt	dash
8	eggs, lightly beaten	8
1 T.	vanilla extract	15 mL

Melt butter with chocolate in top of double boiler over warm water. In large mixing bowl combine sugar replacement, flour and salt; stir in melted chocolate mixture. Add eggs and vanilla extract. Stir just until moistened and blended. Spoon batter into muffin pans lined with paper muffin cups. Bake muffins at 300°F (150°C) for 35 minutes or until muffins test done.

Yield: 36 muffins

Exchange, 1 muffin: ½ bread, 1 fat
Each serving contains: Calories: 78, Carbohydrates: 9 g

Muse Cake

1 med.	orange with rind	1 med.
½ c.	raisins	125 mL
2 c.	flour	500 mL
¼ c.	granulated fructose	60 mL
3 T.	granulated sugar replacement	45 mL
1 oz.	baking chocolate, melted	30 g
¾ c.	buttermilk	190 mL
2	eggs	2
2 T.	butter, softened	30 mL
1 t.	baking soda	5 mL
¼ t.	salt	1 mL

Squeeze juice from orange and set aside. Chop orange rind into small pieces. Combine chopped rind, raisins and 2 T. (30 mL) of the flour in blender. Blend until finely chopped. Transfer to large mixing bowl. Add remaining flour, fructose, sugar replacement, melted chocolate, buttermilk, eggs, butter, baking soda, and salt. Stir to completely blend. Pour batter into well greased 9 × 13 in. (23 × 33 cm) baking pan. Bake at 350°F (175°C) for 40 to 50 minutes or until cake tests done. Remove from oven; immediately pour reserved orange juice over entire surface.

Yield: 24 servings

Exchange, 1 serving: ¾ bread, ½ fat
Each serving contains: Calories: 75, Carbohydrates: 15 g

German Chocolate Cake

A choice for all birthdays.

4 oz.	baking chocolate	120 g
½ c.	water, boiling	125 mL
½ c.	butter	125 mL
½ c.	granulated sugar replacement	125 mL
3 T.	granulated fructose	45 mL
4	egg yolks	4
2 t.	vanilla extract	10 mL
2¼ c.	flour	625 mL
1 t.	baking soda	5 mL
½ t.	salt	2 mL
1 c.	buttermilk	250 mL
4	egg whites, stiffly beaten	4

Melt chocolate in boiling water. Cool. Cream butter, sugar replacement, and fructose until fluffy. Add egg yolks, one at a time, beating well after each addition. Blend in vanilla and chocolate water. Sift flour with baking soda and salt; add alternately with buttermilk to chocolate mixture, beating well after each addition until smooth. Fold in beaten egg whites. Grease three 9 in. (23 cm) baking pans and line them with paper; grease again and lightly flour pans; pour batter into the three pans. Bake at 350°F (175°C) for 25 to 30 minutes or until cakes test done. Remove from pans onto racks, remove paper lining. Cool.

Yield: three 9 in. (23 cm) cakes or 60 servings

Exchange, 1 serving: ½ bread, ½ fat
Each serving contains: Calories: 50, Carbohydrates: 6 g

Sour-Milk Chocolate Cake

A cake superlative.

2 c.	cake flour, sifted	500 mL
1 t.	baking soda	5 mL
¼ t.	salt	1 mL
½ c.	vegetable shortening, softened	125 mL
¼ c.	granulated sugar replacement	60 mL
2 t.	vanilla extract	10 mL
3	egg yolks, beaten	3
2 oz.	baking chocolate, melted	60 g
1 c.	skim milk, soured (see note)	250 mL
3	egg whites, stiffly beaten	3

Sift flour, baking soda and salt together. Cream shortening and sugar replacement until fluffy; add vanilla extract and egg yolks and beat thoroughly. Stir in chocolate. Add sifted dry ingredients and soured milk alternately in small amounts; beat well after each addition. Fold in stiffly beaten egg whites. Pour batter into two 9 in. (23 cm) well greased and floured pans. Bake at 350°F (175°C) for 30 to 35 minutes or until cake tests done.

Note: To sour 1 c. (250 mL) milk, stir in 2 t. (10 mL) vinegar or lemon juice.

Yield: 24 servings (12 servings per cake)

Exchange, 1 serving: ½ bread, 1¼ fat
Each serving contains: Calories: 95, Carbohydrates: 18 g

Marble Cake

Only for rare occasions.

1¾ c.	cake flour	440 mL
2¼ t.	baking powder	12 mL
¼ t.	salt	1 mL
½ c.	vegetable shortening, softened	125 mL
3 T.	granulated sugar replacement	45 mL
2	eggs, well beaten	2
½ c.	skim milk	125 mL
2 t.	vanilla extract	10 mL
1 oz.	baking chocolate, melted	30 g

Sift flour, baking powder and salt together. Cream shortening with sugar replacement until fluffy. Add beaten eggs and mix thoroughly. Add sifted dry ingredients and milk alternately in small amounts, beating well after each addition. Add vanilla extract. Divide batter into two equal parts. Add chocolate to one part of the batter. Drop batter alternately by tablespoons into well greased 8 in. (20 cm) square baking pan. Bake at 350°F (175°C) for 45 to 55 minutes until cake tests done.

Yield: 9 servings

Exchange, 1 serving: 1 bread, 3 fat
Each serving contains: Calories: 218, Carbohydrates: 33 g

Cocoa Spice Cake

The spices make the difference.

2 c.	flour	500 mL
½ c.	cocoa	125 mL
¼ t.	salt	1 mL
1 t.	baking soda	5 mL
2 t.	cinnamon	10 mL
1 t.	cloves	5 mL
½ t.	nutmeg	2 mL
½ c.	vegetable shortening, softened	125 mL
¼ c.	granulated brown sugar replacement	60 mL
3	eggs, separated	3
1 c.	sour cream	250 mL

Sift together 3 times the flour, cocoa, salt, soda and spices. Cream shortening with brown sugar replacement until fluffy. Beat egg yolks thoroughly and add to batter. Add sifted dry ingredients and sour cream alternately in small amounts, beating well after each addition. Beat egg whites until stiff, but not dry, and fold into batter. Pour into greased 9 in. (23 cm) square pan. Bake at 350°F (175°C) for 40 to 50 minutes or until cake tests done.

Yield: 9 servings

Exchange, 1 serving: 1½ bread, 3 fat
Each serving contains: Calories: 242, Carbohydrates: 34 g

Devil's Food Cake

2¼ c.	cake flour	560 mL
¼ c.	granulated sugar replacement	60 mL
2 t.	baking soda	10 mL
1 t.	salt	5 mL
½ c.	cocoa	125 mL
⅔ c.	vegetable shortening, softened	180 mL
1 c.	water	250 mL
2 t.	vanilla extract	10 mL
3	eggs	3

Sift flour, sugar replacement, baking soda, salt, and cocoa together into large mixing bowl. Add shortening, ½ c. (125 mL) of the water and vanilla extract; beat until just moistened. Add remaining water and eggs. Beat until slightly thickened. Pour into well greased and floured 13 × 9 in. (23 × 33 cm) baking pan. Bake at 350°F (175°C) for 40 to 50 minutes or until cake tests done.

Yield: 24 servings

Exchange, 1 serving: ½ bread, 1½ fat
Each serving contains: Calories: 99, Carbohydrates: 13 g

White Cake

1½ c.	cake flour	375 mL
1½ t.	baking powder	7 mL
¼ t.	salt	1 mL
¼ c.	solid shortening	60 mL
½ c.	sorbitol	125 mL
2 t.	clear vanilla flavoring	10 mL
1 t.	water	5 mL
½ c.	2% low-fat milk	125 mL
2	egg whites, stiffly beaten	2

Combine cake flour, baking powder, and salt in a sifter, and then sift into a medium-size bowl. Set aside. Beat shortening, sorbitol, vanilla, and water together until creamy. Add flour mixture and milk alternately beating well after each addition. Fold in stiffly beaten egg whites. Grease an 8 in. (20 cm) cake pan. Line pan with waxed paper and grease again; then flour pan lightly. Spread batter into greased, lined, a floured cake pan. Bake at 350°F (175°C) for 30 to 35 minutes or use toothpick inserted in center comes out dean. Allow to cool. Turn out onto board or plate, and remove waxed paper.

Yield: 10 servings

Exchange, 1 serving: 1 starch/bread, 1 fat
Each serving contains: Calories: 105, Carbohydrates: 12 g

Banana Spice Cake

2¾ c.	sifted all-purpose flour	690 mL
2 t.	baking powder	10 mL
1 t.	baking soda	5 mL
1 t.	salt	5 mL
2 t.	cinnamon	10 mL
1 t.	nutmeg	5 mL
¼ t.	cloves	1 mL
⅔ c.	solid shortening	180 mL
1 c.	granulated sugar replacement	250 mL
2 T.	water	30 mL
1 t.	vinegar	5 mL
2	eggs, well beaten	2
1½ c.	mashed bananas	375 mL
2 t.	vanilla extract	10 mL

Sift flour, baking powder, baking soda, salt, and spices together three times. Set aside. Beat shortening, sugar replacement, water, and vinegar together until fluffy. Add eggs and beat well. Add sifted ingredients and mashed bananas alternately in small amounts to creamed mixture, beating well after each addition. Stir in vanilla. Transfer to greased and floured 13 × 9 in. (33 × 23 cm) cake pan. Bake at 350°F (175°C) for 35 to 45 minutes or until toothpick inserted in center comes out clean.

Yield: 24 servings

Exchange, 1 serving: 1½ starch/bread, ⅔ fat, ⅓ fruit
Each serving contains: Calories: 130, Carbohydrates: 23 g

Orange Rum Cake

1 c.	buttermilk	250 mL
2 T.	granulated fructose	30 mL
1 c.	low-calorie margarine	250 mL
2 T.	grated fresh orange rind	30 mL
2	eggs	2
2½ c.	sifted all-purpose flour	625 mL
2 t.	baking powder	10 mL
1 t.	baking soda	5 mL
½ t.	salt	2 mL
½ c.	orange juice	125 mL
1 T.	lemon juice	15 mL
2 T.	rum	30 mL

Combine buttermilk and granulated fructose. Beat margarine until creamy. Beat in orange rind. Then beat in eggs, one at a time (beating well after each addition). Combine flour, baking powder, baking soda, and salt in a sifter. Sift into a bowl. Add sifted ingredients and sweetened buttermilk alternately in small amounts to creamed mixture, beating until very smooth. Pour batter into a well greased 10 in. (25 cm) tube pan. Bake at 350°F (175°C) for 60 to 70 minutes or until cake tester inserted in center comes out clean. Now combine juices and rum in a small saucepan. Heat to boiling. When cake is done, remove from oven. Slowly pour hot juice mixture over cake in pan. Allow cake to cool; then wrap and refrigerate for 1 or 2 days before serving.

Yield: 30 servings

Exchange, 1 serving: ¾ starch/bread, 1 fat
Each serving contains: Calories: 104, Carbohydrates: 13 g

Almond-Flavored Cake

18	eggs	18
¾ c.	granulated fructose	190 mL
1 t.	vanilla extract	5 mL
½ t.	almond extract	2 mL
2 c.	sifted cake flour	500 mL
¼ c.	butter, melted	60 mL

Combine eggs and fructose in top of double boiler. Beat to blend. Place over simmering water. (Do not allow water to boil!) Continue beating for about 10 or 12 minutes or until very light and fluffy. Remove from heat, and then beat until cool. Beat in vanilla and almond extracts. Fold in cake flour very gradually. Add melted butter and fold well. (Do not stir.) Pour batter into three 9 in. (23 cm) round greased cake pans. Bake at 325°F (165°C) for 30 to 35 minutes or until done. Remove from oven. Remove cakes from pans, and cool completely on racks.

Yield: 30 servings

Exchange, 1 serving: ½ starch/bread, ½ fat, ½ high-fat meat
Each serving contains: Calories: 102, Carbohydrates: 7 g

Apple Walnut Cake

1 qt.	chopped apples	1 L
¼ c.	granulated fructose	60 mL
½ c.	granulated sugar replacement	125 mL
1 t.	lemon juice	5 mL
2 c.	sifted all-purpose flour	500 mL
2 t.	baking soda	10 mL
2 t.	cinnamon	10 mL
1 t.	salt	5 mL
½ c.	liquid shortening	125 mL
2	eggs, well beaten	2
2 t.	vanilla extract	10 mL
½ c.	chopped walnuts	125 mL

Combine chopped apples, fructose, sugar replacement, and lemon juice in a bowl. Toss to coat apples. Set aside for 15 minutes. Sift flour, baking soda, cinnamon, and salt together three times. Beat liquid shortening and eggs together until well mixed. Beat in vanilla. Add sifted ingredients and beat until blended. Add apple mixture and stir very well for at least 2 minutes. Fold in walnuts. Transfer to greased and floured 13 × 9 in. (33 × 23 cm) cake pan. Bake at 350°F (175°C) for 55 to 60 minutes or until toothpick inserted in center comes out clean.

Yield: 24 servings

Exchange, 1 serving: 1 starch/bread, ⅓ fat
Each serving contains: Calories: 86, Carbohydrates: 13 g

Real Sponge Cake

1 c.	sifted cake flour	250 mL
¼ t.	salt	1 mL
1 T.	grated fresh lemon rind	15 mL
1½ T.	fresh lemon juice	21 mL
5	eggs, separated	5
½ c.	sorbitol	125 mL

Sift cake flour and salt together four times. Set aside. Add lemon rind and lemon juice to egg yolks. Beat until very thick. Beat egg whites until very stiff peaks form. Fold sorbitol into egg whites. Then fold in egg yolk mixture. Sift the flour mixture, a fourth of it at a time, over the top of the egg mixture. Gently fold the flour in after each addition. Pour into a 9 in. (23 cm) ungreased tube pan. Bake at 350°F (175°C) for 60 minutes or until done. Invert pan and cool completely. Remove cake from pan.

Yield: 20 servings

Exchange, 1 serving: ¾ starch/bread, fat
Each serving contains: Calories: 83, Carbohydrates: 11 g

Apple Upside-Down Cake

2 T.	low-calorie margarine	30 mL
½ c.	dietetic maple syrup	125 mL
2 large	baking apples	2 large
¼ c.	raisins	60 mL
1½ c.	sifted cake flour	375 mL
3 t.	baking soda	15 mL
½ t.	salt	2 mL
⅓ c.	solid shortening	90 mL
⅓ c.	granulated sugar replacement	90 mL
1 T.	water	15 mL
2	eggs, well beaten	2
1 t.	vanilla extract	5 mL
⅔ c.	water	180 mL

Melt low-calorie margarine in bottom of 9 in. (23 cm) cake pan. Add maple syrup, stirring to mix. Allow to cool. Peel, core, and slice apples; then layer over margarine-syrup mixture in cake pan. Sprinkle with raisins. Combine cake flour, baking soda, and salt in sifter, and sift into bowl. Cream together shortening, sugar replacement and 1 T. (15 mL) water. Beat in eggs and vanilla. Add sifted ingredients and ⅔ c. (180 mL) water alternately in small amounts, beating well after each addition. Pour over apples in pan. Lightly spread to level the batter. Bake at 350°F (175°C) for 45 to 50 minutes or until toothpick inserted in center comes out clean. Turn over onto a serving plate immediately after removing from oven.

Yield: 24 servings

Exchange, 1 serving: ⅔ starch/bread, 1⅓ fat, ¼ fruit
Each serving contains: Calories: 90, Carbohydrates: 11 g

Pineapple Chiffon Cake

2¼ c.	sifted cake flour	560 mL
1 T.	baking powder	15 mL
½ t	salt	2 mL
¾ c.	sorbitol	190 mL
½ c.	liquid vegetable oil	125 mL
5	egg yolks	5
¾ c.	unsweetened pineapple juice	190 mL
8	egg whites	8
¾ t.	cream of tartar	4 mL

Combine cake flour, baking powder, and salt in a sifter. Sift into a large mixing bowl. Add sorbitol. Make a well in the center of flour mixture, and add vegetable oil, egg yolks, and pineapple juice. Beat until mixture becomes very smooth and thick. Now beat egg whites with cream of tartar into very stiff peaks. Pour batter over egg whites in a thin stream. Fold batter gently into egg whites. Transfer to ungreased 10 in. (25 cm) tube pan. Bake at 350°F (175°C) for an hour or until cake tests done. Invert and cool completely. Cut around sides and tube stem. Remove bottom of pan with cake. Carefully cut between cake and pan bottom. Remove cake.

Yield: 24 servings

Exchange, 1 serving: 1 starch/bread, 1 fat
Each serving contains: Calories: 102, Carbohydrates: 14 g

Orange Sunrise Chiffon Cake

7	egg yolks	7
½ c.	sorbitol	125 mL
2 t.	grated fresh orange rind	10 mL
⅓ c.	orange juice	90 mL
1 c.	sifted cake flour	250 mL
7	egg whites	7
1 t.	cream of tartar	5 mL

Beat egg yolks until they become very thick and lemon colored. Beat in ¼ c. (60 mL) of the sorbitol. Beat in orange rind. Add orange juice and cake flour alternately in small amounts to egg-yolk mixture, beating until mixture becomes very smooth and thick. Now beat egg whites and cream of tartar together until soft peaks form. Beat in remaining ¼ c. (60 mL) of the sorbitol. Beat into very firm peaks. Fold egg whites into batter. Pour into 9 in. (23 cm) ungreased tube pan. Bake at 350°F (175°C) for 50 to 60 minutes or until done. Invert and cool completely. Remove cake from pan.

Yield: 24 servings

Exchange, 1 serving: ½ starch/bread
Each serving contains: Calories: 41, Carbohydrates: 7 g

Chocolate Chiffon Cake

4 sq. (1 oz.)	unsweetened chocolate, melted	4 sq. (30 g)
½ c.	boiling water	125 mL
¼ c.	granulated fructose	60 mL
2¼ c.	sifted cake flour	560 mL
¾ c.	sorbitol	190 mL
¼ c.	granulated sugar replacement	60 mL
1 T.	baking powder	15 mL
1 t.	salt	5 mL
½ c.	liquid vegetable oil	125 mL
7	egg yolks	7
¾ c.	cold water	190 mL
1½ T.	vanilla extract	21 mL
7	egg whites	7 mL
½ t.	cream of tartar	2 mL

Blend together melted chocolate, boiling water, and fructose. Allow to cool completely. Sift together cake flour, sorbitol, sugar replacement, baking powder, and salt into a large bowl. Make a well in the center of the flour mixture, and add vegetable oil, egg yolks, cold water, and vanilla. Beat until mixture becomes very smooth and thick. Stir cooled chocolate into mixture. Now beat egg whites and cream of tartar into very stiff peaks. Pour batter over egg whites in a thin stream. Fold batter gently into egg whites. Transfer to ungreased 10 in. (25 cm) tube pan. Bake at 325°F (165°C) for an hour or until cake tests done. Invert and cool completely. Cut around sides and tube stem. Remove bottom of pan with cake. Carefully cut between cake and pan bottom. Remove cake.

Yield: 30 servings

Exchange, 1 serving: 1 starch/bread, 1⅓ fat
Each serving contains: Calories: 123, Carbohydrates: 18 g

Coffee Chiffon Cake

4 t.	instant coffee, powder	20 mL
¾ c.	boiling water	190 mL
2¼ c.	sifted cake flour	560 mL
1 c.	sorbitol	250 mL
¼ c.	granulated sugar replacement	60 mL
1 T.	baking powder	15 mL
1 t.	salt	5 mL
½ c.	liquid vegetable oil	125 mL
5	egg yolks	5
1 t.	vanilla extract	5 mL
2 sq. (1 oz.)	semi-sweet chocolate, grated	2 sq. (30 g)
7	egg whites	7 mL
½ t.	cream of tartar	2 mL

Dissolve coffee powder in boiling water. Cool completely. Sift together cake flour, sorbitol, sugar replacement, baking powder, and salt into a large bowl. Make a well in the center of the flour mixture, and add vegetable oil, egg yolks, and vanilla. Beat until mixture becomes very smooth and thick. Stir in grated chocolate. Now beat egg whites and cream of tartar together into very stiff peaks. Pour batter over egg whites in a thin stream. Fold batter gently into egg whites. Transfer to ungreased 10 in. (25 cm) tube pan. Bake at 325°F (165°C) for 70 minutes or until cake tests done. Invert and cool completely. Cut around sides and tube stem. Remove bottom of pan with cake. Carefully cut between cake and pan bottom. Remove cake.

Yield: 20 servings

Exchange, 1 serving: 1 starch/bread, 1 fat
Each serving contains: Calories: 119, Carbohydrates: 17 g

Vanilla Chiffon Cake

2¼ c.	sifted cake flour	560 mL
1 T.	baking powder	15 mL
1 t.	salt	5 mL
1 c.	sorbitol	250 mL
½ c.	liquid vegetable oil	125 mL
8	egg yolks	8
¾ c.	water	190 mL
2 T.	vanilla extract	30 mL
½ t.	lemon juice	2 mL
8	egg whites	8
½ t.	cream of tartar	2 mL

Combine cake flour, baking powder, and salt in a sifter. Sift into a large mixing bowl. Stir in sorbitol. Make a well in the center of the flour mixture, and add vegetable oil, egg yolks, water, vanilla, and lemon juice. Beat until mixture becomes very smooth and thick. Now beat egg whites and cream of tartar together until very stiff peaks form. Fold egg whites into batter. Transfer to 10 in. (25 cm) ungreased tube pan. Bake at 325°F (165°C) for 55 to 60 minutes or until done. Invert and cool completely. Remove from pan.

Yield: 24 servings

Exchange, 1 serving: 1 starch/bread, ⅓ fat
Each serving contains: Calories: 79, Carbohydrates: 11 g

Best Lemon Chiffon Cake

8	egg yolks	8
⅔ c.	granulated sorbitol	90 mL
2 t.	grated fresh lemon rind	10 mL
2 t.	unsweetened lemon-drink mix	10 mL
⅓ c.	water	90 mL
1 c.	sifted cake flour	250 mL
8	egg whites	8
1 t.	cream of tartar	5 mL

Beat egg yolks until they become very thick and lemon colored. Beat in ⅓ c. (45 mL) of the sorbitol. Beat in lemon rind and lemon-drink mix. Add water and cake flour alternately in small amounts to egg-yolk mixture, beating until mixture becomes very smooth and thick. Now beat egg whites and cream of tartar together until soft peaks form. Beat in remaining ⅓ c. (45 mL) of the sorbitol. Beat into very firm peaks. Fold egg whites into batter. Pour into 9 in. (23 cm) ungreased tube pan. Bake at 325°F (165°C) for 60 to 65 minutes or until done. Invert and cool completely. Remove cake from pan.

Yield: 20 servings

Exchange, 1 serving: ½ starch/bread
Each serving contains: Calories: 43, Carbohydrates: 7 g

Banana Poppy Seed Yolk Cake

3 c.	sifted all-purpose flour	750 mL
1 T.	baking powder	15 mL
1 t.	salt	5 mL
1 t.	banana flavoring	5 mL
12	egg yolks	12
1 c.	mashed bananas	250 mL
¼ c.	hot water	60 mL
1 c.	sorbitol	250 mL
¼ c.	poppy seeds	60 mL

Sift flour and baking powder together four times. Set aside. Add salt and banana flavoring to egg yolks. Beat until very thick. Combine mashed bananas and hot water, stirring to blend. Add sorbitol and bananas alternately in small amounts, to egg yolk mixture, beating until thick after each addition. Fold in poppy seeds. Fold flour mixture, a fourth of it at a time, into batter. Pour into ungreased 10 in. (25 cm) tube pan. Bake at 350°F (175°C) for 60 to 65 minutes or until done. Invert and cool completely. Remove from pan.

Yield: 30 servings

Exchange, 1 serving: 1 starch/bread, ⅓ medium-fat meat
Each serving contains: Calories: 105, Carbohydrates: 18 g

Chocolate Chocolate Chip Cake

3 sq. (1 oz.)	unsweetened chocolate, melted	3 sq. (30 g)
½ c.	boiling water	125 mL
¼ c.	granulated fructose	60 mL
2¼ c.	sifted cake flour	560 mL
¾ c.	sorbitol	190 mL
½ c.	granulated sugar replacement	125 mL
1 T.	baking powder	15 mL
1 t.	salt	5 mL
½ c.	liquid vegetable oil	125 mL
9	egg yolks	9
I c.	cold water	190 mL
1½ T.	vanilla extract	21 mL
9	egg whites	9 mL
½ t.	cream of tartar	2 mL
½ c.	mini chocolate chips	125 mL

Blend together melted chocolate, boiling water, and fructose. Cool completely. Sift together cake flour, sorbitol, sugar replacement, baking powder, and salt into a large bowl. Make a well in the center of the flour mixture, and add vegetable oil, egg yolks, cold water, and vanilla. Beat until mixture becomes very smooth and thick. Stir in cooled chocolate. Now beat egg whites and cream of tartar together into very stiff peaks. Gently fold egg whites into batter. Then fold in chocolate chips. Transfer to ungreased 10 in. (25 cm) tube pan. Bake at 325°F (165°C) for 60 to 70 minutes or until cake tests done. Invert and cool completely. Cut around sides and tube stem. Remove bottom of pan with cake. Carefully cut between cake and pan bottom. Remove cake.

Yield: 30 servings

Exchange, 1 serving: 1 starch/bread, 1⅓ fat
Each serving contains: Calories: 109, Carbohydrates: 16 g

Light White Cake

⅔ c.	soft butter	180 mL
¾ c.	sorbitol	190 mL
1½ t.	clear vanilla flavoring	7 mL
½ t.	almond extract	2 mL
2½ c.	sifted cake flour	625 mL
2½ t.	baking powder	12 mL
⅔ c.	skim milk	180 mL
4	egg whites	4
½ t.	salt	2 mL
½ t.	cream of tartar	2 mL

Cream butter until light and fluffy. Add sorbitol gradually, beating constantly. Continue beating until mixture is light and fluffy. Beat in vanilla flavoring and almond extract. Combine cake flour and baking powder in sifter. Sift a fourth of the flour mixture over the creamed butter, and then beat thoroughly. Add a third of the skim milk, and then beat thoroughly. Add flour mixture and milk alternately, as stated above, beating thoroughly after each addition, Now beat egg whites until frothy. Add salt and cream of tartar. Beat until stiff peaks form. Fold egg whites into batter. Pour batter into two 9 in. (23 cm) pans. Each pan should be greased and lined on the bottom with greased waxed paper. Bake at 375°F (190°C) for 25 to 30 minutes or until done. Cool in pans for 5 minutes. Transfer to racks, peel off paper, and cool completely.

Yield: 30 servings

Exchange, 1 serving: 1 starch/bread, 1 fat
Each serving contains: Calories: 110, Carbohydrates: 13 g

Cream-Filled Chocolate Cake

Cake

¼ c.	granulated sugar replacement	60 mL
3 T.	water	45 mL
2 sq. (1 oz.)	unsweetened chocolate, melted	2 sq. (30 g)
¾ c.	low-calorie margarine	190 mL
½ c.	granulated fructose	125 mL
1 c.	granulated sugar replacement	250 mL
1 t.	vanilla extract	5 mL
4	egg yolks	4
2¼ c.	sifted cake flour	560 mL
1 t.	cream of tartar	5 mL
½ t.	baking soda	2 mL
½ t.	salt	2 mL
1 c.	skim milk	250 mL
4	egg whites, stiffly beaten	4

Combine the ¼ c. (60 mL) sugar replacement and water. Add to melted chocolate and stir to blend. Set aside. Cream margarine. Gradually add the fructose and the 1 c. (250 mL) sugar replacement. Beat until light and fluffy. Add vanilla. Add egg yolks, one at a time, beating well after each addition. Beat in chocolate mixture. Sift dry ingredients together, and add to batter alternately with skim milk. (Begin and end with dry ingredients.) Beat until smooth. Fold stiffly beaten egg whites into batter. Pour batter into three 9 in. (23 cm) round pans. Pans should be greased and their bottoms lined with greased waxed paper. Bake at 350°F (175°C) for 45 to 50 minutes or until done. Cool in pans for 5 minutes. Transfer to racks, peel off paper, and cool completely. Put layers together with Cream Filling.

Cream-Filled Chocolate Cake *(continued)*

Cream Filling

¼ c.	granulated fructose	60 mL
3 T.	all-purpose flour	45 mL
dash	salt	dash
1½ c.	skim milk	375 mL
2	eggs, beaten	2
½ t.	vanilla extract	2

In the top of a double boiler, mix fructose, flour, and salt. Add ½ c. (125 mL) of the skim milk. Stir until smooth. Stir in remaining milk. Cook mixture over boiling water, stirring constantly, until thick and smooth. Add small amount of hot mixture to beaten eggs. Stir to blend. Return to top of double boiler. Cook and stir about 5 minutes longer or until mixture is very thick. Allow to cool; then stir in vanilla. Use to fill and lightly frost cooled cake.

Yield: 30 servings

Exchange, 1 serving: 1 starch/bread, ¼ fat
Each serving contains: Calories: 99, Carbohydrates: 16 g

Magic Devil's Food Cake

5 T.	cocoa powder	75 mL
1	egg yolk	1
1½ c.	skim milk	375 mL
½ c.	low-calorie margarine	125 mL
¾ c.	sorbitol	190 mL
½ c.	granulated sugar replacement	125 mL
1 t.	vanilla extract	5 mL
2	eggs	2
2 c.	sifted all-purpose flour	500 mL
2 t.	baking powder	10 mL
¼ t.	baking soda	1 mL
½ t.	salt	2 mL

Mix cocoa, egg yolk, and 1 c. (250 mL) of the skim milk in a saucepan. Cook over low heat, stirring, until smooth and thickened. Cream margarine until light and fluffy. Create sweetener by combining sorbitol and sugar replacement in a bowl, stirring to mix. Gradually add sweetener to creamed margarine, beating constantly. Continue beating until light and fluffy. Add vanilla and eggs, one at a time, beating well after each addition. Beat in cocoa mixture. Sift dry ingredients together. Add dry ingredients and remaining milk alternately to the creamed mixture. (Begin and end with dry ingredients.) Beat well after each addition. Continue beating until smooth. Pour batter into two 9 in. (23 cm) round layer pans. Pans should be greased and their bottoms lined with greased waxed paper. Bake at 350°F (175°C) for 25 to 30 minutes or until done. Cool in pans for 5 minutes. Turn out onto rack, remove paper, and cool completely.

Yield: 24 servings

Exchange, 1 serving: 1 starch/bread
Each serving contains: Calories: 82, Carbohydrates: 16 g

Golden Butter Cake

½ c.	butter	125 mL
¾ c.	sorbitol	190 mL
½ t.	lemon flavoring	2 mL
dash	mace	dash
1½ c.	sifted cake flour	375 mL
1½ t.	baking powder	7 mL
½ t.	salt	2 mL
4	eggs, well beaten	4

Cream butter until light and fluffy. Gradually add sorbitol to creamed butter. Beat constantly until light and fluffy. Add lemon flavoring and mace. Sift dry ingredients together, and add to creamed mixture alternately with eggs, beating well after each addition. (Begin and end with dry ingredients.) Pour batter into greased and floured 8 in. (20 cm) tube pan or greased and floured 9 × 5 × 3 in. (23 × 13 × 7 cm) loaf pan. Bake at 350°F (175°C) for 50 minutes or until cake tests done. Cool in pan for 5 minutes. Turn out onto rack, and cool completely.

Yield: 16 servings

Exchange, 1 serving: ¾ starch/bread, ¾ fat
Each serving contains: Calories: 81, Carbohydrates: 8 g

Marble Cake

½ c.	solid vegetable shortening	125 mL
1½ c.	granulated sugar replacement	375 mL
2 t.	vanilla extract	10 mL
2 c.	sifted cake flour	500 mL
1 t.	salt	5 mL
2 t.	baking powder	10 mL
½ c.	skim milk	125 mL
4	egg whites, stiffly beaten	4
2 sq. (1 oz.)	unsweetened chocolate, melted	2 sq (30 g)
3 T.	water	45 mL

Cream shortening. Gradually add 1¼ c. (310 mL) of the sugar replacement, beating until light and fluffy. Beat in vanilla. Sift the dry ingredients together. Add dry ingredients alternately with the milk to the creamed mixture. (Begin and end with the dry ingredients.) Fold in the stiffly beaten egg whites. Divide batter in half. Now add remaining sugar replacement to melted chocolate in a saucepan. Blend in water. Cook and stir over low heat until mixture becomes thick. Allow to cool and then blend into half of the batter. Alternate layers of light and chocolate in well greased, waxed-paper lined 9 × 5 × 3 in. (23 × 13 × 7 cm) loaf pan. Cut through layers of batter to produce a marbling effect. Bake at 350°F (175°C) for 60 minutes or until done. Turn out onto rack, remove paper, and cool completely.

Yield: 16 servings

Exchange, 1 serving: 1 starch/bread, 1⅓ fat
Each serving contains: Calories: 128, Carbohydrates: 16 g

Lemon Cream Cake

8 oz.	sugar-free white cake mix	227 g
⅔ c.	water	180 mL
1	egg	1
1 T.	grated lemon zest	15 mL
1 t.	lemon flavoring	5 mL
1 env.	nondairy whipped-topping mix	1 env.
½ c.	water	125 mL
2 t.	cornstarch	10 mL
1 t.	orange flavoring	5 mL
⅛ t.	almond extract	½ mL

Empty cake mix into a bowl. Add ⅔ c. (180-mL) water, egg, lemon zest, and lemon flavoring. Beat for 4 to 5 minutes or until creamy. Transfer to 8 in. (20 cm) greased cake pan. Bake at 350°F (175°C) of 20 to 25 minutes. Allow cake to cool; then remove from pan. In a chilled bowl and using a chilled beater, beat whipped-topping mix and ½ c. (125 mL) water until soft peaks form. Gradually beat in cornstarch and flavorings. Beat to stiff peaks. Frost cake.

Yield: 10 servings

Exchange, 1 serving: 1⅓ starch/bread, 1 fat
Each serving contains: Calories: 132, Carbohydrates: 22 g

Cake de Menthe

8 oz.	sugar-free white cake mix	227 g
½ c.	water	125 mL
3 T.	crème de menthe	45 mL
1	egg white	1

Empty cake mix into a bowl. Add water, crème de menthe, and egg white. Beat for 4 to 5 minutes or until creamy. Transfer to 8 in. (20 cm) greased cake pan. Bake 350°F (175°C) for 20 to 25 minutes. Allow cake to cool; then remove from pan.

Yield: 10 servings

Exchange, 1 serving: 1 starch/bread, 1 fat
Each serving contains: Calories: 104, Carbohydrates: 19 g

Cake de Cacao

8 oz.	sugar-free white cake mix	227 g
½ c.	water	125 mL
2 T.	crème de cacao	30 mL
1 T.	vanilla extract	15 mL
1 t.	cocoa powder	5 mL
1	egg white	1

Empty cake mix into a bowl. Add water, crème de cacao, vanilla, cocoa, and egg white. Beat for 4 to 5 minutes or until creamy. Transfer to 8 in. (20 cm) greased cake pan. Bake at 350°F (175°C) for 20 to 25 minutes. Allow cake to cool; then remove from pan.

Yield: 10 servings

Exchange, 1 serving: 1 starch/bread, 1 fat
Each serving contains: Calories: 102, Carbohydrates: 18 g

Dark-Cherry Chocolate Cake

8 oz.	sugar-free chocolate cake mix	227 g
⅔ c.	water	180 mL
1	egg white	1
½ t.	almond extract	2 mL
¼ c.	chopped dark cherries	60 mL

Empty cake mix into a bowl. Add water, egg white, and almond extract. Beat for 4 to 5 minutes or until creamy. Fold in chopped cherries. Transfer to 8 in. (20 cm) greased cake pan. Bake at 350°F (175°C) for 20 to 25 minutes. Allow cake to cool; then remove from pan.

Yield: 10 servings

Exchange, 1 serving: 1 starch/bread, 1 fat
Each serving contains: Calories: 104, Carbohydrates: 18 g

Pumpkin Carrot Cake

8 oz.	sugar-free white cake mix	227 g
⅓ c.	water	90 mL
⅓ c.	carrot purée*	90 mL
1	egg	1
2 t.	pumpkin-pie spice	10 mL

Empty cake mix into a bowl. Add remaining ingredients. Beat for 4 to 5 minutes or until creamy. Transfer to 8 in. (20 cm) greased cake pan. Bake at 350°F (175°C) for 20 to 25 minutes. Allow cake to cool; then remove from pan.

Yield: 10 servings

Exchange, 1 serving: 1 starch/bread, 1 fat
Each serving contains: Calories: 102, Carbohydrates: 18 g

*Baby food carrot purée can be used.

Chocolate Brandy Cake

8 oz.	sugar-free chocolate cake mix	227 g
⅔ c.	buttermilk	180 mL
1	egg white	1
1 t.	brandy flavoring	2 mL

Empty cake mix into a bowl. Add buttermilk, egg white, and brandy flavoring, Beat for 4 to 5 minutes or until creamy. Transfer to 8 in. (20 cm) greased cake pan. Bake at 350°F (175°C) for 20 to 25 minutes. Allow cake to cool; then remove from pan.

Yield: 10 servings

Exchange, 1 serving: 1 starch/bread, 1 fat
Each serving contains: Calories: 106, Carbohydrates: 18 g

Chocolate Sour Cream Raisin Cake

8 oz.	sugar-free chocolate cake mix	227 g
¼ c.	granulated brown sugar replacement	60 mL
3 T.	granulated sugar replacement	45 mL
1 T.	cornstarch	15 mL
½ c.	low-calorie sour cream	125 mL
1	egg yolk	1
¼ c.	raisins	60 mL
1 t.	vanilla extract	5 mL

Bake cake from mix as directed on package. Allow cake to cool completely. In a small saucepan, mix sugar replacements and cornstarch. Blend in sour cream and egg yolk. Cool and stir over medium heat until mixture thickens and boils. Boil and stir for 1 minute longer. Remove from heat. Stir in raisins and vanilla. Cool completely. Frost cake.

Yield: 10 servings

Exchange, 1 serving: 1 starch/bread, 1 fat
Each serving contains: Calories: 134, Carbohydrates: 19 g

Easy Chocolate Crunch Cake

8 oz.	chocolate cake mix	227 g
⅔ c.	water	180 mL
1	egg white	1
⅓ c.	wheat and barley cereal	90 mL

Empty cake mix into a bowl. Add water and egg white. Beat for 4 to 5 minutes or until creamy. Fold in cereal. Transfer to 8 in. (20 cm) greased cake pan. Bake at 350°F (175°C) for 20 to 25 minutes. Allow cake to cool; then remove from pan.

Yield: 10 servings

Exchange, 1 serving: 1 starch/bread, 1 fat
Each serving contains: Calories: 103, Carbohydrates: 17 g

Carrot Cake

1 c.	liquid shortening	250 mL
2 T.	granulated fructose or granulated sugar replacement	30 mL
4	eggs	4
½ c.	water	125 mL
2 c.	flour	500 mL
1 t.	baking powder	5 mL
1 t.	baking soda	5 mL
2 t.	cinnamon	10 mL
1 t.	nutmeg	5 mL
½ t.	salt	2 mL
½ c.	pecans, chopped	125 mL
3 c.	carrots, grated	750 mL

Beat shortening, sugar replacement and eggs until lemon colored. Add water, flour, baking powder, baking soda, cinnamon, nutmeg, and salt, beating well. Stir in pecans and carrots. Pour into well greased and floured 3 qt. (3 L) tube pan. Bake at 350°F (175°C) for 30 to 40 minutes, or until done.

Microwave: Cook on Medium for 15 to 17 minutes. Allow to rest 5 minutes before removing from pan.

Yield: 16 servings

Exchange, 1 serving with fructose: 1 bread, 3 fat
Each serving contains: Calories: 229

Exchange, 1 serving with sugar replacement: 1 bread, 3 fat
Each serving contains: Calories: 220

Milk Sponge Cake

2	eggs	2
2 T.	granulated sugar replacement or granulated fructose	30 mL
1 c.	cake flour, sifted	250 mL
1 t.	baking powder	5 mL
1 t.	vanilla extract	5 mL
1 t.	margarine	5 mL
½ c.	hot skim milk	125 mL

Beat eggs and sugar replacement; beat in cake flour, baking powder and vanilla. Melt margarine in hot milk and pour into cake batter, beating just to blend. Pour into 9 in. (23 cm) baking dish. Bake at 350°F (175°C) for 30 to 35 minutes, or until done.

Yield: 9 servings

Exchange, 1 serving with sugar replacement: 1 fruit, ½ medium-fat meat
Each serving contains: Calories: 45

Exchange, 1 serving with fructose: 1 fruit, ½ medium-fat meat
Each serving contains: Calories: 48

Walnut Sponge Cake

6	eggs, separated	6
½ c.	cold water	125 mL
½ t.	vanilla extract	3 mL
3 T.	granulated sugar replacement	45 mL
1¼ c.	flour	310 mL
½ t.	cinnamon	3 mL
¼ t.	salt	1 mL
½ c.	walnuts, chopped fine	125 mL
¾ t.	cream of tartar	4 mL

Beat egg yolks until thick and lemon colored. Add water, vanilla, and sugar replacement, beating until light and fluffy. Stir in flour, cinnamon, salt, and walnuts. Beat egg whites until foamy and add cream of tartar, beating until stiff peaks are formed. Gently fold egg yolk mixture into stiffly beaten egg whites. Pour into ungreased 9 in. (23 cm) tube pan. Bake at 325°F (165°C) for 60 to 70 minutes, or until cake springs back when lightly touched with finger. Invert cake in pan over bottle or wire rack and cool 1 hour before removing from pan.

Yield: 20 servings

Exchange, 1 serving: ½ full-fat milk
Each serving contains: Calories: 69

Southern Peach Shortcake

2 c.	sliced peaches	500 mL
2 T.	granulated sugar replacement	30 mL
½ t.	almond extract	2 mL
½ t.	cinnamon	2 mL
1 c.	flour	250 mL
2 t.	baking powder	10 mL
dash	salt	dash
2 T.	liquid vegetable shortening	30 mL
1	egg	1
¼ c.	milk	60 mL

Place peaches in bottom of well greased 8 in. (20 cm) baking dish. Sprinkle with 1 T. (15 mL) of the sugar replacement, the almond extract and cinnamon. Combine flour, remaining 1 T. (15 mL) sugar replacement, baking powder, and salt in mixing bowl. Add shortening, egg and milk, stirring just to mix. Spread evenly over peaches. Bake at 400°F (200°C) for 30 minutes, or until lightly browned. Invert onto serving plate.

Yield: 9 servings

Exchange, 1 serving: 1 bread, ½ fat
Each serving contains: Calories: 102, Carbohydrates: 22 g

Quick Chocolate Walnut-Filled Cake

Cake

2 c.	cake flour	500 mL
½ c.	cocoa	125 mL
3 T.	granulated sugar replacement	45 mL
1 T.	baking powder	15 mL
1¼ c.	milk	310 mL
¼ c.	soft margarine	60 mL
2	eggs	2

Filling

½ c.	all-purpose flour	125 mL
⅓ c.	walnuts, very finely chopped	90 mL
⅓ c.	milk	90 mL
1 t.	granulated sugar replacement	5 mL
1 t.	baking powder	5 mL
1 t.	vanilla extract	5 mL

Combine cake flour, cocoa, sugar replacement and baking powder in sifter. Sift into medium bowl, add remaining ingredients and beat until smooth and creamy. Pour into well greased and floured 3 qt. (3 L) fluted tube pan.

Combine all ingredients in small bowl, mixing with fork until well blended. Spoon in a ring over center of chocolate batter. Do not touch sides of pan with filling. Bake at 350°F (175°C) for 35 minutes, or until done. Cool in pan 20 to 25 minutes, invert onto cooling rack or plate and cool completely. Frost with favorite glaze.

Yield: 24 servings

Exchange, 1 serving: ⅔ bread, ½ lean meat
Each serving contains: Calories: 84, Carbohydrates: 22 g

Apricot Pudding Cake

3	eggs, separated	3
7½ oz. jar	unsweetened apricot purée, baby food	219 g jar
½ t.	almond extract	3 mL
½ c.	milk	125 mL
⅓ c.	flour, sifted	90 mL
2 t.	granulated sugar replacement	10 mL

Beat egg yolks. Add apricot purée, almond extract, milk, flour, and sugar replacement, beating to blend thoroughly. Stiffly beat the egg whites. Gently and completely fold egg yolk mixture into egg whites. Pour mixture into well greased 1 qt. (1 L) baking dish, place dish in pan and add ½ in. (15 mm) water to pan. Bake at 325°F (165°C) for 30 minutes, or until lightly browned and puffy.

Microwave: Cook on Defrost for 15 to 17 minutes. Turn dish a quarter turn every 5 minutes.

Yield: 6 servings

Exchange, 1 serving: 1 bread, ½ fat
Each serving contains: Calories: 113, Carbohydrates: 28 g

Lemon Pudding Cake

3	eggs, separated	3
¼ c.	lemon juice	60 mL
½ c.	milk	125 mL
1 t.	fresh lemon peel, grated	5 mL
2 T.	granulated sugar replacement	30 mL
dash	salt	dash
⅓ c.	flour, sifted	90 mL

Beat egg yolks until creamy. Add lemon juice, milk, lemon peel, sugar replacement, salt, and flour; beat to blend thoroughly. Stiffly beat the egg whites. Gently fold egg yolk mixture into egg whites. Pour mixture into well greased 1 qt. (1 L) baking dish, set dish in pan and add ½ in. (15 mm) water to pan. Bake at 325°F (165°C) for 30 minutes, or until lightly browned and puffy.

Microwave: Cook on Defrost for 15 to 17 minutes. Turn dish a quarter turn every 5 minutes.

Yield: 6 servings

Exchange, 1 serving: ½ bread, ½ medium-fat meat
Each serving contains: Calories: 73, Carbohydrates: 107 g

Rhubarb Cake

2 c.	flour	500 mL
1 c.	2% milk	250 mL
¼ c.	soft margarine	60 mL
1	egg	1
3 T.	granulated sugar replacement	45 mL
1 t.	baking soda	5 mL
1 t.	lemon juice	5 mL
1 t.	vanilla extract	5 mL
dash	salt	dash
1½ c.	rhubarb, cut fine	375 mL

Combine flour, milk, margarine, egg, sugar replacement, baking soda, lemon juice, vanilla, and salt in large mixing bowl. Stir to blend and then fold in rhubarb. Pour into well greased and floured 13 × 9 in. (33 × 23 cm) baking pan. Bake at 350°F (175°C) for 45 minutes, or until done.

Yield: 24 servings

Exchange, 1 serving: ½ bread, ½ fat
Each serving contains: Calories: 60, Carbohydrates: 15 g

Banana Pudding Cake

3	egg yolks	3
2	bananas, very ripe	2
1 t.	vanilla extract	5 mL
½ c.	milk	125 mL
⅓ c.	flour, sifted	90 mL
1 t.	granulated sugar replacement	5 mL
3	egg whites, beaten stiff	3

Beat egg yolks and bananas until well blended. Add vanilla, milk, flour, and sugar replacement, beating to blend thoroughly. Gently and completely fold egg yolk mixture into stiffly beaten egg whites. Pour mixture into well greased 1 qt. (1 L) baking dish, set dish in pan and add ½ in. (15 mm) water to pan. Bake at 325°F (165°C) for 30 minutes, or until lightly browned and puffy.

Microwave: Cook on Defrost for 15 to 17 minutes. Turn dish every 5 minutes.

Yield: 6 servings

Exchange, 1 serving: 1 bread, ½ medium-fat meat
Each serving contains: Calories: 105, Carbohydrates: 34 g

Daisy Cake

9	eggs, separated)	9
2 T.	liquid fructose	30 mL
1½ c.	flour, sifted	375 mL
¾ t.	cream of tartar	4 mL
½ t.	baking powder	2 mL
½ t.	salt	2 mL
2 t.	lemon extract	10 mL

Beat egg whites and fructose until stiff. Beat egg yolks until fluffy and light yellow in color. Combine flour, cream of tartar, baking powder, and salt in sifter. Add alternately with egg yolks to stiffened egg whites, beating continually, and add lemon extract. Pour into 10 in. (25 cm) angel-food cake pan. Bake at 325°F (165°C) for 55 to 60 minutes, or until done.

Yield: 20 servings

Exchange, 1 serving: ½ bread, ½ fat
Each serving contains: Calories: 72, Carbohydrates: 1 g

Cranberry Cake

2 c.	all-purpose flour	500 mL
½ c.	granulated sugar replacement	125 mL
¼ c.	granulated fructose	60 mL
2 t.	baking powder	10 mL
½ t.	salt	2 mL
1 c.	skim milk	250 mL
2	eggs	2
2 T.	solid shortening, softened	30 mL
2 t.	vanilla extract	10 mL
1½ c.	fresh cranberries	375 mL

Combine flour, sugar replacement, fructose, baking powder, and salt in a bowl. Add milk, eggs, shortening, and vanilla. Whisk or beat until smooth and creamy, Stir in cranberries. Transfer to a paper-lined or well greased and floured 9 in. (23 cm) sq. baking pan. Bake at 350°F (175°C) for 35 to 45 minutes or until pick inserted in middle comes out clean.

Yield: 16 servings

Exchange, 1 serving: 1 bread
Each serving contains: Calories: 74, Carbohydrates: 13 g

Buttermilk Cake

½ c.	sifted cake flour	375 mL
½ c.	granulated sugar replacement	125 mL
1 t.	baking powder	5 mL
½ t.	salt	2 mL
¼ t.	baking soda	1 mL
2 T.	solid shortening, softened	30 mL
¼ c.	buttermilk	190 mL
2	egg whites	2
1 t.	vanilla	5 mL

Sift together flour, sugar replacement, baking powder, salt, and baking soda into a medium-sized bowl. Add shortening and ½ c. (125 mL) of the buttermilk. Beat on medium for 2 minutes. Add remaining buttermilk, egg whites, and vanilla. Beat on high for 2 minutes. Transfer batter into an 8 in. (20 cm) round well greased and floured baking pan. Bake at 350°F (175°C) for 22 to 25 minutes or until pick inserted in middle comes out clean. Cool in pan for 5 minutes. Invert onto a cooling rack, and cool completely.

Yield: 10 servings

Exchange, 1 serving: 1 bread
Each serving contains: Calories: 75, Carbohydrates: 12 g

Spice Raisin Cake

⅓ c.	all-purpose flour	340 mL
½ c.	granulated sugar replacement	125 mL
1 T.	granulated fructose	15 mL
2 t.	baking powder	10 mL
1 t.	ground cinnamon	5 mL
¼ t.	ground nutmeg	1 mL
¼ t.	ground cloves	1 mL
¼ t.	ground ginger	1 mL
⅔ c.	skim milk	180 mL
1	egg	1
2 T.	margarine, softened	30 mL
1 t.	vanilla extract	5 mL
½ c.	plumped raisins	125 mL

Combine flour, sugar replacement, fructose, baking powder, cinnamon, nutmeg, cloves, and ginger in a medium-sized bowl. Add milk, egg, margarine, and vanilla. Beat on low for 30 seconds. Then beat on high for 1 to 1½ minutes. Fold in raisins. Transfer batter to a well greased and floured 9 in. (23 cm) round baking pan. Bake at 350°F (175°C) for 25 to 30 minutes or until pick inserted in middle comes out clean. (The all-purpose flour makes this cake a little heavy.

If you prefer a lighter cake, sift the dry ingredients together several times before adding the liquid ingredients.)

Yield: 10 servings

Exchange, 1 serving: 1 bread, 1 fruit
Each serving contains: Calories: 99, Carbohydrates: 17 g

Fructose Chocolate Cake

⅓ c.	granulated fructose	90 mL
1 c.	all-purpose flour	250 mL
¼ c.	unsweetened cocoa powder	60 mL
¾ t.	baking soda	4 mL
¼ t.	cream of tartar	1 mL
¼ c.	solid shortening, softened	60 mL
¾ c.	skim milk	190 mL
1 t.	vanilla extract	5 mL
1	egg	1

Place fructose in a small blender jar. Blend on high for 20 seconds. (Fructose will powder.) Combine flour, fructose, cocoa, baking soda, and cream of tartar in a medium-sized bowl. Stir to mix. Add shortening, milk, and vanilla. Beat on low until blended. Then beat on high for 1½ minutes. Add egg and continue beating on high for 2 more minutes. Transfer batter to a greased and floured 8 or 9 in. (20 or 23 cm) round baking pan. Bake at 350°F (175°C) for 25 to 30 minutes or until pick inserted in middle comes out clean. Allow cake to cool in pan on cooling rack for 10 minutes. Remove from pan. Cool thoroughly on rack.

Yield: 10 servings

Exchange, 1 serving: 1 bread, 1 fat
Each serving contains: Calories: 141, Carbohydrates: 16 g

Fructose White Cake

1⅓ c.	all-purpose flour	340 mL
¼ c.	granulated fructose	60 mL
2 t.	baking powder	10 mL
3 T.	margarine, softened	45 mL
⅓ c.	skim milk	180 mL
1	egg	1
1	vanilla extract	5 mL

Combine flour, fructose, and baking powder in a food processor. Process on high for 30 seconds. Add margarine and process for 30 seconds more. Transfer ingredients to a medium-sized bowl. Add milk, egg, and vanilla. Beat on low for 30 seconds. Then beat on high for 2 minutes. Grease the bottom of an 8 in. (20 cm) round baking pan. (Do not grease the sides of the pan.) Line bottom with waxed paper and grease the waxed paper. Transfer batter to prepared pan. Bake at 350°F (175°C) for 25 to 30 minutes or until pick inserted in middle comes out clean.

Yield: 10 servings

Exchange, 1 serving: 1 bread, ½ fat
Each serving contains: Calories: 109, Carbohydrates: 14 g

Quick Peanut Butter Cake

8 oz.	sugar-free white cake mix	227 g
⅓ c.	water	180 mL
1	egg white	1
⅓ c.	crunchy peanut butter	90 mL

Empty cake mix into a bowl. Add water, egg white, and peanut butter. Blend for 4 to 5 minutes or until creamy. Transfer to 8 in. (20 cm) greased cake pan. Bake at 350°F (175°C) for 20 to 25 minutes. Allow cake to cool, then remove from pan.

Yield: 10 servings

Exchange, 1 serving: 1 starch/bread, 1½ fat
Each serving contains: Calories: 125, Carbohydrates: 18 g

Quick Applesauce Cake

8 oz.	sugar-free white cake mix	227 g
1 c.	unsweetened applesauce	250 mL
1	egg white	1

Empty cake mix into a bowl. Add applesauce and egg white. Blend for 5 to 6 minutes or until creamy. Transfer to 8 in. (20 cm) greased cake pan. Bake at 350°F (175°C) for 20 to 25 minutes. Allow cake to cool; then remove from pan.

Yield: 10 servings

Exchange, 1 serving: 1 starch/bread, 1 fat
Each serving contains: Calories: 110, Carbohydrates: 20 g

Easy Pineapple Cake

8 oz. pkg.	sugar-free yellow cake mix	226 g pkg.
⅔ c.	unsweetened pineapple juice	180 mL

Combine cake mix and half of the pineapple juice in a mixing bowl. Beat on high for 3 minutes. Add remaining juice and continue beating for 3 more minutes. Transfer to an 8 in. (20 cm) wax paper lined or greased and floured cake pan. Bake at 375°F (190°C) for 25 minutes or until tester inserted in middle comes out clean.

Yield: 10 servings

Exchange, 1 serving: 1 bread, ½ fruit, ½ fat
Each serving contains: Calories: 104, Carbohydrates: 20 g

Fast Spice Cake

8 oz. pkg.	sugar-free lemon cake mix	226 g pkg.
1 t.	ground cinnamon	5 mL
½ t.	ground nutmeg	2 mL
¼ t.	ground allspice	1 mL
¼ t.	ground cloves	1 mL
⅔ c.	water	180 mL

Place cake mix in mixing bowl. Add spices to dry ingredients. Add ⅓ c. (90 mL) of the water to the mixture. Beat on high for 3 minutes. Add remaining water and continue beating for 3 more minutes. Transfer to an 8 in. (20 cm) wax-paper lined or greased and floured cake pan. Bake at 375°F (190°C) for 25 minutes or until tester inserted in middle comes out clean.

Yield: 10 servings

Exchange, 1 serving: 1 bread, ½ fat
Each serving contains: Calories: 96, Carbohydrates: 16 g

Chocolate Chocolate Mint Cake

8 oz. pkg.	sugar-free chocolate cake mix	226 g pkg.
⅔ c.	water	180 mL
½ t.	mint flavoring	2 mL
½ c.	mini chocolate mint chips	125 mL
2	egg whites, stiffly beaten	2

Combine cake mix, water, and mint flavoring in a mixing bowl. Beat on medium for 5 to 6 minutes or until batter is thick and creamy. Add chips. Fold in stiffly beaten egg whites. Transfer to a wax-paper lined or greased and floured 8 in. (20 cm) round cake pan. Bake at 350°F (175°C) for 20 to 25 minutes or until tester inserted in middle comes out clean. Cool in the pan for about 10 minutes; then transfer cake to rack. Cool completely.

Yield: 10 servings

Exchange, 1 serving: 1 bread, 1½ fat
Each serving contains: Calories: 133, Carbohydrates: 21 g

Peach Crunch Pie Cake

8 oz. pkg.	sugar-free white cake mix	226 g pkg.
1	egg white	1
⅔ c.	water	180 mL
½ t.	vanilla extract	2 mL
2	peaches, peeled and thinly sliced	2
½ c.	corn flakes	125 mL

Combine cake mix, egg white, water, and vanilla extract in a mixing bowl. Beat on medium for 5 to 6 minutes or until batter is thick and creamy. Transfer to a greased and floured 9 in. (23 cm) pie pan. Lay the thin slices of peaches around the edge of the cake batter in a circular fashion. Crush corn flakes; sprinkle evenly on top of peach slices and batter. Bake at 350°F (175°C) for 15 to 20 minutes or until tester inserted in middle comes out clean. Cool and serve from pie pan.

Yield: 10 servings

Exchange, 1 serving: 1 bread, ½ fat
Each serving contains: Calories: 97, Carbohydrates: 18 g

Sweet Potato Cake

1	egg	1
6 oz. jar	sweet potatoes, baby	170 g jar
½ t.	cinnamon	2 mL
8 oz. pkg.	sugar-free pound cake mix	226 g pkg.
⅔ c.	water	180 mL

Beat egg in a medium-sized mixing bowl until light lemon colored and fluffy. Beat in sweet potatoes and cinnamon. Add cake mix and water alternately in small amounts, beating well after each addition. Beat a minute more. Pour into wax paper lined or greased and floured 8 × 4 × 2 in. (20 × 10 × 5 cm) loaf pan, and bake at 350°F (175°C) for 45 to 50 minutes. Cool cake in pan for 10 minutes. Turn cake out onto rack and cool completely or serve warm.

Yield: 10 servings

Exchange, 1 serving: 1 bread, ½ fat
Each serving contains: Calories: 104, Carbohydrates: 18 g

Heavenly Blueberry Cake

2 pkgs. (8 oz.)	sugar-free yellow cake mix	2 pkgs. (226 g)	
2 env.	unflavored gelatin	2 env.	
½ c.	cold water	125 mL	
2 pkgs. (1 lb.)	Flavorland frozen blueberries, thawed	454 g (2 pkgs.)	
2 c.	prepared nondairy whipped topping	500 mL	
	mint sprigs		

Prepare cake mixes together as directed on package; bake together in one 8 in. (20 cm) square pan, with the bottom lined with wax paper. Cool cake slightly in pan. Carefully release cake from sides of pan by sliding a sharp knife between cake and sides of pan. Transfer to rack, remove wax paper, and cool completely Cut cake into ¼-in. (8 mm) slices. Then cut each slice in half. Lightly grease the 9 in. (23 cm) springform, or loose bottom, pan. Line bottom and sides of springform. pan with cake slices. Soften gelatin in ½ c. (125 mL) of cold water. Heat slightly either in a microwave or on top of the stove. Stir to completely dissolve gelatin. Place thawed blueberries and any juice in a mixing bowl, and slightly crush some of the berries. Stir in softened gelatin and nondairy whipped topping. Pour about a fourth of the berry mixture into the cake-lined pan. Arrange about a third of the remaining cake pieces and crumbs over the berry mixture. Repeat with the next two layers, ending with a layer of the berry mixture. Chill overnight or until completely set. Remove sides of springform, or loose bottom, pan. Place cake with pan bottom on dessert platter. Garnish plate and cake with mint sprigs. Chill until serving time.

Yield: 20 servings

Exchange, 1 serving: 1 bread, ½ fruit, ½ fat
Each serving contains: Calories: 144, Carbohydrates: 25 g

So Good Chocolate Cake

8 oz. pkg.	sugar-free chocolate cake mix	226 g pkg.	
1 T.	unsweetened cocoa powder	15 mL	
1	egg white	1	
⅔ c.	spiced tomato vegetable juice	180 mL	

Combine cake mix, cocoa, and egg white in a mixing bowl. Add vegetable juice. Stir to mix. Beat on high 5 to 6 minutes more or until batter is thick and very creamy. Transfer to a greased and floured 8 in. round cake pan.

Bake at 350°F (175°C) for 20 to 25 minutes. Cool for 10 minutes in the pan. Turn cake out onto a serving plate. Serve warm.

Yield: 10 servings

Exchange, 1 serving: 1 bread, ½ fat
Each serving contains: Calories: 92, Carbohydrates: 17 g

Pineapple Upside-Down Cake

6	pineapple rings, in juice	6
1 T.	margarine	15 mL
¼ c.	Cary's Sugar-Free Maple-Flavored Syrup	60 mL
1 T.	granulated brown sugar replacement	15 mL
1 recipe	Easy Pineapple Cake	1 recipe

Drain juice from pineapple rings. Juice from rings can be used in the preparation of the Easy Pineapple Cake. Melt margarine in an 8 in. (20 cm) round cake pan. Brush melted margarine over sides and bottom of pan. Cut pineapple rings in half and lay them decoratively on the bottom of the pan. Pour maple syrup over pineapple rings; sprinkle with granulated brown sugar replacement. Prepare cake as directed in recipe. Pour batter over pineapple rings. Bake at 375°F (190°C) for 25 minutes or until tester inserted in middle comes out clean. Immediately turn cake out onto a serving plate. Serve warm.

Optional: 1 T. (15 mL) of prepared nondairy whipped topping on each ring to add a pretty and flavorful touch.

Yield: 10 servings

Exchange, 1 serving (without whipped topping): 1 bread, 1 fruit, ½ fat
Each serving contains: Calories: 124, Carbohydrates: 25 g

Black Cherry Upside-Down Cake

2 T.	margarine	30 mL
2 T.	liquid fructose	30 mL
2 c.	Flavorland frozen dark cherries, thawed	500 mL
2 T.	chopped pecans	30 mL
8 oz. pkg.	Featherlight sugar-free chocolate cake mix	226 g pkg.

Melt margarine in an 8 in. (20 cm) round cake pan or skillet. Add liquid fructose and stir until mixed. Add cherries and pecans. Prepare cake mix as directed on package. Pour batter over cherries. Bake at 350°F (175°C) for 25 minutes or until tester inserted in middle comes out clean. Turn cake over onto a dessert tray or platter. Serve warm.

Yield: 10 servings

Exchange, 1 serving: 1 bread, ¼ fruit, 1 fat
Each serving contains: Calories: 137, Carbohydrates: 20 g

Banana Butterscotch Layer Cake

2 pkgs. (8 oz.)	sugar-free yellow cake mix	2 pkgs. (226 g)	
1 pkg.	butterscotch-flavored sugar-free instant pudding mix	1 pkg.	
2 c.	prepared nondairy whipped topping	500 mL	
2	bananas	2	

Prepare cake mixes together as directed on package; bake in two 8 in. (20 cm) round pans, with their sides greased and the bottoms lined with wax paper. Allow to cool. Meanwhile, prepare butterscotch pudding as directed on package. Allow to partially set; then stir in nondairy whipped topping. Place one cake upside down on a cake plate or platter. Frost with a thin layer of pudding topping. Cut each banana into very thin slices. Place one of the sliced bananas between the layers. Add the top cake layer, and frost the top and sides of the cake with pudding topping. Decorate top with remaining banana slices.

Yield: 20 servings

Exchange, 1 serving: 1 bread, ¼ fruit, ½ fat
Each serving contains: Calories: 118, Carbohydrates: 20 g

Strawberry Dream Cake

2 c.	strawberries, rinsed and hulled	500 mL	
1	yeast cake	1	
3 c.	prepared nondairy whipped topping	750 mL	

Reserve 10 of the best strawberries for garnish. Cut the remaining strawberries into thick slices. Cut cake in half horizontally. Place bottom half on a serving dessert plate or platter. Cover with 1 c. (250 mL) of the nondairy whipped topping. Place half of the sliced strawberries on top of the whipped topping. Add top layer of cake. Place remaining sliced strawberries on top of cake. Frost top and sides of cake with remaining whipped topping. Make reserved strawberries into fans by cutting thin lengthwise slices from the tip almost to the stem (do not cut through the stem) and gently fanning out the slices. Place strawberry fans evenly around edge of cake. Chill until serving time.

Yield: 10 servings
Each serving contains: Exchange, 1 serving: 1 bread, ½ fat
Each serving contains: Calories: 135, Carbohydrates: 23 g

Brandy Cake

8 oz. pkg.	no-sugar chocolate cake mix	226 g pkg.
½ c.	buttermilk	125 mL
1	egg	1
2 t.	brandy flavoring	10 mL

Combine all ingredients and blend with an electric mixer on medium speed for 4 minutes. Pour into an 8 or 9 in. (20 or 23 cm) baking pan. Bake at 350°F (175°C) for 25 to 30 minutes or until cake tests done.

Yield: 9 servings

Exchange, 1 serving: 1¼ bread, ½ fat
Each serving contains: Calories: 112, Carbohydrates: 32 g

Cocoa Cake

3 T.	cocoa	45 mL
1½ c.	flour	375 mL
¼ c.	granulated sugar replacement	60 mL
1 t.	baking soda	5 mL
½ t.	salt	2 mL
⅓ c.	liquid shortening	90 mL
1 T.	white vinegar	15 mL
1 T.	vanilla extract	15 mL
1 c.	water	250 mL

Combine all ingredients in large mixing bowl. Beat to blend thoroughly. Pour batter into 9 in. (23 cm) square baking pan. Bake at 350°F (175°C) for 20 to 30 minutes or until cake tests done. Serve warm.

Yield: 9 servings

Exchange, 1 serving: 1 bread, 1½ fat
Each serving contains: Calories: 149, Carbohydrates: 34 g

Peanut Butter Cake

Chocolate and peanut butter made easy.

8 oz. pkg.	sugar-restricted chocolate cake mix	226 g pkg.
½ c.	chunky peanut butter	125 mL

Prepare cake mix as directed on package and add peanut butter. Bake at 375°F (190°C) for 25 minutes or until cake tests done.

Yield: 10 servings

Exchange, 1 serving: 1 bread, 2 fat
Each serving contains: Calories: 169, Carbohydrates: 30 g

Persimmon Mold

⅓ c.	low-calorie margarine	90 mL
1 c.	granulated brown sugar replacement	250 mL
3	eggs	3
1½ c.	sifted all-purpose flour	375 mL
2 t.	baking powder	10 mL
½ c.	skim milk	125 mL
1½ c.	persimmon pulp	375 mL
½ t. each	cinnamon, nutmeg	2 mL each

Beat margarine and brown sugar replacement together until light and fluffy. Add eggs, one at a time, beating well after each addition. Combine flour and baking powder in a bowl. Add flour mixture to eggs alternately with milk, beginning and ending with flour. Fold in persimmon pulp, cinnamon, and nutmeg. Transfer to a 1½ qt. (1½ L) lightly greased baking dish. Place baking dish in a pan of water. (Water should reach halfway up sides of baking dish. Add extra water if needed while baking.) Bake at 325°F (165°C) for 50 to 60 minutes or until custard tests done.

Yield: 10 servings

Exchange, 1 serving: 1 fruit, 1 starch/bread
Each serving contains: Calories: 136, Carbohydrates: 30 g

Strawberry Shortcake

	dough for 1 biscuit	
½ c.	Strawberry Topping	125 mL
¼ c.	fresh strawberries, halved	60 mL
2 T.	low-calorie whipped topping, prepared	30 mL

Bake biscuit as directed on package. Cool, Cut in half. Layer biscuit, half of the Strawberry Topping, and half of the strawberries; repeat. Top with prepared whipped topping.

Yield: 1 serving

Exchange, 1 serving: 1 bread, 1½ fruit
Each serving contains: Calories: 100

Banana Cake Roll

4	eggs, separated	4
10 T.	granulated sugar replacement	150 mL
½ t.	vanilla extract	2 mL
⅔ c.	cake flour, sifted	180 mL
1 t.	baking powder	5 mL
¼ t.	salt	1 mL
	vegetable cooking spray	
1 pkg.	low-calorie banana pudding, prepared	1 pkg.
	chocolate drizzle	

Beat egg yolks until thick and lemon colored; gradually beat in 3 T. (45 mL) of the sugar replacement. Add vanilla extract. Beat egg whites to soft peaks; gradually beat in the remaining sugar replacement; beat until stiff peaks form. Fold yolks into whites. Sift together cake flour, baking powder, and salt. Fold into egg mixture. Spread batter into 15½ × 10½ × 1 in. (39 × 25 × 3 cm) jelly roll pan (coated with vegetable cooking spray and lightly floured). Bake at 375°F (190°C) for 10 to 15 minutes, or until done. Loosen sides and turn out on towel lightly sprinkled with a mixture of flour and sugar replacement. Roll up cake and towel from narrow end. Cool completely; unroll. Spread evenly with prepared banana pudding. Roll up. Frost with chocolate drizzle.

Yield: 10 servings

Exchange, 1 serving: 1 bread, ½ fruit, ¼ milk
Each serving contains: Calories: 62, Carbohydrates: 26 g

Apple Crunch Cake

⅓ c.	Kellogg's bran flakes cereal	90 mL
3 T.	granulated sugar replacement	45 mL
¼ t.	salt	1 mL
¼ t.	ground cinnamon	1 mL
3 T.	margarine	45 mL
1 c.	Kellogg's bran flakes cereal	250 mL
1¼ c.	all-purpose flour	310 mL
2 t.	baking powder	10 mL
½ t.	salt	2 mL
¼ c.	margarine, softened	60 mL
½ c.	granulated sugar replacement	125 mL
1	egg	1
1 t.	lemon peel, grated	5 mL
½ c.	skim milk	125 mL
2½ c.	pared apples, coarsely chopped	625 mL

Stir together first 4 ingredients. Cut in the 3 T. (45 mL) margarine until mixture is crumbly. Set aside to use as a topping. Crush the 1 c. (250 mL) cereal to ½ c. (125 mL). Stir in flour, baking powder and salt. Set aside.

In a large mixing bowl, beat margarine, sugar replacement, egg and lemon peel until light and fluffy. Add flour mixture alternately with milk, mixing well after each addition. Stir in apples. Spread evenly in greased 9 × 9 × 2 in. (23 × 23 × 5 cm) baking pan. Sprinkle evenly with cereal topping. Bake at 375 T (190°C) about 35 minutes or until cake tests done. Cool. Serve with nondairy whipped topping, if desired.

Yield: 16 servings

Exchange, 1 serving: (without whipped topping): 1 bread, 1 fat
Each serving contains: Calories: 105, Carbohydrates: 23 g

Based on a recipe from Kellogg's Test Kitchens.

Coffeecakes

Pineapple Oatmeal Coffeecake

1 c.	quick-cooking oatmeal	250 mL
1 c.	unsweetened pineapple juice	250 mL
2 t.	baking powder	10 mL
½ t.	baking soda	2 mL
1	egg	1
1 c.	all-purpose flour	250 mL
3 env.	aspartame sweetener	3 env.

Combine oatmeal and pineapple juice in a mixing bowl. Stir to mix. Allow to rest for 10 to 15 minutes. Add baking powder, baking soda, and egg. Stir vigorously with a spoon. Then stir in flour. Transfer to a greased 9 in. (23 cm) round baking pan. Bake at 350°F (175°C) for 25 to 35 minutes or until pick inserted in middle comes out clean. Remove from oven. Sprinkle top with aspartame sweetener.

Yield: 16 servings

Exchange, 1 serving: 3¾ bread
Each serving contains: Calories: 66, Carbohydrates: 12 g

Cherry Coffeecake

1 pkg.	dry yeast	1 pkg.
¼ c.	warm water	60 mL
¼ c.	skim milk	190 mL
1 T.	cider vinegar	15 mL
½ c.	granulated sugar replacement	125 mL
2 T.	margarine, softened	30 mL
1	egg	1
1 t.	baking powder	5 mL
½ t.	salt	2 mL
3¼ c.	all-purpose flour	810 mL
1½ c.	fresh or frozen sweet cherries, thawed and drained	375 mL

Dissolve yeast in warm water in a large mixing bowl. Add milk, vinegar, sugar replacement, margarine, egg, baking powder, salt, and 2 c. (500 mL) of the flour. Beat on low until mixture is blended; then mix on medium for 2 minutes. Stir in remaining flour. Transfer to a lightly floured surface, and knead until smooth and elastic (about 5 minutes). Roll dough into a 20 × 6 in. (50 × 15 cm) rectangle. Place on a greased cookie sheet. Cut 2 in. (5 cm) slices on each of the 20 in. (50 cm) sides of the dough.

Cut cherries in quarters. Place cherries lengthwise down the middle of the rectangles. Crisscross sliced strips over cherries. Cover and allow to rise in a warm place until double in size. Bake at 375°F (190°C) for 20 to 22 minutes or until golden brown.

Yield: 22 servings

Exchange, 1 serving: ¼ bread
Each serving contains: Calories: 63, Carbohydrates: 13 g

Cherry Chocolate Coffeecake

2 c.	frozen, unsweetened sweet cherries	500 mL
1½ t.	cornstarch	7 mL
¼ t.	unsweetened black-cherry soft drink mix powder	1 mL
¼ t.	ground nutmeg	1 mL
½ c.	skim milk	125 mL
1 pkg.	dry yeast	1 pkg.
¼ c.	warm water	1 mL
⅔ c.	granulated sugar replacement	180 mL
¼ c.	solid shortening	60 mL
1	egg	1
½ t.	salt	2 mL
⅓ c.	unsweetened baking cocoa	90 mL
2½ c.	all-purpose flour	625 mL
2 T.	margarine, melted	30 mL

Place frozen cherries in a 1 qt. (1 L) microwave measuring cup. Heat in microwave on medium for 2 minutes. Stir and then continue heating on medium for another 2 minutes. Cherries should be thawed but not hot. Use scissors to cut cherries into pieces. (If cherries are hot, allow to cool before stirring in cornstarch.) Stir in cornstarch, soft drink mix powder, and nutmeg. Place back in microwave and cook for 3 to 4 minutes on medium-high or until mixture is very thick and clear. Set aside to cool completely. Meanwhile, pour skim milk in small saucepan. Bring to a boil, remove from heat, and allow to cool. Dissolve the yeast in the warm water. Combine skim milk, yeast mixture, sweetener, shortening, egg, and salt in a large mixing bowl. Combine the cocoa with 1¼ c. (310 mL) of flour in another bowl. Stir to mix. Add to liquid mixture in bowl. Beat on low until mixture is blended and smooth. Add remaining flour and stir until all the flour is incorporated into the dough. Turn out onto a lightly floured surface; then knead for 4 to 5 minutes until dough is smooth and elastic. Place in a greased bowl, turn dough over, cover, and allow to rise until double in size (about 1½ hours). Punch dough down and roll into a 25 × 12 in. (62 × 30 cm) rectangle. Place dough on a well greased cookie sheet. Make 3 in. (7.5 cm) diagonal cuts at 1 in. (2.5 cm) intervals on the 25 in. (62 cm) side of the rectangle with a scissors. Spread cherry filling down the middle of the coffee-cake dough. Crisscross cut strips at an angle over filling, overlapping the strips so that they are about 1 in. (2.5 cm) apart. Cover coffeecake with plastic wrap, then a towel. Allow to rise until double in size (about 45 to 60 minutes). Bake at 350°F (175°C) for 25 to 30 minutes or until done. While warm, brush with melted margarine.

Yield: 18 servings

Exchange, 1 serving: ¾ bread
Each serving contains: Calories: 62, Carbohydrates: 12 g

Easy Apple Coffeecake

1 lb. loaf	frozen bread dough, thawed	500 g loaf
2 T.	margarine, melted	30 mL
¼ c.	granulated brown sugar replacement	60 mL
1 T.	all-purpose flour	15 mL
2 t.	ground cinnamon	10 mL
1 t.	ground nutmeg	5 mL
2 c.	grated peeled apple	500 mL

Divide bread dough in half. Roll each half into an 8 in. (20 cm) square. Place each square on a greased cookie sheet. Brush with melted margarine. Combine brown sugar replacement, flour, cinnamon, and nutmeg in a bowl. Stir to mix. Add grated apple and toss to coat apple. Spoon one half of the apple mixture down the middle of each square. Cut 2 in. (5 cm) strips down two of the sides, towards the apple filling, about 1 in. (2.5 cm) apart. Fold strips alternately, overlapping the filling. Cover and allow coffeecake to rise until double in size. Bake at 350°F (175°C) for 30 to 35 minutes or until golden brown.

Yield: 32 servings

Exchange, 1 serving: ½ bread, ¼ fruit
Each serving contains: Calories: 57, Carbohydrates: 12 g

Crumb Coffeecake

2 c.	all-purpose flour	500 mL
¾ c.	granulated sugar replacement	190 mL
½ t.	ground cinnamon	2 mL
½ t.	ground ginger	2 mL
¼ t.	ground nutmeg	1 mL
½ c.	low-calorie margarine	125 mL
⅓ c.	raisins	90 mL
⅓ c.	walnuts, chopped	90 mL
1	egg, beaten	1
¾ c.	buttermilk	190 mL
1 t.	baking powder	5 mL
½ t.	baking soda	2 mL

Sift the flour twice. In a bowl, combine the sifted flour, sugar replacement, cinnamon, ginger, and nutmeg. Cut in the margarine until the mixture forms crumbs. Remove 1 c. (250 mL) of the mixture and reserve. Stir the raisins and walnuts into the remaining crumb mixture. In another bowl, mix together the egg, buttermilk, baking powder, and baking soda. Stir into the flour mixture just until mixed. Spread half of the reserved crumbs on the bottom of a well-greased 8 in. (20 cm) sq. baking pan. Pour the batter over the crumbs and spread evenly. Sprinkle with the remaining crumbs. Bake at 375°F (190°C) for 40 minutes or until done. Cool in the pan.

Yield: 16 servings

Exchange, 1 serving: 1 bread; ½ fat
Each serving contains: Calories: 107, Carbohydrates: 13 g

Tart Orange Coffeecake

1 pkg.	dry yeast	1 pkg.
¼ c.	warm water	60 mL
12 oz. can	frozen orange juice concentrate, slightly thawed	355 mL can
1	egg	1
½ t.	salt	2 mL
2 c.	all-purpose flour	500 mL
1 T.	solid shortening, melted	15 mL
1 T.	cornstarch	15 mL
2 T.	cold water	30 mL
1 t.	vanilla extract	5 mL

Dissolve the yeast in warm water. Allow to rest for 5 minutes. Pour into medium-sized mixing bowl. Heat ½ c. (125 mL) of the orange juice concentrate just until the chill is off. Pour into yeast mixture. Add egg, salt, and 1 c. (250 mL) of the flour. Beat on low to blend. Then beat on high for 2 minutes. Stir in remaining 1 c. (250 mL) of flour. Beat on low for 1 minute (dough will be soft). Brush about two-thirds of the melted shortening on bottom and sides of a medium-sized bowl. Transfer dough to greased bowl. Brush remaining melted shortening on top of dough. Cover with plastic wrap and then a towel. Allow to rise until double in size. Meanwhile, dissolve cornstarch in cold water. Pour into a saucepan. Add remaining orange juice concentrate. Stir to mix. Cook and stir over medium heat until mixture is very thick. Remove from heat and stir in vanilla. Allow to cool completely. To assemble: Flour your hands and divide dough in half. Press one-half of the dough into the bottom of a greased 9 in. (23 cm) round springform pan, pressing slightly up the sides. Spoon about one-half of the orange juice mixture over the top. Transfer remaining half of dough to a floured surface. Press to flatten dough to a 9 in. (23 cm) round. Place dough round on top of orange juice mixture in pan. Make random indentations in the top of the dough. Spoon remaining orange juice mixture over top. Allow to rise uncovered for 30 to 40 minutes. Place in cold oven. Set oven for 350°F (175°C). Bake for 25 to 30 minutes or until done. Allow coffeecake to cool in pan 10 minutes; then release sides.

Yield: 18 servings

Exchange, 1 serving: ¼ bread
Each serving contains: Calories: 66, Carbohydrates: 14 g

Orange Glazed Coffeecake

Perfect for brunch.

1 pkg.	active dry yeast	1 pkg.
¼ c.	warm water	60 mL
½ c.	warm skim milk, 105–115°F (40–45 c.)	125 mL
½ c.	fresh orange juice, at room temperature	125 mL
3 T.	sugar	45 mL
½ c.	fat-free ricotta cheese	125 mL
1 T.	orange peel, grated	15 mL
½ t.	salt	3 mL
1 large	egg or equivalent egg substitute, lightly beaten	1 large
3½ c.	flour (up to 4 cups)	875 mL
2–3 drops	oil	2–3 drops
1 recipe	Orange Frosting	1 recipe

Put the yeast in a large mixing bowl. Add the warm water and stir. Set aside for 5–10 minutes. The mixture will become foamy. Add all the remaining ingredients except the flour, oil, and icing, and mix together to blend.

By hand or with a heavy duty electric mixer, beat in 2½ cups (625 mL) of the flour, a little at a time. The dough will become stiff. Use a handful of the remaining flour to coat a work board. Turn the batter onto the floured board. Adding more flour as the dough becomes sticky, knead the dough until it becomes smooth and elastic. This will take about 10 minutes.

Put a few drops of oil in the bottom of a large mixing bowl. Put the dough in the bowl and turn it over so it is coated with oil. Cover loosely with a damp dishcloth-damp, not wet. Let the dough rise in a warm place for 2 hours or until doubled. Punch down and knead again for a few minutes on the floured board.

Divide the dough into three equal parts. Use your hands to roll the pieces into three 20 in. (45 cm) strands. Braid. Arrange the braid in a 10 in. (25 cm) round cheesecake or springform pan. Cover with the damp cloth once again and let rise until doubled.

Bake in a preheated 425°F (220°C) oven for 25–30 minutes. Use a sharp knife to loosen the coffeecake from the pan. Remove the cake and cool on a wire rack. Spread Orange Frosting on the cake while it is still somewhat warm. This is best served warm.

Yield: 12 servings

Exchange: 2 starch/bread, ½ fruit
Each serving contains: Calories: 196, Total fat: 0.9 g,
*   Carbohydrates: 39 g, Protein: 6 g, Sodium: 108 mg,*
*   Cholesterol: 19 mg*

Orange Icing

Especially for Orange Glazed Coffeecake or cupcakes.

¼ c.	fruit-only marmalade preserves	60 mL
1 t.	Triple Sec or orange extract	5 mL
½ c.	orange juice	125 mL

Mix all the ingredients together in a small saucepan. Heat gently, stirring constantly until blended.

Yield: ¾ c. (375 mL), or 12 servings

Exchange: free
Each serving contains: Calories: 18, Total fat: 0 g, Carbohydrates: 4 g, Protein: 0.1 g, Sodium: 0 mg, Cholesterol: 0 mg

Prune Streusel Coffeecake

3 T.	all-purpose four	45 mL
2 T.	granulated brown sugar replacement	30 mL
2 t.	ground cinnamon	10 mL
½ c.	Bran Buds cereal	125 mL
3 T.	margarine, softened	45 mL
1 c.	all-purpose flour	250 mL
¾ t.	baking powder	4 mL
¾ t.	baking soda	4 mL
½ t.	salt	2 mL
½ t.	ground cinnamon	2 mL
2 ¾ c.	Bran Buds cereal	190 mL
½ c.	margarine, softened	125 mL
2 T.	granulated sugar replacement	30 mL
2	eggs	2
1 c.	plain low-fat yogurt	250 mL
½ c.	pitted prunes, finely cut	125 mL

For the topping: Measure the first 5 ingredients into a small mixing bowl. Mix with fork or fingers until crumbly. Set aside.

For the cake: Stir together 1 c. (250 mL) flour, baking powder, baking soda, salt, cinnamon and ¾ c. (190 mL) cereal. Set aside. In a large bowl, beat ½ c. (125 mL) margarine and sugar replacement until well blended. Add eggs. Beat well. Stir in yogurt. Add flour mixture, Mixing thoroughly. Spread half the batter evenly in greased 9 in. (23 cm) sq. baking pan. Sprinkle evenly over the batter, half the prunes and then, half the topping. Spread remaining batter over the top and sprinkle batter with the remaining prunes and topping mixture. Bake at 350°F (175°C) about 40 minutes or until done. Serve warm.

Yield: 16 servings

Exchange, 1 serving: 1 bread, ⅔ low-fat milk, ½ fat
Each serving contains: Calories: 180, Carbohydrates: 17 g

Sunshine Stollen

Make the vanilla sugar replacement at least 3 days before you plan to make the stollen.

2 in.	vanilla bean, split	5 cm
1 c.	granulated sugar replacement	250 mL
2½ c.	all-purpose flour	625 mL
2 t.	baking powder	10 mL
½ t.	salt	2 mL
¼ t.	ground mace	1 mL
¼ t.	ground cardamom	1 mL
⅓ c.	almonds, ground	90 mL
½ c.	low-calorie margarine	125 mL
1 c.	low-fat cottage cheese	250 mL
1	egg	1
2 T.	water	30 mL
½ t.	vanilla extract	2 mL
½ t.	rum flavoring	2 mL
⅓ c.	currants	90 mL
⅓ c.	raisins	90 mL
¼ c.	lemon peel	60 mL
2 T.	low-calorie margarine, melted	30 mL

To make the vanilla sugar replacement: Bury the split vanilla bean in 1 c. (250 mL) of granulated sugar replacement in a container. Cover the container tightly. Allow vanilla bean to flavor sugar replacement for at least 3 days at room temperature.

To make the stollen: Combine ½ c. (125 mL) of the vanilla sugar replacement, flour, baking powder, salt, mace, cardamom, and almonds. Cut margarine into the mixture until it resembles coarse crumbs. Blend cottage cheese in a blender until smooth; pour into the flour mixture. Add the egg, water, vanilla, rum flavoring, currants, raisins, and lemon peel; stir to thoroughly mix. Form the dough into a ball. Knead on a lightly floured surface 10 to 12 times or until dough is smooth. Roll dough into an 8 × 10 in. (20 × 25 cm) oval. With the back of your hand, crease the dough just off the middle, parallel to the 10 in. (25 cm) side; fold the smaller section over the larger. Brush with half of the melted margarine. Bake on an ungreased baking sheet at 350°F (175°C) for 45 minutes or until done. Remove stollen from oven and allow to cool. Brush with the remaining melted margarine and sprinkle with 2 T. (30 mL) of the granulated vanilla sugar replacement.

Yield: 20 servings

Exchange, 1 serving: 1 bread, ¾ fat
Each serving contains: Calories: 106, Carbohydrates: 15 g

Blueberry Yogurt Coffeecake

1 pkg.	dry yeast	1 pkg.
¼ c.	lukewarm water	60 mL
⅓ c.	skim milk	90 mL
8 oz.	blueberry low-calorie yogurt	240 g
1¼ t.	granulated fructose	6 mL
2¾ c.	all-purpose flour	690 mL

Dissolve the yeast in warm water; set aside. Scald the skim milk in a medium saucepan. Add the yogurt and stir to dissolve. Stir in the fructose. Allow to cool to lukewarm. When lukewarm, stir in yeast mixture. In the same saucepan, stir in 1 c. (250 mL) of the flour. Beat until smooth. Gradually add remaining flour. Cover and allow to rise for 1½ hours. Turn out onto board and knead until smooth and elastic. (Dough will be soft.) Form into a ball and wrap tightly in plastic. Place in refrigerator overnight. (You might have to punch dough down a second time and rewrap in plastic.) When ready to bake, place dough on a lightly floured surface; cut in half. Roll each half into a small square to fit an 8 in. (20 cm) pan. Place dough in a lightly greased 8 in. (20 cm) sq. pan. Push dough to edges; using your finger, push a small ridge up the sides. Cover and allow to rise until over double in size. Bake at 350°F (175°C) for 25 to 30 minutes or until done.

Yield: 2 coffeecakes or 32 servings

Exchange, 1 serving: ½ bread
Each serving contains: Calories: 29, Carbohydrates: 9 g

Coffee Coconut Cake

1½ c.	all-purpose flour	375 mL
1 t.	baking soda	5 mL
½ t.	salt	2 mL
1 t.	ground cinnamon	5 mL
½ c.	granulated sugar replacement	125 mL
½ c.	Kellogg's All-Bran or Bran Buds cereal	125 mL
1 c.	cold strong coffee	250 mL
¼ c.	vegetable oil	60 mL
1 T.	vinegar	15 mL
½ t.	almond flavoring	2 mL
½ c.	flaked coconut	125 mL

Stir together flour, soda, salt, cinnamon and sugar replacement. Set aside. Measure cereal and coffee into a large bowl. Stir to combine. Let stand about 2 minutes or until cereal softens. Stir in oil, vinegar, almond flavoring, and ⅓ c. (90 mL) of the coconut. Add flour mixture, mixing until well combined. Spread evenly in greased 8 × 8 × 2 in. (20 × 20 × 5 cm) baking pan. Sprinkle remaining coconut over batter. Bake at 350°F (175°C) about 25 minutes or until cake tests done. Serve warm or cool with whipped topping, if desired.

Yield: 12 servings

Exchange, 1 serving (without whipped topping): 1 bread, 1 fat
Each serving contains: Calories: 117

From Kellogg's Test Kitchens

Tortes

Lemon Pistachio Torte

8 oz.	sugar-free white cake mix	227 g
1 T.	grated lemon zest	15 mL
1 t.	lemon flavoring	5 mL
1 pkg.	sugar-free pistachio instant pudding and pie filling★	1 pkg.

Mix cake as directed on package. Beat in lemon zest and lemon flavoring. Bake as directed on package. Cool completely. Cut cake in half horizontally. Chill. Prepare pistachio pudding with 2% milk as directed on package. Cool completely. Frost layers of cake with pistachio pudding. Chill thoroughly before serving.

Yield: 10 servings

Exchange, 1 serving: 1 starch/bread, 1 fat
Each serving contains: Calories: 136, Carbohydrates: 24 g

★four-servings size

Chocolate Rum Torte

¼ c.	boiling water	60 mL
¼ c.	chocolate chips	60 mL
4	eggs, separated	4
3 t.	rum flavoring	15
32	vanilla wafers	32 mL
⅓ c.	water	90 mL

In a saucepan, pour boiling water over chocolate chips and stir to melt chips. Beat egg yolks, one at a time, into the chocolate mixture. Place pan over low heat and cook until thick. Remove from heat and cool completely. Add 1 t. (5 mL) of the rum flavoring. Beat egg whites until stiff. Fold small amount of whites into chocolate mixture to lighten, then fold chocolate mixture into remaining egg whites. In a small cup, dilute the remaining 2 t. (10 mL) rum flavoring with ⅓ c. (90 mL) water. Dip each wafer into flavoring. Place the 16 dipped wafers on bottom of 8 in. (20 cm) springform pan, spread with half of chocolate mixture, top with remaining 16 dipped wafers, spread remaining chocolate mixture over top. Freeze until firm.

Yield: 20 servings

Exchange, 1 serving: ½ bread, ½ fat
Each serving contains: Calories: 55, Carbohydrates: 5 g

Rum Torte

8 oz.	sugar-free white cake mix	227 g
⅓ c.	water	90 mL
⅓ c.	dark Jamaican rum	90 mL
1	egg white	1
¼ c.	skim milk	60 mL
2 T.	dark Jamaican rum	30 mL
1 pkg.	Estee 4-in-1 Frosting Mix	1 pkg.
1 T.	margarine	15 mL
1 c.	prepared nondairy whipped topping	250 mL

Combine cake mix, water, the ⅓ c. (90 mL) rum, and the egg white in a bowl. Beat for 4 or 5 minutes. Transfer to 8 in. (20 cm) round, lightly greased cake pan. Bake at 350°F (175°C) for 20 to 25 minutes. Allow cake to cool and then remove from pan. Cut cake horizontally into two layers. Now combine milk and the 2 T. (30 mL) rum in a saucepan. Over medium heat, gradually add frosting mix. Stir constantly until mixture becomes very thick. Remove from heat and stir in margarine. Allow to cool. Spread a thin coat of frosting and a thin coat of nondairy whipped topping on the bottom layer of the cake. Place top layer of cake on top. Spread with remaining frosting and whipped topping. Chill thoroughly before serving.

Yield: 12 servings

Exchange, 1 serving: 2 starch/bread, 1 fat
Each serving contains: Calories: 175, Carbohydrates: 31 g

Coconut Chocolate Cream Torte

8 oz.	sugar-free chocolate cake mix	227 g
½ c.	unsweetened grated coconut	125 mL
1 c.	prepared nondairy whipped topping	250 mL
⅓ c.	semisweet chocolate chips	90 mL

Combine cake mix and ¼ c. (60 mL) of the coconut in a mixing bowl. Prepare cake as directed on package. Allow cake to cool completely. Cut cake in half horizontally. Spread nondairy whipped topping between layers. Melt chocolate chips in a double boiler, over simmering water. Pour and spread melted chocolate over top of cake. Then sprinkle with remaining grated coconut.

Yield: 10 servings

Exchange, 1 serving: 1 starch/bread, 1 fat
Each serving contains: Calories: 141, Carbohydrates: 21 g

Chantilly Strawberry Torte

¼ c.	Estee 4-in-1 Frosting Mix	60 mL
1 env.	nondairy whipped-topping mix	1 env.
	skim milk	125 mL
8 oz.	sugar-free white cake mix	227 g
1 c.	fresh strawberries	250 mL

Combine frosting mix, nondairy whipped-topping mix, and skim milk in a mixing bowl. With a fork, stir to blend. Place beaters in the bowl and refrigerate for at least an hour. Bake cake in 8 in. (20 cm) round pan as directed on package. Allow cake to cool completely. Slice strawberries lengthwise. Reserve 10 halves for top decoration. Cut cake horizontally into two layers. Beat frosting mix for 5 to 6 minutes or until thick and creamy. Spoon half of frosting mix over the bottom layer of cake. Place cut strawberries on top of frosting. Place top layer of cake on top. Spoon remaining frosting on top and decorate with reserved strawberry halves. Place in freezer. Chill or freeze. If frozen, thaw for 10 minutes before serving.

Yield: 10 servings

Exchange, 1 serving: 2 starch/bread, 1 fat
Each serving contains: Calories: 165, Carbohydrates: 29 g

Duchess Torte

1 loaf	angel food cake, ready-made	1 loaf
1 pkg.	Estee 4-in-1 Frosting Mix	1 pkg.
1 t.	cherry flavoring	5 mL
2 c.	prepared nondairy whipped topping	500 mL
1 c.	pitted dark cherries	250 mL
¼ c.	crushed pineapple, well drained	60 mL
¼ c.	chopped almonds	60 mL

Slice cake into four layers. Prepare frosting mix as directed on package, adding the 1 t. (5 mL) cherry flavoring. Allow frosting to cool. Beat cooled frosting slightly to loosen. Gently fold frosting into the nondairy whipped topping. Reserve ½ c. (125 mL) of the frosting-topping mixture for top of cake. Quarter cherries; then set aside 6 to 10 for top decoration. Fold remaining cherries and the pineapple and almonds into non-reserved frosting-topping mixture. Fill layers. Spread top of cake with reserved frosting; then decorate with reserved cherries. Refrigerate.

Yield: 12 servings

Exchange, 1 serving: 1¾ starch/bread, 1 fat
Each serving contains: Calories: 172, Carbohydrates: 30 g

Raspberry Torte

8 oz.	sugar-free white cake mix	227 g
2 t.	lemon flavoring	10 mL
1 c.	fresh raspberries	250 mL
¾ c.	prepared nondairy whipped topping	190 mL

Mix cake mix and lemon flavoring together. Prepare cake mix as directed on package. Allow cake to cool completely. Cut cake in half horizontally. Fold raspberries into whipped topping. Spread between layers and on top of cake. Chill thoroughly before serving.

Yield: 10 servings

Exchange, 1 serving: 1 starch/bread, 1 fat
Each serving contains: Calories: 115, Carbohydrates: 19 g

Festive Cranberry Torte

2 c.	crushed fresh cranberries	500 mL
2 T.	grated orange peel	30 mL
½ c.	granulated fructose	125 mL
1 loaf	angel food cake, ready-made	1 loaf
3 c.	prepared nondairy whipped topping	750 mL

Combine cranberries, orange peel, and fructose in a saucepan. Stir to mix. Cook over low heat just until boiling. Cool completely. Slice angel food cake loaf into four layers. Spread one-fourth of the nondairy whipped topping on each layer. Spoon one-fourth of the chilled cranberries over the whipped topping. With a spoon or knife, gently swirl the cranberries into the whipped topping. Stack the layers. Refrigerate 2 to 3 hours before serving.

Yield: 12 servings

Exchange, 1 serving: 2 starch/bread, ¼ fruit
Each serving contains: Calories: 172, Carbohydrates: 33 g

Graham Cracker Cake Torte

1 c.	graham cracker crumbs	250 mL
¼ c.	chopped walnuts	60 mL
2 T.	granulated sugar replacement	30 mL
2 T.	granulated fructose	30 mL
1 t.	cinnamon	5 mL
¼ c.	low-calorie margarine, melted	60 mL
8 oz.	sugar-free white cake mix	227 g
⅓ c.	semisweet chocolate chips, melted	90 mL

Mix graham cracker crumbs, walnuts, sugar replacement, fructose, and cinnamon in a bowl. Pour melted margarine over the top of the mixture. Toss to mix. Press half of the mixture into the bottom of an 8 in. (20 cm) square pan. Prepare cake mix as directed on package. Pour half of the cake batter over the crumb mixture in the bottom of the pan. Sprinkle with half of the remaining crumb mixture. Pour remaining batter over crumbs in pan. Sprinkle with remaining crumb mixture. Bake at 350°F (175°C) for 25 to 30 minutes or until torte tests done. While hot, drizzle with melted chocolate chips.

Yield: 12 servings

Exchange, 1 serving: 2 starch/bread, 1 fat
Each serving contains: Calories: 172, Carbohydrates: 31 g

Lemon Torte

1 (9 in.) recipe	Meringue Crust	1 (23 cm.) recipe
4	egg yolks	4
¼ c.	granulated fructose	60 mL
⅛ t.	salt	½ mL
3 T.	grated lemon peel	45 mL
3 T.	lemon juice	45 mL
2 c.	prepared nondairy whipped topping	500 mL

Beat egg yolks in top part of double boiler until they are thick and lemon colored. Beat in fructose gradually. Add salt, 1 T. (15 mL) of the grated lemon peel, and the lemon juice. Cook and stir over simmering water until thick. Cool completely. Spread half of the nondairy whipped topping into the Meringue Crust. Pour the cooled lemon filling over the whipped topping. Decorate top of torte with remaining whipped topping. Then sprinkle with remaining 2 T. (30 mL) of grated lemon peel.

Yield: 8 servings

Exchange, 1 serving: ¾ medium-fat meat, ¼ fruit
Each serving contains: Calories: 85, Carbohydrates: 5 g

Blueberry Cream Torte

8 oz.	sugar-free white cake mix	227 g
1½ c.	fresh blueberries	375 mL
2 T.	granulated fructose	30 mL
1 env.	nondairy whipped-topping mix	1 env.
½ c.	cold water	125 mL

Prepare cake as directed on package in loaf pan. Allow cake to cool completely. Cut cake into 10 even slices. Line the bottom of an 8 in. (20 cm) sq. cake pan with plastic wrap. Cover bottom of plastic-lined pan with five of the cake slices. Crush blueberries; then stir in fructose. Allow to sit at room temperature for 30 minutes. Spoon half of the blueberries over the cake in pan. Combine nondairy whipped-topping mix and water in a bowl. Stir to mix. Place beaters in the bowl and chill for 30 minutes. Beat until thick and creamy, but not into soft peaks. Spoon half of the whipped topping over the blueberries in the pan. Cover with remaining cake slices. Spoon remaining blueberries over cake. Beat remaining whipped topping to soft peaks; then spread it over blueberries. Chill thoroughly before serving.

Yield: 16 servings

Exchange, 1 serving: 1 starch/bread
Each serving contains: Calories: 74, Carbohydrates: 13 g

Grand Marnier Torte

	vegetable spray	
1 c.	low-calorie margarine	250 mL
⅔ c.	granulated fructose	180 mL
4	eggs	4
1 c.	sifted cornstarch	250 mL
1 c.	sifted all-purpose flour	250 mL
1 t.	baking powder	5 mL
2 T.	grated orange rind	30 mL
2 T.	Grand Marnier	30 mL
1 T.	vanilla extract	15 mL

Coat a 10 in. (25 cm) bundt pan with vegetable spray and then set it aside. Cream margarine with fructose in a large bowl for about 10 minutes or until mixture is light and fluffy. Beat in one egg. Gradually add ½ c. (125 mL) of the cornstarch. Beat in second egg. Beat in ½ c. (125 mL) of the flour. Beat in third egg. Beat in remaining ½ c. (125 mL) of the cornstarch. Beat in fourth egg. Combine remaining flour and baking powder; then beat into flour mixture. Beat well. Add orange rind, Grand Marnier, and vanilla. Transfer to greased bundt pan. Bake at 375°F (190°C) for 45 to 55 minutes or until torte tests done. Cool in pan.

Yield: 20 servings

Exchange, 1 serving: 1½ starch/bread
Each serving contains: Calories: 119, Carbohydrates: 21 g

Vienna Torte

	graham cracker crumbs	
1 c.	graham cracker crumbs	250 mL
¼ c.	grated almonds	60 mL
2 T.	granulated sugar replacement	30 mL
2 T.	granulated fructose	30 mL
2 t.	cocoa powder	10 mL
½ t.	cinnamon	2 mL
⅛ t.	cloves	½ mL
¼ c.	low-calorie margarine, melted	60 mL
1 qt.	fresh raspberries	1 L
2 T.	granulated fructose	30 mL
½ c.	water	125 mL
1 T.	cornstarch	15 mL

Mix graham cracker crumbs, almonds, sugar replacement, 2 T. (30 mL) fructose, cocoa, cinnamon, and cloves in a bowl. Pour melted margarine over the top of the mixture. Toss to mix. Press mixture into the bottom and up the sides of a 9 in. (23 cm) springform. pan. Chill. Combine raspberries and 2 T. (30 mL) fructose in a bowl. With a potato masher, mash slightly. Combine water and cornstarch in a saucepan, stirring to blend. Then stir in raspberries. Cook and stir over medium heat until mixture is clear and very thick. Cool slightly. Spread mixture on top of graham crust in pan. Bake at 325°F (165°C) for 20 to 30 minutes. Remove from oven and chill thoroughly. Carefully push bottom of pan up to remove torte.

Yield: 12 servings

Exchange, 1 serving: 1 starch/bread, ½ fat
Each serving contains: Calories: 103, Carbohydrates: 17 g

Cherry Schaum Torte

2	egg whites	2
1 t.	granulated fructose	5 mL
1 t.	white vinegar	5 mL
1 t.	white vanilla extract	5 mL
1 lb. can	sour cherries with juice	450 g can
2 t.	liquid fructose	10 mL
2 t.	cornstarch	10 mL

Crust: Beat egg whites until stiff. Sprinkle granulated fructose on top and beat well. Continue to beat while adding vinegar and vanilla. Beat until egg whites are very stiff and have lost their gloss. Spread into greased 8 in. (20 cm) pie pan. Bake at 250°F (125°C) for 1 hour. Cool completely.

Filling: Drain cherries thoroughly. Combine cherry juice, liquid fructose and cornstarch in saucepan. Cook over medium heat until clear and thickened; remove from heat. Cool slightly. Fold in cherries; cool completely. Pour into cooled crust.

Yield: 6 servings

Exchange, 1 serving: ½ bread
Each serving contains: Calories: 45, Carbohydrates: 5 g

Midnight Torte

½ c.	solid shortening	125 mL
½ c.	granulated sugar replacement	125 mL
2 T.	cold water	30 mL
3	eggs	3
2¼ c.	cake flour	560 mL
⅔ c.	cocoa	180 mL
1¼ t.	baking soda	6 mL
½ t.	baking powder	2 mL
1 t.	salt	5 mL
1⅓ c.	water	340 mL
1 t.	vanilla extract	5 mL
2 t.	almond extract	10 mL
½ c.	Cherry Topping	125 mL
¼ c.	Powdered Sugar Replacement	60 mL

Cream the shortening until fluffy and gradually beat in granulated sugar replacement, 2 T. (30 mL) cold water and eggs, one at a time. Combine cake flour, cocoa, baking soda, baking powder, and salt in sifter. Combine 1⅓ c. (340 mL) water and extracts in bowl or pitcher. Sift flour mixture alternately with water into creamed mixture. Beat until blended. Pour evenly into four 9 in. (23 cm) round cake pans, well greased and floured. Bake at 350°F (175°C) for 15 to 20 minutes, or until done. Remove from pans; cool completely. Spread bottom cake layer with one-third of cherry topping. Add second cake layer and one-third of the topping; repeat. Top with final cake layer. Dust with sifted powdered sugar replacement.

Yield: 20 servings

Exchange, 1 serving: 1 bread
Each serving contains: Calories: 103, Carbohydrates: 30 g

Frankfurt Torte

2½ c.	cake flour	625 mL
dash	salt	dash
⅓ c.	granulated brown sugar replacement	90 mL
1 T.	baking powder	15 mL
¼ c.	margarine	60 mL
2 t.	baking soda	10 mL
2 t.	water	10 mL
¾ c.	buttermilk	190 mL
¼ c.	Powdered Sugar Replacement	60 mL

Combine cake flour, salt, brown sugar replacement and baking powder in bowl. Add margarine; work into crumbs. Reserve 1 c. (250 mL) crumbs for topping. Combine baking soda and water, stirring to dissolve. Add buttermilk and baking soda water to remaining crumbs; stir to completely blend. Pour into 9 × 5 in. (23 × 13 cm) well greased loaf pan and sprinkle with reserved crumbs. Bake at 350°F (175°C) for 50 to 60 minutes, or until done, and then let cool. Sprinkle sifted powdered sugar replacement over top.

Yield: 16 servings

Exchange, 1 serving: 1 bread, ½ fat
Each serving contains: Calories: 88, Carbohydrates: 25 g

Macadamia Torte

This rivals fancy cakes in the best restaurants. No one would guess it's a diabetic recipe.

½ c.	macadamia nuts, chopped fine	125 mL
¼ c.	sugar	60 mL
1 c.	measures-like-sugar saccharin	250 mL
1 t.	baking soda	5 mL
2 c.	flour	500 mL
1 t.	baking powder	5 mL
1 t.	ground ginger	5 mL
1	egg or equivalent egg substitute	1
⅔ c.	canola oil	180 mL
1 c.	nonfat sour cream	250 mL
1 t.	vanilla extract	5 mL
1 t.	butter-flavored extract	5 mL
¼ c.	water	60 mL

Coat a 10-in. (25 cm) tube pan with non-stick cooking spray and sprinkle macadamia nuts evenly in the pan; set aside. Combine the dry ingredients in a large bowl. Combine the wet ingredients. Stir into the dry ingredients until smooth. Pour the batter into the prepared pan. Bake at 350°F (180°C) for 35 to 40 minutes or until a wooden pick inserted comes out clean. Cool 10 to 15 minutes.

Yield: 20 servings

Exchange, 1 serving: 1 bread + 2 fats
Each serving contains: Calories: 153, Carbohydrates: 25 g, Fiber: 0.6 g, Sodium: 99 mg, Cholesterol: 1.6 mg

Passover Chocolate-Nut Torte

This recipe contains no flour or leavening, so it's ideal for Passover—but it's worth making all year long.

½ c.	walnut pieces, coarsely ground	125 mL
½ c.	blanched almonds	125 mL
¼ c.	sugar	60 mL
½ c.	unsweetened cocoa powder	125 mL
3 pkts.	concentrated acesulfame-K	3 pkts.
1 T.	cognac	15 mL
8	large egg whites	8

Put the nuts in a pie pan and bake in a 350°F (180°C) oven for about 10 minutes. Stir the nuts occasionally during toasting—be careful that they don't burn. Cool. Add sugar. Using a food processor, grind until powdery, but do not liquefy. Add the nuts and cocoa, acesulfame-K, and cognac. Pulse on and off until smooth and well combined. In a large bowl, beat the egg whites until stiff but not dry. Fold one quarter of the nut mixture into the egg whites and then fold that mixture into the rest of the nut mixture. Do not mix too much. Gently scrape into a 9-in. (23 cm) springform pan sprayed with non-stick cooking spray. Bake at 350°F (180°C) for 30 minutes. (A toothpick inserted into the center will *not* come out clean.) Cool on a wire rack before removing from the pan. Serve with your favorite whipped topping.

Yield: 12 servings

Exchange, 1 serving: ½ milk + 1 fat
Each serving contains: Calories: 96, Carbohydrates: 8 g, Fiber: 0.63 g, Sodium: 33 mg, Cholesterol: 0 mg

Bridal Torte

An impressive dessert for bridal showers.

⅓ c.	margarine	90 mL
¼ c.	granulated sugar replacement	60 mL
1 oz.	baking chocolate, melted and cooled	30 g
2 t.	vanilla extract	10 mL
2	eggs	2
8	Meringue Nests (see Individual Meringue Nests)	8
8 T.	nondairy whipped topping	120 mL

Cream margarine and sugar replacement until light and fluffy. Blend in baking chocolate and vanilla. Add eggs, one at a time, beating for 5 minutes after each addition. Turn into meringue nests. Chill at least 1 to 2 hours before serving. Top each nest with 1 T. (15 mL) of nondairy whipped topping.

Yield: 8 servings

Exchange, 1 serving: ½ lean meat, 2 fat
Each serving contains: Calories: 110, Carbohydrates: 28 g

Mosaic Chocolate Torte

1 t.	unflavored gelatin	5 mL
1 T.	cold water	15 mL
2 oz.	baking chocolate	60 g
¼ c.	granulated sugar replacement	60 mL
2 T.	sorbitol	30 mL
dash	salt	dash
¼ c.	hot water	60 mL
4	eggs, separated	4
1 t.	vanilla extract	5 mL
1 c.	nondairy whipped topping	250 mL
½	Sponge Cake	½

Soften gelatin in cold water; set aside. Melt baking chocolate in top of double boiler. Add sugar replacement, sorbitol, salt, and hot water. Stir until mixture is well blended. Add softened gelatin and stir until gelatin is completely dissolved. Remove from heat. Add egg yolks, one at a time, beating after every addition. Place pan back over boiling water; cook and stir for 2 more minutes. Remove from heat. Add vanilla extract and stir to mix thoroughly. Cool. Beat egg whites until stiff. Fold into cooled chocolate mixture. Chill until mixture starts to thicken. Fold in prepared nondairy whipped topping. Line bottom and sides of large, decorative mold with thin slices of sponge cake. Alternate layers of chocolate mixture and sponge cake to complete the torte. Chill at least 14 hours.

Yield: 20 servings

Exchange, 1 serving: ¼ fat
Each serving contains: Calories: 40, Carbohydrates: 11 g

Sponge Cake

4	eggs, separated	4
3 T.	granulated sugar replacement	45 mL
½ c.	hot water	125 mL
1½ t.	vanilla extract	7 mL
1½ c.	cake flour, sifted	375 mL
¼ t.	salt	1 mL
¼ t.	baking powder	1 mL

With electric beater, beat egg yolks and sugar replacement until thick and lemon-colored. Beat in hot water and vanilla. Combine cake flour, salt, and baking powder in sifter; sift and stir into the egg yolk mixture. Beat egg whites until stiff and fold into egg yolk mixture. Spoon batter into ungreased 9 in. (23 cm) tube pan. Bake at 325°F (165°C) for 55 to 60 minutes, or until cake is done. Invert pan and allow cake to cool at least 1 hour. Remove from pan.

Yield: 16 servings

Exchange, 1 serving: ½ bread
Each serving contains: Calories: 54, Carbohydrates: 12 g

Chocolate Heaven

½	Sponge Cake	½	
3 oz.	baking chocolate	90 g	
½ c.	skim milk	125 mL	
¼ c.	granulated sugar replacement	60 mL	
4	eggs, separated	4	
2 t.	brandy flavoring	10 mL	
dash	salt	dash	
1 env.	nondairy whipped topping	1 env.	

Line loaf pan with waxed paper. Cover bottom and sides with thin slices of sponge cake (save enough slices to cover top). Melt baking chocolate in top of double boiler; add skim milk and continue cooking and stirring until smooth and well blended. Slightly beat the egg yolks; add sugar replacement and a small amount of chocolate mixture. Stir to thoroughly mix and add to chocolate mixture in the double boiler. Cook until thick and smooth, stirring constantly. Remove from heat; while still hot, fold in stiffly beaten egg whites, brandy flavoring and salt. Cool slightly. Pour chocolate mixture into loaf pan lined with sponge cake. Cover with a layer of the remaining cake slices. Chill for at least 14 hours. Turn out onto a serving plate. Frost with nondairy topping.

Yield: 12 servings

Exchange, 1 serving: ⅓ bread, ½ medium meat, ½ fat
Each serving contains: Calories: 91, Carbohydrates: 21 g

Frostings, Fillings, and Toppings

Fillings, frostings, and sauces are often neglected as an addition to a simple dessert. Yet, easy to make, they can do wonders in dressing up a dip of vanilla ice cream or a slice of plain white cake.

All fruits, fresh or frozen, become a filling or sauce simply by processing them in a food processor or blender. Since sauces are an opportunity to use frozen fruits, there is no need to make them up in advance. To add a little more interest and zip to your sauces, you can use any of the numerous flavorings that are now on the market. For instance, try blending a few sweet cherries with the addition of a small amount of brandy flavoring. Pour this over a slice of cake and your dessert will be beautiful and complete.

Try using the fillings as frosting, the frostings as filling, and the sauces instead of either one, for exciting new dessert treats. Use them for visual interest as well. Place the sauce under or alongside a slice of cake. Or spoon a small amount of frosting, filling, or sauce on top of a custard, pudding, or sliced fresh fruit. Then sprinkle a small amount of special topping on for added flavor, texture, and appeal. Colored cereals or stale cookies crushed to crumbs and nuts ground very fine make good toppings, and instant chocolate pudding can be used as a sauce.

Our frosting recipes give the number of calories, exchanges, etc., per tablespoon. That way you can figure according to how many tablespoons (mL) you are eating.

Strawberry Filling

2 c.	frozen unsweetened strawberries	500 mL
2 T.	water	30 mL
4 t.	cornstarch	20 mL
2 T.	granulated sugar replacement	30 mL

Combine frozen strawberries, water, and cornstarch in a microwave bowl or saucepan. Cook in the microwave on high for 3 to 4 minutes or until mixture is clear and thickened; stir at least once during cooking. Or, on top of the stove, cook in a saucepan on medium heat until mixture is clear and thickened. Remove from microwave or stove, and stir in sugar replacement. Allow to cool until mixture drops from a spoon in large blobs. Spread about two-thirds to three-fourths of the mixture between any number of cake layers. Reserve remaining filling for top decoration.

Yield: 8 servings

Exchange, 1 serving: 1 fruit
Each serving contains: Calories: 11, Carbohydrates: 3 g

Plain and Simple Prune Filling

1 c.	prunes	250 mL
½ t.	cinnamon	2 mL

Place prunes in a saucepan. Cover with water and simmer for 20 to minutes until prunes are tender; then drain. Remove pits and mash with fork or process in food processor or blender. Stir in cinnamon.

Yield: 10 servings

Exchange, 1 serving: ⅓ fruit
Each serving contains: Calories: 26, Carbohydrates: 7 g

Lemon Filling

2 T.	granulated fructose	30 mL
2 T.	cornstarch	30 mL
1¼ c.	evaporated skim milk	310 mL
3 T.	lemon juice	45 mL
1 T.	grated lemon rind	15 mL

Combine fructose and cornstarch in a heavy or non-stick saucepan. Blend in the milk and lemon juice. Cook and stir over medium heat until clear and thickened. Remove from heat and stir in the lemon rind. Cover and cool to room temperature, stirring occasionally.

Yield: 10 servings

Exchange, 1 serving: ½ bread
Each serving contains: Calories: 34, Carbohydrates: 7 g

Almond Filling

5	egg whites	5
dash	salt	dash
2 T.	granulated fructose	30 mL
2 T.	granulated sugar replacement	30 mL
½ t.	ground cinnamon	2 mL
⅓ c.	ground almonds	90 mL

Combine egg whites and salt in a bowl. Beat until stiff. Gradually beat in the fructose and sugar replacement. Beat in cinnamon. Fold in the ground almonds. Refrigerate until ready to use.

Yield: 10 servings

Exchange, 1 serving: negligible
Each serving contains: Calories: 9, Carbohydrates: 1 g

Chocolate Cream Filling

3 c.	skim milk	750 mL
¼ c.	carob powder	60 mL
¼ c.	granulated fructose	60 mL
6 T.	cornstarch	90 mL
½ t.	salt	2 mL
3	eggs, beaten	3
1 T.	margarine	15 mL
2 t.	vanilla extract	10 mL

Combine milk, carob powder, fructose, cornstarch, and salt in a heavy saucepan. Stir to dissolve cornstarch. Cook and stir over medium heat until thick. Cover, reduce heat, and cook 10 minutes longer. Stir a small amount of hot mixture into the beaten eggs. Return egg mixture to saucepan. Cook and stir for about 5 minutes. Remove from heat and stir in margarine until melted. Cover and allow to cool. Stir in vanilla before using.

Yield: 16 servings

Exchange, 1 serving: ⅔ bread, ½ fat
Each serving contains: Calories: 63, Carbohydrates: 8 g

Vanilla Cream Filling

3 c.	skim milk	750 mL
¼ c.	granulated fructose	60 mL
6 T.	cornstarch	90 mL
½ t.	salt	2 mL
3	eggs, beaten	3
1 T.	margarine	15 mL
2 t.	vanilla extract	10 mL

Combine milk, fructose, cornstarch, and salt in a heavy saucepan. Stir to dissolve cornstarch. Cook and stir over medium heat until thick. Covet reduce heat, and cook 10 minutes longer. Stir a small amount of hot mixture into the beaten eggs. Return egg mixture to saucepan. Cook and stir for about 5 minutes. Remove from heat and stir in margarine until melted Cover and allow to cool. Stir in vanilla before using.

Yield: 16 servings

Exchange, 1 serving: ½ bread, ½ fat
Each serving contains: Calories: 56, Carbohydrates: 6 g

Raspberry Filling

1 c.	fresh or frozen unsweetened raspberries	250 mL
2 T.	cornstarch	30 mL
1 T.	granulated sugar replacement	15 mL
¾ c.	evaporated skim milk	190 mL
2 t.	lemon juice	10 mL

Process ½ c. (125 mL) of the raspberries in a food processor or blender until puréed. Combine the cornstarch and sugar replacement in a heavy nonstick saucepan; then gradually add the milk, puréed raspberries, an(lemon juice. Cook and stir over medium heat until clear and thickened Remove from heat and stir in remaining raspberries. Cover and cool to room temperature before using.

Yield: 10 servings

Exchange, 1 serving: ⅓ bread
Each serving contains: Calories: 27, Carbohydrates: 5 g

Raisin Currant Filling

¼ c.	raisins	60 mL
¼ c.	currants	60 mL
¼ c.	cold water	60 mL
1 T.	all-purpose flour	15 mL
1 T.	lemon juice	15 mL
2 t.	grated lemon rind	10 mL

Combine all ingredients in a saucepan. Stir to dissolve flour. Cook over low heat until thick. Remove from heat, and allow to cool before using.

Yield: 10 servings

Exchange, 1 serving: ½ fruit
Each serving contains: Calories: 24, Carbohydrates: 6 g

Spicy Mincemeat Filling

1 c.	raisins	250 mL
¼ c.	cider vinegar	60 mL
2 t.	cornstarch	10 mL
1 t.	ground cinnamon	5 mL
½ t.	ground nutmeg	2 mL
½ t.	ground allspice	2 mL
¼ t.	ground cloves	1 mL

Combine all ingredients in a saucepan. Stir to dissolve cornstarch. Cook and stir over low heat until thick. Remove from heat, and allow to cool before using.

Yield: 10 servings

Exchange, 1 serving: ⅔ fruit
Each serving contains: Calories: 42, Carbohydrates: 11 g

Poppy Seed Filling

½ c.	water	125 mL
¼ c.	granulated fructose	60 mL
¼ c.	ground poppy seeds*	60 mL
⅓ c.	cold water	90 mL
1 T.	cornstarch	15 mL
½ t.	lemon juice	2 mL
¼ t.	ground cinnamon	1 mL
¼ t.	banana or butter rum flavoring	1 mL

Combine the ½ c. of water and the fructose in a small nonstick saucepan. Cook over medium heat, stirring until fructose is dissolved. Bring to a boil and boil for 3 minutes. Reduce heat and add ground poppy seeds. Dissolve cornstarch in the cold water. Add cornstarch solution, lemon juice, and cinnamon to poppy seed mixture. Cook and stir until mixture is thickened. Remove from heat, and stir in flavoring.

Yield: 10 servings

Exchange, 1 serving: ¼ fruit
Each serving contains: Calories: 13, Carbohydrates: 3 g

*I use an electric coffee grinder to grind the poppy seeds, but they can be purchased ground in most Hungarian food stores.

Custard Frosting and Filling

2 c.	water	500 mL
3 T.	cornstarch	45 mL
2 t.	vanilla extract	10 mL
1	egg yolk	1
4.5 oz. box	fructose-sweetened white frosting mix	128 g box
1 T.	any flavoring or extract	15 mL
	food coloring, if desired	

Combine water, cornstarch, vanilla extract, and egg yolk in a nonstick saucepan. Cook and stir over medium heat until mixture is very thick. Transfer to a large, preferably narrow, mixing bowl. Chill thoroughly. Beat in frosting mix and flavoring or extract of your choice. Add food coloring, if desired. Beat until smooth and creamy for spreading.

Yield: 10 servings

Exchange, 1 serving: 1⅓ fruit, ½ fat
Each serving contains: Calories: 74, Carbohydrates: 13 g

Cappuccino Frosting

1 t.	unflavored gelatin	5 mL
2 T.	cold water	30 mL
3 T.	granulated fructose	45 mL
2 T.	instant coffee powder	30 mL
½ t.	ground cinnamon	2 mL
1 env.	nondairy whipped topping powder	1 env.
½ c.	skim milk	125 mL
1 t.	vanilla extract	5 mL

Sprinkle gelatin over cold water in a small saucepan. Allow to soften for 1 minute. Stir over low heat until gelatin is dissolved. Stir in fructose, instant coffee powder, and cinnamon. Stir until all ingredients are dissolved. Remove from heat and allow to cool to lukewarm. Combine nondairy topping powder and skim milk in a large, preferably narrow, bowl. Whip into soft peaks. Slowly beat in vanilla and lukewarm gelatin mixture. Beat to stiff peaks. Do not overbeat.

Yield: 20 servings

Exchange, 1 serving: ¼ bread
Each serving contains: Calories: 21, Carbohydrates: 2 g

Maple Icing

2	egg whites	2
2 T.	Cary's Sugar-Free Maple-Flavored Syrup	30 mL
1 t.	maple flavoring	5 mL

Beat egg whites until stiff. Beating constantly, slowly pour maple syrup into egg whites. Beat in maple flavoring.

Yield: 10 servings

Exchange, 1 serving: negligible
Each serving contains: Calories: 5, Carbohydrates: 1 g

Caramel-Flavored Frosting

1 box	butterscotch-flavored sugar-free to-cook pudding mix	1 box	
2 c.	water	500 mL	
1	egg white	1	

Combine butterscotch pudding mix and water in a saucepan. Cook and stir over medium heat until mixture comes to a full boil. Pour into mixing bowl and cool completely until set. Beat egg white until stiff. Beat egg white into cooled pudding just before using.

Yield: 10 servings

Exchange, 1 serving: negligible
Each serving contains: Calories: 9, Carbohydrates: 1 g

Peanut Butter Frosting

⅔ c.	creamy peanut butter	180 mL
⅓ c.	granulated brown sugar replacement	90 mL
¼ c.	skim milk	60 mL

Cream peanut butter with the brown sugar replacement. Gradually beat in the milk. Beat to spreading consistency.

Yield: 10 servings

Exchange, 1 serving: ⅓ bread, 1½ fat
Each serving contains: Calories: 97, Carbohydrates: 3 g

Seven-Minute Frosting

½ c.	granulated sugar replacement	125 mL
2	egg whites	2
½ t.	cream of tartar	2mL
¼ c.	cold water	60 mL
2 t.	vanilla extract	10 mL

Simmer a small amount of water in the bottom of a double boiler. In the top of the boiler, combine sugar replacement, egg whites, cream of tartar, and the cold water. Set over the simmering water. Beat the egg white mixture on high for 6 to 7 minutes or until very thick. Add the vanilla extract and beat a minute longer or until frosting is thick enough to spread.

Yield: 10 servings

Exchange, 1 serving: negligible
Each serving contains: Calories: 3, Carbohydrates: 1 g

Peach Melba Frosting

1 t.	unflavored gelatin	5 mL
2 T.	cold water	30 mL
2 T.	granulated fructose	30 mL
1 env.	nondairy whipped topping powder	1 env.
½ c.	skim milk	125 mL
1 t.	vanilla extract	5 mL
3	fresh peaches, peeled and puréed	3
1 c.	fresh raspberries	250 mL

Sprinkle gelatin over cold water in a small saucepan. Allow to soften for 1 minute. Stir over low heat until gelatin is dissolved. Stir in fructose until dissolved. Remove from heat and allow to cool to lukewarm. Combine nondairy topping powder and skim milk in a large, preferably narrow, bowl. Whip into soft peaks. Slowly beat in vanilla, lukewarm gelatin mixture, and peach purée. Beat to stiff peaks. Fold in raspberries.

Yield: 20 servings

Exchange, 1 serving: ⅓ fruit
Each serving contains: Calories: 30, Carbohydrates: 4 g

Semisweet Carob Frosting

¼ c.	carob powder	60 mL
2 T.	cornstarch	30 mL
1 T.	granulated fructose	15 mL
dash	salt	dash
½ c.	boiling water	125 mL
2 t.	vegetable oil	10 mL
1 t.	vanilla extract	5 mL

Combine carob powder, cornstarch, fructose, and salt in a small saucepan Add boiling water. Stir to blend. Place over medium heat, and stir and cook until thick. Remove from heat. Stir in vegetable oil and vanilla thoroughly. Frost cake while frosting is still warm.

Yield: 10 servings

Exchange, 1 serving: ⅓ bread
Each serving contains: Calories: 26, Carbohydrates: 4 g

Orange Frosting

1 c.	orange juice	250 mL
2 T.	cornstarch	30 mL
1 T.	granulated fructose	15 mL
dash	salt	dash
2 t.	vegetable oil	10 mL
1 t.	lemon extract	5 mL
½ t.	grated orange rind	2 mL

Combine orange juice, cornstarch, fructose, and salt in a small saucepan Place over medium heat, and stir and cook until thick. Remove from heat. Stir in vegetable oil, lemon extract, and orange rind. Frost cake while frosting is still warm.

Yield: 10 servings

Exchange, 1 serving: ½ fruit
Each serving contains: Calories: 27, Carbohydrates: 4 g

Milk Chocolate Frosting

¼ c.	carob powder	60 mL
2 T.	cornstarch	30 mL
1 T.	granulated fructose	15 mL
dash	salt	dash
½ c.	hot low-fat milk	125 mL
1 t.	vanilla extract	5 mL

Combine carob powder, cornstarch, fructose, and salt in a small saucepan. Add hot milk. Place over medium heat, and stir and cook until thick. Remove from heat. Stir in vanilla. Frost cake while frosting is still warm.

Yield: 10 servings

Exchange, 1 serving: ⅓ bread
Each serving contains: Calories: 23, Carbohydrates: 5 g

Burnt-Sugar Frosting

1 c.	water	250 mL
2 T.	cornstarch	30 mL
2 T.	granulated fructose	30 mL
2 t.	burnt sugar flavoring	10 mL
¼ c.	fructose-sweetened white frosting mix	60 mL

Combine water, cornstarch, and fructose in a saucepan. Stir to dissolve cornstarch. Cook and stir over medium heat until mixture is very thick, about 4 to 5 minutes. Remove from heat. Stir in flavoring. Allow to cool slightly Beat in frosting mix.

Yield: 10 servings

Exchange, 1 serving: ½ fruit
Each serving contains: Calories: 31, Carbohydrates: 7 g

Orange Sauce

¼ c.	granulated sugar replacement	60 mL
2 T.	cornstarch	30 mL
1½ c.	fresh or frozen orange juice	375 mL
1 t.	grated orange peel	5 mL

Combine sugar replacement and cornstarch in a heavy or nonstick sauce pan. Slowly blend in the orange juice. Cook and stir over medium heat until clear and thickened. Remove from heat, cool to room temperature, and stir in orange peel. Store in refrigerator.

Yield: 10 servings

Exchange, 1 serving: ¼ fruit
Each serving contains: Calories: 21, Carbohydrates: 5 g

Caramel Sauce

1 box	butterscotch-flavored sugar-free to-cook pudding mix	1 box
3 c.	water	750 mL

Combine pudding mix and water in a saucepan. Bring to a boil, stirring to dissolve. Boil 1 minute longer. Remove from heat. Serve hot or cold.

Yield: 10 servings

Exchange, 1 serving: negligible
Each serving contains: Calories: 8, Carbohydrates: 1 g

Crushed Pineapple Sauce

¼ c.	unsweetened pineapple juice	60 mL
1 T.	cornstarch	15 mL
2 T.	granulated fructose	30 mL
20 oz. can	unsweetened crushed pineapple in juice	560 g can

Combine pineapple juice and cornstarch in a saucepan. Stir to dissolve cornstarch. Stir in fructose and canned crushed pineapple with its juice. Stir and cook over medium heat until the sauce is thickened.

Yield: 10 servings

Exchange, 1 serving: ½ fruit
Each serving contains: Calories: 27, Carbohydrates: 7 g

Fast Apricot Sauce

1 c.	all-natural apricot preserves	250 mL
⅓ c.	water	90 mL
½ t.	lemon juice	2 mL
¼ t.	brandy flavoring	1 mL

Combine apricot preserves and water in a saucepan. Bring to a boil. Simmer for 1 minute. Remove from heat, and stir in lemon juice and brandy flavoring. Serve hot or cold.

Yield: 10 servings

Exchange, 1 serving: 1 fruit
Each serving contains: Calories: 57, Carbohydrates: 13 g

Fresh Ginger Sauce

1½ c.	boiling water	375 mL
1 T.	grated fresh ginger	15 mL
¼ c.	granulated sugar replacement	60 mL
¼ c.	granulated fructose	60 mL
2 T.	cornstarch	30 mL
1 t.	lemon juice	5 mL

Combine boiling water and fresh ginger in a measuring cup or bowl. Cover and allow to cool to room temperature. Combine sugar replacement, fructose, and cornstarch in a heavy or nonstick saucepan. Slowly blend in the ginger water and lemon juice. Cook and stir over medium heat until clear and thickened. Store in refrigerator.

Yield: 10 servings

Exchange, 1 serving: ¼ fruit
Each serving contains: Calories: 15, Carbohydrates: 4 g

Peach Sauce

29 oz. can	sliced peaches in juice	822 g can
1 t.	vanilla or almond extract	5 mL

Pour peaches with juice and extract into a food processor or blender. Process into a purée. Serve cold or warm.

Yield: 10 servings

Exchange, 1 serving: ⅓ fruit
Each serving contains: Calories: 22, Carbohydrates: 6 g

Chocolate-Flavored Sauce

¼ c.	carob powder	60 mL
1 T.	granulated fructose	15 mL
1 T.	cornstarch	15 mL
½ c.	skim milk	125 mL
½ c.	evaporated skim milk	125 mL
1 t.	vanilla extract	5 mL

Combine carob powder, fructose, and cornstarch in a heavy or nonstick saucepan. Slowly add skim milk and evaporated skim milk. Blend well. Cook and stir over medium heat until mixture is thick and smooth. Remove from heat, and stir in vanilla. Cover and cool before serving.

For Chocolate Mocha Sauce: Add 2 t. (10 mL) of instant coffee powder to the fructose-cornstarch mixture.

Yield: 10 servings

Exchange, 1 serving: ⅓ bread
Each serving contains: Calories: 30, Carbohydrates: 6 g

Chocolate Orange Sauce

¼ c.	carob powder	60 mL
1 T.	granulated fructose	15 mL
1 T.	cornstarch	15 mL
1 c.	skim milk	250 mL
2 T.	orange-flavored liqueur	30 mL
1 t.	grated orange peel	5 mL

Combine carob powder, fructose, and cornstarch in a heavy or nonstick saucepan. Slowly add skim milk and blend well. Cook and stir over medium heat until mixture is thick and smooth. Remove from heat, and stir in the orange-flavored liqueur and orange peel. Cover and cool before serving.

Yield: 10 servings

Exchange, 1 serving: ⅓ skim milk
Each serving contains: Calories: 25, Carbohydrates: 5 g

Prune Purée as Fat Replacement

2 c.	prunes, stewed	500 mL stewed
¼ c.	unsweetened apple juice	60 mL
1 T.	flavoring (vanilla extract or lemon extract or liquer)	15 mL

Use a food processor to purée all the ingredients. Store the mixture in the refrigerator. Use it as a fat substitute in cooking.

Yield: 1¼ c. (310 mL)

Exchange: free
Each serving of G c. (60 mL) contains: Calories: 13,
*   Fiber: 0.45 g, Sodium: 0.4 mg, Cholesterol: 0 mg*

Lemon Curd

As good as the expensive version in the fancy container.

⅓ c.	fresh lemon juice	90 mL
1 T.	cornstarch dissolved in 2 T. (30 mL) water	15 mL
7 pkts.	concentrated acesulfame-K	7 pkts.
¼ c.	egg substitute	60 mL
2 t.	vanilla extract	10 mL

Put the lemon juice, cornstarch, and acesulfame-K into a small saucepan and whisk together over medium-low heat. Cook gently until the mixture starts to thicken.

In a separate container heat the egg substitute and add it to a small amount of the thickened lemon mixture. Then whisk this mixture into the rest of the lemon mixture in the saucepan. Add the vanilla extract and cook over medium-low heat for one minute.

Yield: 1 c. (250 mL)

Exchange: free
Each serving of 1 T. (15 mL) contains: Calories: 5, Carbohydrates: 2 g, Fiber: trace, Sodium: 9 mg, Cholesterol: 0 mg

Banana Frosting

We used the banana cream pie-flavored fat-free, sugar-free yogurt in this recipe, but you can try other flavors as well. Just change the extract to match the yogurt.

4 oz.	nonfat cream cheese	125 mL
4 oz.	banana cream pie-flavored fat-free, sugar-free (½ container) yogurt	125 mL
½ t.	vanilla extract	2 mL
½ t.	banana extract	2 mL
1 T.	aspartame	15 mL

Use an electric mixer to combine all ingredients until smooth.

Yield: 16 servings of 1 c. (250 mL)

Exchange: free
Each serving of 1 T. (15 mL) contains: Calories: 9, Carbohydrates: 3 g, Fiber: 0 g, Sodium: 38 mg, Cholesterol: 1 mg

Glaze to Add Sweetness to Cakes and Muffins

This trick comes from aspartame cookbooks.

15 pkts.	concentrated aspartame	15 pkts.
3 T.	boiling water	45 mL
½ t.	cinnamon	2 mL

Blend and drizzle over cakes and cookies as they come out of the oven or brush on with pastry brush to coat more evenly. You may want to use a fork first to poke holes in the pastry to help the glaze penetrate.

Yield: 8 servings

Exchange: free
Each serving contains: Calories: 0, Carbohydrates: 4 g, Fiber: 0 g, Sodium: 0 mg, Cholesterol: 0 mg

Applesauce Frosting

A healthy topping that's also easy to make.

4 oz.	nonfat cream cheese	170 mL
1 t.	vanilla extract	5 mL
2 T.	unsweetened applesauce	30 mL
1 T.	concentrated aspartame	15 mL
1 T.	nonfat milk	15 mL

Combine all ingredients and beat with an electric mixer until smooth and creamy.

Yield: 1 c. (250 mL)

Exchange: free
Each serving of 1 T. (15 mL) contains: Calories: 9, Carbohydrates: 2 g, Fiber: trace, Sodium: 36 mg, Cholesterol: 1 mg

Rich Chocolate Frosting

Very satisfying.

½ c.	unsweetened cocoa powder	125 mL
⅓ c.	measures-like-sugar saccharin	90 mL
½ c.	nonfat buttermilk	125 mL
1 t.	vanilla extract	5 mL
1 T.	measures-like sugar aspartame	15 mL

Combine cocoa and saccharin in a saucepan and whisk in a small amount of buttermilk. Slowly whisk in the remaining buttermilk. Heat over medium heat, whisking constantly. Bring to a boil. Boil for 2 minutes, stirring constantly. When it is thick, remove from heat and stir in vanilla extract and aspartame.

Yield: 1 c. (250 mL)

Exchange: free
Each serving of 1 T. (15 mL) contains: Calories: 10, Carbohydrates: 4 g, Fiber: 0 g, Sodium: 49 mg, Cholesterol: 0 mg

Chocolate Frosting

The low-fat version is very nice but does not keep as attractively as high-fat frosting.

1 c.	nonfat cottage cheese	250 mL
2 T.	nonfat cream cheese	30 mL
½ t.	vanilla extract	2 mL
½ t.	chocolate extract	2 mL
1 T.	concentrated aspartame	15 mL
1 T.	unsweetened cocoa powder	15 mL

Combine all ingredients in a food processor or blender. Frost just before serving.

Yield: 1 c.

Exchange: free
Each serving of 1 T. (15 mL) contains: Calories: 14.5, Carbohydrates: 1 g, Fiber: 0 g, Sodium: 223 mg, Cholesterol: 3 mg

Creamy Frosting

A rich, creamy frosting with lemon peel to brighten the flavor.

1 pkg.	nonfat cream cheese	1 pkg.
¼ c.	nonfat yogurt, no sugar added	60 mL
1 T.	aspartame	15 mL
1 t.	dried lemon peel	5 mL
1 t.	vanilla extract	5 mL

Combine all the ingredients and beat with an electric mixer until creamy.

Yield: ¾ c. (190 mL)

Exchange: free
Each serving of 1 T. (15 mL) contains: Calories: 19, Carbohydrates: 3 g, Fiber: 0 g, Sodium: 93 mg, Cholesterol: 2.7 mg

Creamy Cocoa Frosting

This frosting is great on the Chocolate Tube Cake or on the Chocolate Muffins.

4 oz.	nonfat cream cheese	120 g
3 T.	skim milk	45 mL
2 t.	concentrated aspartame	10 mL
2 T.	unsweetened cocoa powder	30 mL
1 t.	cornstarch	5 mL
1 t.	vanilla extract	5 mL

Soften the cream cheese in a microwave oven for about 30 seconds. Whisk together the remaining ingredients until smooth. Whisk in the cream cheese.

Yield: 8 servings

Exchange: free
Each serving contains: Calories: 21, Carbohydrates: 5 g, Fiber: 0 g, Sodium: 79 mg, Cholesterol: 2.1 mg

Light Cocoa Frosting

Quick and very satisfying.

1 env.	sugar-free whipped topping mix	1 env.
1 T.	unsweetened cocoa powder	15 mL
½ c.	ice water	125 mL
1 t.	vanilla extract	5 mL

If possible, chill bowl and beaters of an electric mixer. Then combine all ingredients and beat for 4–5 minutes.

Makes enough to frost top and middle of large cake.

Yield: 1 c. (250 mL)

Exchange: 1 fat
Each serving of 1 T. (15 mL) contains: Calories: 34, Carbohydrates: 1 g, Fiber: 0 g, Sodium: 22 mg, Cholesterol: 0 mg

Wonderful Whipped Cream Substitute

Don't cheat on the time for processing the cottage cheese!

1 c.	nonfat cottage cheese	250 mL
1 t.	concentrated aspartame	5 mL
½ t.	vanilla extract	2 mL

Process the cottage cheese in a food processor for a full 2 minutes. Add aspartame and vanilla extract and process for another minute. Store in the refrigerator up to a few days.

Yield: 1 c. (250 mL)

Exchange: free
Each serving of 2 T. (30 mL) contain: Calories: 11.5, Carbohydrates: 1 g, Fiber: 0 g, Sodium: 0 mg, Cholesterol: 1 mg

Peach Shortcake Topping

You can serve this over a shortcake-type biscuit, hot milk sponge cake, angel cake, dessert waffles, or crepes.

4	peaches	4
1½ T.	fresh lemon juice	22 mL
1 t.	concentrated aspartame	5 mL
¼ t.	cinnamon	1 mL

Drop the peaches into boiling water for two minutes to loosen skins. Remove them from hot water; peel, and slice. Place the peaches in a bowl sprinkle with lemon juice, aspartame, and cinnamon. Stir to combine.

Yield: 6 servings

Exchange: free
Each serving contains: Calories: 25, Fiber: trace, Sodium: trace, Cholesterol: 0 mg

Granola Topping

If you like a crunchy topping on frozen yogurt or other desserts, make up some granola topping and keep it on hand. This is also the recipe we used for our Granola Cheesecake.

3 c.	oatmeal	750 mL
½ c.	wheat germ	125 mL
⅔ c.	sliced unsalted almonds (optional)	180 mL
1 T.	safflower oil	15 mL
2 T.	molasses	30 mL
½ c.	unsweetened apple juice	125 mL

Mix the oatmeal, wheat germ, and almonds in a lasagna or jelly-roll pan. Heat the remaining ingredients in a saucepan and stir to combine. Drizzle this over the oatmeal mixture, then use a spatula to push the mixture around in the pan until evenly coated. Bake in a 325°F (160°C) oven for about 30 minutes. Then mix again and bake for 10 minutes. The longer you cook it, the crunchier the granola gets. Makes 4½ c. (1.125 L).

Yield: 70 T. (15 mL)

Exchange: free
Each serving of 1 T. (15 mL) contains: Calories: 12, Fiber: trace, Sodium: 16 mg, Cholesterol: 0 mg

Blueberry Topping

This is a great topping for plain yogurt, ice cream, crepes, and waffles. You'll be glad to have it on hand. If it seems too thick, heat it a little before serving.

12 oz. pkg.	frozen whole blueberries, no sugar added, thawed	250 mL pkg.	
1 T.	cornstarch	15 mL	
½ c.	fruit-only blueberry jam	125 mL	

Put 8 oz. (80 mL) of blueberries in a food processor or blender along with the cornstarch and jam. Process until the mixture is liquid and well blended. Pour into a small saucepan. Cook over low heat, stirring constantly until thickened and bright. Remove from the heat. Add the reserved blueberries. Stir. Serve warm or cold. Keeps well in the refrigerator.

Yield: 1½ c. (375 mL)

Exchange, 1 serving: ½ fruit
Each serving of T. (15 mL) contains: Calories: 56, Carbohydrates: 5 g, Fiber: 0.2 g, Sodium: trace, Cholesterol: 4 mg

Crunchy Topping for Iced Desserts

Yes, it is unusual to top desserts with chickpeas. But they're good, and they're rich in fiber!

15 oz. can	chickpeas	425 g can
6 pkts.	concentrated acesulfame-K	6 pkts.
4 t.	cinnamon	20 mL
1 t.	vanilla extract	5 mL
½ t.	nutmeg	2 mL
2 T.	measures-like-sugar aspartame	30 mL

Drain the liquid from a can of chickpeas and pour the chickpeas into a saucepan. Cover with water and add acesulfame-K, cinnamon, and vanilla extract. Cook over medium heat for half an hour. Let cool. Drain off the cooking liquid. Place the chickpeas in a single layer on a large flat pan or cookie sheet with a rim, a pan that has been coated with non-stick cooking spray. Bake in a preheated 375°F (190°C) oven for an hour. Then combine the nutmeg and aspartame in a paper bag. Put the chickpeas into the bag and shake to coat them. Store in an airtight container in the refrigerator for serving over iced desserts.

Yield: 2 c. (500 mL) or 8 servings

Exchange: free
Each serving of 2 T. (30 mL) contains: Calories: 21.75, Carbohydrates: 8 g, Fiber: trace, Sodium: 54 mg, Cholesterol: 0 mg

Maple Walnut Topping

This is wonderful over frozen desserts. Be careful to note what form of sweetener is in various syrups.

1 c.	pancake syrup with no sugar added	250 mL
1 t.	butter-flavored extract	5 mL
½ t.	concentrated aspartame	2 mL
⅓ c.	walnuts, chopped	90 mL

Combine all the ingredients in a small bowl and whisk together. To serve hot, heat, but only briefly (for a few seconds) in a microwave oven.

Yield: 21 servings per 1⅓ c. (340 mL)

Exchange: free
Each serving contains: Calories: 18, Carbohydrates: 11 g, Fiber: 1 g, Sodium: 20 mg, Cholesterol: 0 mg

Nonfat Whipped Topping

Make this just before serving. Karin likes to chill it during dinnertime.

⅓ c.	nonfat milk	90 mL
⅓ c.	instant dry milk solids	90 mL
2 t.	fructose	10 mL
½–1 t.	vanilla	2–5 mL

Put a bowl with nonfat milk in the freezer until ice crystals begin to form, about 15–20 minutes. Chill the beaters. With an electric mixer at high speed, beat the nonfat dry milk solids into the nonfat milk for 2 minutes, until soft peaks form. Add the fructose and vanilla extract and beat about 2 additional minutes. Use within 20 minutes to avoid the cream separating.

Yield: 24 servings

Exchange: free
Each serving of 1 T. (15 mL) contains: Calories: 8, Fiber: 0 g, Sodium: 10 mg, Cholesterol: trace

Bittersweet Sauce

This is fabulous drizzled over cream puffs or an angel food cake or any time you want a not-too-sweet chocolaty sauce.

3 T.	unsweetened cocoa powder	45 mL
1 T.	flour	15 mL
1½ c.	nonfat milk	375 mL
2 T.	margarine or butter (optional)	30 mL
3 pkts.	concentrated acesulfame-K	3 pkts.
1 t.	vanilla extract	5 mL

Combine the cocoa and flour in the top of a double boiler. Add the milk slowly, stirring until the mixture is free of lumps. Cook over boiling water stirring until the mixture is thick and smooth. Remove from the heat and stir in the margarine or butter. Let cool for 15 minutes. Add the acesulfame-K and vanilla extract. Stir. Serve.

Yield: 24 servings

Exchange: free
Each serving of 1 T. (15 mL) contains: Calories: 8, Carbohydrates: 3 g, Fiber: trace, Sodium: 12 mg, Cholesterol: trace

Chocolate Sauce

Very good over any dessert.

2 T.	unsweetened cocoa powder	30 mL
2 T.	cornstarch	30 mL
pinch	salt (optional)	pinch
¾ c.	water	190 mL
1 oz.	nonfat cream cheese	30 g
2 t.	vanilla extract	10 mL
2 t.	concentrated aspartame	10 mL

Combine the first three ingredients in a saucepan. Add the water and cream cheese. Use a wire whisk to stir, and cook until thickened. Turn off the heat. Add the vanilla extract and aspartame. Stir well to combine.

Yield: 1 c. (250 mL)

Exchange: free
Each serving of 1 T. (15 mL) contains: Calories: 7, Fiber: 0 g, Sodium: 13 mg, Cholesterol: trace

Rum Sauce

This adds a rich taste to plain puddings, plain frozen desserts, or over plain cake.

1 c.	nonfat frozen yogurt, no sugar added	250 mL
1 t.	rum extract	5 mL

Allow the yogurt to defrost. Whisk in the rum extract until it's well blended and smooth. Store in the refrigerator.

Yield: 1 c. (250 mL)

Exchange: free
Each serving of 1 T. (15 mL) contains: Calories: 10, Carbohydrates: 1 g, Fiber: 0 g, Sodium: 9 mg, Cholesterol: 0 mg

Low-Low-Calorie Syrup

1 env.	unflavored gelatin	1 env.
2½ c.	water	625 mL
2 T.	cocoa	30 mL
3 pkg.	aspartame sweetener	3 pkg.

Sprinkle gelatin over water in saucepan and allow to soften for 5 minutes. Bring to boil and stir in cocoa. Allow to cool. Add aspartame and stir to completely dissolve. Place in refrigerator. Stir occasionally to keep cocoa in suspension.

Yield: 2 c. (500 mL)

Exchange, full recipe: 1 bread, 1 fat
Full recipe contains: Calories: 120

For a richer sauce, add ½ c. (125 mL) dry milk powder.

Yield: 2 c. (500 mL)

Exchange, full recipe: ½ bread, 2 nonfat milk, 1 fat
Full recipe contains: Calories: 240, Carbohydrates: 90 g

Instant Chocolate Syrup

| 1 | Instant Drink Mix | 1 |
| 1 c. | hot water | 250 mL |

Combine ingredients and stir to dissolve completely. Chill or use hot.

Yield: 1 c. (250 mL)

Exchange, 1 serving: 6 low-fat milk
Each serving contains: Calories: 480

Chocolate Marshmallow Frosting

2 env.	unflavored gelatin	2 env.
¾ c.	water	190 mL
3 T.	cocoa	45 mL
3 T.	granulated sugar replacement	45 mL
1 T.	white vanilla extract	15 mL
2	egg whites	2

Sprinkle gelatin over water in saucepan; allow to soften for 5 minutes. Cook and stir over medium heat until gelatin is dissolved. Remove from heat and cool to the consistency of thick syrup. Add cocoa, sugar replacement and vanilla, stirring to blend. Beat egg whites into soft peaks. Very slowly, trickle a small stream of gelatin mixture into egg whites, beat until all gelatin mixture is blended. Continue beating until light and fluffy.

Yield: Frosts sides and tops of two 9 in. (23 cm) layers or one 9 × 13 in. (23 × 33 cm) cake or 30 cupcakes

Exchange, 1 serving: negligible
Each serving contains: Calories: negligible, Carbohydrates: 5 g

Nut Frosting

A frosting which complements all cakes.

1	egg	1
⅓ c.	granulated brown sugar replacement	90 mL
2 t.	vanilla extract	10 mL
⅓ c.	semisweet chocolate chips	90 mL
½ c.	walnuts, chopped	125 mL

Combine egg, brown sugar replacement, and vanilla in bowl. Beat with an electric mixer until thick. Stir in chocolate chips and walnuts. Spoon and spread over hot cake or cupcakes. Place in 350°F (175°C) oven for 10 minutes. Remove and cool.

Yield: 24 servings

Exchange, 1 serving: ½ fat
Each serving contains: Calories: 31, Carbohydrates: 5 g

Chocolate Whipped Topping

1 env.	nondairy topping mix	1 env.
2 T.	cocoa	30 mL
dash	salt	dash
½ t.	vanilla extract	2 mL
½ c.	ice water	125 mL
2 T.	Powdered Sugar Replacement	30 mL

Combine topping mix, cocoa and salt in mixing bowl; stir to blend. Add vanilla and water, and beat until soft peaks form. Gradually, add sugar replacement and beat until mixture is stiff.

Yield: 2 c. (500 mL)

Exchange, one serving of 1 T. (15 mL): negligible
Each serving contains: Calories: 11, Carbohydrates: 4 g

Smooth-as-Silk Frosting

1 env.	unflavored gelatin	1 env.
½ c.	water	125 mL
⅓ c.	granulated brown sugar replacement	90 mL
2	egg whites, stiffly beaten	2
1 t.	vanilla extract	5 mL

Sprinkle gelatin over water in saucepan; allow to soften for 5 minutes. Bring to a boil. Add brown sugar replacement and stir to dissolve. Remove from heat; cool to the consistency of thin syrup. Beating constantly, pour syrup in a thin stream into beaten egg whites. Beat in vanilla.

Yield: Frosts sides and tops of any size cake.

Exchange, 1 serving: negligible
Each serving contains: Calories: negligible, Carbohydrates: 11 g

Cherry Yogurt Frosting

1	egg white	1
2 T.	cherry yogurt	30 mL

Beat egg white to soft peaks; gradually add the yogurt. Beat to stiff peaks. Spread on 8 or 9 in. (20 or 23 cm) cake. Serve immediately.

Yield: 9 servings

Exchange, 1 serving: negligible
Each serving contains: Calories: negligible, Carbohydrates: 1 g

Caramel Fluff Frosting

1 env.	nondairy topping mix	1 env.
½ c.	skim milk	125 mL
¼ c.	granulated brown sugar replacement	60 mL
1 t.	vanilla extract	5 mL

Combine all ingredients in a chilled bowl. Beat into stiff peaks.

Yield: 2 c. (500 mL) or 20 servings

Exchange, 1 serving: 16 bread
Each serving contains: Calories: 9, Carbohydrates: 4 g

Plain Chocolate Frosting

1 c.	skim evaporated milk	250 mL
2 T.	cornstarch	30 mL
¼ c.	granulated sugar replacement	60 mL
2 oz.	baking chocolate, melted	60 g
1 t.	vanilla extract	5 mL
dash	salt	dash
3 T.	water	45 mL

Combine all ingredients in top of double boiler. Cook, stirring constantly, over boiling water until thick. Cool. Beat to spreading consistency.

Yield: Frosts 9 × 13 in. (23 × 33 cm) cake or 24 servings

Exchange, 1 serving: ¼ bread, ¼ fat
Each serving contains: Calories: 25, Carbohydrates: 5 g

Crème Semisweet Chocolate Frosting

¼ c.	semisweet chocolate chips	60 mL
2 T.	butter	30 mL
¼ c.	skim evaporated milk	60 mL
½ recipe	marshmallow crème	½ recipe

Melt chocolate chips and butter in top of double boiler over boiling water. Gradually add evaporated milk and stir until smooth. Allow to cool to room temperature. Add marshmallow crème and beat until smooth.

Yield: Frosts sides and tops of 8 or 9 in. (20 or 23 cm) layer cake

Exchange, 1 serving: ½ fat
Each serving contains: Calories: 19, Carbohydrates: 3 g

Pure Juice Jellies or Toppings

1 c.	fruit juice (unsweetened)	250 mL
1 T.	granulated sugar replacement	15 mL
1 T.	low-calorie pectin	15 mL

Apple Juice

Exchange, 1 T. (15 mL): ⅓ fruit
Each serving contains: Calories: 10, Carbohydrates: 55 g

Cranberry Juice (unsweetened)

Exchange, 1 serving: negligible
Each serving contains: Calories: negligible, Carbohydrates: 12 g

Grapefruit Juice

Exchange, 1 T. (15 mL): ¼ fruit
Each serving contains: Calories: 8, Carbohydrates: 10 g

Grape Juice

Exchange, 1. T. (15 mL): ⅓ fruit
Each serving contains: Calories: 13, Carbohydrates: 10 g

Pineapple Juice

Exchange, 1 T. (15 mL): ⅓ fruit
Each serving contains: Calories: 9, Carbohydrates: 12 g

Combine ingredients in saucepan and bring to a boil. Boil for 2 minutes, remove from heat, and let cool slightly. Pour mixture into serving dish or jelly jar; chill.

Microwave: Follow directions, using large bowl. Cook on High.

Yield: ⅓ c. (189 mL)

Strawberry Preserves or Topping

1 c.	fresh or frozen strawberries (unsweetened)	250 mL
1 t.	low-calorie pectin	5 mL
1 t.	granulated sugar replacement	5 mL

Place strawberries in top of double boiler, and mash slightly. Cook over boiling water until soft and juicy, crushing berries against sides of double boiler. Add pectin and sugar replacement, blending thoroughly. Cook until medium thick. Remove from heat and allow to cool slightly. Pour preserves into a jar or bowl. Preserves can also be made with blueberries or raspberries.

Microwave: Place strawberries in glass bowl; cover. Cook on High for 4 minutes, or until soft and juicy, crushing berries against sides of bowl. Add pectin and sugar replacement; blend in thoroughly. Cook on High for 30 seconds.

Yield: ⅔ c. (180 mL)

Exchange, 2 T. (30 mL): ¼ fruit
Each serving contains: Calories: 7, Carbohydrates: 4 g

Cherry Jelly or Topping

1 c.	sour cherries	250 mL
1 c.	water	250 mL
3 T.	granulated sugar replacement	45 mL
1 T.	low-calorie pectin	15 mL

Rinse cherries and remove the stems. Combine cherries and water in saucepan. Bring to boil, reduce heat, and simmer 5 minutes. Strain; reserve juice. Add sugar replacement and pectin to 1 c. (250 mL) of juice, adding extra water, if necessary, to make up the juice. Stir to completely blend and return to heat. Bring back to boil, boil for 1 minute and then remove from heat. Cool slightly. Pour into serving dish or jelly jar; chill.

Microwave: Follow directions using large bowl. Cook on High.

Yield: ¾ c. (190 mL)

Exchange, 1 T. (15 mL): ¼ fruit
Each serving contains: Calories: 8, Carbohydrates: 6 g

Pecan Topping

½ c.	granulated brown sugar replacement	125 mL
½ c.	finely chopped pecans	125 mL
¼ c.	all-purpose flour	60 mL
¼ c.	low-calorie margarine	60 mL

Combine all ingredients. Toss and stir with a fork until completely mixed.

Yield: 8 servings

Exchange, 1 serving: 1⅔ fat
Each serving contains: Calories: 75, Carbohydrates: 3 g

Caramelized-Pecan Topping

⅔ c.	coarsely chopped pecans	180 mL
2 T.	low-calorie margarine	30 mL
⅓ c.	granulated fructose	90 mL

Place pecans in small skillet over medium heat and toast slightly. Add margarine and allow to melt. Stir in fructose. Allow to cool. Stir until mixture becomes thick. Pour out onto waxed paper and allow to cool.

Yield: 8 servings

Exchange, 1 serving: ½ fruit, 1½ fat
Each serving contains: Calories: 97, Carbohydrates: 7 g

Coconut Topping

2	egg whites, slightly beaten	2
2 T.	granulated sugar replacement	30 mL
⅓ c.	unsweetened grated coconut	90 mL

Combine egg whites and sugar replacement in a medium-size mixing bowl. Beat until soft peaks form. Fold in coconut. Spoon topping onto top of cool pie filling. Spread gently with the back of the spoon. Broil on bottom rack of oven for 5 to 6 minutes. Watch carefully because this topping tends to burn.

Yield: 8 servings

Exchange, 1 serving: negligible
Each serving contains: Calories: 11, Carbohydrates: negligible

Ginger-Crumb Topping

12	gingersnaps	12
2 T.	all-purpose flour	30 mL
1 T.	hot water	15 mL

Break gingersnaps and place in blender. Blend into fine crumbs. Combine gingersnap crumbs and flour in a bowl. Stir to mix. Add hot water and stir until mixture turns to crumbs.

Yield: 8 servings

Exchange, 1 serving: ½ starch/bread
Each serving contains: Calories: 40, Carbohydrates: 11 g

Brazil Nut Topping

⅓ c.	coarsely chopped Brazil nuts	180 mL
1 T.	granulated fructose	15 mL
⅓ c.	graham cracker crumbs	90 mL

Toast Brazil nuts in a small skillet over low heat until lightly browned. Sprinkle with fructose. Shake pan to coat nuts. Stir in graham cracker crumbs. Remove from heat and allow to cool.

Yield: 8 servings

Exchange, 1 serving: ⅓ starch/bread, ⅓ fat
Each serving contains: Calories: 102, Carbohydrates: 5 g

Estee's Fudgy Fructose Frosting

1 c.	fructose	250 mL
⅔ c.	skim milk	180 mL
2 T.	cornstarch	30 mL
2 sq. (1 oz.)	unsweetened chocolate	2 sq. (30 g)
2 T.	margarine (corn oil)	30 mL
1 t.	vanilla extract	5 mL

Mix fructose, skim milk, and cornstarch together in saucepan until cornstarch dissolves. Add chocolate and cook over medium heat until chocolate melts and mixture thickens and bubbles. Remove from heat. Add margarine and vanilla, stirring until creamy. Spread over cake.

Yield: 20 servings

Exchange, 1 serving: 1 fruit, ½ fat
Each serving contains: Calories: 70, Carbohydrates: 12 g

Estee's Cream Cheese Frosting

8 oz.	cream cheese	240 g
¼ c.	margarine (corn oil)	60 mL
½ c.	fructose	125 mL
½ t.	vanilla extract	2 mL

Beat cream cheese, margarine, and fructose together in mixer until smooth. Add vanilla, if desired, and continue beating until creamy. Spread over cake.

Yield: 20 servings

Exchange, 1 serving: ⅓ fruit, 1 fat
Each serving contains: Calories: 80, Carbohydrates: 5 g

Lemon Crumb Topping

½ c.	all-purpose flour	125 mL
¼ c.	granulated sugar replacement	60 mL
2 t.	grated lemon peel	10 mL
¼ c.	cold low-calorie margarine	60 mL

Combine flour, sugar replacement, and lemon peel in a mixing bowl. Toss to mix. Cut cold margarine into lemon mixture until mixture turns to crumbs.

Yield: 8 servings

Exchange, 1 serving: negligible
Each serving contains: Calories: 26, Carbohydrates: 5 g

Oatmeal Crumb Topping

½ c.	quick-cooking oatmeal (uncooked)	125 mL
⅓ c.	granulated brown sugar replacement	90 mL
2 T.	granulated fructose	30 mL
¼ c.	all-purpose flour	60 mL
¼ c.	cold low-calorie margarine	60 mL

Combine oatmeal, brown sugar replacement, fructose, and flour in a bowl. Stir to mix. Cut cold margarine into mixture until mixture turns to crumbs.

Yield: 8 servings

Exchange, 1 serving: ½ starch/bread, ½ fat
Each serving contains: Calories: 70, Carbohydrates: 7 g

Raisin Topping

3 slices	white bread	3 slices
⅓ c.	raisins	90 mL
2 t.	all-purpose flour	10 mL
1 T.	granulated fructose	15 mL

Cut crusts from bread and allow bread to dry completely. Break bread into pieces and place in a blender. Blend into coarse crumbs. Toss raisins in flour. Add to bread crumbs in blender. Blend until mixed and raisins are slightly chopped. Then blend in fructose.

Yield: 8 servings

Exchange, 1 serving: ¼ starch/bread, ½ fruit
Each serving contains: Calories: 51, Carbohydrates: 12 g

Decorative Frosting

¼ c.	solid shortening, soft	60 mL
½ t.	white vanilla extract	2 mL
¾ c.	Powdered Sugar Replacement	190 mL
1 T.	milk	15 mL

Cream together shortening and vanilla until light and fluffy. Stir in powdered sugar replacement and milk until mixture is well blended. If frosting is too stiff, add a few drops of milk. Tint as desired. Make flowers with a pastry tube on waxed paper. Allow to harden in freezer and then quickly transfer onto the cake.

Yield: ½ c. (125 mL)

Exchange, full recipe: 3 bread, 10 fat
Full recipe contains: Calories: 638, Carbohydrates: 178 g

Butter Frosting

2 c.	skim milk	500 mL
5 T.	flour	75 mL
⅓ c.	butter	90 mL
⅓ c.	granulated sugar replacement	90 mL
1 T.	vanilla extract	15 mL
1	egg white, beaten stiff	1

Combine milk and flour in saucepan. Cook and stir over low heat until a thick sauce results. Cool completely. Combine butter, sugar replacement and vanilla in mixing bowl, beating until fluffy. Add sauce mixture and beat until consistency of whipped cream. Fold in stiffly beaten egg white.

Yield: Frosts sides and tops of two 9 in. (23 cm) layers or 30 cupcakes

Exchange, ⅛ recipe: ½ bread, 1 fat
⅛ recipe contains: Calories: 110, Carbohydrates: 23 g

Coconut Pecan Frosting

1 c.	evaporated skimmed milk	250 mL
⅓ c.	granulated sugar replacement	90 mL
1	egg	1
1 T.	flour	15 mL
2 T.	margarine	30 mL
2 t.	vanilla extract	10 mL
¾ c.	unsweetened coconut	190 mL
⅓ c.	pecans, chopped	90 mL

Combine milk, sugar replacement, egg, flour and margarine in saucepan. Cook and stir on low heat until mixture thickens and then remove from heat. Stir in vanilla, coconut and pecans; let cool slightly. Spread over cake while warm.

Yield: Frosts two 9 in. (23 cm) layers or 13 × 9 in. (33 × 23 cm) cake

Exchange, full recipe: ⅛ bread, 1 fat
Full recipe contains: Calories: 54, Carbohydrates: 8 g

Jelly Frosting

½ c.	juice jelly, see Pure Juice Jellies	125 mL
2	egg whites	2
2 t.	granulated sugar replacement	10 mL

Combine juice jelly, egg whites and sugar replacement in top of double boiler; place over boiling water. Beat constantly until mixture thickens and holds stiff peaks. Remove from boiling water; continue to beat until smooth and of spreading consistency.

Yield: Frosts sides and tops of two 9 in. (23 cm) layers or 30 cupcakes

Exchange, 1 serving: Negligible
Each serving contains: Calories: 4, Carbohydrates: 3 g

Crumb Topping

⅓ c.	flour	90 mL
1 T.	granulated sugar replacement	15 mL
1 T.	liquid shortening	15 mL
½ t.	cinnamon	2 mL
¼ t.	nutmeg	1 mL

Combine all ingredients in mixing bowl, blender or food processor. Work until crumbly.

Yield: ⅓ c. (90 mL)

Exchange, full recipe: 2 bread, 3 fat
Full recipe contains: Calories: 265, Carbohydrates: 86 g

Sweet Whipped Topping

1 env.	low-calorie whipped topping mix	1 env.
½ c.	ice cold water	125 mL
2 T.	Powdered Sugar Replacement	30 mL

Whip together topping mix and water until soft peaks form. Gradually add sugar replacement; whip until stiff.

Yield: 2 c. (500 mL)

Exchange, 1 T. (15 mL): negligible
Each serving contains: Calories: 9, Carbohydrates: 1 g

Spiced Whipped Topping

1 env.	low-calorie whipped topping mix	1 env.	
dash each	nutmeg, cinnamon, allspice	dash each	
½ c.	ice cold water	125 mL	
1 T.	Powdered Sugar Replacement	15 mL	

Combine topping mix and spices in mixing bowl; add water. Beat mixture until soft peaks form. Gradually add sugar replacement; beat to stiff peaks.

Yield: 2 c. (500 mL)

Exchange, 1 T. (15 mL): negligible
Each serving contains: Calories: 9, Carbohydrates: 1 g

Fruit-Flavored Whipped Topping

1 env.	low-calorie whipped topping mix	1 env.	
1 env.	unsweetened fruit drink mix	1 env.	
½ c.	ice cold water	125 mL	
2 T.	Powdered Sugar Replacement	30 mL	

Combine topping mix and soft drink mix in mixing bowl. Stir to blend; add water. Beat until soft peaks form. Gradually add sugar replacement; beat to stiff peaks.

Yield: 2 c. (500 mL)

Exchange, 1 T. (15 mL): negligible
Each serving contains: Calories: 9, Carbohydrates: 2 g

Coffee Whipped Topping

1 env.	low-calorie whipped topping mix	1 env.	
½ c.	ice cold water	125 mL	
1 T.	Powdered Sugar Replacement	15 mL	

Whip together topping mix and coffee until soft peaks form. Gradually add sugar replacement; beat to stiff peaks.

Yield: 2 c. (500 mL)

Exchange, 1 T. (15 mL): negligible
Each serving contains: Calories: 9, Carbohydrates: 1 g

Vanilla Glaze

¼ c.	cold water	60 mL	
2 t.	cornstarch	10 mL	
dash	salt	dash	
⅓ c.	granulated sugar replacement	90 mL	
1 t.	vanilla extract	5 mL	

Blend cold water and cornstarch and pour into small saucepan. Add salt. Boil until clear and thickened; remove from heat. Add sugar replacement and vanilla, stirring to dissolve, and cool.

Yield: ¼ c. (60 mL)

Exchange: negligible
Each serving contains: Calories: negligible, Carbohydrates: 80 g

Apple Glaze

1 c.	apple juice	250 mL
½ c.	water	125 mL
1 t.	cornstarch	5 mL
2 t.	liquid sugar replacement	10 mL
1 t.	margarine	5 mL

Combine juice, water and cornstarch in saucepan. Cook and stir until mixture is clear and slightly thickened; remove from heat. Add sugar replacement and margarine. Serve hot or cold.

Yield: 1¼ c. (310 mL)

Exchange, ¼ c. (60 mL): ½ fruit
Each serving contains: Calories: 30, Carbohydrates: 8 g

Dry Milk Glaze

½ c.	nonfat dry milk powder	125 mL
2 t.	granulated sugar replacement	10 mL
1 t.	vanilla extract	5 mL
1 T.	cold water	15 mL

Combine dry milk and sugar replacement in food processor or blender. Blend to fine powder, pour into small bowl, and add vanilla and water. Stir with fork until well blended. If glaze hardens too quickly, add a few drops of cold water. Stir to blend.

Yield: ½ c. (125 mL)

Exchange, full recipe: 1½ bread
Full recipe contains: Calories: 120, Carbohydrates: 96 g

Rhubarb Sauce

1 lb.	fresh or frozen rhubarb	454 g
¾ c.	water	190 mL
1 t.	cornstarch	5 mL
¼ c.	cold water	60 mL
¾ c.	granulated sugar replacement	190 mL
dash	salt (optional)	dash

Combine rhubarb and the ¾ c. (190 mL) of water in a saucepan or microwavable bowl. Cook until rhubarb is tender, stirring occasionally. Or microwave on high for 2 minutes; then reduce to medium until rhubarb is tender (about 6 to 7 minutes). Dissolve cornstarch in the ¼ c. (60 mL) of cold water. Stir into rhubarb mixture. Stir in the sweetener. If desired, add the dash of salt. Cook and stir until mixture has lost its cloudy look. Serve warm or chilled.

Yield: 6 servings

Exchange, 1 serving: negligible
Each serving contains: Calories: negligible, Carbohydrates: negligible

Orange Cranberry Sauce

1 pkg. (12 oz.)	fresh cranberries, cleaned	1 pkg. (340 g)	
½ c.	granulated fructose	125 mL	
½ c.	orange juice concentrate, undiluted	125 mL	

Combine all ingredients in a saucepan. Cook until mixture comes to a boil, stirring occasionally. Reduce heat and boil gently until all cranberries have "popped." Serve warm or chilled.

Yield: 6 servings, with granulated fructose

Exchange, 1 serving: 1 fruit
Each serving contains: Calories: 64, Carbohydrates: 16 g

Blackberry Sauce

1 lb. pkg.	frozen, unsweetened blackberries, thawed	453 g pkg.	
1 T.	all-natural orange marmalade	15 mL	
1 t.	fresh lemon juice	5 mL	
2 env.	aspartame sweetener	2 env.	

Combine all ingredients in a food processor or blender. Process or blend into a purée. Strain sauce through a fine sieve to remove seeds. Transfer to a serving bowl. Cover and refrigerate.

Yield: 4 servings

Exchange, 1 serving: 1 fruit
Each serving contains: Calories: 54, Carbohydrates: 15 g

Strawberry Sauce

1 qt.	fresh or unsweetened frozen strawberries, thawed	1 L	
3 env.	aspartame sweetener	3 env.	
1 t.	orange juice	5 mL	
1 t.	fresh lemon juice	5 mL	

Combine all ingredients in a food processor or blender. Process or blend into a purée. Transfer to a serving bowl. Cover and refrigerate.

Yield: 4 servings

Exchange, 1 serving: 1 fruit
Each serving contains: Calories: 52, Carbohydrates: 13 g

Raspberry Sauce

12 oz. pkg.	frozen, unsweetened red raspberries	340 g pkg.	
½ t.	cornstarch	2 mL	
5 env.	aspartame sweetener	5 env.	

Thaw raspberries. Transfer raspberries and their juice to a saucepan. Stir in the cornstarch. Cook over medium heat until mixture comes to a full boil and the mixture is clear. Remove from heat. Cool until you can place your hand comfortably on the bottom of the pan. Stir in the aspartame sweetener. Serve warm or chilled.

Yield: 6 servings

Exchange, 1 serving: ⅓ fruit
Each serving contains: Calories: 43, Carbohydrates: 9 g

Brandy Sauce

1 c.	cool water	250 mL
2 t.	cornstarch	10 mL
2 T.	granulated sugar replacement	30 mL
or		
6 env.	aspartame sweetener	6 env.
¾ t.	brandy extract	4 mL

In a saucepan, dissolve the cornstarch in the cool water. Bring to a boil. Reduce heat and boil gently for 5 minutes. Remove from heat, and cool slightly. Stir in sweetener and the brandy extract. If desired, tint a light shade of brown with food coloring. This is a good sauce to use on top of the Cinnamon Apple Cheesecake.

Yield, 1 c. (250 mL)

Exchange, full recipe: negligible
Full recipe contains: Calories: negligible, Carbohydrates: negligible

Apricot Lemon Sauce

1 c.	apricot nectar	250 mL
1 T.	cornstarch	15 mL
3 T.	fresh lemon juice	45 mL
1 t.	grated lemon peel	5 mL
2 env.	aspartame sweetener	2 env.

Combine apricot nectar and cornstarch in a small saucepan. Stir to dissolve cornstarch. Bring to a boil. Cook and stir until mixture is smooth and thick. Stir in lemon juice and lemon peel. Remove from heat. Allow to cool until pan can be set comfortably on the palm of your hand. Stir in aspartame sweetener. This sauce is especially good for fresh berries or on plain cake.

Yield: 4 servings

Exchange, 1 serving: 1 fruit
Each serving contains: Calories: 59, Carbohydrates: 14 g

Custard Sauce

3	egg yolks	3
2 T.	granulated sugar replacement	30 mL
dash	salt	dash
1 c.	skim milk	250 mL
½ t.	vanilla extract	2 mL
1 c.	prepared nondairy whipped topping	250 mL

Slightly beat egg yolks. Combine the beaten egg yolks with the sugar replacement and salt in a saucepan. Gradually stir in the skim milk. Cook and stir over low heat until mixture thickens and coats the spoon. Remove from heat and pour into a bowl. Stir in the vanilla. Chill thoroughly. Fold in the nondairy whipped topping.

Yield: 8 servings

Exchange, 1 serving: ½ low-fat milk
Each serving contains: Calories: 57, Carbohydrates: 3 g

Toasted Coconut Sauce

½ c.	unsweetened, grated coconut	125 mL
1 c.	skim milk	250 mL
2 t.	cornstarch	10 mL
½ t.	vanilla extract	2 mL
½ t.	coconut flavoring	2 mL
3 env.	aspartame sweetener	3 env.

Place coconut in a small nonstick saucepan over medium heat. Cook and stir until all the coconut is a dark tan. Combine milk and cornstarch in a measuring cup or bowl. Stir to dissolve cornstarch, Pour into toasted coconut. Continue cooking over medium heat until mixture just begins to thicken. Pour mixture through a fine sieve into a bowl to remove coconut. Return coconut liquid to the saucepan. Cook and stir until mixture is thickened to a light syrup. Remove from heat. Stir in vanilla and coconut flavoring. Cool until pan can comfortably be placed in the palm of your hand. Stir in aspartame sweetener.

Yield: 4 servings

Exchange, 1 serving: ½ low-fat milk
Each serving contains: Calories: 63, Carbohydrates: 6 g

Egg White Sweet Wash

| 1 | egg white | 1 |
| ⅓ c. | granulated sugar replacement | 90 mL |

Beat egg white to very soft peaks, beat in sugar replacement, and then brush on desired surface.

Yield: enough for large coffeecake or 12 to 18 rolls

Exchange: negligible
Each serving contains: Calories: negligible, Carbohydrates: negligible

Frosting Glaze

| ¼ c. | sugar-free white frosting mix | 60 mL |
| 7 t. | boiling water | 35 mL |

Combine the frosting mix and boiling water in a small narrow bowl or cup. Beat with a small wire whisk or fork until mixture is smooth. Dampen a pastry brush, and brush glaze over desired surface.

Yield: enough for large coffeecake or 12 to 18 rolls

Exchange: negligible
Each serving contains: Calories: negligible, Carbohydrates: negligible

Egg Yolk Glaze

1	egg yolk	1	
2 T.	water	30 mL	

Beat egg yolk and water until light and fluffy. Brush on desired surface.

Yield: enough for large coffeecake or 12 to 18 rolls

Exchange: negligible
Each serving contains: Calories: negligible, Carbohydrates: negligible

Powdered Fructose Icing or Filling

8 T.	Powdered Fructose	120 mL
½ t.	vanilla extract	2 mL
1 T.	plain low-fat yogurt	15 mL
1	egg white	1

Combine powdered fructose, vanilla, and yogurt in a small bowl. Beat to blend. Beat egg white to firm peaks. Very slowly add fructose mixture to beaten egg white.

Yield: 10 servings

Exchange, 1 serving: 1 fruit
Each serving contains: Calories: 53, Carbohydrates: 7 g

Powdered-Sugar Replacement

½ c.	nonfat dry milk powder	125 mL
½ c.	cornstarch	125 mL
¼ c.	granulated sugar replacement	60 mL

Combine all ingredients in a blender. Process on high until powdered.

Yield: 1 c. (250 mL)

Exchange, ¼ c. (60 mL): ½ skim milk, ½ bread
Each serving contains: Calories: 81, Carbohydrates: 13 g

Powdered Fructose

1 c.	granulated fructose	250 mL
⅓ c.	cornstarch	90 mL

Combine fructose and cornstarch in a blender container. Process on high for 30 to 45 seconds or until mixture appears like powdered sugar. Do not overprocess or mixture will become liquid and sticky.

Yield: 24 T. (360 mL)

Exchange, 1 T. (15 mL): 1 fruit
Each serving contains: Calories: 62, Carbohydrates: 8 g

Raspberry Purée

Raspberry purée is great between layers of napoleons or topping cream puffs or just on nonfat, unsweetened yogurt. You're only limited by your imagination.

1 c.	raspberries (fresh or frozen without sugar)	250 mL

Purée the raspberries in a food processor. Spoon into a sieve; with the spoon, push the juice through to remove the seeds. Sweeten to taste with artificial sweetener such as aspartame or acesulfame-K.

Yield: 1 c. (250 mL)

Exchange: free
Each serving of 2 T. (30 mL) contains: Calories: 8, Carbohydrates: 2 g, Fiber: 0.75 g, Sodium: 0 mg, Cholesterol: 0 mg

Vanilla Gloss

¼ c.	cold water	60 mL
2 t.	cornstarch	10 mL
dash	salt	dash
⅓ c.	sugar replacement	90 mL
1 t.	vanilla extract	5 mL

Blend cold water and cornstarch. Pour into small saucepan. Add salt. Boil until clear and thickened. Remove from heat. Add sugar replacement and vanilla extract. Stir to dissolve. Cool.

Yield: ¼ c. (60 mL)

Exchange: negligible
Each serving contains: Calories: negligible, Carbohydrates: 80 g

Candies and Fudge

Basic Crème Center

3 oz.	cream cheese, softened	90 g
1 c.	Powdered Sugar Replacement	250 mL
2 T.	water	30 mL
1 t.	vanilla extract	5 mL

Beat cream cheese until fluffy. Stir in sugar replacement, water and vanilla extract. (Dough may be divided into parts and different flavorings and/or food color added to each part as suggested in various recipes.) Knead or work with the hand until dough is smooth. Use as directed in the recipes.

Yield: 1 c. (250 mL)

Exchange, full recipe: 4 fruit, 6 fat
Full recipe contains: Calories: 600, Carbohydrates: 28 g

Quick No-Cook Fondant

Easy—and I like easy.

7 oz.	low-calorie white frosting mix	200 g
2 T.	margarine	30 mL
1 to 2 T.	water	30 to 60 mL

Combine frosting mix and margarine in food processor or bowl. Work with steel blade or spoon until mixture is well blended. (Add very small amounts of water if needed.) Mixture will be very stiff at first; work and knead until mixture is well blended and smooth. Use as directed in recipe.

Yield: 1 c. (2.50 mL)

Exchange, full recipe: 7 bread, 16 fat
Full recipe contains: Calories: 1,200, Carbohydrates: 188 g

Fast Holiday Drops

1 env.	unflavored gelatin	1 env.
⅔ c.	skim milk	180 mL
30	soda crackers, crumbed	30
½ c.	pecans, chopped fine	125 mL
1 t.	vanilla extract	5 mL
⅓ c.	creamy peanut butter	90 mL
⅓ c.	mini chocolate chips	90 mL

Soak gelatin in milk for 5 minutes; heat and stir until gelatin is dissolved and mixture boils. Remove from heat and quickly add remaining ingredients. Beat with a wooden spoon until mixture is thick enough to drop from a teaspoon onto waxed paper. Makes 24 drops. Refrigerate until firm.

Yield: 24 drops

Exchange, 1 drop: ½ bread, 1 fat
Each serving contains: Calories: 76, Carbohydrates: 4 g

Out-of-Bounds Candy Bars

Coconut and chocolate—a popular American combination.

1¼ c.	unsweetened coconut	310 mL
1½ c.	milk	125 mL
2 t.	unflavored gelatin	10 mL
1 t.	cornstarch	5 mL
1 t.	white vanilla extract	5 mL
1 recipe	semisweet dipping chocolate	1 recipe

Combine ¼ c. (60 mL) of the coconut, the milk, gelatin and cornstarch in blender; blend until smooth. Pour into small saucepan, cook and stir over medium heat until slightly thickened. Remove from heat and stir in vanilla and remaining coconut. Form into 8 bars, allow to firm and cool completely. Dip in chocolate.

Yield: 8 bars

Exchange, 1 bar: ⅔ full-fat milk, 1 fat
Each serving contains: Calories: 133, Carbohydrates: 13 g

Rum Rounds

⅓ c.	Quick No-Cook Fondant	90 mL
1 t.	rum flavoring	5 mL
1 oz.	white dietetic chocolate coating	30 g

Stir fondant and rum flavoring until completely blended. Divide mixture in half. Form into two 5½ × ½ in. (14 × 1.3 cm) rolls. Cut into ¼ in. (6 mm) round discs. Place on plate and refrigerate until firm. Melt white dietetic chocolate coating in small custard cup over simmering water. Using two forks, dip rounds one at a time. Pick rounds out of the melted chocolate and place on waxed paper to dry. Refrigerate until very firm. Remove chocolate coating from heat; reserve. When rounds are firm, re-melt any remaining chocolate and re-dip rounds.

Yield: 34 rounds

Exchange, 1 round: ⅓ fat
Each serving contains: Calories: 17, Carbohydrates: negligible

Chocolate Pudding Squares

A candy for pudding fans.

3 env.	unflavored gelatin	3 env.
1 c.	cold water	250 mL
2 T.	cocoa	30 mL
1 oz.	paraffin wax, grated	30 g
2 T.	flour	30 mL
1 c.	skim milk	250 mL
3 T.	margarine	45 mL

Combine unflavored gelatin and cold water in bowl; stir to mix. Set aside. Combine cocoa, wax, flour and skim milk in heavy saucepan; cook and stir until wax has melted and mixture is thick and smooth. Add softened gelatin. Cook and stir until mixture is thick. Remove from heat and add margarine. Stir to completely dissolve. Pour into lightly greased 9 in. (23 cm) sq. pan.

Refrigerate until completely set. Cut into 1 in. (2.5 cm) squares. Refrigerate.

Yield: 81 pieces

Exchange, 1 piece: negligible
Each serving contains: Calories: 3, Carbohydrates: 2 g

Date Surprise

You may tint white chocolate with small amount of food coloring.

50	dates, pitted	50
100	salted peanuts, whole	100
2 oz.	white dietetic chocolate coating	60 g
¼ oz.	paraffin wax	8 g

Remove any stem ends from dates. Carefully open each date and stuff with two whole peanuts. Place on a plate and refrigerate until cool. Melt white coating and paraffin wax in a small jar or dish over simmering water. Using two forks, dip each date, one at a time, until completely coated. Place on waxed paper to firm. Store in refrigerator.

Yield: 50 pieces

Exchange, 1 piece: ½ bread
Each serving contains: Calories: 45, Carbohydrates: 9 g

Fancy Prunes

Choose soft prunes for this candy

48	dried prunes	48
24	walnut halves	24
¼ c.	Basic Crème Center	60 mL
½ recipe	semisweet dipping chocolate	½ recipe

Slit sides of prunes and carefully remove the pits. Break walnut halves in half lengthwise. Wrap equal amounts of crème center around each section of walnut. Stuff a covered walnut into each prune cavity. Place on waxed paper on a plate. Refrigerate. Allow to chill at least 4 hours or overnight. When cold, dip in the chocolate. Place on waxed paper until firm. Store in refrigerator.

Yield: 48 pieces

Exchange, 1 piece: ½ bread
Each serving contains: Calories: 35, Carbohydrates: 9 g

Triple C Treat

40	Bing cherries	40
1 c.	unsweetened coconut, grated	250 mL
½ c.	skim milk	125 mL
2 t.	unflavored gelatin	10 mL
2 t.	cornstarch	10 mL
2 t.	coconut flavoring	10 mL
1 oz.	dietetic chocolate coating	30 g
1 oz.	white dietetic dipping chocolate	30 g

Carefully pit the cherries. Set in refrigerator to chill. Combine unsweetened coconut, skim milk, gelatin, cornstarch and coconut flavoring in saucepan and stir to blend. Set aside for 5 minutes to allow gelatin to soften. Cook and stir over low heat until mixture is very thick. Remove from heat and allow to cool. Divide in half. Form 40 pea-size balls of the coconut mixture and push one ball into each cherry center. Cover cherries with remaining coconut mixture. Place on plate and refrigerate to firm. Melt chocolate coating in small custard cup and dip one-half of each cherry. Place on waxed paper to harden. Melt white chocolate in another custard cup and dip the other side of each cherry. Place on waxed paper to harden. Store in refrigerator.

Yield: 40 pieces

Exchange, 1 piece: ¼ bread
Each serving contains: Calories: 20, Carbohydrates: 3 g

Apricot Nuggets

Elegant candy to delight your guests.

1 env.	unflavored gelatin	1 env.
¼ c.	water	60 mL
1½ c.	dried apricots	375 mL
1 T.	flour	15 mL
2 T.	orange peel, grated	30 mL
1 t.	vanilla extract	5 mL
2 oz.	dietetic chocolate coating, melted	60 g

Sprinkle gelatin over water; allow to soften for 5 minutes. Heat and stir until gelatin is completely dissolved. Combine apricots, flour, orange peel in blender or food processor and work until finely chopped. Add apricot mixture to gelatin. Add vanilla extract and stir to completely blend. Line with plastic wrap or waxed paper an 8 in. (20 cm) sq. pan. Spread fruit mixture evenly into pan and set aside until cool and completely firm. Turn out onto a cutting board. Cut into 1 in. (2.5 cm) squares. Place on plate in refrigerator until chilled. Dip in melted dietetic chocolate.

Yield: 64 nuggets

Exchange, 1 nugget: ¼ bread
Each serving contains: Calories: 14, Carbohydrates: 2 g

Sweet Chocolate-Covered Pineapple

⅓ c.	Quick No-Cook Fondant	90 mL
18	bite-size pineapple tidbits in their own juice	18
1 oz.	dietetic chocolate coating	30 g

Drain pineapple tidbits thoroughly. Place on paper towel, drain for 10 to 15 minutes and pat until slightly dry. Form 1 t. (5 mL) of fondant mixture around each pineapple tidbit. Place on plate and refrigerate until firm. Melt chocolate coating in a small custard cup over simmering water. Using two forks, dip each pineapple bit, one at a time, in the chocolate. Remove and place on waxed paper and allow to harden. Store in refrigerator.

Yield: 18 pieces

Exchange, 1 piece: ⅓ fruit, ½ fat
Each serving contains: Calories: 32, Carbohydrates: 6 g

Raisin Balls

1 env.	unflavored gelatin	1 env.
¼ c.	apple juice	60 mL
2 c.	raisins	500 mL
2 T.	flour	30 mL
½ c.	walnuts, finely chopped	125 mL
½ c.	semisweet chocolate chips	125 mL
¼ oz.	paraffin wax	8 g

Sprinkle gelatin over apple juice; allow to soften for 5 minutes. Heat and stir until gelatin is completely dissolved. Combine raisins and flour in a mixing bowl; toss to completely coat. Stir in walnuts. Add raisin mixture to apple gelatin. Stir to thoroughly blend. Remove from heat and allow to cool. Form into 30 balls. Refrigerate until firm. Melt chocolate chips and wax in small pan or bowl over simmering water. Dip chilled raisin balls in chocolate. Place on waxed paper until firm. Store in refrigerator.

Yield: 30 balls

Exchange, 1 ball: ½ bread, ½ fat
Each serving contains: Calories: 56, Carbohydrates: 13 g

Mint Mounds

⅓ c.	Quick No-Cook Fondant	90 mL
½ t.	wintergreen flavoring	2 mL
2 drops	green food coloring	2 drops
1 oz.	dietetic chocolate coating	30 g
¼ oz.	paraffin wax	8 g

Combine fondant, flavoring and food coloring; mix until color is completely blended in fondant. Cover a ½ t. (2 mL) spoon with plastic wrap, press a small amount of fondant mixture into plastic on spoon to make a mound. Remove and place on plate. Repeat with remaining fondant. Refrigerate until firm. Melt dietetic chocolate coating and wax in a small custard cup over simmering water. Remove and discard plastic wrap from mounds. Using two forks, dip mounds one at a time. Pick mounds out of melted chocolate and place on waxed paper to dry.

Yield: 26

Exchange, 1 mound: ½ fat
Each serving contains: Calories: 22, Carbohydrates: 3 g

Fudge Candy

13 oz. can	skim evaporated milk	385 mL can
3 T.	cocoa	45 mL
¼ c.	butter	60 mL
1 T.	granulated sugar replacement	15 mL
dash	salt	dash
1 t.	vanilla extract	5 mL
2½ c.	unsweetened cereal crumbs	625 mL
¼ c.	nuts, very finely chopped	60 mL

Combine milk and cocoa in saucepan; cook and beat over low heat until cocoa is dissolved. Add butter, sugar replacement, salt and vanilla. Bring to a boil; reduce heat and cook for 2 minutes. Remove from heat; add cereal crumbs and work in with wooden spoon. Cool 15 minutes. Divide in half; roll each half into a tube 8 in. (20 cm) long. Roll each tube in finely chopped nuts. Wrap in waxed paper; chill overnight. Cut into ¼ in. (6 mm) slices.

Yield: 64 slices

Exchange, 2 slices: ½ bread, ½ fat
Each serving contains: Calories: 60

Butterscotch-Chocolate Fudge

13 oz. can	skim evaporated milk	385 g can
1 c.	water	250 mL
¼ c.	cornstarch	60 mL
3 T.	granulated sugar replacement	45 mL
½ c.	chocolate chips	125 mL
½ c.	butterscotch chips	125 mL
1 t.	vanilla extract	5 mL
½ c.	walnuts, chopped	125 mL

Combine evaporated milk, water, cornstarch, sugar replacement, chocolate chips and butterscotch chips in saucepan. Cook and stir over medium heat until mixture thickens and chips are melted. Cool. Stir in vanilla extract. Beat with an electric mixer until light. Stir in walnuts. Turn into buttered 9 in. (23 cm) sq. baking dish. Spread evenly. Cool and cut in 1 in. (2.5 cm) squares.

Yield: 81

Exchange, 1 square: ¼ bread, ¼ fat
Each serving contains: Calories: 21, Carbohydrates: 3 g

French Fudge

Do you like fudge extra rich?

13 oz. can	skim evaporated milk	385 g can
2 T.	cornstarch	30 mL
1 T.	liquid sugar replacement	15 mL
½ c.	chocolate chips	125 mL
3 oz.	cream cheese, softened	90 g
1½ t.	vanilla extract	7 mL

Combine evaporated milk, cornstarch, sugar replacement and chocolate chips in saucepan. Cook and stir until mixture is thick and chocolate chips are melted. Whip cream cheese until light and fluffy. Beat in chocolate-milk mixture. Stir in vanilla extract. Turn into buttered 8 in. (20 cm) sq. baking dish. Chill until firm. Cut into 1 in. (2.5 cm) squares. Store in refrigerator.

Yield: 64 pieces

Exchange, 1 piece: ¼ bread
Each serving contains: Calories: 18, Carbohydrates: 2 g

Maple-Pecan Centers

⅓ c.	Quick No-Cook Fondant	90 mL
½ t.	maple flavoring	2 mL
¼ c.	pecans, finely chopped	60 mL
1 oz.	dietetic chocolate coating	30 g

Combine fondant and maple flavoring in bowl and mix until completely blended. Work in the pecans. Set aside until mixture is slightly firm. Form into 20 small balls. Place on plate in refrigerator until firm. Melt chocolate coating in small custard cup over simmering water. Dip each ball in chocolate; set on waxed paper to harden.

Yield: 20 pieces

Exchange, 1 piece: ¼ bread, ½ fat
Each serving contains: Calories: 38, Carbohydrates: 4 g

Mock Turtles

18	pecan halves	18
½ c.	cold water	125 mL
1 env.	unflavored gelatin	1 env.
½ c.	skim milk	125 mL
1 T.	granulated sugar replacement	15 mL
½ t.	maple flavoring	2 mL
1 oz.	dietetic chocolate coating	30 g

Place a pecan half in bottom of petit four cup. Place petit four cup into small nut cup or mini muffin tin. (This is to keep the petit four cup in shape.) Combine cold water and gelatin in saucepan; allow to rest for 5 minutes. Cook and stir over medium heat until mixture comes to full boil; boil for 2 minutes. Remove from heat. Stir in milk, sugar replacement and maple flavoring to thoroughly blend. Set aside until mixture is the consistency of thick syrup. Spoon 2 t. (10 mL) of maple mixture over pecan in petit four cup. Chill until firm. Melt chocolate coating in small custard cup over simmering water. Divide melted chocolate evenly among the 18 petit four cups. Store in refrigerator.

Yield: 18

Exchange, 1 turtle: ¼ bread
Each serving contains: Calories: 16, Carbohydrates: 2 g

Peanut Favorites

1 env.	unflavored gelatin	1 env.
¼ c.	skim milk	60 mL
½ c.	chunky peanut butter	125 mL
¾ c.	unsalted peanuts, chopped	190 mL
½ c.	no-sugar wheat flakes	125 mL
2 oz.	dietetic chocolate coating	60 g
¼ oz.	paraffin wax	8 g

Soak gelatin in cold milk in saucepan, allow to soften for 5 minutes. Add peanut butter. Cook and stir over medium heat until peanut butter is melted and mixture is very hot. Remove from heat and allow to cool slightly. Stir in peanuts and wheat flakes. Form into 28 fingerlike shapes. Place on a plate and refrigerate until cool and set. Melt chocolate coating and wax in small pan or bowl over simmering water. Dip peanut fingers, one at a time. Place on waxed paper to cool.

Yield: 28 fingers

Exchange, 1 finger: ¼ bread, 1 fat
Each serving contains: Calories: 63, Carbohydrates: 4 g

Marble Creams

9	graham crackers	9
1 c.	cold water	250 mL
2 pkg.	unflavored gelatin	2 pkg.
2 T.	flour	30 mL
2 T.	cornstarch	30 mL
½ t.	cream of tartar	2 mL
⅓ c.	dietetic maple syrup	90 mL
¼ t.	baking soda	1 mL
⅓ c.	chocolate chips	90 mL

Arrange graham crackers in the bottom of a greased 9 in. (23 cm) sq. baking dish. Set aside. Combine cold water and gelatin in a saucepan; allow to soften for 5 minutes. Stir in flour, cornstarch, cream of tartar and maple syrup. Cook and stir over medium heat until mixture is very thick. Remove from heat and beat in baking soda. Cool slightly, pour mixture over graham crackers. Sprinkle with chocolate chips. With the tip of a knife, carefully swirl melting chips into maple mixture. Refrigerate until firm. With a sharp knife, cut into 1 in. (2.5 cm) squares.

Yield: 81 squares

Exchange, 2 squares: ¼ bread
Each serving contains: Calories: 17, Carbohydrates: 4 g

Walnut Riches

1 recipe	Basic Crème Center	1 recipe
2 t.	brandy flavoring	10 mL
¼ c.	mini chocolate chips	60 mL
2 oz.	dietetic chocolate coating	60 g
¼ oz.	paraffin wax	8 g
35	walnut halves, roasted	35

Combine crème center dough and brandy flavoring in a mixing bowl. Work with your hands until mixture is well blended. Work in chocolate chips. Divide mixture into 70 small pieces and form into desired shapes. Place on plate and refrigerate until firm. Melt chocolate coating and wax in a small custard cup over simmering water. Using two forks, dip each shape one at a time in the chocolate. Remove and place on waxed paper. Break each walnut in half lengthwise and place each of these walnut quarters lengthwise on each candy. Cool.

Yield: 70 pieces

Exchange, 1 piece: ½ fat
Each serving contains: Calories: 22, Carbohydrates: 1 g

Candy and Then Some

1 env.	unflavored gelatin	1 env.
¼ c.	water	60 mL
½ c.	dried apricots	125 mL
½ c.	dates, chopped	125 mL
½ c.	white raisins	125 mL
½ c.	dried apples	125 mL
¼ c.	pecans	60 mL
¼ c.	walnuts	60 mL
2 T.	flour	30 mL
2 t.	brandy flavoring	10 mL
1 recipe	Semisweet Dipping Chocolate	1 recipe

Soak gelatin in water for 5 minutes; heat and stir until gelatin is dissolved. Combine remaining ingredients in food processor and work with an on/off method until fruits are finely chopped. Stir into gelatin mixture until completely coated. Form into 40 balls. Place on plate and refrigerate until firm. Dip in Semisweet Dipping Chocolate.

Yield: 40 balls

Exchange, 1 ball: 1 fruit
Each serving contains: Calories: 40, Carbohydrates: 6 g

Molded Candies

¼ c.	solid white shortening	60 mL
2 T.	water	30 mL
1 c.	Powdered Sugar Replacement	250 mL

Beat shortening and water until fluffy; stir in sugar replacement. Knead until smooth. Continue as follows for individual molds.

Apples: Flavor with 2 t. (10 mL) unsweetened drink mix. Mold into apple shapes; brush lightly with diluted red food color. Use whole clove for stem.

Banana: Flavor with 1 t. (5 mL) banana oil and knead in 3 drops of yellow food color. Mold into banana shapes.

Orange: Flavor with 1 t. (5 mL) orange oil and knead in 2 drops of red and 1 drop of yellow food color. Mold into orange shapes. Use whole clove for stem.

Strawberry: Flavor with 2 t. (10 mL) strawberry flavoring or rose water and knead in 3 drops of red food color or desired amount. Mold into strawberry shapes, pricking each with toothpick to create seed holes. Push small green satin decoration into top for stem. (Satin decorations can be purchased at craft stores.)

Yield: 20 molded fruits

Exchange, 1 fruit: ⅓ fruit, ½ fat
Each serving contains: Calories: 36, Carbohydrates: 11 g

Butter Rum Patties

5 c.	puffed rice, unsweetened	1250 mL
3 T.	granulated sugar replacement	45 mL
2	egg whites	2
2 t.	butter rum flavoring	10 mL
1 t.	vanilla extract	5 mL

Pour rice into blender and work into a powder. Pour into large bowl or food processor and add remaining ingredients. Work with wooden spoon or steel blade until mixture is completely blended; mixture will be sticky. Form into 20 patties. Place patties on an ungreased cookie sheet and bake at 300°F (150°C) for 15 to 20 minutes, or until surface feels dry.

Yield: 20 patties

Exchange, 1 patty: ¼ bread
Each serving contains: Calories: 23, Carbohydrates: 8 g

Cream Cheese Mints

3 oz. pkg.	softened cream cheese	90 g pkg.
1 c.	Powdered Sugar Replacement	250 mL
2 T.	water	30 mL
½ to 1 t.	mint flavoring	2 to 5 mL
	food color as desired	

Beat cream cheese until fluffy. Stir in sugar replacement, water, flavoring and food color. (Dough may be divided into parts and different flavorings and food color added to each part.) Knead or work with the hand until dough is smooth. Roll into small marble-size balls, press each ball firmly into cavity of mold, and unmold onto waxed paper.

Yield: 60 pieces

Exchange, 5 pieces: ⅓ fruit, ½ fat
Each serving contains: Calories: 50, Carbohydrates: 18 g

Butter Mints

¼ c.	soft margarine	60 mL
2 T.	evaporated milk	30 mL
1 t.	butter flavoring	5 mL
1 c.	Powdered Sugar Replacement	250 mL

Cream together margarine, milk and butter flavoring until fluffy. Stir in sugar replacement. Knead or work with hands until smooth, roll into small marble-size balls and press each ball firmly into mold. Unmold onto waxed paper.

Yield: 45 pieces

Exchange, 3 pieces: ⅓ low-fat milk
Each serving contains: Calories: 56, Carbohydrates: negligible

Chocolate Butter Creams

3 oz. pkg.	softened cream cheese	90 g pkg.	
2 T.	skim milk	30 mL	
1½ t.	white vanilla extract	7 mL	
1 c.	Powdered Sugar Replacement	250 mL	
1 recipe	Semisweet Dipping Chocolate	1 recipe	

Beat cream cheese, milk and vanilla until fluffy; stir in powdered sugar replacement. Form into 30 balls and dip each one in chocolate.

Yield: 30 creams

Exchange, 1 cream: ¼ low-fat milk
Each serving contains: Calories: 31, Carbohydrates: 8 g

Double Fudge Balls

⅓ c.	soft margarine	90 mL	
3 T.	evaporated skimmed milk	45 mL	
dash	salt	dash	
1 t.	vanilla extract	5 mL	
¼ c.	cocoa	60 mL	
1 c.	Powdered Sugar Replacement	250 mL	
1 recipe	Semisweet Dipping Chocolate	1 recipe	

Cream together margarine, milk, salt and vanilla until fluffy. Stir in cocoa and sugar replacement. Knead or work with hands until dough is smooth, and form dough into 60 small balls. Dip balls in chocolate, cool completely; dip again and cool.

Yield: 60 balls

Exchange, 1 ball: ⅓ bread, ½ fat
Each serving contains: Calories: 50, Carbohydrates: 4 g

Chocolate-Coated Cherries

1 recipe	Butter Mints	1 recipe	
30	Bing cherries (with pits and stems)	30	
½ recipe	Semisweet Dipping Chocolate	½ recipe	

Wrap Butter Mint dough around each cherry; chill slightly. Dip in chocolate and dry completely.

Yield: 30 cherries

Exchange, 1 cherry: ¼ bread, ¼ fat
Each serving contains: Calories: 31, Carbohydrates: 2 g

Dried Apple Snack

1	apple	1	

Peel, core and slice apple very thinly. Place on cookie rack. Bake at 200°F (100°C) for 1 hour (soft and chewy); 1½ hours (very chewy); or 2 hours (crisp).

Yield: 1 serving

Exchange, 1 serving: 1 fruit
Each serving contains: Calories: 20, Carbohydrates: 22 g

Jell Jots

3 env.	unflavored gelatin	3 env.
½ c.	cold water	125 mL
1¾ oz. pkg.	low-calorie jelly pectin	49.6 g pkg.
1½ c.	water	375 mL
1 T.	liquid sugar replacement	15 mL
1½ t.	lemon juice	7 mL
1 t.	fruit oil	5 mL
or 2 t.	fruit flavoring	10 mL
	food color	
	flour or cornstarch	

Combine gelatin and ½ c. (125 mL) cold water in bowl, stirring to mix, and set aside. Combine pectin and 1½ c. (375 mL) water in saucepan; cook and stir over medium-high heat until boiling. Cook and stir 12 minutes longer and then remove from heat. Add soaked gelatin, stirring until gelatin completely dissolves. Add sugar replacement, lemon juice, fruit oil and food color; stir to mix. Using teaspoon, fill holes in prepared pan (see below) with this mixture. Allow to set completely. Remove jots to strainer; shake off excess flour or cornstarch. (If jot mixture becomes hard, reheat slightly to liquefy.)

To prepare pan: Half fill 13 × 9 × 2 in. (33 × 23 × 5 cm) pan with flour or cornstarch. Place a thimble on finger and make holes in flour to bottom of pan.

Yield: 150 pieces

Exchange, 50 pieces: 1 bread
Each serving contains: Calories: 80, Carbohydrates: 25 g

Butter Sticks

7 large	shredded wheat biscuits	7 large
½ c.	crunchy peanut butter	125 mL
3 T.	granulated sugar replacement	45 mL
2	egg whites	2
1 T.	flour	15 mL
1 T.	water	15 mL
1 t.	baking powder	5 mL
1 t.	vanilla extract	5 mL
1 recipe	Semisweet Dipping Chocolate	1 recipe

Break biscuits into large bowl or food processor. Add peanut butter, sugar replacement, egg whites, flour, water, baking powder and vanilla. Work with wooden spoon or steel blade until mixture is completely blended; mixture will be sticky. Form into 16 sticks and place them on an ungreased cookie sheet. Bake at 400°F (200°C) for 10 minutes, or until surface feels hard. Remove; cool slightly. Dip in chocolate.

Yield: 16 sticks

Exchange, 1 stick: ⅔ bread
Each serving contains: Calories: 115, Carbohydrates: 10 g

Cookie Brittle

½ c.	margarine	125 mL
2 t.	vanilla extract	10 mL
1 t.	salt	5 mL
3 T.	granulated sugar replacement	45 mL
2 c.	flour, sifted	500 mL
1 c.	semisweet chocolate chips	250 mL
½ c.	walnuts, chopped fine	125 mL

Combine margarine, vanilla, salt, and sugar replacement in mixing bowl or food processor; beat until smooth. Stir in flour, chocolate chips, and walnuts. Press into ungreased 15 × 10 in. (39 × 25 cm) pan. Bake at 375°F (190°C) for 25 minutes. Remove from oven, score into 2 × 1 in. (5 × 2.5 cm) pieces and cool completely. Break into candy pieces.

Yield: 60 pieces

Exchange, 1 piece: ½ fat, ⅓ bread
Each serving contains: Calories: 48, Carbohydrates: 6 g

Sugared Pecans

½ c.	water	250 mL
¼ c.	granulated sugar replacement	60 mL
¼ c.	granulated brown sugar replacement	60 mL
1 c.	pecan halves	250 mL

Combine water and sugar replacements in saucepan, stirring to dissolve. Bring to boil, and boil for 3 minutes. Stir in pecans until completely coated; remove pan from heat. Allow pecans to rest in sugar water for 2 to 3 minutes. Remove with slotted spoon and cool completely.

Yield: 1 c. (250 mL)

Exchange, 1 serving: 1 fat
Each serving contains: Calories: 48, Carbohydrates: 119 g

Orange Walnuts

1 t.	unflavored gelatin	5 mL
½ c.	orange juice	125 mL
¼ c.	granulated sugar replacement	60 mL
1 t.	orange rind	5 mL
½ t.	vanilla extract	2 mL
1 c.	walnut halves	250 mL

Sprinkle gelatin over orange juice; allow to rest 5 minutes to soften. Cook and stir over medium heat until gelatin is dissolved. Stir in sugar replacement and orange rind. Bring to a boil, boil for 2 minutes and remove from heat. Cool slightly. Stir in vanilla; stir in walnuts until completely coated. Allow walnuts to rest in juice 10 minutes. Remove with slotted spoon and cool completely.

Yield: 1 c. (250 mL)

Exchange, 1 serving: 1 fat
Each serving contains: Calories: 50, Carbohydrates: 84 g

Crunch Nuts

7 large	shredded wheat biscuits	7 large
3 T.	granulated sugar replacement	45 mL
2 t.	almond extract	10 mL
2	egg whites	2

Crumble biscuits into blender; work into a powder. Combine with remaining ingredients in large mixing bowl or food processor. Work with wooden spoon or steel blade until completely blended; mixture will be sticky. Cover and refrigerate 1 hour. Form into walnut-size balls, place on ungreased cookie sheet and bake at 400°F (200°C) for 10 minutes.

Yield: 40 pieces

Exchange, 1 piece: ¼ bread
Each serving contains: Calories: 17, Carbohydrates: 2 g

Coconut Macaroons

1 c.	evaporated skimmed milk	250 mL
2 t.	granulated sugar replacement	10 mL
3 c.	unsweetened coconut, shredded	750 mL

Combine milk and sugar replacement in large bowl, stirring until sugar replacement dissolves. Add coconut and stir until coconut is completely moistened. Drop by teaspoonfuls onto greased cookie sheets, 2 to 3 in. (5 to 7 cm) apart. Bake at 350°F (175°C) for 15 minutes, or until tops are lightly browned. Remove from pan immediately.

Yield: 48 drops

Exchange, 1 drop: ¼ fruit, ½ fat
Each serving contains: Calories: 31, Carbohydrates: 3 g

Coconut Candy

1¼ c.	unsweetened coconut, grated	310 mL
½ c.	milk	125 mL
2 t.	unflavored gelatin	10 mL
1 t.	cornstarch	5 mL
1 t.	white vanilla extract	5 mL
1 recipe	Semisweet Dipping Chocolate	1 recipe

Combine ¼ c. (60 mL) of the coconut and the milk, gelatin, and cornstarch in a blender, and blend until smooth. Pour into small saucepan; cook and stir over medium heat until slightly thickened. Remove from heat and stir in vanilla and remaining coconut. Form into 16 patties, and allow to cool completely. Dip into chocolate.

Yield: 16 candies

Exchange, 1 candy: ⅓ whole milk, ½ fat
Each serving contains: Calories: 66, Carbohydrates: 4 g

Crunch Candy

6 large	shredded wheat biscuits	6 large
1 t.	unflavored gelatin	5 mL
¾ c.	cold milk	190 mL
½ c.	creamy peanut butter	125 mL
1 recipe	Semisweet Dipping Chocolate	1 recipe

Break shredded wheat biscuits into small pieces. Set aside. Soak gelatin in ¼ c. (60 mL) of the cold milk; set aside. Combine peanut butter and remaining milk in top of a double boiler and place over hot (not boiling) water. Cook and stir until smooth. Add soaked gelatin; then cook and stir until gelatin is completely dissolved and smooth. Fold reserved shredded wheat pieces into peanut butter mixture. Drop by teaspoonfuls onto lightly greased waxed paper. Allow to firm and cool; then dip in chocolate.

Yield: 32 candies

Exchange, 1 candy: ⅓ whole milk
Each serving contains: Calories: 44, Carbohydrates: 4 g

Semisweet Dipping Chocolate (for Candy)

1 c.	nonfat dry milk powder	250 mL
⅓ c.	unsweetened cocoa	90 mL
2 T.	grated paraffin wax	30 mL
½ c.	water	250 mL
1 T.	vegetable oil	15 mL
1 T.	liquid fructose	15 mL

Combine milk powder, cocoa, and wax in a food processor or blender; process or blend to a soft powder. Transfer into the top of a double boiler and add the water, stirring to blend. Add vegetable oil. Place over hot (not boiling) water. Cook and stir until wax pieces are completely melted and mixture is thick, smooth, and creamy. Remove double boiler from heat. Stir in liquid fructose. Allow to cool slightly. Dip candies according to recipe in cookbook or your recipe. Shake off excess chocolate. Place on very lightly greased waxed paper, and allow candies to cool completely. (If candies cannot be removed easily, slightly warm a cookie sheet in the oven, lay the waxed paper with candies on warmed cookie sheet, and remove them. Store in cool place.)

Yield: 1 c. (250 mL)

Exchange, full recipe: 3 low-fat milk
Full recipe contains: Calories: 427, Carbohydrates: 30 g

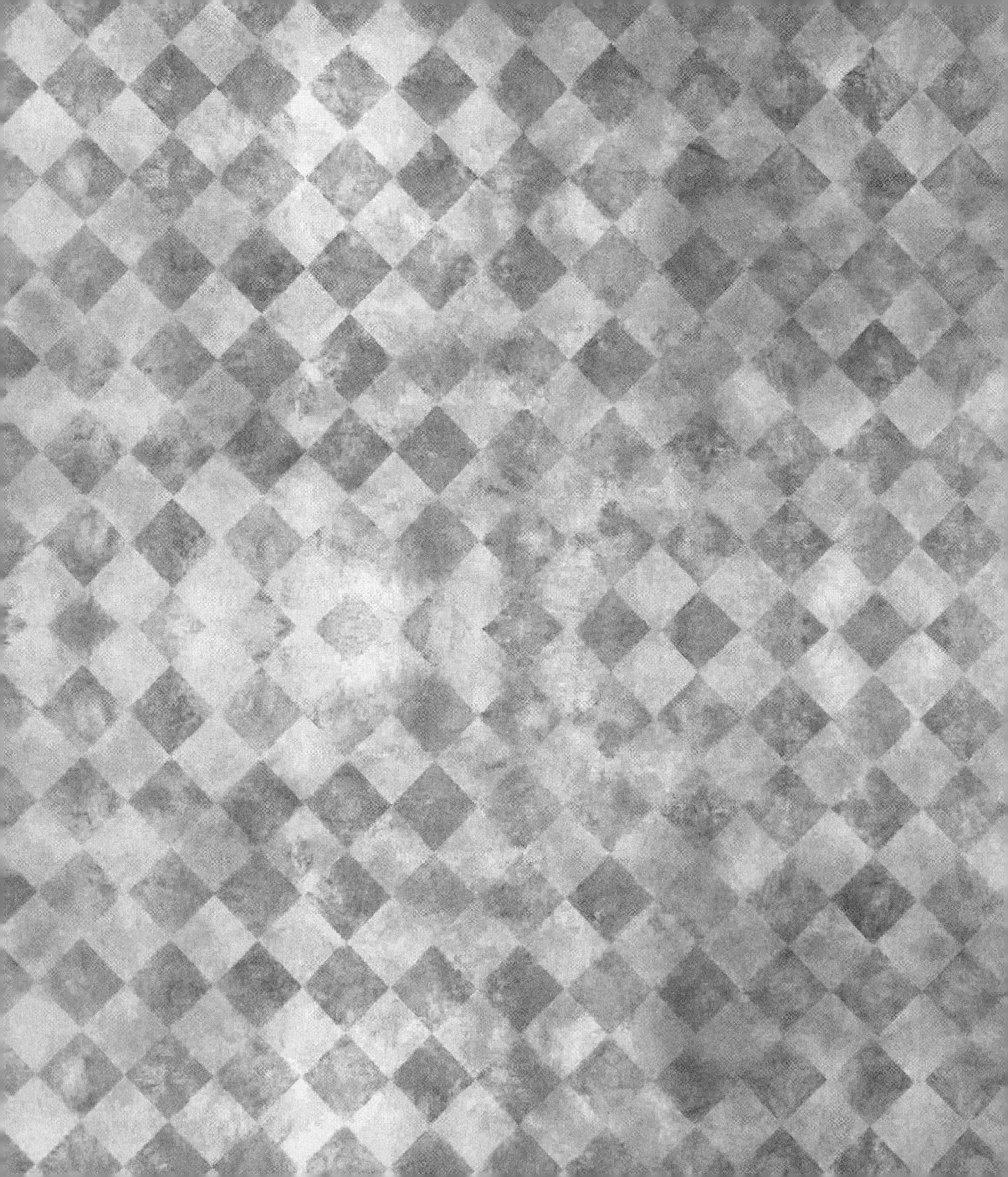

Brownies and Bars

Chocolate-Mint Brownies

1 c.	flour	250 mL
½ t.	baking powder	2 mL
¼ t.	salt	1 mL
½ c.	vegetable shortening, softened	125 mL
½ c.	granulated sugar replacement	125 mL
3 T.	fructose	45 mL
3	eggs	3
2 oz.	baking chocolate, melted	60 g
1 T.	mint flavoring	15 mL
⅔ c.	no-sugar white frosting mix	165 mL
	green food coloring	
	hot water	
1 T.	chocolate sprinkles or jimmies	15 mL

Sift flour, baking powder, and salt together. Cream shortening, sugar replacement and fructose; beat in eggs, melted chocolate, and mint flavoring. Spread batter in two 8 in. (20 cm) greased pans. Bake at 325°F (165°C) for 25 to 30 minutes. Cool. Combine no-sugar frosting mix with a few drops of green food coloring and enough hot water to make frosting soft enough to spread. Spread on brownies; sprinkle tops with chocolate sprinkles. Cut into 1 × 2 in. (2.5 × 5 cm) bars.

Yield: 64 bars

Exchange, 1 bar: ¼ bread, ¾ fat
Each serving contains: Calories: 41, Carbohydrates: 6 g

Chocolate Pudding Brownies

⅓ c.	margarine, melted	90 mL
1 pkg.	reduced-calorie chocolate pudding mix	1 pkg.
2	eggs	2
1 t.	vanilla	15 mL
3 T.	water	45 mL
½ c.	flour	125 mL
¼ t.	baking powder	2 mL
⅓ c.	walnuts	90 mL

In medium-size bowl, combine margarine, pudding mix, eggs, vanilla, and water. Beat to thoroughly mix. Add sifted flour and baking powder; stir until well blended. Fold in walnuts. Spread evenly into a greased 8 in. (20 cm) sq. pan. Bake at 350°F (175°C) for 15 minutes or until done. Cut into 2 in. (5 cm) squares.

Yield: 16 brownies

Exchange, 1 brownie: ½ bread, 1 fat
Each serving contains: Calories: 78, Carbohydrates: 5 g

Butterscotch-Chocolate Brownies

½ c.	margarine, melted	125 mL
1 env.	reduced-calorie butterscotch pudding mix	1 env.
1 env.	reduced-calorie chocolate pudding mix	1 env.
2	eggs	2
2 t.	vanilla	10 mL
⅓ c.	water	90 mL
1 c.	cake flour, sifted	250 mL
1½ t.	baking powder	7 mL

Combine margarine, pudding mixes, eggs, vanilla, and water in medium size bowl; beat to blend thoroughly. Add cake flour and baking powder and continue beating until smooth and creamy. Pour into greased 8 in. (20 cm) sq. pan. Bake at 350°F (175°C) for 20 minutes or until done. Cut into 2 in. (5 cm) squares.

Yield: 16 brownies

Exchange, 1 brownie: ⅔ bread, 1½ fat
Each serving contains: Calories: 94, Carbohydrates: 10 g

Walnut Cubes

Crust

¾ c.	flour	250 mL
¼ c.	cocoa	60 mL
2 T.	granulated sugar replacement	30 mL
½ c.	butter	125 mL

Center Filling

2	eggs, well beaten	2
½ c.	granulated sugar replacement	125 mL
½ c.	unsweetened coconut, grated	125 mL
½ c.	walnuts, chopped	125 mL
2 T.	flour	30 mL
¼ t.	baking powder	1 mL
½ t.	salt	2 mL
1 t.	vanilla extract	5 mL

Frosting

1 c.	Powdered Sugar Replacement	250 mL
3 T.	cocoa	45 mL
2 T.	butter, melted	30 mL
2 T.	orange juice	30 mL
1 t.	orange rind, grated	5 mL
	water	

Combine flour, cocoa and granulated sugar replacement; work in the butter. Spread mixture in the bottom of a greased 9 in. (23 cm) pan. Bake at 350°F (175°C) for 15 minutes.

Combine center filling ingredients and stir to completely mix. Spread over crust. Return to oven and bake 25 minutes longer. Cool slightly.

Combine frosting ingredients and enough water to make a thick spreading paste, then spread on top of warm filling. Cool. Cut into 1 in. (2.5 cm) squares.

Yield: 81 cubes

Exchange, 2 cubes: ¼ bread, 1 fat
Each serving contains: Calories: 80, Carbohydrates: 12 g

Hawaiian Coconut Bars

Crust

1 c.	flour sifted	250 mL
3 T.	granulated brown sugar replacement	45 mL
¼ t.	salt	1 mL
¼ c.	margarine	60 mL
1 T.	water	15 mL

Topping

½ c.	flour	125 mL
½ t.	baking powder	2 mL
dash	salt	dash
1	egg	1
½ c.	granulated brown sugar replacement	125 mL
¼ c.	sorbitol	60 mL
1 T.	vanilla extract	15 mL
½ c.	mini chocolate chips	125 mL
½ c.	unsweetened coconut, shredded	125 mL
½ c.	unsweetened pineapple, crushed and well drained	125 mL

To prepare crust, blend flour, brown sugar, and salt together, then cut in margarine. Work in water. Press into bottom of greased 13 × 9 in. (33 × 23 cm) pan. Bake at 350°F (175°C) for 10 minutes or until lightly browned.

To prepare topping, sift together the flour, baking powder and salt. Beat egg; gradually add brown sugar replacement and sorbitol. Add flour mixture, vanilla, mini chocolate chips, coconut, and pineapple. Spread on top of crust. Bake at 350°F (175°C) for 35 to 40 minutes or until mixture is set. Cool slightly, cut into 1 × 3 in. (2.5 × 7.5 cm) bars.

Yield: 39 bars

Exchange, 1 bar: ⅓ bread, ½ fat
Each serving contains: Calories: 46, Carbohydrates: 10 g

Delight Bar Cookies

1¾ c.	flour	440 mL
1 t.	baking powder	5 mL
½ t.	cloves, ground	2 mL
⅓ c.	cocoa	90 mL
⅓ c.	granulated brown sugar replacement	90 mL
¼ c.	sorbitol	60 mL
4	eggs, well beaten	4
1 c.	dried apricots, finely chopped	250 mL
¼ c.	walnuts, chopped	60 mL
	Powdered Sugar Replacement	

Sift flour, baking powder, cloves, and cocoa together. Gradually, beat brown sugar replacement, and sorbitol into eggs. Add dry ingredients. Fold in apricots and walnuts. Spread in three, greased 9 in. (23 cm) sq. pans. Bake at 350°F (175°C) for 25 to 30 minutes. Dust lightly with powdered sugar replacement. Cut into 1 × 3 in. (2.5 × 7.5 cm) bars.

Yield: 81 bars

Exchange, 1 bar: ¼ bread, ¼ fat
Each serving contains: Calories: 20, Carbohydrates: 4 g

Frosted Coffee Creams

½ c.	vegetable shortening	125 mL
¼ c.	granulated brown sugar replacement	60 mL
¼ c.	granulated sugar replacement	60 mL
1 oz.	baking chocolate, melted	30 g
2	eggs	2
1½ c.	flour	375 mL
¼ t.	salt	1 mL
½ t.	baking soda	2 mL
½ t.	baking powder	2 mL
½ t.	nutmeg	2 mL
½ c.	cold strong coffee	125 mL
½ t.	vanilla extract	2 mL
7 oz. pkg.	no-sugar white frosting mix	198 g pkg.
¼ c.	hot coffee	60 mL

Cream shortening; add sugar replacements and continue beating. Beat in melted chocolate and eggs until fluffy. Sift together flour, salt, baking soda, baking powder, and nutmeg. Add to creamed mixture alternately with cold coffee. Add vanilla extract. Spread in greased 15½ × 10½ in. (39 × 25 cm) pan. Bake at 350°F (175°C) 20 to 25 minutes. Cool. Pour frosting mix into mixing bowl; gradually add hot coffee. Beat until smooth. Spread on cooled dough. Cut into 1½ in. (4 cm) squares.

Yield: 70 squares

Exchange, 1 square: ¼ bread, ¾ fat
Each serving contains: Calories: 43, Carbohydrates: 6 g

Afternoon Tea Brownies

1 c.	cake flour	250 mL
½ t.	salt	2 mL
1 t.	baking powder	5 mL
2 T.	cocoa	30 mL
1 oz.	baking chocolate, melted	30 g
¼ c.	vegetable shortening	60 mL
3	eggs	3
½ c.	granulated sugar replacement	125 mL
½ c.	skim milk	125 mL
½ c.	pecans, toasted and ground	125 mL

Sift flour, salt, baking powder and cocoa together. Pour melted chocolate over shortening and stir until completely blended. Beat eggs until thick and lemon-colored; gradually add sugar replacement. Add chocolate mixture and small amount of flour mixture. Beat to thoroughly blend. Add remaining flour mixture alternately with the milk.

Fold in the pecans. Spread in two 8 in. (20 cm) greased and paper-lined pans. Bake at 325°F (165°C) for 17 to 20 minutes. Cut into 1 × 2 in. (2.5 × 5 cm) bars.

Yield: 64 bars

Exchange, 2 bars: ⅓ bread, 1 fat
Each serving contains: Calories: 54, Carbohydrates: 8 g

Goodlies

The name for this treat is an inside joke. In our home, whenever we taste foods that everyone likes, we call them "goodlies." Ages 8 to 80 love them.

1 c.	cake flour	250 mL
⅓ c.	granulated sugar replacement	90 mL
2½ c.	oatmeal	625 mL
1 c.	margarine, softened	256 mL
¾ c.	chocolate topping	190 mL

Combine cake flour, sugar replacement, and oatmeal in a bowl; cut in margarine until all ingredients are blended into a crumbly dough. Press one-half of the dough into the bottom of a 11 × 7 in. (27 × 17 cm) well greased pan. Spread ½ c. (125 mL) of the chocolate topping over the entire surface. Sprinkle with remaining dough and gently press the top dough. Drizzle with remaining chocolate topping. Bake at 350°F (175°C) for 25 to 30 minutes. Cool slightly. Cut into 1 in. (2.5 cm) squares.

Yield: 77 squares

Exchange, 1 square: ¼ bread, ½ fat
Each serving contains: Calories: 32, Carbohydrates: 5 g

Date Brownies

¾ c.	cake flour	190 mL
½ t.	baking powder	2 mL
dash	salt	dash
½ c.	dates, finely chopped	125 mL
½ c.	vegetable shortening, softened	125 mL
½ c.	granulated sugar replacement	125 mL
2	eggs	2
2 t.	vanilla extract	10 mL
1 oz.	baking chocolate, melted	30 g
	Powdered Sugar Replacement	

Sift flour, baking powder, and salt together. Stir chopped dates into flour mixture. Cream shortening and gradually add sugar replacement. Beat until light and fluffy. Continue beating and add eggs and vanilla extract. Beat in chocolate. Stir in flour-date mixture. Spread evenly in a greased 8 in. (20 cm) pan. Bake at 350°F (175°C) for 25 to 30 minutes. Cool and dust lightly with powdered sugar replacement. Cut into 1 × 2 in. (2.5 × 5 cm) bars.

Yield: 32 bars

Exchange, 1 bar: ⅓ bread, 1 fat
Each serving contains: Calories: 54, Carbohydrates: 10 g

Pineapple-Nut Brownies

1 c.	flour	250 mL
½ t.	baking powder	2 mL
¼ t.	baking soda	1 mL
¼ t.	salt	1 mL
½ c.	margarine	125 mL
1 oz.	baking chocolate	30 g
½ c.	granulated sugar replacement	125 mL
2	eggs, beaten	2
8 oz. can	crushed, canned pineapple, drained	227 g can
1 t.	almond extract	5 mL
⅓ c.	walnuts, chopped	90 mL

Sift flour, baking powder, baking soda, and salt together. In the top of a double boiler, melt margarine and baking chocolate; blend in sugar replacement. Remove from heat. Beat in eggs, pineapple, and almond extract. Stir in flour mixture until well blended. Fold in walnuts. Pour into a greased 8 in. (20 cm) sq. pan. Bake at 350°F (175°C) for 30 to 35 minutes. Cool and cut into 1 × 2 in. (2.5 × 5 cm) bars.

Yield: 32 bars

Exchange, 1 bar: ⅓ bread, 1 fat
Each serving contains: Calories: 60, Carbohydrates: 8 g

Café-au-Lait Squares

4 envs.	unflavored gelatin	4 envs.
1 c.	skim milk	250 mL
1½ c.	strong coffee	375 mL
6 T.	semisweet chocolate chips (use low-fatchips, if available)	90 mL
6 pkgs.	saccharin or acesulfame-K sugar substitute	6 pkgs.
1½ t.	vanilla extract	8 mL

Put the unflavored gelatin into a medium mixing bowl. Add the skim milk. Stir and set aside. In a small saucepan, bring the coffee to a boil. Pour over the gelatin. Stir until the gelatin is completely dissolved. Add the other ingredients. Coat an 8 in. (20 cm) sq. baking pan with non-stick vegetable spray. Pour the batter into the pan. Chill until firm. Cut into 9 squares.

Yield: 9 squares

Exchange, 1 square: ½ high fat meat; ½ fruit
Each serving contains: Calories: 81, Total fat: 3 g, Carbohydrates: 10 g, Protein: 4 g, Sodium: 27 mg, Cholesterol: 0 mg

English Toffee Squares

A sweet and nutty taste.

1 t.	salt	5 mL
1 t.	cinnamon	5 mL
2 c.	cake flour	500 mL
¾ c.	butter	190 mL
½ c.	granulated sugar replacement	125 mL
1 oz.	baking chocolate, melted	30 g
1	egg yolk	1
2 t.	vanilla extract	10 mL
½ c	pecans, finely chopped	125 mL
1	egg white	1

Sift together salt, cinnamon, and flour. Cream butter and sugar replacement. Beat in baking chocolate and egg yolk. Add sifted dry ingredients and mix. Add vanilla extract and pecans. Mix well, press dough into a greased 14 × 10 in. (35 × 25 cm) cookie sheet. Beat egg white until frothy. Spread egg white over dough in pan. Bake at 375°F (190°C) for 25 minutes. Cut into 2 in. (5 cm) squares.

Yield: 35 squares

Exchange, 1 square: ⅓ bread, 1 fat
Each serving contains: Calories: 74, Carbohydrates: 10 g

Black Forest Bars

16 oz. can	sour cherries, pitted	454 g can
8 oz. pkg.	no-sugar chocolate cake mix	266 g pkg.
2 T.	granulated sugar replacement	30 mL

Drain cherries very well. Combine cake mix, cherries and sugar replacement in mixing bowl. Stir to blend thoroughly. Spread batter in well greased 9 in. (23 cm) pan. Bake at 375°F (190°C) for 20 to 25 minutes. Cut into 1 × 1½ in. (2.5 × 4 cm) bars.

Yield: 54 bars

Exchange, 1 bar: ¼ bread
Each serving contains: Calories: 20, Carbohydrates: 4 g

Blond Brownies

8 oz. pkg.	no-sugar white cake mix	226 g pkg.
2	eggs	2
2 T.	granulated brown sugar replacement	30 mL
2 T.	water	30 mL
¼ c.	mini chocolate chips	60 mL
¼ c.	peanut butter chips	60 mL

Combine cake mix, eggs, brown sugar replacement and water in mixing bowl. Beat at medium speed until well blended and thickened. Fold in chips. Pour batter into two, greased and papered 8 in. (20 cm) pans. Bake at 375°F (190°C) for 12 to 15 minutes or until brownies test done. Cut into 2 in. (5 cm) squares.

Yield: 32 squares

Exchange, 1 square: ¼ bread, ½ fat
Each serving contains: Calories: 56, Carbohydrates: 8 g

Pistachio Bars

8 oz. pkg.	sugar-restricted chocolate cake mix	226 g pkg.
⅓ c.	hot water	90 mL
⅓ c.	pistachio nuts, finely chopped	90 mL

Combine all ingredients and stir to completely blend. Spread batter evenly in a greased and papered 8 in. (20 cm) pan. Bake at 350°F (175°C) for 20 to 25 minutes. Cool slightly; cut into 1 in. (2.5 cm) squares.

Yield: 32 squares

Exchange, 1 square: ⅓ bread, ¼ fat
Each serving contains: Calories: 35, Carbohydrates: 6 g

Chinese Chews

¼ c.	cake flour	190 mL
¾ t.	baking powder	4 mL
3 T.	granulated sugar replacement	45 mL
⅛ t.	salt	1 mL
1 c.	dates, finely chopped	250 mL
1 c.	walnuts, finely chopped	250 mL
¼ c.	water	60 mL

Sift together cake flour, baking powder, sugar replacement, and salt. Add dates and walnuts. Slowly add water and stir to make a soft dough. Spread in well greased 8 in. (20 cm) sq. pan. Bake at 350°F (175°C) for about 40 minutes. Score into 1 in. (2.5 cm) squares while warm.

Yield: 64 cookies

Exchange, 1 cookie: ⅓ bread
Each serving contains: Calories: 24, Carbohydrates: 5 g

Cherry Bars

Crust

1 c.	flour	250 mL
⅓ c.	butter	90 mL
2 T.	Powdered Sugar Replacement	30 mL

Filling

½ c.	sour cherries, fresh or well drained	125 mL
2	eggs	2
¼ c.	granulated brown sugar replacement	60 mL
½ c.	unsweetened coconut, grated	125 mL
2 T.	flour	30 mL
½ t.	baking powder	2 mL
½ t.	salt	2 mL
1 t.	vanilla extract	5 mL

Combine ingredients. Work with pastry blender or food processor until mixture is the texture of coarse crumbs. Press into bottom of 13 × 9 in. (33 × 23 cm) lightly greased cookie sheet. Bake at 350°F (175°C) for 12 to 15 minutes. Cool.

Pit and chop cherries. Beat eggs, and stir in chopped cherries and remaining ingredients until well blended. Pour over baked crust, spreading evenly. Bake at 350°F (175°C) for 25 minutes, or until set. Cool slightly. While warm, cut into 48 bars with a sharp knife.

Yield: 48 cookies

Exchange, 2 cookies: ⅓ bread, 1 fat
Each serving contains: Calories: 62, Carbohydrates: 10 g

Currant Bars

½ c.	low-calorie margarine	125 mL
¼ c.	granulated fructose	60 mL
1 t.	finely grated lemon peel	5 mL
1	egg	1
1	egg white	1
1¼ c.	all-purpose flour	310 mL
¼ t.	baking powder	1 mL
⅓ c.	currants	90 mL
¼ c.	sliced almonds	60 mL
2 t.	aspartame sweetener	10 mL

Beat margarine until light and fluffy. Scrape down bowl; then add fructose and beat for at least 1 minute. Mixture should be creamy. Beat in lemon peel and egg. Beat in egg white. Combine flour and baking powder in a bowl; stir to mix. Add to creamed mixture, and beat until completely blended. Lightly spray a 13 × 9 in. (33 × 23 cm) cookie sheet or pan with vegetable-oil spray. Transfer cookie dough to pan. Spread evenly over bottom of pan. To ease spreading, dampen a knife in a glass of hot water. Sprinkle surface of dough with currants and almonds; press them into the dough. Bake at 350°F (175°C) for 12 to 13 minutes. Remove pan from oven. Sprinkle with aspartame sweetener. Cut into 35 bars. Cool in pan on a rack. Remove bars from pan when cool.

Yield: 35 bars

Exchange, 1 bar: ⅓ bread, ½ fat
Each serving contains: Calories: 56, Carbohydrates: 5 g

Mixed Fruit Squares

1 c.	all-purpose flour	250 mL
1 c.	quick-cooking oatmeal	250 mL
⅓ c.	granulated fructose	90 mL
¼ t.	baking soda	1 mL
½ c.	soft margarine	125 mL
¾ c.	cold water	190 mL
1 T.	cornstarch	15 mL
1 c.	unsweetened dried mixed fruit	250 mL

Combine flour, oatmeal, fructose, and baking soda in a large mixing bowl; stir to mix. Cut in the margarine until mixture is coarse crumbs. Remove ½ c. (125 mL) and set aside. Press remaining crumbs into an ungreased 9 in. (23 cm) shiny baking pan. Combine cold water and cornstarch in a small saucepan. Stir to blend. Add mixed dried fruit. Stir and cook over medium heat until mixture is thick and bubbly. Spread over crumb layer in pan. Sprinkle reserved crumbs over fruit mixture. Lightly press top crumbs into fruit layer. Bake at 350°F (175°C) for 30 minutes. Cool in pan on a wire rack. Cut into 25 squares.

Yield: 25 squares

Exchange, 1 square: 1 bread
Each serving contains: Calories: 89, Carbohydrates: 14 g

Lemon Poppy Seed Bars

2 c.	pancake mix	500 mL
8 oz. carton	lemon yogurt	224 g carton
2	eggs	2
¼ c.	cooking oil	60 mL
2 T.	poppy seeds	30 mL

Combine pancake mix, lemon yogurt, eggs, and cooking oil in a mixing bowl. Mix until blended. Beat for 2 more minutes. Stir in poppy seeds. Pour into a greased 13 × 9 in. (33 × 23 cm) baking pan. Bake at 350°F (175°C) for 25 to 30 minutes or until toothpick inserted in middle comes out clean. Cut into 32 bars.

Yield: 32 bars

Exchange, 1 bar: ⅓ bread, ⅓ fat
Each serving contains: Calories: 42, Carbohydrates: 5 g

Spiced Fruit Bars

⅓ c.	low-calorie margarine	90 mL
¼ c.	creamy peanut butter	60 mL
1¼ c.	all-purpose flour	310 mL
¼ c.	granulated fructose	60 mL
8 oz. pkg.	light cream cheese, softened	227 g pkg.
1 T.	water	15 mL
2 T.	all-purpose flour	30 mL
1 t.	ground cinnamon	5 mL
½ t.	ground nutmeg	2 mL
3	egg whites	3
½ c.	unsweetened dried mixed fruit, finely chopped	125 mL

Combine margarine and peanut butter in a medium-size mixing bowl. Beat to blend. Add half of the ¼ c. (310 mL) of flour and the ¼ c. (60 mL) of fructose. Beat well (mixture will stick to the beaters of the mixer). Push mixture from beaters, and add remaining flour. Beat until mixture is fine crumbs. Transfer to a 13 × 9 in. (33 × 23 cm.) ungreased, shiny baking pan. Bake at 350°F (175°C) for 15 minutes or until surface is lightly browned. Meanwhile, combine cream cheese, water, the 2 T. (30 mL) of flour, cinnamon, and nutmeg in a mixing bowl. (The same bowl can be used.) Beat until well blended. Add the egg whites; beat until thoroughly combined. Stir in the mixed fruit. Pour over the baked dough. Return to oven, and bake for 15 more minutes or until cream cheese mixture is set. Remove from oven to cooling rack. Cool completely. Cut into 48 bars.

Yield: 48 bars

Exchange, 1 bar: ⅓ bread, ¼ fat
Each serving contains: Calories: 32, Carbohydrates: 5 g

Rice Bars with Chocolate Chips

¼ c.	cold water	60 mL
1 env.	unflavored gelatin	1 env.
1 T.	granulated fructose	15 mL
1 T.	granulated sugar replacement	15 mL
2 T.	margarine	30 mL
1	egg white	1
6 c.	crisp rice cereal	1500 mL
½ c.	mini chocolate chips	125 mL

In a microwavable bowl or saucepan, sprinkle the gelatin over the cold water; then allow the gelatin to soften for 5 minutes. Heat until gelatin is completely dissolved. Remove from heat. Add fructose, sugar replacement, and margarine. Stir to dissolve fructose and melt margarine. Allow mixture to cool to a thick syrup. Beat egg white to soft peaks. Continue beating the egg white, and pour the gelatin mixture in a thin stream into it. (Mixture will not fluff up.) Place rice cereal in a large bowl. Thoroughly fold egg white gelatin mixture into cereal. Fold in chocolate chips. Transfer to a lightly greased 13 × 9 in. (33 × 23 cm.) cake pan. Cool. Cut into 24 bars.

Yield: 24 bars

Exchange, 1 bar: ⅓ bread
Each serving contains: Calories: 23, Carbohydrates: 4 g

Walnut Rice Bars

¼ c.	cold water	60 mL
1 env.	unflavored gelatin	1 env.
1 T.	granulated fructose	15 mL
1 T.	granulated sugar replacement	15 mL
2 T.	margarine	30 mL
1	egg white	1
6 c.	crisp rice cereal	1500 mL
½ c.	coarsely chopped walnuts	125 mL

In a microwavable bowl or saucepan, sprinkle the gelatin over the cold water; then allow the gelatin to soften for 5 minutes. Heat until gelatin is completely dissolved. Remove from heat. Add fructose, sugar replacement, and margarine. Stir to dissolve fructose and melt margarine. Allow mixture to cool to a thick syrup. Beat egg white to soft peaks. Continue beating the egg white, and pour the gelatin mixture in a thin stream into it. (Mixture will not fluff up.) Place rice cereal in a large bowl. Thoroughly fold egg white gelatin mixture into cereal. Fold in walnuts. Transfer to a lightly greased 13 × 9 in. (33 × 23 cm) cake pan. Cool. Cut into 24 bars.

Yield: 24 bars

Exchange, 1 bar: ⅓ bread, ¼ fat
Each serving contains: Calories: 29, Carbohydrates: 3 g

Date Custard Bars

Base

¼ c.	margarine	60 mL
1 c.	all-purpose flour	250 mL

Filling

2	eggs	2
1 T.	granulated fructose	15 mL
3 T.	granulated sugar replacement	45 mL
1 t.	vanilla extract	5 mL
½ c.	finely chopped dates	125 mL
1 T.	all-purpose flour	15 mL
⅛ t.	baking powder	½ mL

Base: Cut margarine into flour in a bowl until mixture crumbles. Press crumb mixture into an ungreased 7 × 11 in. (17 × 27 cm) baking pan. Bake at 350°F (175°C) for 12 to 15 minutes, or until lightly browned.

Filling: Beat eggs in a bowl until light and lemon-colored. Gradually beat in fructose, sugar replacement, and vanilla extract. Combine dates and flour in a bowl; then flip or stir to cover all date pieces lightly with the flour. Stir dates and baking powder into custard mixture. Spread mixture over baked base. Return to oven, and continue baking for 20 minutes more, or until surface is lightly tanned. Cool on rack. Cut into 45 bars.

Yield: 45 bars

Exchange, 1 bar: ⅓ bread, ⅓ fat
Each serving contains: Calories: 41, Carbohydrates: 3 g

Butterscotch Bars

1 c.	all-purpose flour	250 mL
1 t.	baking powder	5 mL
dash	salt	dash
¼ c.	melted margarine	60 mL
½ c.	granulated brown sugar replacement	125 mL
1	egg	1
1 t.	vanilla extract	5 mL
1 t.	liquid butter flavoring	5 mL

Sift together flour, baking powder, and salt. Set aside. Combine margarine and brown sugar replacement in a bowl. Beat or stir to blend. Add egg, vanilla extract, and liquid butter flavoring. Mix well. Gradually stir flour mixture into margarine mixture. Lightly grease an 8 × 8 in. (20 × 20 cm) baking pan with vegetable oil spray. Spread mixture into bottom of pan. Bake at 350°F (175°C) for 30 minutes, or until top springs back when touched. Cool in pan on cooling rack. Cut into 36 bars.

Yield: 36 bars

Exchange, 1 bar: ¼ bread
Each serving contains: Calories: 22, Carbohydrates: 2 g

Oatmeal Applesauce Bars

Filling

2 T.	margarine	30 mL
¾ c.	unsweetened applesauce	190 mL
1 t.	vanilla extract	5 mL
1 t.	apple-pie spices	5 mL
2 t.	cornstarch	10 mL

Base

½ c.	margarine	125 mL
¼ c.	fructose	60 mL
2 T.	granulated sugar replacement	30 mL
1	egg	1
1 t.	vanilla extract	5 mL
1 t.	apple-pie spices	5 mL
¾ c.	all-purpose flour	190 mL
½ t.	baking soda	2 mL
2 c.	quick-cooking oatmeal	500 mL

Filling: Combine margarine, applesauce, vanilla extract, apple-pie spices, and cornstarch in a saucepan. Stir to completely dissolve cornstarch. Place saucepan over medium heat, and stir until mixture comes to a full rolling boil. Remove from heat. Stir occasionally until mixture has cooled.

Base: Cream margarine, fructose, and sugar replacement. Beat in egg, vanilla extract, and apple-pie spices. Add flour and baking soda. Beat well. Blend in 1¾ c. (440 mL) of the oatmeal. Press three-fourths of the base mixture into the bottom of a 9 × 9 in. (23 × 23 cm) shiny baking pan. Spread with cooled applesauce filling. Add remaining ¼ c. (60 mL) of the oatmeal to the remaining base mixture. Crumb with a fork or with your hands. Sprinkle crumb mixture over cookie surface. Bake at 350°F (175°C) for 25 to 30 minutes. Cool on cooling rack. Cut into 36 bars.

Yield: 36 bars

Exchange, 1 bar: ½ bread, ¾ fat
Each serving contains: Calories: 73, Carbohydrates: 9 g

Oatmeal Chocolate Bars

Filling

2 T.	margarine	30 mL
½ c.	semisweet chocolate chips	125 mL
¾ c.	evaporated milk	190 mL
1 T.	chocolate flavoring	15 mL
2 t.	cornstarch	10 mL

Base

½ c.	margarine	125 mL
¼ c.	fructose	60 mL
2 T.	granulated sugar replacement	30 mL
1	egg	1
1 t.	vanilla extract	5 mL
1 c.	all-purpose flour	250 mL
½ t.	baking soda	2 mL
2 c.	quick-cooking oatmeal	500 mL

Filling: Combine margarine, chocolate chips, evaporated milk, chocolate flavoring, and cornstarch in saucepan. Stir to completely dissolve cornstarch. Place saucepan over medium heat, and stir until mixture comes to a full rolling boil. Remove from heat. Stir occasionally until mixture has cooled.

Base: Cream margarine, fructose, and sugar replacement. Beat in egg and vanilla extract. Add flour and baking soda. Beat well. Blend in ¾ c. (440 mL) of the oatmeal. Press three-fourths of the base mixture into the bottom of a 9 × 9 in. (23 × 23 cm) shiny baking pan. Spread with cooled chocolate filling. Add remaining ¼ c. (60 mL) of the oatmeal to the remaining base mixture. Crumb with a fork or your hands. Sprinkle crumb mixture over cookie surface. Bake at 350°F (175°C) for 25 to 30 minutes. Cool on cooling rack. Cut into 36 bars.

Yield: 36 bars

Exchange, 1 bar: ½ bread, ¾ fat
Each serving contains: Calories: 72, Carbohydrates: 8 g

Butterscotch Brownies

1 c.	all-purpose flour	250 mL
1 t.	baking powder	5 mL
dash	salt	dash
¼ c.	melted margarine	60 mL
½ c.	granulated brown sugar replacement	125 mL
1	egg	1
1 t.	vanilla extract	5 mL
1 t.	liquid butter flavoring	5 mL
2 oz.	semisweet baking chocolate	58 g
2 T.	margarine	30 mL

Sift together flour, baking powder, and salt. Set aside. Combine the ¼ c. (60 mL) of melted margarine and brown sugar replacement in a bowl. Beat or stir to blend. Add egg, vanilla extract, and liquid butter flavoring. Mix well. Gradually stir flour mixture into margarine mixture. Lightly grease an 8 × 8 in. (20 × 20 cm) baking pan with vegetable oil spray. Spread mixture into bottom of pan. Bake at 350°F (175°C) for 30 minutes, or until top springs backed when touched. Cool in pan on cooling rack. Melt semisweet baking chocolate and the 2 T. (30 mL) of margarine in a small saucepan over low heat. Cool slightly; then pour and spread over top. Allow to cool. Cut into 36 brownies.

Yield: 36 brownies

Exchange, 1 brownie: ¼ bread, ¼ fat
Each serving contains: Calories: 29, Carbohydrates: 2 g

Lemon Coconut Bars

Base

¼ c.	margarine	60 mL
1 c.	all-purpose flour	250 mL

Filling

2	eggs	2
1 T.	granulated fructose	15 mL
3 T.	granulated sugar replacement	45 mL
1 t.	vanilla extract	5 mL
¾ c.	unsweetened coconut*	190 mL
⅛ t.	baking powder	½ mL

Lemon Icing

¼ c.	granulated fructose	60 mL
3 T.	granulated sugar replacement	45 mL
1 T.	cornstarch	15 mL
2 t.	aspartame sweetener	5 mL
1 t.	grated lemon rind	5 mL
	lemon juice	

Base: Cut margarine into flour in a bowl until mixture crumbles. Press crumb mixture into an ungreased 7 × 11 in. (17 × 27 cm) baking pan. Bake at 350°F (175°C) for 12 to 15 minutes, or until lightly browned.

Filling: Beat eggs in a bowl until light and lemon-colored. Gradually beat in fructose, sugar replacement, and vanilla extract. Stir in coconut and baking powder. Spread mixture over baked base. Return to oven, and continue baking for 20 minutes more, or until surface is lightly tanned. Cool on rack.

Icing: Combine fructose, sugar replacement, cornstarch, and aspartame sweetener in a small food-blender container. Blend, turning the blender from High to off for about 10 seconds. Pour mixture into a small mixing bowl. Add lemon rind. Stir in just enough lemon juice to make mixture smooth and of a thick liquid consistency. Drizzle over cooled base and filling; then cut into 45 bars.

Yield: 45 bars

Exchange, 1 bar: ¼ bread, ¼ fat
Each serving contains: Calories: 29, Carbohydrates: 2 g

*Unsweetened coconut can be bought at most health food stores.

Cherry Vanilla Bars

8 oz. pkg.	pound cake mix, fructose-sweetened	227 g pkg.
3 T.	low-fat cherry vanilla yogurt	45 mL
1	cherry flavoring	5 mL
1	egg white	1
2 T.	chopped dried cherries*	30 mL

Combine cake mix, yogurt, cherry flavoring, and egg white in a bowl. Stir to mix thoroughly. Fold in dried cherries. Spread evenly in the bottom of a 9 × 9 in. (23 × 23 cm) baking pan. Bake at 350°F (175°C) for 20 to 25 minutes. Allow to cool in pan. Cut into 36 bars.

Yield: 36 bars

Exchange, 1 bar: 1⅓ bread
Each serving contains: Calories: 27, Carbohydrates: 4 g

*Chopped dried cherries can be bought at health food stores.

Cinnamon Brownies

2 c.	all-purpose flour	500 mL
½ c.	granulated sugar replacement	125 mL
¼ c.	granulated fructose	60 mL
1 t.	baking soda	5 mL
dash	salt	dash
¾ t.	ground cinnamon	4 mL
1 c.	margarine	250 mL
1 c.	water	250 mL
3 T.	baking cocoa	45 mL
½ c.	buttermilk	125 mL
2	eggs	2
2 t.	vanilla extract	10 mL

Sift together flour, sugar replacement, fructose, baking soda, salt, and cinnamon. Combine margarine, water, and baking cocoa in a saucepan. Cook over low heat until margarine is melted. Beat cocoa mixture into dry flour mixture. Add buttermilk, eggs, and vanilla extract. Beat for 2 minutes. Grease a 15 × 10 in. (39 × 25 cm) jelly-roll pan. Pour brownie mixture into pan, spreading evenly. Bake at 350°F (175°C) for 25 minutes, or until top springs back when lightly touched. Cool slightly in pan before cutting into 50 brownies.

Yield: 50 brownies

Exchange, 1 brownie: ⅓ bread
Each serving contains: Calories: 37, Carbohydrates: 4 g

Pear Bars

16 oz. can	pears in juice	454 g can
2 c.	all-purpose flour	500 mL
¾ c.	granulated sugar replacement	190 mL
⅓ c.	granulated fructose	90 mL
2 t.	baking soda	10 mL
2	eggs	2
¼ c.	margarine, softened	60 mL

Drain juice from pears into a large mixing bowl; reserve juice. Cut pears into chunks, and place into bowl with juice. Add flour, sugar replacement, fructose, baking soda, eggs, and margarine. Beat well, at least 2 minutes. Pour batter into a greased 13 × 9 in. (33 × 23 cm) baking pan. Bake at 350°F (175°C) for 30 to 35 minutes or until toothpick inserted in middle comes out clean. Cool. Cut into 32 bars.

Yield: 32 bars

Exchange, 1 bar: ½ bread, ¼ fat
Each serving contains: Calories: 45, Carbohydrates: 7 g

Pineapple Oatmeal Bars

Base

1 c.	quick-cooking oatmeal	250 mL
½ c.	all-purpose flour	125 mL
2 T.	granulated fructose	30 mL
¼ t.	baking soda	1 mL
dash	salt	dash
⅓ c.	margarine	90 mL

Filling

8 oz. can	crushed pineapple in juice	227 g can
1 T.	cornstarch	15 mL
3 T.	granulated sugar replacement	45 mL
¼ c.	low-fat milk	60 mL
1	egg yolk	1
1 t.	pineapple flavoring	5 mL

Base: Combine oatmeal flour, fructose, baking soda, and salt in a mixing bowl. Cut and work margarine into dry mixture until mixture is in small crumbs. Lightly grease a 11 × 7 in. (17 × 27 cm) baking pan with vegetable oil spray. Press three-fourths of the mixture into the bottom the pan. Reserve remaining base for topping.

Filling: Combine pineapple with juice, cornstarch, sugar replacement, milk, and egg yolk in a saucepan. Cook over medium heat, stirring constantly, until mixture is thick. Remove from heat. Stir in pineapple flavoring. Pour filling over base. Sprinkle with reserved base. Bake at 375°F (190°C) for 30 minutes, or until topping is set. Cool in pan on rack. Cut into 40 bars.

Yield: 40 bars

Exchange, 1 bar: ⅓ bread
Each serving contains: Calories: 22, Carbohydrates: 3 g

Great Banana Bars

Base

1 c.	all-purpose flour	250 mL
¼ c.	margarine	60 mL

Filling

2	very ripe bananas	2
2	eggs	2
1 t.	vanilla extract	5 mL
1 T.	all-purpose flour	15 mL
	Optional: banana flavoring	

Base: Cut margarine into flour until mixture crumbles. Press crumb mixture into an ungreased 7 × 11 in. (17 × 27 cm) baking pan.

Filling: Place bananas in a medium-size mixing bowl. Using an electric mixer, mash bananas until creamy. Add eggs and beat thoroughly. Beat in vanilla extract and flour. If desired, add banana flavoring. Pour mixture over base. Bake at 350°F (175°C) for 25 minutes. Cool on rack. Cut into 40 bars.

Yield: 40 bars

Exchange, 1 bar: ⅓ fruit, ¼ fat
Each serving contains: Calories: 25, Carbohydrates: 4 g

Apricot Bars

Filling

16 oz. can	apricot halves in juice	454 g can
1 T.	white grape juice concentrate	15 mL
2 T.	granulated sugar replacement	30 mL
1 T.	cornstarch	15 mL
1 t.	almond flavoring	5 mL
1 drop	red food coloring	1 drop
1 drop	yellow food coloring	1 drop

Base

½ c.	quick-cooking oatmeal	125 mL
½ c.	all-purpose flour	125 mL
¼ c.	margarine	60 mL

Filling: Drain ½ c. (125 mL) of the juice from the apricots into a small saucepan. Thoroughly drain remaining apricots. Reserve apricot halves. Add grape juice concentrate, sugar replacement, and cornstarch to saucepan. Stir to thoroughly dissolve cornstarch. Place over medium heat, and cook until mixture comes to a full boil, stirring constantly. Boil for 5 minutes, stirring constantly. Remove from heat. Add almond flavoring and food coloring. Set aside to cool.

Base: Combine oatmeal, flour, and margarine in a bowl. Cut and work margarine into dry mixture until mixture is in small crumbs. Lightly grease an 8 × 8 in. (20 × 20 cm) baking pan with vegetable oil spray. Press mixture into the bottom of the pan. Bake at 350°F (175°C) for 10 minutes. Remove from oven. Place apricot halves over entire surface of base. Pour apricot filling over surface. Return to oven, and bake for 35 minutes or until filling is set. Cool on rack. Cut into 36 bars.

Yield: 36 bars

Exchange, 1 bar: ⅓ fruit, ¼ fat
Each serving contains: Calories: 29, Carbohydrates: 4 g

Old Fashioned Apple Bars

1 c.	all-purpose flour	250 mL
1 t.	baking powder	5 mL
1 t.	ground cinnamon	5 mL
½ t.	baking soda	2 mL
½ t.	ground nutmeg	2 mL
¼ t.	ground cloves	1 mL
⅔ c.	margarine	165 mL
½ c.	granulated sugar replacement	125 mL
¼ c.	granulated fructose	60 mL
2	eggs	2
1 c.	diced pared apples	250 mL
¾ c.	quick-cooking oatmeal	190 mL
⅓ c.	chopped walnuts	90 mL

Sift together flour, baking powder, cinnamon, baking soda, nutmeg, and cloves; set aside. Cream margarine, sugar replacement, and fructose in a mixing bowl, using an electric mixer at Medium speed. Add eggs, one at a time, beating well after each addition. Gradually add dry ingredients to creamed mixture, beating well after each addition, using an electric mixer at Low speed. Stir in diced apples, oatmeal, and walnuts. Spread batter into a greased 9 × 13 in. (23 × 33 cm.) baking pan. Bake at 350°17 (175°C) for 25 to 30 minutes or until top springs back when touched. Cool in pan on rack. Cut into 48 bars.

Yield: 48 bars

Exchange, 1 bar: ¼ bread, ½ fat
Each serving contains: Calories: 46, Carbohydrates: 3 g

Banana Oat Bran Squares

2	very ripe bananas	2
1	egg, slightly beaten	1
3 T.	granulated sugar replacement	45 mL
1 t.	vanilla extract	5 mL
½ c.	all-purpose flour	125 mL
1 c.	oat bran flour	250 mL
1 t.	baking powder	5 mL
¼ t.	baking soda	1 mL
⅓ c.	coarsely chopped walnuts	90 mL

Slightly whip bananas in a bowl. Add beaten egg, sugar replacement, and vanilla. Beat just until blended. Stir in flours, baking powder, and baking soda thoroughly. Spray a 9 × 9 in. (23 × 23 cm) baking pan with vegetable oil spray. Spread batter into the bottom of the pan. Sprinkle with the walnuts. Bake at 350°F (175°C) for 18 to 25 minutes or until toothpick inserted in middle comes out clean. Remove from oven, cool on rack, and cut into 36 squares.

Yield: 36 squares

Exchange, 1 square: ⅓ bread
Each serving contains: Calories: 23, Carbohydrates: 5 g

Popular Raspberry Bars

½ c.	margarine	125 mL
¼ c.	granulated sugar replacement	60 mL
¼ c.	granulated fructose	60 mL
1 t.	almond flavoring	5 mL
1	egg	1
1 c.	all-purpose flour	250 mL
½ c.	quick-cooking oatmeal	125 mL
½ t.	baking powder	2 mL
dash each	salt and ground cloves	dash each
½ c.	all-fruit raspberry preserves	125 mL

Beat margarine, sugar replacement, and fructose together until well blended. Beat in almond flavoring and egg. Mix together flour, oatmeal, baking powder, salt, and cloves. Stir into creamed mixture. Spread half of the mixture on the bottom of a greased 9 × 9 in. (23 × 23 cm) baking pan. Spread with the raspberry preserves. Drop remaining batter by teaspoonfuls onto the top of the preserves. Bake at 350°F (175°C) for 25 minutes. Cut into 36 bars. Serve warm.

Yield: 36 bars

Exchange, 1 bar: ⅓ bread, ½ fat
Each serving contains: Calories: 46, Carbohydrates: 5 g

Yogurt Brownie Bars

8 oz. pkg.	brownie mix, fructose-sweetened	227 g pkg.
3 T.	low-fat plain yogurt	5 mL
½ t.	vanilla extract	2 mL
1	egg white	1

Combine brownie mix, yogurt, vanilla, and egg white in a bowl. Stir to mix thoroughly. Spread evenly in the bottom of a 9 × 9 in. (23 × 23 cm) baking pan. Bake at 350°F (175°C) for 20 to 25 minutes. Allow to cool in pan. Cut into 36 bars.

Yield: 36 bars

Exchange, 1 bar: ½ bread, ½ fat
Each serving contains: Calories: 50, Carbohydrates: 8 g

Granola Bars

1 c.	low-fat granola	250 mL
1 c.	quick-cooking oatmeal	250 mL
½ c.	all-purpose flour	125 mL
1	large egg	1
1	egg white	1
¼ c.	liquid fructose	60 mL
⅓ c.	cooking oil	90 mL
3 T.	granulated brown sugar replacement	45 mL

Combine granola, oatmeal, and flour in a mixing bowl. Stir to blend. Combine egg and egg white in a small bowl or cup. Beat until well blended. Pour into cereal mixture. Add liquid fructose, cooking oil, and brown sugar replacement. Stir thoroughly until the mixture is completely coated with liquid. Completely line an 8 × 8 in. (20 × 20 cm) baking pan with foil. (You'll use this foil to remove cookie mixture from pan.) Grease foil with a vegetable oil spray. Press cookie mixture into the bottom of the pan. Bake at 325°F (165°C) for 30 to 35 minutes, or until lightly browned around the edges. Remove pan from oven. Remove foil with cookie mixture from pan to a rack. Cool. Cut into 25 bars.

Yield: 25 bars

Exchange, 1 bar: ⅔ bread
Each serving contains: Calories: 47, Carbohydrates: 9 g

Lemon Cream Bars

Base

⅓ c.	margarine	90 mL
2 T.	granulated sugar replacement	30 mL
1 c.	all-purpose flour	250 mL

Filling

2	eggs	2
2 T.	all-purpose flour	30 mL
¼ c.	granulated fructose	60 mL
3 T.	granulated sugar replacement	45 mL
3 T.	fresh lemon juice	45 mL
2 t.	finely shredded lemon peel	10 mL
¼ t.	baking powder	2 mL

Base: Combine margarine and sugar replacement in a mixing bowl. Beat to blend. Beat in flour until mixture is crumbly. Press into the bottom of an 8 × 8 in. (20 × 20 cm) baking pan. Bake at 350°F (175°C) for 15 to 17 minutes, or until lightly browned. Remove from oven.

Filling: Combine eggs, flour, fructose, sugar replacement, lemon juice, lemon peel, and baking powder in a mixing bowl. Beat for 2 minutes. Pour over base layer. Return to oven, and bake about 20 minutes more, or until set. Cool on rack. Cut into 25 bars.

Yield: 25 bars

Exchange, 1 bar: ⅓ bread, ½ fat
Each serving contains: Calories: 48, Carbohydrates: 4 g

Prune Bars

¼ c.	margarine	60 mL
1 c.	all-purpose flour	250 mL
½ t.	ground cinnamon	2 mL
2 T.	granulated fructose	30 mL
2 T.	granulated sugar replacement	30 mL
½ c.	orange juice	125 mL
1	egg	1
½ t.	baking powder	2 mL
¼ t.	baking soda	1 mL
½ c.	snipped dried pitted prunes	125 mL

Beat margarine with an electric mixer on High for 30 seconds. Add ½ c. (125 mL) of the flour, cinnamon, fructose, sugar replacement, ¼ c. (60 mL) of the orange juice, egg, baking powder, and baking soda; then continue beating for 1 minute more, or until thoroughly blended. Beat in remaining ½ c. (125 mL) of flour and remaining orange juice. Stir in snipped prunes. Spread cookie batter into the bottom of a 7 × 11 in. (17 × 27 cm) ungreased baking pan. Bake at 350°F (175°C) for 25 minutes, or until toothpick inserted in middle comes out clean. Cool on rack. Cut into 40 bars.

Yield: 40 bars

Exchange, 1 bar: ⅓ bread, ¼ fat
Each serving contains: Calories: 30, Carbohydrates: 3 g

Chocolate and Vanilla Layered Bars

1½ c.	all-purpose flour	375 mL
¼ t.	salt	1 mL
¾ c.	margarine	190 mL
¾ c.	granulated sugar replacement	190 mL
⅓ c.	granulated fructose	90 mL
3	eggs	3
1 t.	vanilla extract	5 mL
1½ oz.	unsweetened chocolate, melted and cooled	43 g

Sift together flour and salt; set aside. Beat margarine, sugar replacement, and fructose until creamy. Add eggs, one at a time, beating well after each addition. Beat in vanilla. Gradually stir flour mixture into creamed mixture. Blend well. Spread two-thirds of the batter on the bottom of a greased 9 in. (23 cm) baking pan. Stir melted chocolate into the remaining cookie batter. Spread chocolate batter evenly over vanilla batter. Bake at 350°F (175°C) for 35 minutes, or until toothpick inserted in middle comes out clean. Allow to cool in pan. Cut into 36 bars.

Yield: 36 bars

Exchange, 1 bar: ⅓ bread, ½ fat
Each serving contains: Calories: 46, Carbohydrates: 5 g

Fig Bars

1½ c.	all-purpose flour	375 mL
¾ c.	Kretschmer wheat germ	190 mL
¼ c.	sugar	60 mL
1½ t.	orange rind, grated	7 mL
¼ t.	salt	1 mL
½ c.	margarine	125 mL
¾ c.	orange juice, divided	190 mL
8 oz.	moist-pack figs	240 g

Combine flour, ½ c. (125 mL) of the wheat germ, sugar, orange rind, and salt in bowl. Stir well to blend. Cut in margarine with pastry blender until mixture looks like fine crumbs. Add ¼ c. (60 mL) of the orange juice, a little at a time, mixing lightly with fork. With your hands, shape into a firm ball. Trim stems from figs. Purée figs in blender container with remaining ½ c. (125 mL) orange juice for 30 seconds. Stir in remaining ¼ c. (60 mL) wheat germ.

Roll out dough into a 14 × 12 in. (35.6 × 30.5 cm) rectangle on a lightly floured cloth-covered board. Cut lengthwise into 3 4-in. (10 cm)wide strips. Place on ungreased baking sheets. Spoon about ⅓ c. (90 mL) of the filling on each strip to within ½ in. (13 mm) of the long edges. Fold dough over to cover filling. Press long edges together with tines of fork. Bake at 350°F (175°C) for 17 to 20 minutes until golden. Remove from baking sheet. Cool on rack. Slice diagonally into 1 in. (2.5 cm) wide strips.

Yield: 36 cookies

Exchange, 1 cookie: ½ bread, ⅓ fruit
Each serving contains: Calories: 45, Carbohydrates: 6 g

With the courtesy of Kretschmer Wheat Germ/International Multifoods.

Date Sandwich Bars

2 c.	pitted dates, snipped	500 mL
1 c.	water	250 mL
1 t.	orange rind, grated	5 mL
2 T.	orange juice	30 mL
1 t.	lemon juice	5 mL
1½ c.	all-purpose flour	375 mL
1½ c.	uncooked oatmeal	375 mL
2 T.	brown sugar replacement	30 mL
1 t.	baking powder	5 mL
½ t.	salt	2 mL
¾ c.	butter	190 mL

Combine dates, water, rind, and juices in a saucepan. Blend well. Cook over low heat, stirring occasionally, until thickened, about 10 minutes. Cool while preparing crumb mixture. Measure flour into a large bowl. Add all remaining ingredients except butter. Stir well to blend. Cut in butter with pastry blender until particles are the size of small peas. Spread half of the crumb mixture in a greased 13 × 9 × 2 in. (33 × 23 × 5 cm) pan. Press down. Spread cooled date filling evenly over mixture in pan. Cover with remaining crumb mixture. Pat down lightly. Bake at 375°F (190°C) for 25 to 30 minutes until golden brown. Cool in pan on rack. Cut into bars.

Yield: 3 dozen bars

Exchange, 1 bar: 1½ fruit, 1 fat
Each serving contains: Calories: 97, Carbohydrates: 11 g

Buttermilk Brownies

2 c.	all-purpose flour	500 mL
¼ c.	granulated fructose	60 mL
¼ c.	granulated sugar replacement	60 mL
1 t.	baking soda	5 mL
dash	salt	dash
¾ c.	margarine	190 mL
1 c.	water	250 mL
⅓ c.	unsweetened baking cocoa	90 mL
2	eggs	2
½ c.	buttermilk	125 mL
2 t.	vanilla extract	10 mL

Combine flour, fructose, sugar replacement, baking soda, and salt in a mixing bowl. Combine margarine, water, and cocoa in a saucepan. Cook and stir over medium heat until mixture begins to boil. Remove from heat. Pour chocolate mixture into flour mixture. Using an electric mixer, beat batter until thoroughly blended. Add eggs, buttermilk, and vanilla extract. Beat for 1 minute. Grease and flour a 15 × 10 in. (39 × 25 cm) jelly-roll pan. Pour batter into pan, and spread evenly on the bottom. Bake at 350°F (175 °C) for 25 minutes, or until toothpick inserted in middle comes out clean. Cut into 50 brownies.

Yield: 50 brownies

Exchange, 1 brownie: ¼ bread, ⅓ fat
Each serving contains: Calories: 51, Carbohydrates: 4 g

Gingerbread Bars

1 c.	all-purpose flour	250 mL
¾ c.	whole wheat flour	190 mL
⅔ c.	granulated sugar replacement	180 mL
1 T.	baking powder	15 mL
½ t.	ground ginger	2 mL
¼ t.	salt	1 mL
¼ t.	ground cloves	1 mL
2	eggs	2
⅔ c.	low-fat milk	180 mL
¼ c.	cooking oil	60 mL
3 T.	molasses*	45 mL

Combine flours, sugar replacement, baking powder, ginger, salt, and cloves in a mixing bowl. Stir to mix. Add eggs, milk, and oil. Beat to blend thoroughly. Beat in molasses. Beat 1 to 2 minutes more. Pour into a greased 13 × 9 in. (33 × 23 cm) baking pan. Bake at 350°F (175°C) for 25 to 30 minutes, or until toothpick inserted in middle comes out clean. Cool. Cut into 32 bars.

Yield: 32 bars

Exchange, 1 bar: ⅓ bread, ⅓ fat
Each serving contains: Calories: 47, Carbohydrates: 5 g

*Because the recipe for these bars calls for molasses, check with your doctor or dietician before baking or eating this dessert.

Orange Oat Bars

1 c.	quick-cooking oatmeal	250 mL
1 c.	orange juice	250 mL
2 c.	uncooked oat bran	500 mL
⅔ c.	all-purpose flour	180 mL
½ c.	nonfat dry milk	125 mL
2 t.	baking powder	10 mL
½ t.	baking soda	2 mL
dash	salt	dash
⅓ c.	granulated sugar replacement	90 mL
⅓ c.	granulated fructose	90 mL
¼ c.	vegetable oil	60 mL
2	eggs	2
2 t.	vanilla extract	10 mL

Soak oatmeal in orange juice in a large bowl for at least 15 minutes. Combine oat bran, flour, dry milk, baking powder, baking soda, and salt in a large mixing bowl. Stir sugar replacement, fructose, oil, eggs, and vanilla into the soaked oatmeal. Then stir oat bran-flour mixture into the oatmeal mixture. Turn into a greased 13 × 9 in. (33 × 23 cm) baking pan. Bake at 425°F (220°C) for 25 to 35 minutes, or until a toothpick inserted in middle comes out clean. Cool. Cut into 54 bars.

Yield: 54 bars

Exchange, 1 bar: ½ bread, ¼ fat
Each serving contains: Calories: 47, Carbohydrates: 7 g

Puddings and Creams

Before baking puddings in the oven, put them into separate little "custard" dishes and bake them in a hot water bath. The separate little dishes cook faster and the hot water bath also helps prevent the pudding from developing a rubbery texture, an unfortunate tendency of egg whites and egg substitutes. Low-fat dishes in general benefit from a hot water bath to bake in.

Grape-Nuts Pudding I

This classic dessert is like the ones delicatessens and diners offer for dessert.

2 c.	skim milk	500 mL
½ c.	egg substitute	125 mL
4 pkts.	concentrated acesulfame-K	4 pkts.
pinch	salt (optional)	pinch
1 t.	vanilla extract	5 mL
1 t.	almond extract	5 mL
½ t.	cinnamon	2.5 mL
⅓ c.	Grape-Nuts cereal	90 mL
¼ c.	golden raisins	60 mL

Heat the milk over hot water in the top of a double boiler. In a bowl, whisk together the egg substitute, acesulfame-K, salt, extracts, and spices. Pour the hot milk slowly over the egg mixture, stirring constantly with a wire whisk. Stir in the Grape-Nuts and raisins. Pour the mixture into eight ovenproof custard cups that have been coated with non-stick vegetable cooking spray.

Place these in a large pan. Pour hot water into the pan to the top of the outside of the custard cups. Place this pan in a preheated 350°F (180°C) oven and bake about an hour. A knife inserted in the center of each pudding should come out clean. Serve warm or chilled.

Yield: 8 servings

Exchange, 1 serving: 1 milk
Each serving contains: Calories: 65, Carbohydrates: 15 g, Fiber: trace, Sodium: 94 mg, Cholesterol: 1 mg

Grape-Nuts Pudding II

This is a light and airy sort of Grape-Nuts pudding.

4	egg whites	4
½ c.	nonfat sour cream	125 mL
12 pkts.	concentrated acesulfame-K	12 pkts.
1 T.	sugar	15 mL
2 t.	grated lemon peel	15 mL
½ c.	egg substitute	125 mL
2 c.	skim milk	500 mL
½ c.	Grape-Nuts cereal	125 mL
⅓ c.	flour	90 mL
½ c.	fresh lemon juice	60 mL
pinch	nutmeg	pinch

Use an electric mixer to beat the egg whites until stiff peaks form. Set them aside. Then use the electric mixer to combine the sour cream with the acesulfame-K, sugar, and lemon peel. Beat until fluffy. Beat in the egg substitute. Then add the milk, cereal, flour, and lemon juice. Stir in a small amount of beaten egg whites to lighten the mixture. Then use a rubber spatula to fold in the remaining egg whites. Pour the mixture into a large ovenproof baking dish that has been coated with non-stick cooking spray and sprinkled with nutmeg. Place this dish in a larger pan filled with hot water. Bake in a preheated 350°F (180°C) oven for 1¼ hours.

Yield: 16 servings

Exchange, 1 serving: ½ milk
Each serving contains: Calories: 51, Carbohydrates: 13 g, Fiber: trace, Sodium: 77 mg, Cholesterol: 1.5 mg

Bread Pudding

This bread pudding is low in calories and exchanges but still has the genuine bread-pudding taste.

½ loaf	"light" sourdough bread	½ loaf
12 oz. can	evaporated skim milk	375 mL can
½ c.	unsweetened applesauce	125 mL
1 t.	vanilla extract	5 mL
½ c.	skim milk	125 mL
8 pkts.	acesulfame-K	8 pkts.
⅓ c.	raisins	90 mL
½ t.	cinnamon	2 mL
4	egg whites	4

Cut the bread slices into cubes; place them on a cookie sheet coated with non-stick cooking spray. Place the tray in a preheated 350°F (180°C) oven for 10 minutes. Combine all the other ingredients and add the bread. Toss well and place in an ovenproof baking dish that has been sprayed with nonstick vegetable cooking spray. Place this baking dish in a large pan of water filled nearly to the top of the baking dish, and place the pan in a preheated 350°F (180°C) oven. Bake for 40 minutes. Serve hot or cold.

Yield: 8 servings

Exchange, 1 serving: 1½ breads
Each serving contains: Calories: 109, Carbohydrates: 40 g, Fiber: 4 g, Sodium: 128 mg, Cholesterol: trace

Raspberry Pudding

Raspberries are a natural for low-fat, low-sugar cooking because they add such a nice flavor. They also help to cover up any taste of artificial sweeteners.

½ loaf	"light" sourdough bread	½ loaf
12 oz.	can evaporated skim milk	354 mL
½ c.	unsweetened applesauce	125 mL
1 t.	vanilla extract	5 mL
½ c.	skim milk	125 mL
1 T.	sugar	15 mL
8 pkts.	concentrated acesulfame-K	8 pkts.
½ c.	egg substitute	125 mL
½ c.	raspberries	125 mL

Cut the bread into large cubes. Put the cubes into an ovenproof baking dish that has been coated with non-stick cooking spray. Use a food processor to combine the other ingredients; pour the mixture over the cubes. Let it sit a few minutes so the bread soaks in some of the wet mixture. Place the baking dish in a large pan of hot water nearly to the top of the baking dish. Bake in a preheated 350°F (180°C) oven for 35 minutes. Serve hot or cold.

Yield: 8 servings

Exchange, 1 serving: 1½ breads
Each serving contains: Calories: 111, Carbohydrates: 34 g, Fiber: 4 g, Sodium: 162 mg, Cholesterol: trace

Indian Pudding

As good as any restaurant dessert. If you require a topping, try ¼ cup of frozen, no-sugar-added, low-fat or nonfat vanilla yogurt.

3½ c.	skim milk	875 mL
½ c.	cornmeal	125 mL
2 T.	molasses	30 mL
¼ c.	diet pancake syrup (sugar-free and fructose-free if either elevates your blood sugar)	125 mL
2 pkts.	concentrated acesulfame-K	2 pkts.
2 t.	margarine or butter	10 mL
1 t.	vanilla extract	5 mL
1 t.	cinnamon	5 mL
1 t.	ginger	5 mL
½ t.	nutmeg	2 mL
pinch	salt (optional)	pinch
⅛ t.	baking soda	½ mL
¾ c.	egg substitute	190 mL

Heat 2½ c. (625 mL) of milk in a saucepan; bring to a boil. While this is heating, combine ½ c. (125 mL) milk and the cornmeal with a wire whisk. When the milk boils, pour in the cornmeal-milk mixture and cook over medium heat. Stir with a wire whisk and cook for approximately 10 minutes or until the mixture is thickened. Remove from the heat and stir in the molasses, pancake syrup, acesulfame-K, margarine, vanilla extract, spices, and baking soda.

In a separate bowl, use a wire whisk to beat the egg substitute; pour a little of the hot cornmeal into the egg and beat together. Then pour the beaten egg into the larger pan and whisk together.

Pour the mixture into a ½ gallon (2 L) ovenproof baking dish that has been coated with non-stick cooking spray. Set it in a pan of hot water that comes halfway up the side of the dish. Pour the remaining ½ c. (125 mL) of milk over the top, but do not stir it in. Bake in a preheated 275°F (140°C) oven for approximately 2½ hours.

Yield: 10 servings

Exchange, 1 serving: 1 bread
Each serving contains: Calories: 88, Carbohydrates: 28 g, Fiber: trace, Sodium: 95 mg, Cholesterol: 1 mg

Scandinavian Pudding

This is a variation of klappgrot, the traditional Scandinavian dessert.

6 oz.	frozen apple juice concentrate	180 g
2½ c.	water	625 mL
4 T.	farina	60 mL
8 oz.	pineapple juice, unsweetened (from a can of crushed pineapple)	240 g

Mix the apple juice and water in a saucepan. Bring to a rapid boil. Stir the mixture while gradually adding the farina. Cook gently for five minutes or so and remove from the heat. Beat by hand or with an electric mixer until the mixture is smooth. Fold in the pineapple. Pour into individual pudding dishes; chill.

Yield: 6 servings

Exchange, 1 serving: 1 fruit
Each serving contains: Calories: 88, Carbohydrates: 81 g, Fiber: trace, Sodium: 33 mg, Cholesterol: 0 mg

Lemon Cake Pudding

This is a tangy, moist cake that you can proudly present at a social event. The beaten egg whites make it rise high.

1 T.	margarine or butter, melted	15 mL
2 T.	sugar	30 mL
10 pkts.	concentrated acesulfame-K	10 pkts.
1 t.	vanilla extract	5 mL
⅓ c.	egg substitute	90 mL
⅓ c.	lemon juice	90 mL
2 t.	grated lemon peel	10 mL
¼ c.	flour	90 mL
1 c.	nonfat milk	250 mL
2 drops	yellow food coloring (optional)	2 drops
2	egg whites	2
⅛ t.	cream of tartar	½ mL

Use an electric mixer to beat together the melted margarine, sugar, acesulfame-K, vanilla extract, and egg substitute until smooth. Then add the lemon juice, lemon peel, flour, milk, and food coloring, if desired. Be sure it's well blended.

In a separate bowl, using clean, dry beaters, beat the egg whites until stiff. Add the cream of tartar and beat until stiff. Add a small amount to the lemon batter to lighten it. Then use a rubber spatula to gently fold the remaining egg whites into the batter. Pour it into an ovenproof baking dish that has been coated with non-stick cooking spray. Put this dish into a larger oven pan that has hot water in it. Put it into a preheated 350°F (180°C) oven for 40 minutes. Serve hot or cold.

Yield: 8 servings

Exchange, 1 serving: ½ milk
Each serving contains: Calories: 59, Carbohydrates: 17 g, Fiber: trace, Sodium: 50 mg, Cholesterol: trace

Hawaiian Custard

2 c.	skim milk	500 mL
6 pkts.	concentrated acesulfame-K	6 pkts.
⅓ c.	tapioca	90 mL
¼ c.	egg substitute	60 mL
1 T.	cold water	15 mL
1 c.	drained, unsweetened crushed pineapple	250 g

Heat the milk over boiling water in the top of a double boiler. Add the acesulfame-K and tapioca and bring to a boil, stirring occasionally. (If you do not have a double boiler, stir constantly to avoid burning the milk.) With an electric mixer, beat the egg substitute, add cold water, and beat again. Pour the hot mixture over the egg mixture, then return it to the top of a double boiler and cook a moment, stirring constantly. When smooth and thick, beat in the crushed pineapple. Chill thoroughly and serve in dessert cups.

Yield: 8 servings

Exchange, 1 serving: 1 fruit
Each serving contains: Calories: 62, Carbohydrates: 12 g, Fiber:
trace, Sodium: 50 mg, Cholesterol: 1 mg

Thanksgiving Pudding

This pudding is so low in calories and fat, it's easy to fit in with any meal.

15 oz. can	pumpkin	425 g can
2 t.	pumpkin pie spice	10 mL
2 t.	olive oil	10 mL
1 T.	fructose	15 mL
2 t.	vanilla extract	10 mL
7 pkts.	concentrated acesulfame-K	7 pkts.
1 c.	skim milk	250 mL
4	egg whites	4

Put the pumpkin, pumpkin pie spice, olive oil, fructose, vanilla extract, and acesulfame-K into a mixing bowl; use a wire whisk to mix completely.

In a small saucepan heat the milk just to the boiling point. Whisk into the pumpkin mixture. In a separate small bowl use an electric mixer to heat the egg whites. Fold the egg whites into the pumpkin-milk mixture. Be sure it is well mixed.

Pour the mixture into 10 separate custard cups that have been coated with non-stick cooking spray. Place the filled custard cups into one very large or two medium ovenproof pans. Carefully pour boiling water into the baking pan(s), taking care that water doesn't spill into the filled cups.

Bake in a preheated 375°F (190°C) oven for 35 minutes. A knife inserted in the center of each custard should come out clean. Chill before serving.

Yield: 10 servings

Exchange, 1 serving: ½ bread
Each serving contains: Calories: 43, Carbohydrates: 8 g, Fiber: 2 g,
Sodium: 35 mg, Cholesterol: trace

Tapioca Pudding

Very creamy and satisfying.

3 c.	skim milk	750 mL
¼ c.	quick-cooking (instant) tapioca	125 mL
¼ t.	salt (optional)	1 mL
¼ c.	egg substitute	60 mL
1	egg white, beaten	1
1 t.	vanilla extract	5 mL
2½ t.	concentrated aspartame	7 mL

Whisk together the milk, tapioca, salt (optional), egg substitute, and beaten egg white in the top of a double boiler. Heat the water in the lower part to boiling. Cover the top part and cook for five minutes while stirring. Remove from the heat; add the vanilla extract and aspartame. The pudding will thicken as it cools.

Yield: 6 servings

Exchange, 1 serving: 1 bread
Each serving contains: Calories: 79, Carbohydrates: 16 g, Fiber: 0, Sodium: 93 mg, Cholesterol: 2 mg

Creamed Apple Tapioca

Luscious and sweet, this is a very satisfying dessert.

2 T.	tapioca	30 mL
3 c.	skim milk	750 mL
½ c.	egg substitute	125 mL
6 pkts.	concentrated acesulfame-K	6 pkts.
6	apples	6
1 t.	nutmeg	5 mL
1 t.	cinnamon	5 mL

Cook the tapioca in the milk until it reaches a full boll. Then add the beaten egg substitute and acesulfame-K; stir and remove at once from the heat. Peel and quarter the apples, put them in a casserole dish, and sprinkle them with spices, stirring to coat evenly. Pour the tapioca mixture over them and bake at 325°F (160°C) for 45 minutes or until the apples are soft.

Yield: 6 servings

Exchange, 1 serving: 2 breads
Each serving contains: Calories: 147, Carbohydrates: 35 g, Fiber: 4 g, Sodium: 106 mg, Cholesterol: 2 mg

Chocolate Pudding

This recipe is so easy. You are sure to prefer it to boxed pudding. It's much lower in sodium too.

¼ c.	sugar	60 mL
3 pkts.	concentrated acesulfame-K	3 pkts.
2 T.	unsweetened cocoa powder	30 mL
3 T.	cornstarch	45 mL
2 c.	nonfat milk	500 mL
1 t.	vanilla extract	5 mL

Combine the sugar, acesulfame-K, cocoa, and cornstarch in a saucepan. Add about ½ c. (125 mL) milk. Stir with a wire whisk until dissolved and the mixture is smooth. Add the remaining milk and vanilla extract. Cook, stirring occasionally until thick, about 5 minutes. Cool before serving.

Yield: 4 servings

Exchange, 1 serving: 1 bread + ½ fruit
Each serving contains: Calories: 118, Carbohydrates: 32 g, Fiber: trace, Sodium: 81 mg, Cholesterol: 2 mg

Creamy Pudding

Our diabetic friends were really impressed with this pudding, especially those who are the most careful about restricting calories and fat.

8 oz. can	crushed pineapple, unsweetened	240 mL can	
1 pkg.	unflavored gelatin	1 pkg.	
¼ c.	water	60 mL	
1 T.	concentrated aspartame	15 mL	
1 t.	vanilla extract	5 mL	
1 c.	nonfat milk	250 mL	

Drain the liquid from the canned pineapple into a saucepan; sprinkle the gelatin over it to soften. Bring to a boil and stir until dissolved. Use a blender or food processor to combine with all the other ingredients. Pour into individual dishes. Chill until set.

Yield: 8 servings

Exchange, 1 serving: ½ milk
Each serving contains: Calories: 31, Carbohydrates: 8 g, Fiber: trace, Sodium: 17 mg, Cholesterol: trace

Grapefruit Snow Pudding

This is a tart, light pudding that's perfect after a heavy meal.

1 env.	unsweetened gelatin	1 env.
¼ c.	cold water	60 mL
¼ c.	boiling water	60 mL
¼ c.	orange juice	60 mL
1 T.	lemon juice	15 mL
¾ c.	grapefruit, chopped	190 mL
4 pkts.	concentrated acesulfame-K	4 pkts.
2	egg whites	2
1	grapefruit, cut into sections (optional)	1

Soak the gelatin in the cold water for about five minutes; add the boiling water, then add the acesulfame-K. Stir to dissolve the gelatin. Add the fruit juices and grapefruit, cut in small pieces. Cool, and when the gelatin begins to stiffen, beat until frothy. In another bowl, beat the egg whites until stiff. Fold them into the grapefruit mixture. Turn into a bowl and chill. When serving, garnish with sections of grapefruit.

Yield: 6 servings

Exchange: free
Each serving contains: Calories: 27, Carbohydrates: 8 g, Fiber: trace, Sodium: 18 mg, Cholesterol: 0 mg

Lemon Pudding

Sometimes your main meal has used up your quota of calories and exchanges. A very light dessert such as this can satisfy the emotional need to have some sweet ending to a meal.

1 env.	unflavored gelatin, unsweetened	1 env.
2 T.	cold water	30 mL
½ c.	boiling water	125 mL
1½ c.	nonfat buttermilk	375 mL
2 t.	lemon rind	10 mL
2 t.	lemon juice	10 mL
2 t.	concentrated aspartame	10 mL
2 drops	yellow food coloring (optional)	2 drops

In a large mixing bowl, sprinkle the gelatin over the cold water to soften. Let sit for a few minutes. Pour boiling water over it and stir until completely dissolved. Add the remaining ingredients and whisk together. Pour into five individual pudding dishes that have been sprayed very lightly with nonstick cooking spray. The pudding may be served in the individual dishes or unmolded onto separate plates. This can be served plain or dressed up with a little fresh cut-up fruit. If you keep plain frozen strawberries in your freezer, you can take out one to garnish each serving.

Yield: 5 servings

Exchange, 1 serving: ½ milk
Each serving contains: Calories: 31, Carbohydrates: 5 g, Fiber: 0, Sodium: 39 mg, Cholesterol: 1.2 mg

Caramel Pudding

This pudding can be unfolded onto separate little dishes for a fancier look. If you wish, spread a thin layer of fruit purée over the top of the pudding, or do what they do in restaurants: Spread the purée directly onto the serving plate and unfold the molded pudding on it.

1 env.	unflavored gelatin	1 env.
2 T.	cold water	30 mL
¼ c.	boiling water with 1 t. (5 mL) coffee granules dissolved in it	60 mL
1 t.	vanilla extract	5 mL
1½ c.	skim milk	375 mL
8 oz.	fat-free, sugar-free, light "Cream Caramel" flavored yogurt	250 g
1 t.	aspartame	5 mL

Sprinkle the gelatin over the cold water; allow it to soften. Add the coffee dissolved in the boiling water and whisk well until the gelatin is completely dissolved. Put the remaining ingredients into a food processor. Blend until smooth. Add the coffee and gelatin mixture and mix well. Pour into individual custard cups that have been coated with nonstick cooking spray. Chill until set.

Yield: 8 servings

Exchange, 1 serving: ½ milk
Each serving contains: Calories: 32, Carbohydrates: 8 g, Fiber: 0, Sodium: 43 mg, Cholesterol: 1.3 mg

Pineapple Mousse

Karin's mother served this at a dinner party that included diabetic and nondiabetic friends. It was a great success, and it's so quick to make.

20 oz. can	pineapple, packed in juice, drained	625 mL can	
2 T.	fructose	30 mL	
1 c.	evaporated skim milk, chilled	250 mL	
1 env.	unflavored gelatin	1 env.	
1 T.	lemon juice	15 mL	

Purée the pineapple in a blender or food processor. Add the fructose; stir. Set aside. In a mixing bowl, whip the evaporated milk until thick and creamy. In the top of a double boiler, sprinkle the gelatin over the lemon juice. Let stand 3–5 minutes. Stir over hot water until dissolved. Stir the gelatin into the whipped milk. Fold the pineapple mixture into the milk. Spoon into dessert dishes. Chill until set.

Yield: 16 servings

Exchange, 1 serving: 1 milk
Each serving contains: Calories: 51, Carbohydrates: 7 g, Fiber: trace, Sodium: 85 mg, Cholesterol: 0 mg

Yogurt Molds

Make one of the fruit toppings from this book to pour over your yogurt. Add a dollop of your favorite whipped topping.

2 env.	flavored gelatin	2 env.	
3 T.	water	45 mL	
2 c.	nonfat plain yogurt, chilled	500 mL	
2 t.	strawberry extract	10 mL	
1 t.	almond extract	5 mL	

In the top of a double boiler, sprinkle the gelatin over the water and let it stand for 1–5 minutes, until softened. Stir until dissolved. Heat over boiling water. Whisk into the yogurt. Add strawberry and almond extracts. Mix well. Then pour into individual dessert dishes. Chill until set.

Yield: 4 servings

Exchange, 1 serving: 1 milk
Each serving contains: Calories: 64, Carbohydrates: 12 g, Fiber: 0, Sodium: 76 mg, Cholesterol: 0 mg

Maple Custard

3	eggs	3	
½ c.	dietetic maple syrup	125 mL	
2 t.	maple flavoring	10 mL	
dash	salt	dash	
2 c.	2% milk	500 mL	

Beat eggs with maple syrup, flavoring, and salt until mixture becomes foamy and well blended. Scald the milk. Gradually beat milk into egg mixture. Transfer mixture to six custard cups. Place custard cups in a pan of hot water. Bake at 350°F (175°C) for 35 to 40 minutes. Custard is done when tip of a knife inserted in center comes out clean. Chill thoroughly before serving.

Yield: 6 servings

Exchange, 1 serving: ½ medium-fat meat, ½ low-fat milk
Each serving contains: Calories: 92, Carbohydrates: 8 g

Cinnamon-Apple Custard

3	eggs	3
dash	salt	dash
2 large	apples	2 large
2 t.	lemon juice	10 mL
2 t.	cinnamon	10 mL
½ t.	nutmeg	2 mL
2 c.	skim milk	500 mL
⅓ c.	granulated sugar replacement	90 mL
1 T.	granulated fructose	15 mL

Beat eggs with salt until foamy and well blended. Peel, core, and chop apples. Sprinkle with lemon juice, cinnamon, and nutmeg. Toss to completely mix. Scald the milk. Remove from heat and stir in sugar replacement and fructose. Gradually beat milk into egg mixture. Divide the apple mixture evenly among eight custard cups. Pour egg-milk mixture over the apple mixture. Place custard cups in a pan of hot water. Bake at 350°F (175°C) for 35 to 40 minutes. Custard is done when tip of a knife inserted in center comes out clean. Chill thoroughly before serving.

Yield: 8 servings

Exchange, 1 serving: ½ medium-fat meat, ½ fruit
Each serving contains: Calories: 89, Carbohydrates: 7 g

Hot Fudge Pudding

1 c.	flour	250 mL
3 T.	granulated sugar replacement	45 mL
½ t.	baking soda	2 mL
¼ t.	salt	1 mL
3 1 oz. sqs.	bitter chocolate	3 30 g sqs.
2 T.	white vinegar	30 mL
⅓ c.	skim milk	90 mL
2 T.	liquid shortening	30 mL
2 T.	granulated brown sugar replacement	30 mL
1¾ c.	boiling water	440 mL

Sift flour, granulated sugar replacement, baking soda, and salt into medium mixing bowl. Melt 1 square of the bitter chocolate. Add vinegar, milk, shortening, and the melted chocolate to flour mixture; stir to blend. Pour into well greased 8 in. (20 cm) sq. baking dish, and sprinkle with brown sugar replacement. Add remaining chocolate to the boiling water; heat until chocolate is melted. Pour chocolate-water mixture over pudding batter, and bake at 350°F (175°C) for 45 minutes. Serve warm from baking dish.

Yield: 10 servings

Exchange, 1 serving: 1 bread, 1 fat
Each serving contains: Calories: 105

Baked Plum Pudding

2	eggs	2
1	egg white	1
3 T.	granulated sugar replacement	45 mL
¼ c.	liquid shortening	60 mL
1 c.	unsweetened plum purée (baby food)	250 mL
1 c.	flour	250 mL
1 t.	baking soda	5 mL
½ t.	cinnamon	2 mL
¼ t.	nutmeg	1 mL
3 T.	skim milk	45 mL
2 T.	lemon juice	30 mL

Beat eggs and egg white until soft and fluffy; beat in sugar replacement, shortening, and plum purée. Combine flour, baking soda, cinnamon and nutmeg in sifter. Combine milk and lemon juice in cup. Sift flour mixture alternately with milk mixture into plum mixture. Fold gently to mix completely. Pour into well greased 9 in. (23 cm) sq. baking dish. Bake at 350°F (175°C) for 20 to 30 minutes, or until firm.

Yield: 9 servings

Exchange, 1 serving: 1 bread, 1 fat
Each serving contains: Calories: 144, Carbohydrates: 20 g

Apricot Pudding

⅓ c.	unsweetened apricot purée (baby food)	90 mL
1 t.	baking soda	5 mL
1	egg, beaten	1
½ c	milk	125 mL
1 t.	lemon juice	5 mL
½ t.	almond extract	2 mL
1 T.	margarine, melted	15 mL
1 c.	flour, sifted	250 mL
2 T.	granulated sugar replacement	30 mL
dash	salt	dash

Combine apricot purée and baking soda in small mixing bowl; allow to rest 5 minutes. Combine remaining ingredients in large mixing bowl, add purée, and beat well to blend. Pour into well greased 8 in. (20 cm) square baking dish, and bake at 350°F (175°C) for 1 hour. Allow to cool slightly before serving.

Yield: 8 servings

Exchange, 1 serving: 1 bread, ½ fat
Each serving contains: Calories: 90, Carbohydrates: 18 g

Rhubarb Sponge Pudding

2 T.	margarine	30 mL
2 T.	granulated brown sugar replacement	30 mL
1 qt.	rhubarb, cut into 1 in. (2.5 cm) pieces	1 L
2	egg yolks	2
2 T.	granulated sugar replacement	30 mL
1 c.	flour	250 mL
½ t.	salt	2 mL
½ t.	baking powder	2 mL
½ c.	water	125 mL
1 t.	vanilla extract	5 mL
2	egg whites, stiffly beaten	2

Melt margarine in small saucepan, add brown sugar replacement, and stir to blend. Spread mixture into bottom of 13 × 9 in. (33 × 23 cm) baking dish, and place rhubarb pieces evenly over the margarine mixture. Combine egg yolks and sugar replacement, beating until light and fluffy. Combine flour, salt, and baking powder in sifter; beat alternately with water and vanilla into egg yolks. Fold egg yolk mixture completely into stiffly beaten egg whites and pour batter over rhubarb, spreading it out evenly. Bake at 350°F (190°C) for 45 minutes. Turn upside down on serving plate, and serve warm or cold.

Yield: 12 servings

Exchange, 1 serving: ½ bread, ½ fat
Each serving contains: Calories: 69, Carbohydrates: 8 g

Hasty Pudding

Cake

2 T.	margarine	30 mL
2 t.	granulated brown sugar replacement	10 mL
1 c.	flour, sifted	250 mL
1½ t.	baking powder	7 mL
¼ t.	salt	1 mL
½ c.	skim milk	125 mL
½ c.	raisins	25 mL

Cream together margarine and sugar replacement. Combine flour, baking powder and salt, and add alternately with milk to creamed mixture. Fold in raisins. Pour batter into well greased 8 in. (20 cm) baking dish.

Syrup

1 T.	flour	15 mL
2 c.	cold water	500 mL
2 T.	granulated brown sugar replacement	30 mL
2 t.	margarine	10 mL
1 t.	vanilla extract	5 mL

Combine flour and water in saucepan; cook and stir over medium heat until slightly thickened. Remove from heat. Add sugar replacement, margarine and vanilla, stirring to mix. Pour over cake batter, and bake at 350°F (175°C) for 45 minutes.

Yield: 9 servings

Exchange, 1 serving: 1 bread, 1 fruit, 1 fat
Each serving contains: Calories: 84, Carbohydrates: 18 g

Whipped Banana Yogurt

½ c.	fresh or frozen (reconstituted) orange juice	125 mL
	peel of 1 orange, grated	
4	bananas, cut into 1 in. (2.5 cm) pieces	4
2 t.	fresh lemon juice	10 mL
1 c.	plain low-fat yogurt	250 mL
2	egg whites	2

Combine orange juice and orange peel in small saucepan; cook and stir over medium heat until peel is tender. Let cool; refrigerate. Combine banana pieces and lemon juice in mixing bowl or food processor. Whip to purée; add orange juice and mix together. Add yogurt and whip just to blend. Pour into 8 in. (20 cm) round cake pan and freeze until firm.

Remove from freezer and let mixture soften slightly, just until it can easily be spooned out of pan. Place in mixing bowl or food processor; mix until smooth and fluffy. With machine running, add egg whites and mix thoroughly. Return to cake pan and freeze. Remove from freezer and allow to soften slightly. Turn into mixing bowl or food processor and whip until soft, light and smooth. Spoon into individual dishes and serve immediately.

Yield: 8 servings

Exchange, 1 serving: 1 bread
Each serving contains: Calories: 73, Carbohydrates: 19 g

Lemon Custard

1 pkg.	vanilla-flavored sugar-free instant pudding mix	1 pkg.
2 c.	low-fat milk	500 mL
1 T.	fresh lemon juice	15 mL
2 t.	grated lemon rind	10 mL
1	egg yolk, slightly beaten	1

Combine pudding mix, milk, lemon juice, and lemon rind in a nonstick saucepan. Cook and stir until mixture just comes to a boil. Stir a small amount of pudding mixture into beaten egg; then return to saucepan. Continue cooking until mixture comes to full boil. Remove from heat. Pour into large dessert dish or four smaller dishes or margarita glasses.

Yield: 4 servings

Exchange, 1 serving: 1 low-fat milk
Each serving contains: Calories: 100, Carbohydrates: 12 g

Coconut Custard

1 pkg.	vanilla-flavored sugar-free instant pudding mix	1 pkg.
2 c.	low-fat milk	500 mL
⅔ c.	unsweetened coconut flakes, toasted	180 mL
1	egg yolk, slightly beaten	1

Combine pudding mix, milk, and ½ c. (125 mL) of the toasted coconut in a saucepan. Cook and stir until mixture just comes to a boil. Pour a small amount of mixture into beaten egg yolk; then return to saucepan. Cook until mixture comes to a full boil. Cover with wax paper and allow to cool slightly. Spoon into six dessert dishes. Top with remaining toasted coconut. Refrigerate to chill thoroughly.

Yield: 6 servings

Exchange, 1 serving: ½ low-fat milk, 1 fat
Each serving contains: Calories: 110, Carbohydrates: 9 g

True Chocolate Custard

2 c.	skim milk	500 mL
1 T.	vegetable oil	15 mL
1 t.	vanilla extract	5 mL
2 oz.	semisweet chocolate, chopped	57 g
6	egg yolks	6
2 T.	granulated fructose	30 mL

Combine skim milk, vegetable oil, and vanilla in a saucepan. Bring to a simmer. Remove from heat; stir in chocolate until melted and mixture is smooth. Whisk egg yolks and fructose in a medium bowl. Very slowly whisk egg yolk mixture into hot chocolate. Cool to room temperature, stirring occasionally. Position a rack in the middle of the oven. Preheat oven to 300°F (150°C). Place six custard cups in a shallow baking pan. Evenly divide the chocolate mixture between the cups. Fill baking pan with enough hot water to come halfway up the sides of the custard cups. Bake until custards are just set, about 35 to 40 minutes. Cool or serve warm.

Yield: 6 servings

Exchange, 1 serving: 1 skim milk, 1 fat
Each serving contains: Calories: 150, Carbohydrates: 11 g

Hot Peach Pudding

1 lb.	dried peaches	454 g
3 c.	water	750 mL
1 pkg.	vanilla-flavored sugar-free instant pudding mix	1 pkg.

Rinse peaches under cool water. Combine peaches and 3 c. (750 mL) of the water in a saucepan. Cook until tender; then remove peaches, cool, and cut into pieces. Continue cooking peach water until reduced to about 1 c. (250 mL); then return peaches to pan. Meanwhile, prepare pudding mix as directed on package. Allow to thicken for 10 minutes. Add hot peaches and peach juice. Serve hot.

Yield: 4 servings

Exchange, 1 serving: 1 fruit
Each serving contains: Calories: 58, Carbohydrates: 12 g

Orange Cream Custard

1 pkg.	vanilla-flavored sugar-free instant pudding mix	1 pkg.
1 c.	low-fat milk	250 mL
1 c.	orange juice	250 mL
1	egg, separated	1
4	orange sections	4

Combine pudding mix, milk, and orange juice in a saucepan. Cook and stir over medium heat just until mixture comes to a boil. Meanwhile, slightly beat the egg yolk. Pour a small amount of pudding mixture into the egg yolk, stir, and return mixture to saucepan. Continue cooking until mixture comes to a full boil. Remove from heat, cover with wax paper, and cool slightly. Spoon into four dessert glasses. Refrigerate and chill until firm. Beat egg white until stiff. Just before serving, garnish with whipped egg white and orange section.

Yield: 4 servings

Exchange, 1 serving: 1 low-fat milk, ⅓ fat
Each serving contains: Calories: 126, Carbohydrates: 16 g

Maple Raisin Pudding

½ c.	raisins	125 mL
2 c.	water	500 mL
¼ t.	maple flavoring	1 mL
1 pkg.	vanilla-flavored sugar-free instant pudding mix	1 pkg.
4 T.	prepared nondairy whipped topping	60 mL

Combine raisins and water in a nonstick saucepan. Bring to a boil. Remove from heat; cool to room temperature. Stir in maple flavoring. Drain raisin water into a bowl. Add pudding mix, stirring as directed on package.

Spoon into dessert dishes or wine glasses in three layers: raisins, maple pudding, and a dab of dairy topping.

Yield: 4 servings

Exchange, 1 serving: 1¼ fruit
Each serving contains: Calories: 83, Carbohydrates: 20 g

Chocolate Polka-Dot Pudding

1 pkg.	chocolate-flavored sugar-free instant pudding mix	1 pkg.
¼ c.	mini chocolate chips	60 mL

Make pudding mix as directed on package. Chill until set. Fold in chocolate chips. Spoon into dessert dishes.

Yield: 4 servings

Exchange, 1 serving: 1 skim milk, 1 fat
Each serving contains: Calories: 135, Carbohydrates: 17 g

Creamy Pumpkin Pudding

1 c.	puréed pumpkin	250 mL
¾ c.	water	190 mL
1 pkg.	butterscotch-flavored sugar-free instant pudding mix	1 pkg.

Combine pumpkin and water in a saucepan or microwave bowl. Heat on high until boiling. Remove from heat and chill thoroughly. Whisk or beat in pudding mix. Spoon into four dessert dishes.

Yield: 4 servings

Exchange, 1 serving: 1 fruit
Each serving contains: Calories: 50, Carbohydrates: 13 g

Prune Whip

2 jars (4 oz.)	baby prunes	2 jars (113 g)
2 t.	lemon juice	10 mL
2	egg whites	2
dash	salt	dash
¼ c.	granulated sugar replacement	60 mL

Combine strained prunes and lemon juice in a small bowl; stir to mix. Beat the egg whites and salt to soft peaks. Gradually add the sugar replacement; beat to stiff peaks. Fold prune mixture into stiffly beaten egg whites. Spoon into four sherbet or dessert glasses. Chill.

Yield: 4 servings

Exchange, 1 serving: 1 fruit
Each serving contains: Calories: 56, Carbohydrates: 13 g

Pineapple Bread Pudding

9 oz. can	crushed pineapple, in juice	256 g can
2 c.	soft white bread crumbs	500 mL
2 c.	skim milk	500 mL
¼ t.	salt	1 mL
2	eggs, beaten	2
21	granulated fructose	30 mL

Drain pineapple juice into a measuring cup; add enough water to the juice to make ¼ c. (60 mL) of liquid. Combine crushed pineapple, pineapple liquid, and remaining ingredients in a large bowl. Fold to blend. Pour into a 1½ qt. (1½ L) baking dish. Bake at 325 °F (165 °C) for about 45 minutes or until set.

Yield: 6 servings

Exchange, 1 serving: ½ bread, 1 fruit, ⅓ skim milk
Each serving contains: Calories: 128, Carbohydrates: 19 g

Chocolate Fudge Rice Pudding

1 pkg.	chocolate-flavored sugar-free instant pudding mix	1 pkg.
1½ c.	cold cooked rice	325 mL
6 sprigs	mint leaves (optional)	6 sprigs

Prepare pudding as directed on package. Chill to completely set. Fold in cooked rice. Spoon into six dessert glasses. Refrigerate to keep cold. Just before serving, garnish with mint leaves.

Yield: 6 servings

Exchange, 1 serving: ⅔ bread, ½ low-fat milk
Each serving contains: Calories: 116, Carbohydrates: 21 g

Thanksgiving Pumpkin Mousse

A light finish for a turkey dinner.

1¼ c.	skim milk	310 mL
1 c.	pumpkin pie filling	250 mL
¼ t.	cinnamon	2 mL
¼ t.	nutmeg	2 mL
¼ t.	ginger	2 mL
1 pkg.	butterscotch-flavored sugar-free instant pudding mix	1 pkg.
1¼ c.	water	310 mL
1 c.	frozen low-fat nondairy whipped topping	250 mL

In a mixing bowl, combine the milk, pumpkin, cinnamon, nutmeg, and ginger. Add the pudding mix and water and mix with a wire whisk or electric mixer until blended. Add the whipped topping and gently but thoroughly combine. Spoon into individual dessert dishes and chill 2–3 hours before serving.

Yield: 6 servings

Exchange, 1 serving: 1 starch/bread
Each serving contains: Calories: 101, Total fat : 2 g, Carbohydrates: 19 g, Protein: 3 g, Sodium: 157 mg, Cholesterol: 1 mg

Ricotta Cheese Pudding

A pudding for grown-ups—rich and very special.

1 lb.	fat-free ricotta cheese	450 g
2 T.	frozen low-fat nondairy whipped topping	30 mL
2 T.	Triple Sec	30 mL
1 t.	aspartame sweetener	5 mL
2 oz.	diabetic chocolate candy bar, coarsely chopped	55 g
¼ c.	Not-Too-Sweet Chocolate Sauce	60 mL

Process the ricotta in a blender or food processor until smooth. Add the whipped topping, Triple Sec, and aspartame. Blend again. Transfer to a mixing bowl. Fold in the chocolate. Cover the bowl and refrigerate it for one hour before serving. Serve with chocolate sauce.

Yield: 4 servings

Exchange, 1 serving: 1½ milk
Each serving contains: Calories: 139, Total fat: 1 g, Carbohydrates: 16 g, Protein: 14 g, Sodium: 88 mg, Cholesterol: 12 mg

Not-Too-Sweet Chocolate Sauce

Stores well refrigerated, but warm gently before serving.

3 T.	unsweetened cocoa powder	45 mL
1 T.	flour	15 mL
1½ c.	skim milk	375 mL
2 T.	butter or margarine	0 mL
3 t.	sugar substitute	15 mL
1 t.	vanilla extract	5 mL
½ t.	butter extract	3 mL

Combine the cocoa powder and flour in the top of a double boiler. Add the milk. Stir until free of lumps. Cook over boiling water, stirring until thick and smooth. Remove from heat. Stir in the butter. Cool for 15 minutes. Stir in the sugar substitute, vanilla extract, and butter extract. Serve over pudding or frozen treats.

Yield: 24 servings

Exchange: free
Each serving contains: Calories: 18, Total fat: 1 g, Carbohydrates: 2 g, Protein: 0.7 g, Sodium: 19 mg, Cholesterol: 3 mg

Lemon Sponge Pudding

This is an adaptation of one of my Grandmother Lily's favorites.

1 T.	flour	15 mL
2 T.	sugar	30 mL
3 pkgs.	saccharin or acesulfame-K sugar substitute	3 pkgs.
2 T.	lemon juice	30 mL
1½ t.	lemon peel	8 mL
2 large	eggs, separated	2 large
1 c.	skim milk	250 mL

In a mixing bowl, combine flour, sugar, sugar substitute, lemon juice, and lemon peel. Mix. In another bowl, beat the egg yolks at high speed until lemon colored. Add the yolks to the flour mixture. Blend well. Beat the egg whites until stiff. Fold them into the custard mixture. Pour the pudding into a casserole coated with non-stick cooking spray. Put the casserole in a pan of hot water in a preheated 350°F (180°C) oven. Bake for 35–40 minutes. The top will be lightly browned.

Yield: 4 servings

Exchange, 1 serving: 1 milk
Each serving contains: Calories: 95, Total fat: 3 g, Carbohydrates: 12 g, Protein: 6 g, Sodium: 66 mg, Cholesterol: 107 mg

Quick (Microwave) Custard

When I first made this I couldn't believe how quick custard could be.

1½ c.	skim milk	375 mL
3 large	eggs, or equivalent egg substitute	3 large
2 T.	sugar	30 mL
3 pkgs.	saccharin	3 pkgs.
1 t.	vanilla	5 mL
¼ t.	nutmeg	2 mL

Pour the milk into a glass measuring cup and put it in the microwave on high for three minutes. In a mixing bowl, stir together the eggs, sugar, sugar substitute, and vanilla. Gradually stir in the hot milk. Pour into a glass baking dish. Sprinkle nutmeg on top. Cook on defrost in the microwave for 10 minutes. The custard will become more firm as it sets.

Yield: 4 servings

Exchange, 1 serving: 1 milk; ½ fat
Each serving contains: Calories: 117, Total fat: 4 g, Carbohydrates: 12 g, Protein: 8 g, Sodium: 98 mg, Cholesterol: 161 mg

Microwave Vanilla Pudding

Perfect for a lazy day dessert. A spoonful of Not-Too-Sweet Chocolate Sauce makes it extra special.

3 T.	sugar	45 mL
2 T.	cornstarch	30 mL
2 c.	skim milk	500 mL
1 large	egg or equivalent egg substitute	1 large
1 t.	butter or margarine	5 mL
2 t.	vanilla	10 mL
2 pkgs.	sugar substitute	2 pkgs.

Put the sugar and cornstarch in a 4 c. (1 L) glass mixing bowl. Mix in the skim milk. Cook on high in the microwave for 5–7 minutes. Stop a few times to stir during the process. The mixture will be smooth and thick. Beat the egg in a small bowl. Mix in a few spoonfuls of the hot milk mixture. Turn the egg mixture into the thickened milk. Mix well. Return to the microwave and cook on roast or medium for a minute or two. Stop and stir during the process. Remove from the microwave. Stir in the butter, vanilla, and sugar substitute.

Yield: 4 servings

Exchange, 1 serving: 1 starch/bread; ½ milk
Each serving contains: Calories: 126, Total fat: 2 g, Carbohydrates: 20 g, Protein: 6 g, Sodium: 91 mg, Cholesterol: 58 mg

Rhubarb Bread Pudding

1 qt.	diced rhubarb	1 L
3½ c.	dry bread cubes	875 mL
1 c.	granulated sugar replacement	250 mL
¼ c.	margarine, melted	60 mL
2 T.	granulated fructose	30 mL
½ t.	ground nutmeg	2 mL
½ t.	ground cinnamon	2 mL
¼ t.	ground allspice	1 mL

Combine all ingredients in a bowl. Toss to mix. Transfer to a well greased 2 qt. (2 L) casserole dish. Cover and bake at 375°F (190°C) for 45 minutes; then uncover and continue baking another 10 minutes or until set. Serve warm.

Yield: 8 servings

Exchange, 1 serving: 1⅓ bread, 1 fat
Each serving contains: Calories: 148, Carbohydrates: 21 g

Great Lakes Pudding

Pudding

3 c.	wide noodles, uncooked	750 mL
2	eggs, beaten	2
½ c.	low-calorie cottage cheese	125 mL
⅓ c.	sour cream	90 mL
¼ c.	granulated sugar replacement	60 mL
¾ c.	skim milk	190 mL
1 oz.	baking chocolate, melted	30 g
1 T.	margarine	15 mL
1 t.	vanilla extract	5 mL

Topping

½ c.	unsweetened cornflakes	125 mL
1 T.	margarine, melted	15 mL
1 t.	granulated sugar replacement	5 mL

Cook noodles in boiling water until tender. Drain, rinse and cool thoroughly. Set aside. In large bowl, combine eggs, cottage cheese, sour cream, and sugar replacement and stir until smooth. Add skim milk, melted chocolate, margarine, and vanilla extract. Mix thoroughly. Stir in noodles and blend well. Cover and refrigerate overnight. Pour noodle mixture into a greased 8 in. (20 cm) baking dish. Combine topping ingredients in mixing bowl and lightly stir to blend. Sprinkle evenly over pudding. Bake at 350°F (175°C) for 40 to 50 minutes until topping is golden brown. Serve warm.

Yield: 9 servings

Exchange, 1 serving: 1 bread, 1 high-fat meat
Each serving contains: Calories: 164, Carbohydrates: 25 g

Pouding de Riz

Adapted from a Haitian rice pudding.

4	egg yolks	4
3 T.	granulated sugar replacement	45 mL
dash	salt	dash
1½ t.	vanilla extract	7 mL
1 qt.	skim milk, hot	1 L
1½ c.	cooked rice	375 mL
½ c.	semisweet chocolate chips	25 mL
4	egg whites	4
3 pkg.	aspartame sweetener	3 pkg.

In a mixing bowl, beat egg yolks with the sugar replacement and salt until pale yellow in color and slightly thickened. Stir in 1 teaspoon (5 mL) of the vanilla. Stir egg yolk mixture into the hot milk and cook, stirring, until custard coats the spoon. *Be careful not to let mixture boil.* Add rice and chocolate chips; stir to completely mix. Pour into greased 1 qt. (1 L) baking dish. Bake at 350°F (175°C) for 10 minutes. Meanwhile, beat egg whites until stiff but not dry. Beat in aspartame sweetener. Stir in the remaining vanilla extract. Remove pudding from oven, spread the egg white mixture over the pudding. Place pudding back in oven, bake for 5 minutes more or until meringue is slightly brown.

Yield: 8 servings

Exchange, 1 serving: 1 medium-fat milk, 1 fruit
Each serving contains: Calories: 176, Carbohydrates: 47 g

Regal Custard

5 T.	granulated sugar replacement	70 mL
3 c.	skim milk, hot	750 mL
8	egg yolks	8
1½ t.	vanilla extract	7 mL
3 T	cream de cacao	45 mL
6	egg whites	6

Add 2 T. (30 mL) of the sugar replacement to skim milk and stir to dissolve. Beat egg yolks until frothy; gradually beat in hot milk mixture. Add vanilla extract. Pour into a well-greased 2 qt. (2 L) baking dish. Bake at 350°F (175°C) for 35 to 45 minutes or until a knife comes out clean. Remove from oven. Pour cream de cacao over the surface. Beat egg whites until stiff and gradually beat in the remaining 3 T. (45 mL) of the sugar replacement and vanilla extract. Spread half the meringue over the custard. Decorate with remaining meringue by pressing it through a pastry tube or dropping it from a teaspoon. Return to oven and bake for 12 to 15 minutes or until meringue is a delicate brown.

Yield: 12 servings

Exchange, 1 serving: ⅓ bread, ½ high-fat meat
Each serving contains: Calories: 74, Carbohydrates: 12 g

Chocolate Custard with "Snow" Mounds

2 c.	skim milk	500 mL
¼ c.	skim evaporated milk	60 mL
2 T.	granulated sugar replacement	30 mL
½	vanilla bean, split	½
4	eggs, separated	4
2 T.	sorbitol	30 mL
1 oz.	baking chocolate, melted	30 g

In a large saucepan, combine skim milk, evaporated milk, sugar replacement and vanilla bean. Bring to a simmer. Beat egg whites until stiff and gradually beat in the sorbitol to make a smooth meringue. Drop meringue by tablespoons into the simmering milk mixture, turning each mound over two or three times as it poaches. Poach for about 3 minutes. (Do not overcrowd pan when poaching.) Remove meringues and drain on a towel. Stir melted chocolate into custard mixture. Beat egg yolks and gradually pour hot milk mixture over them. Stir continuously. Pour mixture back into saucepan. Return saucepan to low heat on stove. Stir until custard thickens. Pour custard into 6 individual serving dishes. Top with meringue mounds.

Yield: 8 servings

Exchange, 1 serving: ½ high-fat meat, ⅓ nonfat milk
Each serving contains: Calories: 86, Carbohydrates: 12 g

Aladdin's Cream

Smooth and creamy, a treat for the whole family.

1	egg	1
⅓ c.	granulated sugar replacement	90 mL
2 oz.	baking chocolate, melted	60 g
½ c.	skim milk	125 mL
2 t.	unsalted butter, melted	10 mL
1 c.	all-purpose flour	250 mL
1 T.	baking powder	15 mL
¼ t.	salt	1 mL
1 t.	vanilla extract	5 mL

Beat egg and granulated sugar replacement until well blended and frothy. Add baking chocolate, milk, butter, flour, baking powder, salt, and vanilla extract. Beat until thoroughly blended and smooth. Pour into a well greased 1½ qt. (1½ L) mold or baking dish. Place a rack in a large saucepan on top of the stove. Add boiling water to level of the rack. Place mold with pudding on rack. Cover saucepan and keep water boiling over low heat to steam the cream. Cook for 1½ hours or until cream is set.

Yield: 14 servings

Exchange, 1 serving: ½ bread, ¾ fat
Each serving contains: Calories: 68, Carbohydrates: 15 g

French Cream

The little extra work is well worth the trouble.

3 T.	granulated sugar replacement	45 mL
3 T.	cocoa	45 mL
2 T.	all-purpose flour	30 mL
3	egg yolks	3
1	egg	1
dash	salt	dash
1 c.	skim milk, hot	250 mL
1 t.	vanilla extract	5 mL
1 T.	margarine	15 mL
1 T.	almond paste	15 mL
1 T.	coconut, finely grated	15 mL

In the top of a double boiler combine sugar replacement, cocoa, flour, egg yolks, egg, and salt. Stir in skim milk. Cook and stir over simmering water until cream is smooth and thick. Remove from heat and stir in vanilla extract, margarine, almond paste, and coconut. Pour into 4 individual serving dishes. Serve hot.

Yield: 4 servings

Exchange, 1 serving: ¾ high-fat milk, ⅓ fat
Each serving contains: Calories: 140, Carbohydrates: 25 g

Fructose Custard

The vanilla bean gives it that special flavor.

2 c.	skim milk	500 mL
3 T.	liquid fructose	45 mL
3 T.	cocoa	45 mL
1	vanilla bean, split	1
4	egg yolks	4

Combine milk, liquid fructose, and cocoa in saucepan. Stir to completely mix. Add vanilla bean. Heat to the scalding point, stirring often; remove from heat. In a separate bowl, beat egg yolks until thick. Remove vanilla bean from the chocolate-milk mixture. Very gradually beat the hot milk into the egg yolks. Pour the mixture into the saucepan. Continue cooking and stirring over very low heat until the custard thickens. Pour into 4 individual custard cups. Chill.

Yield: 4 servings

Exchange, 1 serving: ½ bread, 1 medium-fat meat
Each serving contains: Calories: 115, Carbohydrates: 22 g

C & C Tureen

Chestnuts and chocolate—an unbeatable combination.

1 lb.	chestnuts	500 g
⅓ c.	sweet butter	90 mL
2 oz.	German chocolate, grated	60 g
2 T.	granulated sugar replacement	30 mL
1 t.	vanilla extract	5 mL

With a sharp knife slit shells of the chestnuts on convex side. Put chestnuts in a saucepan with enough water to cover, bring to a boil and simmer for 5 minutes. Remove pan from heat and remove chestnuts, one by one. Remove shells and inner skins while the nuts are still hot. Return peeled nuts to boiling water and cook for 20 minutes or until tender. Drain and place nuts in blender; blend into a purée.

Combine chestnut purée, butter, chocolate, sugar replacement and vanilla extract in bowl and stir to completely mix. Press mixture firmly into a greased paper-lined loaf pan. Chill 6 to 8 hours or overnight. Unmold the loaf onto a serving plate; cut into thin slices. Serve on chilled plates.

Yield: 8 servings

Exchange, 1 serving: ¾ bread, 3 fat
Each serving contains: Calories: 182, Carbohydrates: 35 g

Chocolate Bread Pudding

Ol'-fashioned—but now with chocolate!

½ c.	chocolate chips	125 mL
3 c.	skim milk	750 mL
2	eggs	2
½ t.	salt	2 mL
⅓ c.	granulated sugar replacement	90 mL
2 t.	vanilla extract	10 mL
8 slices	dry bread	8 slices

Melt the chocolate chips in 1 c. (250 mL) of the skim milk over medium heat. Stir in the remaining milk. Set aside. Beat eggs until frothy; add salt, sugar replacement, and vanilla extract. Beat well. Stir egg mixture into chocolate-milk mixture. Trim crusts from bread and cut slices into small cubes. Drop cubes into greased 1½ qt. (1½ L) casserole or baking dish. Pour chocolate mixture over the bread cubes; be sure to saturate all the cubes. Set casserole in pan of hot water. Bake at 350°F (175°C) for 1 hour or until pudding is completely set. Serve warm or cold.

Yield: 14 servings

Exchange, 1 serving: 1 bread, ½ fat
Each serving contains: Calories: 99

Pioneer Cornstarch Cream

2 oz.	baking chocolate	60 g
3 c.	skim milk	750 mL
½ c.	granulated sugar replacement	125 mL
¼ c.	cornstarch	60 mL
¼ t.	salt	1 mL
¼ c.	water	60 mL
2 t.	vanilla extract	10 mL
1 T.	margarine	15 mL

Melt baking chocolate in top of double boiler over simmering water; add skim milk. Stir until well blended. In shaker bottle or bowl combine the sugar replacement, cornstarch and salt with water. Shake or stir to blend well. Add to chocolate-milk mixture in double boiler. Cook and stir until thickened. Cook 20 minutes longer. Remove from heat, add vanilla extract and margarine. Spoon into serving dishes and press waxed paper directly to cream surface. Chill. Remove paper before serving.

Yield: 8 servings

Exchange, 1 serving: ¾ bread, 1 fat
Each serving contains: Calories: 103, Carbohydrates: 28 g

New England Baked Chocolate Custard

3	eggs	3
3 T.	dietetic maple syrup	45 mL
2 c.	skim milk	500 mL
1 oz.	baking chocolate, melted	30 g
1 t.	vanilla extract	5 mL

Beat eggs until foamy and light. Add dietetic maple syrup, skim milk, melted chocolate and vanilla extract; beat until thoroughly mixed. Pour the custard mixture into 4 individual custard cups. Set the cups in a pan of hot water which comes halfway up the sides of the custard cups. Bake at 350°F (175°C) for 35 to 40 minutes or until knife inserted in center of custard comes out clean. Serve hot or cold.

Yield: 4 servings

Exchange, 1 serving: 1 bread, 1 high-fat meat
Each serving contains: Calories: 166, Carbohydrates: 25 g

Cherry Bread Pudding

A good way to use up slightly stale bread.

1 c.	bread crumbs from 3 slices of Italian bread or 6 slices of French bread, toasted and then crumbled	250 mL
1 c.	skim milk	250 mL
1 lb.	ripe cherries, pitted	450 g
½ c.	fruit-only cherry preserves, no added sugar	125 mL
½ c.	sliced almonds, toasted (optional)	125 mL
1 t.	sugar	5 mL
1 c.	fat-free sour cream	250 mL

Crumble the toast into a medium mixing bowl. Add the milk. Stir. Add the cherries and most of the almonds. Reserve a few tablespoons (about 30 mL) of almonds for topping. Coat a 6 c. (1.5 L) baking dish with nonstick vegetable cooking spray. Pour the toast mixture into the prepared baking dish and top with the almonds, if you are using them. Sprinkle 1 t. (5 mL) of sugar on top. Bake in a preheated 350°F (180°C) oven for 35–45 minutes. Serve each with a dollop of sour cream.

Yield: 6 servings

Exchange, 1 serving: 2 starch/bread; 1 fruit
Each serving contains: Calories: 200, Total fat: 2 g, Carbohydrates: 40 g, Protein: 6 g, Sodium: 181 mg, Cholesterol: 1 mg

Raisin Rice Pudding

1 pkg.	low-calorie rice pudding	1 pkg.
½ c.	raisins	125 mL

Prepare rice pudding as directed on package. Soak raisins in warm water for 1 hour. Drain thoroughly. Add raisins to rice pudding.

Yield: 5 servings, ½ c. (125 mL) each

Exchange, 1 serving: ½ bread, ½ milk, ½ fruit
Each serving contains: Calories: 100, Carbohydrates: 18 g

Rhubarb Pudding

1 qt.	rhubarb, cut in pieces	1 L
1 c.	water	250 mL
2 T.	cornstarch	30 mL
1 t.	sugar replacement	5 mL

Cut rhubarb into pieces. Place rhubarb in saucepan. Add water. Cook rhubarb until tender. Mix cornstarch with small amount of cold water; add to rhubarb. Cook until thickened. Remove from heat; add sugar replacement. Stir until dissolved.

Microwave: Place rhubarb in large bowl. Add water. Cook on High for 4 minutes, or until tender. Mix cornstarch with small amount of cold water; add to rhubarb. Cook on High for 1 to 2 minutes, or until thickened.

Yield: 6 servings

Exchange, 1 serving: ⅛ fruit, ⅛ bread
Each serving contains: Calories: 22, Carbohydrates: 6 g

Rice Pudding

4 c.	water	1 L
¾ c.	Stone-Buhr long grain brown rice	190 mL
½ c.	granulated sugar replacement	125 mL
¼ c.	golden raisins	60 mL
¼ c.	margarine	60 mL
3 in.	vanilla bean	7 cm
3 in.	cinnamon stick	7 cm
3 c.	skim milk	750 mL
½ c.	fresh apricots, chopped	125 mL
3	eggs, separated	3
¼ t.	cream of tartar	1 mL

Bring water to a boil. Add rice and boil for 20 minutes. Drain rice in a sieve. Place rice. sugar replacement, raisins, 2 T. (30 mL) of the margarine, vanilla bean, cinnamon stick, and milk in a saucepan. Bring to a boil, cover and cook over low heat, stirring occasionally, for about 1¼ hours or until most of the milk is absorbed. Stir in remaining margarine. Spread out in a pan and cool. Remove the vanilla and cinnamon pieces from the rice and mix in apricots and egg yolks. In a bowl, beat the egg whites with the cream of tartar until soft peaks form. Fold gently into rice mixture. Pour into a mold and place in a pan of hot water. Bake at 325°F (165°C) for 1 hour. Remove from oven and let stand at room temperature for 1 hour before serving.

Yield: 8 servings

Exchange, 1 serving: 1½ fruit, ½ full-fat milk
Each serving contains: Calories: 142, Carbohydrates: 35 g

Based on a recipe with the compliments of Arnold Foods Company, Inc.

Sweet Potato Pudding

A favorite at our home on holidays.

4	eggs	4
2 c.	skim milk	500 mL
3 c.	sweet potatoes, peeled and grated	750 mL
3 T.	butter	45 mL
1¼ c.	granulated brown sugar replacement	310 mL
¼ c.	wheat germ	60 mL
½ t.	ground cinnamon	2 mL
¼ t.	ground cloves	1 mL
¼ t.	ground allspice	1 mL
¼ t.	salt	1 mL

Beat eggs until light and fluffy. Add remaining ingredients and stir to mix well. Pour into a well greased baking dish. Bake at 325°F (165°C) for 30 minutes or until set and top is lightly browned.

Yield: 10 servings

Exchange, 1 serving: 1 bread, ½ high-fat meat
Each serving contains: Calories: 129, Carbohydrates: 114 g

Apple Indian Pudding

1 qt.	2% milk	1 L
½ c.	cornmeal	125 mL
⅓ c.	liquid fructose	90 mL
⅓ c.	granulated brown sugar replacement	310 mL
1 t.	salt	5 mL
1 t.	ground cinnamon	5 mL
¼ t.	ground ginger	1 mL
2	apples	2
1 c.	skim milk	250 mL

Bring milk to a boil. Slowly stir in the cornmeal and cook until thickened. Remove from heat. Stir in fructose, sugar replacement, salt, cinnamon and ginger. Core and thinly slice the apples. Layer cornmeal mixture alternately with apple slices in well greased casserole. Pour skim milk over entire mixture. Bake at 275°F (135°C) for 1 hour.

Yield: 10 servings

Exchange, 1 serving: 1 bread, ¾ fruit
Each serving contains: Calories: 97, Carbohydrates: 35 g

Yogurt Tortoni

2 8 oz. cartons	plain yogurt	2 227 g cartons
1 c.	applesauce	250 mL
½ t.	vanilla extract	2 mL
¾ c.	Kretschmer wheat germ	190 mL
⅓ c.	walnuts, finely chopped	90 mL
1 T.	honey	15 mL

Combine yogurt, applesauce, and vanilla. Stir well to blend. Mix wheat germ, walnuts, and honey together. Reserve ¼ c. (60 mL) wheat germ mixture for the topping. Add remaining wheat germ mixture to yogurt mixture. Blend well. Spoon into paper-lined muffin-pan cups. Top with reserved wheat germ mixture. Pat in lightly. Freeze for at least 2 hours or overnight. Let stand at room temperature for 15 to 20 minutes before serving.

Yield: 9 servings

Exchange, 1 serving: 1 bread, ¼ fat
Each serving contains: Calories: 84, Carbohydrates: 10 g

With the courtesy of Kretschmer Wheat Germ/International Multifoods.

Banana Pecan Frozen Dessert

1 pt.	nonfat sugar-free vanilla frozen dessert, ice cream, or frozen yogurt	500 mL
1	very ripe banana, mashed	1
¼ c.	chopped pecans	60 mL

Allow frozen dessert to thaw slightly. Beat in the mashed banana and chopped pecans. Pack in a freezer container or bowl. Cover and freeze until firm.

Yield: 6 servings

Exchange for frozen dessert, 1 serving: ¾ bread
Each serving contains: Calories: 58, Carbohydrates: 11 g

Exchange for ice cream, 1 serving: 1½ bread, ¼ fat
Each serving contains: Calories: 92, Carbohydrates: 22 g

Exchange for frozen yogurt, 1 serving: 1 bread
Each serving contains: Calories: 72, Carbohydrates: 13 g

Toasted-Hazelnut Frozen Dessert

| ½ c. | hazelnuts | 125 mL |
| 1 pt. | nonfat sugar-free vanilla frozen dessert, ice cream, or frozen yogurt | 500 mL |

Place hazelnuts in a single layer on a baking sheet. Bake at 350°F (175°C) for 15 minutes or until lightly toasted. Cool slightly and rub off the very loose skins. (It's not necessary to rub all the skin off.) Chop hazelnuts. Cool. Allow frozen dessert to thaw slightly. Mix hazelnuts into the frozen dessert. Pack in a freezer container or bowl. Cover and freeze until firm.

Yield: 6 servings

Exchange for frozen dessert, 1 serving: 1 bread, ½ fat
Each serving contains: Calories: 105, Carbohydrates: 11 g

Exchange for ice cream, 1 serving: 1¼ bread, 2 fat
Each serving contains: Calories: 150, Carbohydrates: 22 g

Exchange for frozen yogurt, 1 serving: 1 bread, 1½ fat
Each serving contains: Calories: 128, Carbohydrates: 12 g

Frozen Dessert with Raspberry–Grand Marnier Sauce

10 oz. bag	frozen red raspberries	250 g bag
1½ T.	Grand Marnier	21 mL
6 T.	prepared nondairy whipped topping	90 mL
1 pt.	nonfat sugar-free vanilla frozen dessert, ice cream, or frozen yogurt	500 mL

Thaw and drain raspberries. Select six of the best raspberries for garnish and refrigerate. Place remaining raspberries in a bowl, and carefully fold in Grand Marnier. Cover and chill thoroughly.

To serve: Divide frozen dessert of your choice evenly between six serving glasses. Spoon raspberries and liqueur over frozen dessert. Top with 1 T. (15 mL) of the nondairy whipped topping. Garnish with reserved raspberries.

Yield: 6 servings

Exchange for frozen dessert, 1 serving: 1¼ bread, ½ fruit
Each serving contains: Calories: 86, Carbohydrates: 16 g

Exchange for ice cream, 1 serving: 1 bread, ½ fruit, 1 fat
Each serving contains: Calories: 131, Carbohydrates: 27 g

Exchange for frozen yogurt, 1 serving: 1 bread, ½ fat
Each serving contains: Calories: 109, Carbohydrates: 17 g

Apricot Cream

1 lb. can	apricot halves in juice	454 g can
4 oz. jar	baby apricots	113 g jar
2 c.	prepared nondairy whipped topping	500 mL

Drain apricot halves and place in a food processor or blender. Process to semi-purée stage. Transfer to a bowl; stir in baby food apricot puree and ½ c. (250 mL) of the nondairy whipped topping. Freeze for 3 to 4 hours overnight. Cut frozen apricot mixture into pieces, and reprocess in a food processor to a frozen slush. Occasionally, stop machine to push mixture down. Return to freezer and chill again. About 2 or 3 hours before serving check hardness of mixture; if necessary, return to processor and process until smooth. To serve: Divide the mixture evenly between eight serving glasses. Top with remaining whipped topping.

Yield: 8 servings

Exchange, 1 serving: ½ fruit, 1 fat
Each serving contains: Calories: 79, Carbohydrates: 12 g

Strawberry Ice Cake

14	graham cracker squares	14
¼ c.	melted margarine	60 mL
1 env.	unflavored gelatin	1 env.
¼ c.	cold water	60 mL
1 pkg.	sugar-free strawberry gelatin	1 pkg.
1 c.	boiling water	250 mL
2 c.	fresh strawberries	500 mL
2 c.	prepared nondairy whipped topping	500 mL
1	egg white, beaten stiff	1

Crush graham crackers into fine crumbs; then add margarine and stir to mix. Line bottom and sides of a 9 in. (23 cm) pie pan or springform pan with the crumb mixture. Sprinkle the unflavored gelatin over the top of the cold water. Allow to soften for several minutes. Dissolve strawberry gelatin in the boiling water. Stir unflavored gelatin into strawberry gelatin and stir to dissolve gelatin. Cool completely. Cut strawberries in half. Select 16 of the prettiest halves for garnish, and reserve. Fold strawberries and nondairy whipped topping into the gelatin mixture thoroughly. Fold in egg white, leaving a few white streaks. Transfer to crumb-lined pan. Refrigerate until set or overnight. To serve, remove from springform pan. Transfer to serving plate and decorate with reserved strawberry halves.

Yield: 10 servings

Exchange, 1 serving: 1 bread, 1 fat
Each serving contains: Calories: 128, Carbohydrates: 11 g

Raspberries with Peach Sauce

16 oz. pkg.	frozen peach slices	454 g pkg.
3 T.	granulated fructose	45 mL
⅓ c.	cold water	90 mL
2 t.	lemon juice	10 mL
1 t.	vanilla extract	5 mL
½ c.	low-fat plain yogurt	125 mL
2 c.	fresh raspberries	500 mL

Combine frozen peach slices, fructose, water, lemon juice, and vanilla extract in a food processor. Process until mixture is a slush. Add yogurt and process until smooth. Arrange about two-thirds to three-fourths of the raspberries in four stemmed glasses or cups. Spoon the peach slush over the top of the raspberries. Garnish with remaining fresh raspberries.

Yield: 4 servings

Exchange, 1 serving: 1 fruit
Each serving contains: Calories: 58, Carbohydrates: 15 g

Frozen Cottage Cheese Torte

14	graham cracker squares	14
¼ c.	melted margarine	60 mL
2 env.	unflavored gelatin	2 env.
½ c.	cold water	125 mL
2	eggs, separated	2
½ c.	granulated fructose	125 mL
¼ c.	granulated sugar replacement	60 mL
dash	salt	dash
½ c.	skim milk	125 mL
16 oz. carton	low-fat cottage cheese	454 g carton
½ t.	vanilla extract	2 mL
2 c.	prepared nondairy whipped topping	500 mL

Crush graham crackers into fine crumbs; then add margarine and stir to mix. Line bottom and sides of a 9 in. (23 cm) spring-form pan with the crumb mixture. Chill. Sprinkle gelatin over cold water and allow to soften for several minutes. Beat egg yolks slightly; then pour into nonstick saucepan or top of double boiler. Stir in fructose, sugar replacement, salt, and milk. Cook and stir over medium heat until mixture is thick and coats a spoon. Cool. Stir in cottage cheese and vanilla extract. Beat cottage cheese mixture until light and fluffy. Beat egg whites until stiff. Fold egg whites into cottage cheese mixture. Fold nondairy whipped topping into cottage cheese mixture. Transfer to a graham crust. Freeze for 8 to 10 hours or overnight.

Yield: 10 servings

Exchange, 1 serving: 1 bread, 1 fat
Each serving contains: Calories: 163, Carbohydrates: 16 g

Three Fruit Parfait

1 c.	frozen strawberries, thawed	250 mL
1 pt.	nonfat sugar-free dairy dessert (any flavor)	500 mL
1 c.	frozen blueberries, thawed	250 mL
1	banana, sliced thin	1

Distribute about two-thirds to three-fourths of the thawed strawberries between six stemmed glasses or cups. Distribute half of the dairy dessert equally between the glasses. Top each with one-sixth cup of the blueberries. Spoon remaining dairy dessert evenly into the glasses. Distribute the sliced banana between the glasses. Top with the reserved strawberries.

Yield: 6 servings

Exchange, 1 serving: 1 fruit
Each serving contains: Calories: 63, Carbohydrates: 15 g

Sweet Cherry O'Lee

1½ c.	cold water	375 mL
1 T.	cornstarch	15 mL
¼ t.	vanilla extract	1 mL
1 t.	unsweetened cherry drink mix	5 mL
2 c.	vanilla ice cream	500 mL
2 c.	frozen sweet cherries, thawed	500 L

Combine cold water and cornstarch in a saucepan. Stir to dissolve cornstarch. Cook and stir over medium heat until mixture comes to a boil. Continue boiling for 3 minutes, stirring occasionally. Remove from heat, and stir in vanilla extract. Cool to lukewarm; then stir in cherry drink mix. Place ⅓ c. (90 mL) of ice cream in each of the six glasses. (Wine glasses are very pretty to use.) Top each with ⅓ c. (90 mL) of the thawed sweet cherries. Distribute the warm cherry sauce evenly between the glasses.

Yield: 6 servings

Exchange, 1 serving: 1 bread, ½ fat
Each serving contains: Calories: 109, Carbohydrates: 17 g

Frosty 'nilla

4 c.	skim milk	1000 mL
¼ c.	granulated fructose	60 mL
1 t.	vanilla extract	5 mL

Combine ingredients in a mixing bowl or measuring cup. Stir to dissolve fructose. Pour into an ice cream maker. Freeze as directed by ice cream-maker manufacture You can pack Frosty 'Nilla in a freezer container for later use. It freezes very hard in a normal freezer.

Yield: 8 servings

Exchange, 1 serving: ½ skim milk, ⅓ fruit
Each serving contains: Calories: 57, Carbohydrates: 9 g

Summer Strawberry Blaster

1 pkg.	sugar-free strawberry gelatin	1 pkg.
1 c.	boiling water	250 mL
1 c.	cold skim milk	250 mL

Dissolve the strawberry gelatin in the boiling water. Allow to cool to lukewarm. Stir in cold skim milk. (If water is hot, milk will appear to curdle.) Pour into a flat cake pan. Freeze. Break into pieces and process in a food processor or blender into a slush. Serve in disposable plastic V-shaped coffee-liner cups.

Yield: 6 servings

Exchange, 1 serving: negligible
Each serving contains: Calories: 15, Carbohydrates: 1 g

Great Grape Blaster

1 pkg.	sugar-free grape gelatin	1 pkg.
1 c.	boiling water	250 mL
1 c.	cold purple grape juice	250 mL

Dissolve the grape gelatin in the boiling water. Allow to cool to lukewarm. Stir in cold grape juice. Pour into a flat cake pan. Freeze. Break into pieces and process in a food processor or blender into a slush. Serve in disposable plastic V-shaped coffee-liner cups.

Yield: 6 servings

Exchange, 1 serving: ⅓ fruit
Each serving contains: Calories: 23, Carbohydrates: 6 g

Rum Modia Ice Cream

½ gal.	vanilla ice cream	1064 g
9 oz.	semisweet chocolate, finely chopped	255 g
3 T.	instant coffee powder	45 mL
¼ c.	dark rum	60 mL

Soften the ice cream in the refrigerator until it can be whipped with an electric beater. Melt the semisweet chocolate in a double boiler over warm water, stirring occasionally. Allow to cool slightly. Dissolve the instant coffee in the rum. Transfer the ice cream to a large mixing bowl. Whip the ice cream on low, slowly pour the cooled melted chocolate into the ice cream, and continue beating until chocolate is completely incorporated. Gradually pour in coffee-rum mixture, and continue beating. Transfer ice cream to a covered freezer container. Freeze for several hours before serving. If ice cream becomes solid, allow to soften slightly in refrigerator before serving.

Yield: 16 servings

Exchange, 1 serving: 1 bread, 3 fat
Each serving contains: Calories: 210, Carbohydrates: 16 g

Limey Lime Blaster

1 pkg.	sugar-free lime gelatin	1 pkg.	
1 c.	boiling water	250 mL	
1 c.	cold limeade	250 mL	

Dissolve the lime gelatin in the boiling water. Allow to cool to lukewarm. Stir in cold limeade. Pour into a flat cake pan. Freeze. Break into pieces and process in a food processor or blender into a slush. Serve in disposable plastic V-shaped coffee-liner cups.

Yield: 6 servings

Exchange, 1 serving: negligible
Each serving contains: Calories: 17, Carbohydrates: 5 g

White Chocolate Ice Cream with Fresh Peaches

½ gal.	vanilla ice cream	1064 g
8 oz.	white dietetic chocolate, chopped fine	227 g
2 jars (4 oz.)	baby peaches	2 jars (113 g)
2	fresh peaches	2

Soften the ice cream in the refrigerator until it can be whipped with an electric beater. Melt the white chocolate in a double boiler over warm water, stirring occasionally. Allow to cool slightly. Transfer the ice cream to a large mixing bowl. Whip the ice cream on Low, slowly pour the cooled melted chocolate into the ice cream, and continue beating until chocolate is completely incorporated. Gradually pour in peach purée, and continue beating until smooth. Transfer ice cream to a covered freezer container. Freeze for several hours before serving. If ice cream becomes solid, allow to soften slightly in refrigerator before serving. Just before serving, peel, pit, and slice the peaches. Use sliced peaches as garnish.

Yield: 16 servings

Exchange, 1 serving: 1 bread, 2½ fat
Each serving contains: Calories: 193, Carbohydrates: 15 g

Fresh Raspberry Ice Cream

½ gal.	vanilla ice cream	1064 g
1 qt.	fresh raspberries	1 L
1 T	granulated fructose	15 mL

Soften the ice cream in the refrigerator until it can be whipped with an electric beater. Wash and clean the raspberries. Transfer to a medium-sized bowl. With a fork, slightly crush raspberries. Sprinkle with fructose. Stir, cover, and allow to rest 30 minutes. Transfer the ice cream to a large mixing bowl. Whip the ice cream on low until smooth. Fold in the crushed raspberries, allowing the raspberries to marbleize the ice cream. Transfer ice cream to a covered freezer container. Freeze for several hours before serving. If ice cream becomes solid, allow to soften slightly in refrigerator before serving.

Yield: 16 servings

Exchange, 1 serving: 1 bread, 1 fruit, 1 fat
Each serving contains: Calories: 185, Carbohydrates: 28 g

Toasted Walnut and Chocolate Chip Ice Cream

½ gal.	vanilla ice cream	1064 g
1 c.	English walnut pieces	250 mL
½ c.	semisweet mini chocolate chips	125 mL

Let the ice cream soften in the refrigerator until it can be whipped with an electric beater. Meanwhile, place walnuts in a nonstick frying pan. Place over medium-low heat, shaking pan occasionally to toast the walnuts. Remove from heat and allow to cool completely. Transfer the ice cream to a large mixing bowl. Whip the ice cream on low until smooth. Fold in the toasted walnuts and chocolate chips. Transfer ice cream to a covered freezer container. Freeze for several hours before serving. If ice cream becomes solid, allow to soften slightly in refrigerator before serving.

Yield: 16 servings

Exchange, 1 serving: 1 bread, 3 fat
Each serving contains: Calories: 213, Carbohydrates: 17 g

Swedish Citrus Fromage

This is so fast and easy to "whip" up, and your friends and family will love it. It's especially good after spaghetti and meatballs.

2 t.	unflavored, unsweetened gelatin	10 mL
2 T.	water	30 mL
2 T.	freshly squeezed orange juice	30 mL
1 T.	fresh lemon juice	15 mL
1 t.	grated orange rind	5 mL
4	eggs, separated	4
2 T.	sugar (optional)	30 mL
3 pkts.	concentrated acesulfame-K	3 pkts.

In a small saucepan, combine the gelatin and water. Let stand for five minutes, then cook over low heat, stirring until the gelatin dissolves. Set aside to cool. Mix in the orange juice, lemon juice, and orange rind. Beat the egg yolks and sugar together until thick and light. Add the gelatin mixture and the acesulfame-K and beat. In a separate bowl, beat the egg whites until stiff. Use a rubber spatula to fold gently into the other gelatin mixture. The mixture will be evenly yellow when it is well combined. Spoon into six dessert dishes.

Yield: 6 servings

Exchange, 1 serving: 1 fat
Each serving contains: Calories: 58, Carbohydrates: 6 g, Fiber: trace, Sodium: 47 mg, Cholesterol: 183 mg

Apricot Peanut Butter Dessert

1 pkg.★	sugar-free lemon gelatin	1 pkg.★
2 c.	hot water	500 mL
16	apricot halves, in their own juice	16
⅓ c.	creamy peanut butter	90 mL
¼ c.	chopped dates	60 mL
2 T.	chopped walnuts	30 mL

Dissolve gelatin in the hot water; then chill to the consistency of egg whites. Drain apricots. Combine peanut butter, dates, and walnuts. Mix well. Divide peanut butter mixture evenly among the cavities of the apricots; then press halves together. Place an apricot into a mold or dessert dish. Fill mold or dessert dish with the lemon gelatin. Chill until firm.

Yield: 8 servings

Exchange, 1 serving: 1 fruit, 1 fat
Each serving contains: Calories: 119, Carbohydrates: 15 g

★four-servings size

Sparkling Fruit Dessert

1 pkg.*	sugar-free lime gelatin	1 pkg.*
2 c.	hot water	500 mL
1	orange	1
1 c.	pineapple chunks, in their own juice	250 mL
1 c.	peach slices, in their own juice	250 mL
16	seedless green grapes	16

Dissolve lime gelatin in hot water. Chill until the consistency of egg whites. Peel and section orange, removing seeds and membrane. Drain pineapple and peaches thoroughly. Reserve four peach slices. Add orange sections, pineapple chunks, and remaining peach slices to gelatin. Transfer to a mold or eight dessert dishes. Chill until firm. Now cut reserved peach slices in half crosswise. Decorate each serving with a half peach slice and two grapes.

Yield: 8 servings

Exchange, 1 serving: ½ fruit
Each serving contains: Calories: 25, Carbohydrates: 8 g

*four-servings size

Black-Cherry Dessert

1 qt.	black cherries	1 L
2 c.	water	500 mL
1 pkg.*	sugar-free cherry gelatin	1 pkg.*
½ c.	chopped blanched almonds	125 mL
¾ c.	prepared nondairy whipped topping	180 mL

Pit black cherries. Combine cherries and water in a saucepan. Cook over low heat until cherries are just tender. Drain thoroughly, reserving liquid. Measure liquid and add enough water to make 2 c. (500 mL). Heat liquid to boiling. Remove from heat; then stir in gelatin. Stir to dissolve. Chill until mixture is the consistency of egg whites. Then fold in cooked cherries and almonds. Transfer to dessert dishes, mold, or serving dish. Chill until firm. Decorate with nondairy whipped topping before serving.

Yield: 6 servings

Exchange, 1 serving: ⅔ fruit, 1½ fat
Each serving contains: Calories: 101, Carbohydrates: 10 g

*four-servings size

Pineapple Smoothie

16 oz. can	crushed pineapple, in its own juice	459 g can
1 env.	unflavored gelatin	1 env.
½ c.	cold water	125 mL
1 small	apple, grated	1 small
¼ c.	chopped hazelnuts	60 mL

Combine crushed pineapple and unflavored gelatin in a saucepan. Allow gelatin to soften for 5 minutes. Bring to a boil, stirring to dissolve gelatin. Remove from heat. Stir in cold water. Chill until mixture is the consistency of egg whites. Stir in grated apple. Transfer to four dessert dishes. Sprinkle with hazelnuts. Chill until firm.

Yield: 4 servings

Exchange, 1 serving: ⅔ fruit, ⅓ fat
Each serving contains: Calories: 77, Carbohydrates: 10 g

Peach-Yogurt Dessert

1 env.	unflavored gelatin	1 env.	
1 c.	hot peach juice	250 mL	
10 oz. pkg.	frozen unsweetened peach slices	300 g pgk.	
8 oz.	vanilla yogurt	240 g	

Dissolve gelatin in peach juice. Add frozen peaches. Stir peaches and allow them to thaw. Stir in yogurt. Transfer to six dessert dishes or a serving dish. Chill until firm.

Yield: 6 servings

Exchange, 1 serving: ½ fruit, ⅓ skim milk
Each serving contains: Calories: 65, Carbohydrates: 11 g

Grape Supreme

2 c.	white grape juice	500 mL
1 env.	unflavored gelatin	1 env.
1 c.	seedless white grapes	250 mL
1 c.	seedless red grapes	250 mL

Sprinkle gelatin over grape juice in a saucepan. Allow to soften for 5 minutes. Bring to a boil, stirring until gelatin is dissolved. Chill until the consistency of egg whites. Fold in grapes. (If grapes are large, just cut them in half.) Transfer to serving dish. Chill until firm.

Yield: 6 servings

Exchange, 1 serving: 1⅓ fruit
Each serving contains: Calories: 78, Carbohydrates: 20 g

Sparkling Orange Dessert

1 env.	unflavored gelatin	1 env.
1½ c.	water	375 mL
1 env.	unsweetened orange drink mix	1 env.
1 T.	granulated fructose	15 mL
1 c.	mandarin orange slices	250 mL

Sprinkle gelatin over water in a saucepan. Allow gelatin to soften for 5 minutes. Bring to a boil, stirring to dissolve gelatin. Remove from heat. While hot, stir in orange-drink mix and fructose. Chill until the consistency of egg whites. Stir in mandarin orange slices. Transfer to four dessert dishes. Chill until firm.

Yield: 4 servings

Exchange, 1 serving: ½ fruit
Each serving contains: Calories: 37, Carbohydrates: 8 g

Lemon-Fluff Dessert

1 pkg.*	sugar-free lemon gelatin	1 pkg.*	
2 c.	prepared nondairy whipped topping	500 mL	
	sprigs of mint		

Prepare lemon gelatin as directed on package. When the gelatin is firm, beat with an electric mixer. Then beat in nondairy whipped topping. Transfer to 10 dessert glasses or serving dishes. Chill until firm. Decorate with mint sprigs just before serving.

Yield: 10 servings

Exchange, 1 serving: negligible
Each serving contains: Calories: negligible, Carbohydrates: negligible

*four-servings size

Cocktail Sour Cream Supreme

1 pkg.*	sugar-free lime gelatin	1 pkg.*	
½ t.	salt	2 mL	
2 c.	hot water	500 mL	
½ c.	low-calorie salad dressing	125 mL	
½ c.	low-calorie sour cream	125 mL	
1 lb. can	fruit cocktail, in its own juice	457 g can	

Dissolve gelatin and salt in hot water. Stir in salad dressing and sour cream. Chill until the consistency of egg whites. Drain fruit cocktail thoroughly. Fold fruit cocktail into thickened gelatin mixture. Chill until firm.

Yield: 8 servings

Exchange, 1 serving: 1 fat, ¼ fruit
Each serving contains: Calories: 56, Carbohydrates: 4 g

*four-servings size

Cranberry Mellow Dessert

1 env.	unflavored gelatin	1 env.	
2 c.	cranberry fruit cocktail	500 mL	
1 c.	mandarin orange slices	250 mL	
1 c.	mini marshmallows	250 mL	

Sprinkle gelatin over cranberry fruit cocktail in saucepan. Allow to soften for 5 minutes. Bring to boiling, stirring to dissolve gelatin. Chill until mixture is the consistency of egg whites. Then fold in orange slices and marshmallows. Transfer to serving dish. Chill until firm.

Yield: 8 servings

Exchange, 1 serving: 1 fruit
Each serving contains: Calories: 50, Carbohydrates: 17 g

Tart Lime Dessert

1 env.	unflavored gelatin	1 env.	
1 c.	water	250 mL	
6 oz. can	frozen limeade	177 g can	
1 env.	nondairy whipped topping mix	1 env.	

Sprinkle gelatin over water in a saucepan. Allow to soften for 5 minutes. Heat to boiling, stirring to dissolve gelatin. Remove from heat; then stir in limeade until thawed. Add extra water to make 2 c. (500 mL) of liquid. Allow to cool but not set. Meanwhile, chill a bowl and electric beaters. Measure ½ c. (125 mL) of the lime liquid into the chilled bowl; then add the nondairy whipped-topping mix. Beat until thoroughly mixed. Place in freezer of refrigerator, and chill thoroughly. Place remaining lime liquid in refrigerator to set. Beat lime-whipped topping mixture until stiff peaks form. (Re-chill if necessary.) Fold set lime gelatin and lime whipped topping mixture together. Transfer to serving dish.

Yield: 8 servings

Exchange, 1 serving: 1 fruit
Each serving contains: Calories: 51, Carbohydrates: 13 g

Orange-Sherbet Dessert

1 pkg.★	sugar-free orange gelatin	1 pkg.★	
½ c.	hot water	125 mL	
2 c.	orange sherbet	500 mL	

Dissolve gelatin in hot water. Stir in orange sherbet until melted. Pour into four individual serving dishes. Chill until firm.

Yield: 4 servings

Exchange, 1 serving: 1 starch/bread
Each serving contains: Calories: 96, Carbohydrates: 13 g

★four-servings size

Peanut Butterscotch Delight

1 env.	unflavored gelatin	1 env.
1½ c.	water	375 mL
½ c.	chunky peanut butter	125 mL
1 pkg.*	sugar-free butterscotch instant pudding and pie filling	1 pkg.*

Sprinkle gelatin over water in saucepan. Allow to soften for 5 minutes. Bring to a boil, stirring to dissolve gelatin. Remove from heat; then stir in peanut butter until melted. Chill until gelatin mixture is the consistency of egg whites. Chill until firm. Prepare pudding as directed on package. When both the gelatin and the pudding are firm, layer the pudding and the gelatin into eight dessert dishes, starting with pudding and ending with gelatin. Chill until firm.

Yield: 8 servings

Exchange, 1 serving: 1 starch/bread, 1 fat
Each serving contains: Calories: 105, Carbohydrates: 13 g

*four-servings size

Black Walnut Bavarian

1 env.	unflavored gelatin	1 env.
¼ c.	cold water	60 mL
3	egg yolks	3
2 T.	granulated sugar replacement or granulated fructose	30 mL
¼ t.	salt	1 mL
¾ c.	skim milk	190 mL
1 t.	vanilla extract	5 mL
½ c.	black walnuts (chopped fine)	125 mL
1 c.	low-calorie whipped topping (prepared)	250 mL

Combine gelatin and cold water in small cup; set aside 10 minutes to soften. Beat egg yolks, sugar replacement and salt in top of double boiler, and place top of double boiler over hot (not boiling) water. Stir in milk and cook over simmering water until mixture thickens; remove from heat. Stir in softened gelatin until completely dissolved, and add vanilla and black walnuts. Remove top of double boiler from heat and let cool completely. Fold in topping, spoon into serving dishes or mold, and chill thoroughly.

Yield: 6 servings

Exchange, 1 serving with sugar replacement: ½ full-fat milk, 1 fat
Each serving contains: Calories: 129, Carbohydrates: 15 g

Exchange, 1 serving with fructose: ½ high-fat meat, ⅓ fruit, 1 fat
Each serving contains: Calories: 141, Carbohydrates: 15 g

Maple Bavarian

1 env.	unflavored gelatin	1 env.
2 T.	cold water	30 mL
½ c.	low-calorie maple syrup	125 mL
3	egg yolks, beaten	3
2 T.	granulated sugar replacement	30 mL
dash	salt	dash
1 c.	skim milk	190 mL
1 t.	rum flavoring	5 mL
2 c.	low-calorie whipped topping (prepared)	500 mL

Sprinkle gelatin over cold water in small cup and set aside to soften. Combine maple syrup, beaten egg yolks, sugar replacement, salt, and milk in top of double boiler. Cook and stir over simmering (not boiling) water until mixture thickens. (*Do not allow bottom of pan to touch water.*) Add softened gelatin, stir to dissolve completely, and remove from heat. Stir in rum flavoring. Remove top of double boiler from heat. When mixture has cooled completely, fold it into the topping. Scoop into serving dishes or mould; chill thoroughly.

Yield: 8 servings

Exchange, 1 serving: ⅓ low-fat milk
Each serving contains: Calories: 76, Carbohydrates: 26 g

Coconut Bavarian

1 env.	unflavored gelatin	1 env.
2 T.	cold water	30 mL
1½ c.	skim milk	375 mL
½ c.	unsweetened coconut	125 mL
1 t.	white vanilla extract	5 mL
1 c.	low-calorie whipped topping (prepared)	250 mL

Combine gelatin and cold water in small cup; set aside 10 minutes to soften. Combine milk and coconut in blender, whip on High for 2 minutes, and pour into saucepan. Stir and cook over low heat just to boiling, but *do not boil.* Remove from heat. Stir in softened gelatin, until completely dissolved, and add the vanilla. Cool completely and fold coconut mixture into topping.

Yield: 6 servings

Exchange, 1 serving: ⅓ full-fat milk
Each serving contains: Calories: 64, Carbohydrates: 16 g

Bavarian Deluxe

1 env.	unflavored gelatin	1 env.
2 T.	cold water	30 mL
4	egg yolks	4
2 T.	granulated sugar replacement	30 mL
dash	salt	dash
¼ c.	evaporated skim milk	60 mL
¼ c.	water	60 mL
1 env.	low-calorie whipped topping mix (prepared)	1 env.

Combine gelatin and 2 T. (30 mL) cold water in small cup; set aside 10 minutes to soften. Combine egg yolks, sugar replacement and salt in top of double boiler, beating with electric beater or wire whisk until well blended. Place top of double boiler over hot (not boiling) water, and beat in milk and ¼ c. (60 mL) water. Cook and stir over simmering water until mixture thickens, remove from heat, and stir in gelatin until dissolved. Remove top of double boiler from heat; cool until almost set. Fold egg mixture into topping, spoon into serving dishes or mold, and chill thoroughly.

Yield: 6 servings

Exchange, 1 serving: ½ high-fat meat, 1 fat
Each serving contains: Calories: 93, Carbohydrates: 11 g

Quick Gelatin

1 qt.	cold water	1 L
2 env.	unflavored gelatin	2 env.
1 env.	any flavor unsweetened drink mix	1 env.
2 T.	granulated sugar replacement	30 mL

Sprinkle unflavored gelatin over 1 c. (250 mL) of the cold water and allow to rest 10 minutes to soften. Place over medium heat; bring to boil. Cook and stir until gelatin is completely dissolved. Combine drink mix, sugar replacement and remaining 3 c. (750 mL) of water in mixing bowl, stirring to blend. Add gelatin mixture and stir to blend completely. Refrigerate until firm.

Yield: 4 c. (1 L)

Exchange: negligible
Each serving contains: Calories: negligible, Carbohydrates: 43 g

Raspberry Dream

1 env.	unflavored gelatin	1 env.
2 T.	cold water	30 mL
½ c.	boiling water	125 mL
2 t.	liquid sugar replacement	10 mL
dash	salt	dash
3 oz. pkg.	cream cheese, softened	90 g pkg.
3 c.	fresh raspberries	750 mL
	cold water	

Sprinkle gelatin over 2 T. (30 mL) cold water in small cup; set aside 10 minutes to soften. Combine boiling water and softened gelatin in mixing bowl, stirring until gelatin is completely dissolved. Add sugar replacement and salt and stir to blend. Beat cream cheese and 2 T. (30 mL) of gelatin mixture until creamy and then spoon cheese mixture into bottom of a 4 c. (1000 mL) wet mold. Refrigerate until set. Mash 2 c. (500 mL) of the raspberries, adding enough cold water to make 1½ c. (375 mL), and stir into remaining gelatin mixture. Refrigerate until consistency of egg whites. Fold in remaining cup (125 mL) whole raspberries, pour into mold over cream cheese and refrigerate until set. Unmold.

Yield: 6 servings

Exchange, 1 serving: 1 fruit, 1 fat
Each serving contains: Calories: 88, Carbohydrates: 10 g

Lemon Bisque

1½ c.	graham cracker crumbs	375 mL
1 env.	low-calorie lemon gelatin	1 env.
1¼ c.	boiling water	310 mL
2 T.	lemon juice	30 mL
2 T.	granulated sugar replacement or granulated fructose	30 mL
1 env.	low-calorie whipped topping mix (prepared)	1 env.
½ c.	walnuts, chopped fine	125 mL

Spread graham cracker crumbs on bottom of 9 in. (23 cm) baking dish and press down to tighten crumbs; refrigerate. Dissolve lemon gelatin in boiling water and add lemon juice and sugar replacement. Chill mixture until congealed. Beat until fluffy. Fold lemon mixture and nuts into topping. Pour mixture into baking dish; refrigerate 3 hours or overnight.

Yield: 9 servings

Exchange, 1 serving with sugar replacement: 1 fruit, 1 fat
Each serving contains: Calories: 127, Carbohydrates: 19 g

Exchange, 1 serving with fructose: 1 fruit, 1 fat
Each serving contains: Calories: 133, Carbohydrates: 19 g

Lemon Snow

1 env.	unflavored gelatin	1 env.
¼ c.	cold water	60 mL
½ c.	boiling water	125 mL
3 T.	granulated sugar replacement or granulated fructose	45 mL
¼ c.	fresh lemon juice	60 mL
2 t.	fresh lemon rind, grated	10 mL
3	egg whites, beaten stiff	3

Sprinkle gelatin over cold water in mixing bowl; set aside for 10 minutes to soften. Add boiling water and stir until gelatin is completely dissolved, and add sugar replacement, lemon juice and rind. Stir to thoroughly blend. Cool until mixture is consistency of unbeaten egg whites. With an electric beater, whip lemon mixture until frothy. Fold beaten egg whites into lemon mixture. Spoon into 6 serving dishes; refrigerate until set.

Yield: 6 servings

Exchange, 1 serving with sugar replacement: negligible
Each serving contains: Calories: 8, Carbohydrates: 9 g

Exchange, 1 serving with fructose: ½ fruit
Each serving contains: Calories: 26, Carbohydrates: 9 g

Lemon Gelatin

1 env.	unflavored gelatin	1 env.
¼ c.	cold water	60 mL
1¼ c.	boiling water	375 mL
4 t.	liquid sugar replacement	20 mL
dash	salt	dash
⅓ c.	fresh lemon juice	90 mL
1 t.	fresh lemon rind, grated	5 mL

Sprinkle gelatin over cold water in small cup; set aside 10 minutes to soften. Combine boiling water and softened gelatin in a 2 c. (500 mL) mixing bowl, stirring until gelatin is completely dissolved. Add sugar replacement, salt, lemon juice and rind; stir to completely blend. Refrigerate until set.

Yield: 2 c. (500 mL)

Exchange: negligible
Each serving contains: Calories: negligible, Carbohydrates: 35 g

Pecan Whip

1 env.	unflavored gelatin	1 env.
¼ c.	cold water	60 mL
3	eggs, separated	3
2 T.	granulated sugar replacement	30 mL
dash	salt	dash
¾ c.	skim milk	190 mL
2 t.	vanilla extract	10 mL
½ c.	pecans, ground fine	125 mL
½ t.	cream of tartar	2 mL

Sprinkle gelatin on top of water in small cup; set aside 10 minutes to soften. Beat egg yolks until frothy in top of double boiler. Add sugar replacement, salt, and milk, beating well. Place top of double boiler over simmering (not boiling) water. (*Do not allow bottom of pan to touch water.*) Cook and stir until mixture coats spoon, and then stir in softened gelatin until it is completely dissolved. Stir in 1 t. (5 mL) of the vanilla and the pecans. Remove top of double boiler from heat and let cool completely. Combine egg whites, cream of tartar and remaining 1 t. (5 mL) of vanilla, beating until very stiff, and fold into cooled pecan mixture. Spoon into serving dishes.

Yield: 6 servings

Exchange, 1 serving: ½ high-fat meat, ⅓ fruit, 1 fat
Each serving contains: Calories: 112

Mocha Mounds

1 env.	unflavored gelatin	1 env.
2 T.	cold water	30 mL
1¼ c.	strong boiling coffee	310 mL
1 oz. sq.	bitter chocolate, melted	30 g sq.
1 T.	liquid sugar replacement	15 mL
3	egg whites, beaten stiff	3
8 T.	low-calorie whipped topping (prepared)	120 mL

Sprinkle gelatin over cold water in mixing bowl; set aside 10 minutes to soften. Add boiling coffee and stir to completely dissolve gelatin. Stir in melted chocolate and sugar replacement until completely blended. Cool mixture to consistency of unbeaten egg whites. With electric beater, beat mocha mixture until frothy. Fold stiffly beaten egg whites into the mixture. Spoon into 8 serving dishes; refrigerate until set. Before serving, top with 1 T. (15 mL) topping.

Yield: 8 servings

Exchange, 1 serving: ½ fat
Each serving contains: Calories: 39, Carbohydrates: 6 g

Peach Rice Dessert

6	peach halves, peeled	6	
½ c.	orange juice	125 mL	
1½ t.	unflavored gelatin	7 mL	
2 c.	cold cooked rice	500 mL	
dash	salt	dash	
1 c.	low-calorie whipped topping (prepared)	250 mL	

Place each peach half in individual mold or custard cup. Combine orange juice and gelatin in saucepan, cooking over medium heat until gelatin is dissolved. Add cooked rice and salt, stirring to blend completely. Fold in topping, pour over peach halves, and chill until set. Unmold.

Yield: 6 servings

Exchange, 1 serving: 2 fruit, ½ fat
Each serving contains: Calories: 122, Carbohydrates: 79 g

Bing Cherry Soufflé

1 env.	unflavored gelatin	1 env.	
¾ c.	water	190 mL	
2 c.	Bing cherries, pitted	500 mL	
1 T.	lemon juice	15 mL	
2 T.	granulated sugar replacement	30 mL	
3	egg whites, beaten stiff	3	
2 c.	low-calorie whipped topping (prepared)	500 mL	

Sprinkle gelatin over water in saucepan and allow to soften for 10 minutes. Chop 1 c. (250 mL) of the cherries. Add cherries, lemon juice, and sugar replacement to gelatin mixture, and bring to a boil. Cool and stir 5 minutes; refrigerate to thick syrup stage. Fold in remaining cherries. Thicken until firm but not solid. Fold in beaten egg whites, then the topping. Spoon into soufflé dish; refrigerate till set.

Yield: 8 servings

Exchange, 1 serving: ½ fruit, 1 fat
Each serving contains: Calories: 58, Carbohydrates: 17 g

Rhubarb Soufflé

1 qt.	rhubarb, chopped	1 L
¼ c.	water	60 mL
¼ c.	granulated sugar replacement, or granulated fructose	60 mL
1 t.	strawberry flavoring	5 mL
1 env.	unflavored gelatin	1 env.
2 T.	cold water	30 mL
3	egg whites	3
1 t.	vanilla extract	5 mL
2 c.	low-calorie whipped topping (prepared)	500 mL

Combine rhubarb and ¼ c. (60 mL) water in saucepan. Cook and stir over medium heat until rhubarb is very soft; remove from heat. Stir in sugar replacement and strawberry flavoring. Sprinkle gelatin over 2 T. (30 mL) cold water; set aside 10 minutes to soften. Stir gelatin into hot rhubarb until gelatin is completely dissolved. Set aside to completely cool. Beat egg whites and vanilla until very stiff and fold into cooled rhubarb mixture. Fold topping into rhubarb mixture. Fit a 2 in. (5 cm) waxed paper collar around a 1½ qt. (1½ L) soufflé dish. Spoon rhubarb mixture into dish. Refrigerate until set (at least 8 hours). Remove collar and serve.

Yield: 6 servings

Exchange, 1 serving with sugar replacement: ⅓ lean meat
Each serving contains: Calories: 50, Carbohydrates: 23 g

Exchange, 1 serving with fructose: ⅓ lean meat, ½ fruit
Each serving contains: Calories: 70, Carbohydrates: 23 g

Raspberry Cream Gelatin

The sour cream makes this very mousse-like. Save a few raspberries to garnish with mint leaves for a "company" look.

1 pkg.	sugar-free raspberry gelatin mix	1 pkg.
1 c.	boiling water	250 mL
½ c.	fat-free sour cream	125 mL
½ c.	cold water	125 mL
½ c.	frozen raspberries, thawed	125 mL

Put the gelatin powder in a large mixing bowl. Add the boiling water and stir until the powder is dissolved. Add the sour cream and cold water. Stir to mix. Arrange the raspberries in four dessert bowls. Pour the gelatin mixture over the raspberries. Chill until set, about 3–4 hours.

Yield: 4 servings

Exchange, 1 serving: ½ starch/bread
Each serving contains: Calories: 31, Total fat: 0.1 g, Carbohydrates: 7 g, Protein: 2 g, Sodium: 83 mg, Cholesterol: 0 mg

Strawberry Yogurt Dessert

The yogurt adds a creamy texture.

1 pkg.	sugar-free strawberry gelatin mix	1 pkg.
¾ c.	boiling water	185 mL
½ c.	cold water	125 mL
	ice cubes	
1 c.	fat-free yogurt, plain or vanilla	250 mL
½ c.	fresh strawberries, hulled and sliced	125 mL
4	mint leaves (optional)	4

Put the gelatin powder into a large mixing bowl. Add the boiling water and stir until the gelatin is dissolved. Put the cold water into a 2 c. (500 mL) measure. Add enough ice cubes until the measuring cup is 1¼ c. (310 mL) full. Put the cold water and ice into a food processor. Add the gelatin mixture. Blend until the ice cubes almost disappear. Add the yogurt and blend again. Distribute the strawberry slices on four dessert dishes. Pour the yogurt and gelatin mixture over the fruit. Chill for 1–2 hours. Top with your favorite white topping and garnish with mint leaves and strawberry slices, if desired.

Yield: 4 servings

Exchange, 1 serving: ½ fruit
Each serving contains: Calories: 40, Total fat: 0.1 g, Carbohydrates: 8 g, Protein: 0.6 g, Sodium: 100 mg, Cholesterol: 2 mg

Ginger-Strawberry Cooler

Ginger is a flavor favored by people who live in tropical climates because it's cooling. Try making this easy dessert or snack for the hottest days.

1 pkg.	sugar-free strawberry-kiwi gelatin mix	1 pkg.
1 c.	boiling water	250 mL
¼ t.	ground ginger	2 mL
1 c.	sugar-free ginger ale	250 mL
½ c.	fresh strawberries or frozen no-sugar-added, thawed and then sliced	125 mL

Put the gelatin powder into a large mixing bowl. Add the boiling water and ginger. Stir until the gelatin is dissolved. Add the ginger ale and mix. Arrange the strawberries in four dessert bowls. Pour the gelatin mixture over the strawberries. Chill for 3–4 hours. Top with your favorite white topping, if desired.

Yield: 4 servings

Exchange: free
Each serving contains: Calories: 10, Total fat: 0.1 g, Carbohydrates: 3 g, Protein: 0.6 g, Sodium: 57 mg, Cholesterol: 0 mg

Strawberry Layered Dessert

Although this recipe calls for sugar-free, fat-free ice cream, you can use sugar-free, fat-free frozen yogurt instead.

1 pkg.	sugar-free strawberry-banana gelatin mix	1 pkg.
¾ c.	boiling water	185 mL
½ c.	cold water	125 mL
	ice cubes	
½ c.	sugar-free low-fat vanilla ice cream	125 mL
½ c.	fresh strawberries, hulled and sliced	125 mL

Put the gelatin powder into a large mixing bowl. Add the boiling water and stir until dissolved. Put the cold water into a 2 c. (500 mL) measure. Add enough ice cubes until the measuring cup is 1¼ c. (310 mL) full. Put the cold water and ice into a food processor. Add the gelatin mixture. Blend until the ice cubes almost disappear. Divide this gelatin mixture in half. Add the ice cream to one half and the strawberries to the other. Mix until smooth. In each of four individual dessert dishes, spoon a layer of fruit mixture. Spoon a creamy layer on top. Chill until set. This will take an hour or so. Top with your favorite white topping.

Yield: 4 servings

Exchange, 1 serving: ½ fruit
Each serving contains: Calories: 22, Total fat: 0.1 g, Carbohydrates: 6 g, Protein: 0.6 g, Sodium: 66 mg, Cholesterol: 0 mg

Strawberry-Banana Cubes

Kids love these. For special effects use cookie cutters.

1 pkg.	sugar-free strawberry-banana gelatin mix	1 pkg.
¾ c.	boiling water	185 mL
¾ c.	cold water	185 mL
1 med.	banana, sliced	1 med.
½ c.	fresh strawberries, sliced (optional)	125 mL

Put the strawberry-banana gelatin powder into a large mixing bowl. Add the boiling water and stir until the powder is dissolved. Add the cold water and stir. Arrange the fruit in an 8 × 8 in. (20 × 20 cm) brownie pan. Pour the gelatin over the fruit. Chill for 3–4 hours until the mixture sets. Cut into cubes and arrange the cubes in a circle around the edge of the plate. Optional: Place fresh fruit or a dash of your favorite white topping in the center.

Yield: 4 servings

Exchange, 1 serving: ½ fruit
Each serving contains: Calories: 36, Total fat: 0.2 g, Carbohydrates: 10 g, Protein: 0.9 g, Sodium: 58 mg, Cholesterol: 0 mg

Pear and Banana Gelatin Dessert

If you like your fruit floating in gelatin, let it begin to set for 20–30 minutes and then stir in the fruit and nuts. No one in my house minds the fruit at the bottom.

1 pkg.	sugar-free strawberry-banana gelatin mix	1 pkg.
1 c.	boiling water	250 mL
½ t.	rum-flavored extract	3 mL
1 c.	cold water	250 mL
½ c.	fresh pears, sliced, or canned pears, drained	125 mL
½ c.	bananas, sliced	125 mL
2 T.	walnuts, chopped fine (optional)	30 mL

Put the gelatin powder into a large mixing bowl. Add the boiling water and rum extract. Stir until the gelatin is dissolved. Add the cold water and mix. Arrange the fruit and the nuts (if used) in four individual dessert bowls. Pour the gelatin mixture over the fruit. Chill until firm, about 3–4 hours. Top with your favorite white topping, if desired.

Yield: 4 servings

Exchange, 1 serving: ⅔ fruit
Each serving contains: Calories: 43, Total fat: 0.2 g, Carbohydrates: 12 g, Protein: 0.9 g, Sodium: 59 mg, Cholesterol: 0 mg

Lime and Banana Gelatin Dessert

If you want the bananas to "float," wait to add them after the gelatin has started to jell.

1 pkg.	sugar-free lime gelatin mix	1 pkg.
1 c.	boiling water	250 mL
½ c.	cold water	125 mL
½ c.	fat-free sour cream	125 mL
1 med	banana, sliced	1 med

Put the gelatin powder into a large mixing bowl. Add the boiling water and stir until the powder is dissolved. Add the cold water and the sour cream and stir until the sour cream is completely blended. Arrange the banana slices in four dessert dishes. Pour the gelatin mixture over the bananas. Chill for 3–4 hours.

Yield: 4 servings

Exchange, 1 serving: ½ starch/bread
Each serving contains: Calories: 50, Total fat: 0.1 g, Carbohydrates: 12 g, Protein: 2 g, Sodium: 83 mg, Cholesterol: 0 mg

Orange Cottage Cheese Dessert

Not too sweet. My mother loves this dessert.

1 pkg.	sugar-free orange gelatin mix	1 pkg.
1 c.	boiling water	250 mL
1 c.	cold water	125 mL
1 c.	fat-free small curd cottage cheese	125 mL
2 c.	orange sections, diced	500 mL

Put the gelatin powder into a large mixing bowl. Add the boiling water. Stir until the gelatin dissolves. Add the cold water. Stir. Place the gelatin mixture into a food processor or blender. Add the cottage cheese. Blend until the mixture is smooth. Pour into four dessert dishes. Chill 3–4 hours. Garnish with the diced orange sections just before serving.

Yield: 4 servings

Exchange, 1 serving: 1 milk
Each serving contains: Calories: 79, Total fat: 0.1 g, Carbohydrates: 16 g, Protein: 8 g, Sodium: 209 mg, Cholesterol: 5 mg

Creamy Melon Gelatin Dessert

I make this when I have a leftover melon or cantaloupe.

1 pkg.	sugar-free lime gelatin mix	1 pkg.
1 c.	boiling water	250 mL
½ c.	sugar-free low-fat vanilla ice cream	125 mL
½ c.	cold water	125 mL
½ c.	cantaloupe or honeydew melon pieces, fresh or frozen	125 mL

Put the gelatin powder into a large mixing bowl. Add the boiling water and stir until the gelatin is dissolved. Add the ice cream and cold water. Stir to mix. Arrange the pieces of melon in four dessert dishes. Pour the gelatin mixture over the fruit. Chill 3–4 hours.

Yield: 4 servings

Exchange, 1 serving: ½ fruit
Each serving contains: Calories: 23, Total fat: 0.1 g, Carbohydrates: 7 g, Protein: 0.7 g, Sodium: 68 mg, Cholesterol: 0 mg

"Creamsicle" Gelatin

Do you love creamsicles? This recipe will get you close in taste for very few calories!

1 pkg.	sugar-free orange gelatin mix	1 pkg.
1 c.	boiling water	250 mL
½ c.	vanilla sugar-free low-fat ice cream	125 mL
½ c.	cold water	125 mL
¼ c.	orange sections	60 mL

Put the gelatin powder into a large mixing bowl. Add the boiling water and stir until the powder is dissolved. Add the ice cream and cold water. Stir to mix. Pour into four dessert bowls. Chill until firm, 3–4 hours. Garnish with orange sections.

Yield: 4 servings

Exchange, 1 serving: ½ fruit
Each serving contains: Calories: 22, Total fat: 0 g, Carbohydrates: 6 g, Protein: 0.6 g, Sodium: 66 mg, Cholesterol: 0 mg

Easy Chocolate Ice Cream

½ c.	skim milk	125 mL
¼ c.	semisweet chocolate chips	60 mL
1 env.	nondairy topping mix	1 env.

Heat milk and chocolate chips just to boiling, stirring constantly to dissolve chips. Refrigerate until mixture is very cold. Add topping mix. Beat until mixture is thick and fluffy. Pour into freezer box or tray and freeze until firm.

Yield: 2 c. (500 mL)

Exchange, ½ c. (125 mL): 1 bread, ⅔ fat
Each serving contains: Calories: 97, Carbohydrates: 13 g

Ice Cream Clones

1 recipe	Easy Chocolate Ice Cream	1 recipe
20	Cream Puff Pastry mini cream puffs	20

Prepare Easy Chocolate Ice Cream but do not freeze. Scoop mixture into pastry bag with a large tube. Squeeze mixture into the mini cream puffs. Freeze.

Yield: 20 clones

Exchange, 1 clone: ⅓ bread
Each serving contains: Calories: 21

Chocolate Mint Gelatin

A lean and flavorful dessert.

¼ c.	cocoa	60 mL
3 T.	granulated sugar replacement	45 mL
1 env.	unflavored gelatin	1 env.
1 c.	boiling water	250 mL
½ c.	plain nonfat yogurt	125 mL
2 t.	mint extract	10 mL
½ t.	vanilla extract	2 mL
½ c.	cold water	125 mL
1 c.	nondairy whipped topping	250 mL

Combine cocoa, sugar replacement, and gelatin in medium-sized mixing bowl. Stir to mix. Pour boiling water over mixture and stir to completely dissolve ingredients. Stir in yogurt, extracts and cold water. Pour into 2 c. (500 mL) decorative mold. Chill until set. Unmold and decorate with nondairy whipped topping.

Yield: 6 servings

Exchange, 1 serving: ½ nonfat milk
Each serving contains: Calories: 48, Carbohydrates: 19 g

Mocha Dessert

½ c.	chocolate chips	125 mL
2 c.	hot coffee	500 mL
1 env.	unflavored gelatin	1 env.
1 env.	nondairy topping mix	1 env.

In a medium-sized mixing bowl, dissolve the chocolate chips and gelatin in the hot coffee. Cool. Stir in non-dairy whipped topping powder until it is completely blended. Place mixing bowl in a larger bowl of ice. Beat with a whip or electric mixer until mixture is slightly fluffy. Divide into 8 sherbet or dessert glasses. Chill until completely set.

Yield: 8 servings

Exchange, 1 serving: ⅔ bread, 1 fat
Each serving contains: Calories: 71, Carbohydrates: 11 g

Split Parfaits

No one can resist these.

2 c.	fresh strawberries	500 mL
2 T.	sorbitol	30 mL
2 c.	Easy Chocolate Ice Cream	500 mL
1½	bananas, sliced	1½

Mash strawberries. Stir in sorbitol and set aside for 20 minutes. Place 2 T. (30 mL) of mashed strawberries in bottom of 6 parfait glasses. Add ⅓ c. (90 mL) of ice cream and one sixth of banana slices to glasses. Top each glass with equal amounts of remaining strawberries.

Yield: 6 servings

Exchange, 1 serving: ⅔ bread, 1 fruit, ⅓ fat
Each serving contains: Calories: 108, Carbohydrates: 19 g

Sweet Chocolate Turban

2 env.	unflavored gelatin	2 env.
½ c.	cold water	125 mL
⅓ c.	granulated sugar replacement	90 mL
2 T	liquid fructose	30 mL
½ c.	chocolate chips	125 mL
2½ c.	buttermilk	625 mL
1 c.	Chocolate Whipped Topping	250 mL

Sprinkle the gelatin on top of cold water in a saucepan. Allow to soften for 5 minutes. Cook and stir over low heat until the gelatin is completely dissolved. Remove from heat and add sugar replacement, fructose and chocolate chips. Stir until blended. Stir in buttermilk. Mix thoroughly. Pour into a lightly greased turban mold or decorative ice cream mold. Refrigerate until firm, about 3 to 4 hours. Unmold onto a well-chilled serving plate. Decorate around the edge with chocolate whipped topping.

Yield: 6 servings

Exchange, 1 serving: 1 bread, 1 fat
Each serving contains: Calories: 117, Carbohydrates: 36 g

Mocha Ice Cream

A bittersweet treat.

2	eggs	2
2	egg yolks	2
3 T.	granulated sugar replacement	45 mL
2 T.	sorbitol	30 mL
2 c.	2% milk	500 mL
1 T.	cornstarch	15 mL
2 oz.	baking chocolate, melted	60 g
2 T.	very strong coffee	30 mL
1 c.	nondairy whipped topping	250 mL

Beat egg and egg yolks in bowl; add sugar replacement and sorbitol and beat until thick and creamy. Combine milk and cornstarch in saucepan; stir to thoroughly mix. Heat until mixture is about to boil and is slightly thickened. Remove from heat and pour over egg mixture in a steady stream. Beat thoroughly to blend. Return mixture to saucepan, cook and stir over low heat until custard thickens. *Do not allow to boil.* Stir in melted chocolate and strong coffee. Place hot saucepan in bowl over ice cubes, to speed the cooling process. When cool to the touch, fold in whipped topping. Chill and freeze. As it hardens, push the sides of the mixture to the center. When nearly set, scrape mixture into large mixing bowl. Beat well. Pack and freeze.

Yield: 8 servings

Exchange, 1 serving: ½ bread, ⅓ high-fat meat
Each serving contains: Calories: 122, Carbohydrates: 19 g

Frozen Chocolate Banana Yogurt

Quick and easy.

1	very ripe banana	1
2 T.	cocoa	30 mL
8 oz.	plain yogurt	226 g

Combine banana, cocoa, and yogurt in blender or food processor. Blend until smooth. Turn into two dessert dishes. Freeze until firm.

Yield: 2 servings

Exchange, 1 serving: 1 nonfat milk, ⅔ bread
Each serving contains: Calories: 132, Carbohydrates: 130 g

Cool Chocolate Gelatin

A fast perfection while you do other chores.

1 env.	unflavored gelatin	1 env.
½ c.	cold water	125 mL
1½ c.	2% chocolate milk	375 mL

Sprinkle gelatin over water; allow to soften for 5 minutes. In microwave or on top of the stove bring mixture to boiling. Allow to cool slightly. Stir in chocolate milk. Pour into 4 dessert dishes. Chill.

Yield: 4 servings

Exchange, 1 serving: ⅔ low-fat milk
Each serving contains: Calories: 70, Carbohydrates: 13 g

Cool Chocolate Custard Ice Cream

4	egg yolks	4
3 T.	granulated sugar replacement	45 mL
1 c.	2% milk	250 mL
2 oz.	baking chocolate, melted	60 g
2 c.	nondairy whipped topping	500 mL

In a medium-sized mixing bowl beat the egg yolks with the sugar replacement until light and fluffy. Heat milk just to boiling. Pour hot milk over egg yolk mixture, beating constantly. Beat in melted chocolate. Return mixture to saucepan. Cook and stir over low heat until mixture thickens. Remove from heat and cool. Beat slightly with electric mixture to loosen. Fold prepared nondairy whipped topping into custard. Chill or freeze.

Yield: 8 servings

Exchange, 1 serving: ⅔ low-fat milk, 1 fat
Each serving contains: Calories: 112, Carbohydrates: 17 g

Spanish Delight

1	cinnamon stick	1
¼ t.	ground nutmeg	2 mL
dash	ground cloves	dash
dash	ground ginger	dash
2 c.	water	500 mL
1 env.	unflavored gelatin	1 env.
½ c.	chocolate chips	125 mL
3 T.	granulated sugar replacement	45 mL

Combine cinnamon stick, nutmeg, cloves, and ginger with water in saucepan. Bring to a boil, reduce heat and simmer for 5 minutes. Remove from heat. Remove cinnamon stick. Add unflavored gelatin, chocolate chips, and sugar replacement. Stir to dissolve completely. Refrigerate until completely set.

Yield: 4 servings

Exchange, 1 serving: 1 bread, 1 fat
Each serving contains: Calories: 110, Carbohydrates: 26 g

Fudge Almandine Mousse

6	egg yolks	6
3 T.	liquid fructose	45 mL
2 c.	nondairy whipped topping	500 mL
7	egg whites	7
⅓ c.	almonds, toasted and ground	90 mL
½ c.	chocolate chips, ground	125 mL
1 T.	rum flavoring	15 mL

Beat egg yolks until pale and creamy. Pour liquid fructose over yolks and beat until thick. Fold in nondairy whipped topping. Beat egg whites and salt until stiff. Fold into mixture. Fold in ground almonds and chocolate chips. Pile into decorate mold and freeze. Allow to soften 15 minutes in refrigerator before unmolding. Unmold onto serving plate. Sprinkle with rum flavoring.

Yield: 10 servings

Exchange, 1 serving: ⅔ high-fat meat, 1 fruit
Each serving contains: Calories: 125, Carbohydrates: 15 g

Chocolate Yogurt Ice

3 c.	crushed ice	750 mL
8 oz.	plain nonfat yogurt	226 g
2 oz.	baking chocolate, melted	60 g
3 T.	granulated sugar replacement	45 mL
4 T.	nondairy whipped topping	60 mL

Combine all ingredients in food processor or blender. Whip until thoroughly blended but not melted. Pour into 4 tall glasses. Place in freezer until mixture is slightly frozen. Stir, top with 1 T. (15 mL) nondairy whipped topping and serve.

Yield: 4 servings

Exchange, 1 serving: ⅝ full-fat milk
Each serving contains: Calories: 134, Carbohydrates: 19 g

Chocolate Buttermilk Ice

A German specialty.

1 qt.	buttermilk	1 L
2 oz.	baking chocolate, melted	60 g
3 T.	granulated sugar replacement	45 mL

Mix all ingredients thoroughly in a large mixing bowl. Pour into a freezer tray or metal baking dish. Freeze until mushy and slightly frozen around the edges of the tray. Return to large mixing bowl and beat until the mixture is light. Pile into 6 individual sherbet dishes and freeze until ready to serve.

Yield: 6 servings

Exchange, 1 serving: 1 medium-fat milk
Each serving contains: Calories: 116, Carbohydrates: 17 g

Christmas Dessert

An elegant dessert. Make it in advance.

4	egg yolks	4
⅓ c.	granulated sugar replacement	90 mL
1	cream de cacao	15 mL
4	egg whites	4
⅓ c.	pecans, finely ground	90 mL
1 env.	nondairy topping mix	1 env.
½ c.	skim milk	125 mL
3 drops	green food coloring	3 drops

Cook egg yolks, sugar replacement, and cream de cacao over low heat in the top of a double boiler until thick; cool. Beat egg whites until stiff. Fold egg whites into cooled custard mixture. Fold in chopped pecans. Beat topping mix with skim milk and green food coloring until stiff. Fold into custard mixture. Turn into well-chilled 1½ qt. (1½ L) serving dish. Refrigerate or freeze.

If frozen, allow to set at room temperature 15 minutes before serving.

Yield: 10 servings

Exchange, 1 serving: ½ high-fat meat, ½ fruit
Each serving contains: Calories: 73, Carbohydrates: 11 g

Pineapple au Chocolat

Something for one.

2	pineapple slices, drained	2
1	large lettuce leaf	1
2 T.	chocolate topping	30 mL
1 T.	nondairy whipped topping	15 mL

Place pineapple slices on lettuce leaf, drizzle with chocolate topping. Top with whipped topping.

Yield: 1 serving

Exchange, 1 serving: 35 bread, 1 fruit
Each serving contains: Calories: 88, Carbohydrates: 25 g

Chocolate Bombe

1 recipe	Easy Chocolate Ice Cream	1 recipe
1 c.	vanilla ice cream	250 mL
1 c.	nondairy whipped topping	250 mL
¼ c.	almonds, toasted and finely chopped	60 mL

Chill a 1 qt. (1 L) metal mold in the freezer. With a chilled spoon, quickly spread chocolate ice cream over bottom and sides of mold. Freeze firm. Stir the vanilla ice cream just to soften. Quickly spread over chocolate layer, covering completely. Freeze firm. Fold toasted almonds into whipped topping. Pile into center of mold, smoothing the top. Cover with plastic wrap or foil. Freeze 6 to 8 hours or overnight. Peel off cover, invert mold onto chilled plate. Cover mold with a damp warm towel; lift off mold. Refreeze or serve.

Yield: 14 servings

Exchange, 1 serving: ½ bread, ⅔ fat
Each serving contains: Calories: 65, Carbohydrates: 6 g

Piña Colada Cooler

2 c.	unsweetened pineapple juice	500 mL
¼ c.	unsweetened flaked coconut	60 mL
¼ c.	cold water	60 mL
2 t.	rum flavoring	10 mL

Combine all ingredients in a bowl. Stir to mix. Pour into ice-cream maker. Freeze to desired consistency, following manufacturer's directions.

Yield: 4 servings

Exchange, 1 serving: 1 fruit, ½ fat
Each serving contains: Calories: 87, Carbohydrates: 16 g

Chocolate-Coffee Cream

2 c.	skim milk	500 mL
2 T.	low-calorie instant chocolate-drink mix	30 mL
2 t.	instant coffee, powder	10 mL

Heat milk in the top of a double boiler. Add chocolate-drink mix and instant coffee. Stir to completely dissolve. Cool thoroughly. Pour into ice-cream maker. Freeze to desired consistency, following manufacturer's directions.

Yield: 4 servings

Exchange, 1 serving: ⅔ skim milk
Each serving contains: Calories: 60, Carbohydrates: 8 g

Cooling Stinger

3 c.	skim milk	750 mL
2 T.	brandy flavoring	30 mL
1 T.	wintergreen flavoring	15 mL

Combine all ingredients in a bowl. Stir to mix. Pour into ice-cream maker. Freeze to desired consistency, following manufacturer's directions.

Yield: 4 servings

Exchange, 1 serving: ¾ skim milk
Each serving contains: Calories: 68, Carbohydrates: 9 g

Pink-Petunia Cream

1 qt.	2% milk	1 L
1 env.	nondairy whipped topping mix	1 env.
1 T.	cherry flavoring	15 mL
1	egg white, stiffly beaten	1

Combine milk, whipped-topping mix, and cherry flavoring in a bowl. Stir to blend thoroughly. Fold in stiffly beaten egg white. Pour into ice cream maker, and freeze according to manufacturer's directions.

Yield: 8 servings

Exchange, 1 serving: ¾ low-fat milk
Each serving contains: Calories: 92, Carbohydrates: 10 g

Long Island Freeze

1 qt.	buttermilk	1 L
3 T.	brandy flavoring	45 mL
3 T.	low-calorie instant chocolate-drink mix	45 mL
1 t.	vanilla extract	5 mL
⅓ c.	mini chocolate chips	90 mL

Combine buttermilk, brandy flavoring, chocolate-drink mix, and vanilla in a bowl. Stir to mix. Pour into ice-cream maker, and freeze according to manufacturer's directions. Halfway through freezing, add chocolate chips.

Yield: 8 servings

Exchange, 1 serving: ½ starch/bread, ½ skim milk
Each serving contains: Calories: 101, Carbohydrates: 13 g

Apricot-Brandy Freeze

1 qt.	2% milk	1 L
2 jars (4½ oz.)	puréed baby peaches	2 jars (126 g)
2 env.	aspartame low-calorie sweetener	2 env.
2 t.	brandy flavoring	10 mL

Combine all ingredients in a bowl. Stir to blend. Pour into ice-cream maker, and freeze according to manufacturer's directions.

Yield: 8 servings

Exchange, 1 serving: ½ low-fat milk, ½ fruit
Each serving contains: Calories: 86, Carbohydrates: 12 g

Angel-Tip Cooler

2 c.	skim milk	500 mL
1 T.	clear vanilla flavoring	30 mL
1 t.	cornstarch	5 mL

Combine all ingredients in the top of a double boiler. While stirring, cook over simmering water until mixture is slightly thickened. Cool completely. With a rotary beater or electric mixer, beat until slightly fluffy. Turn into ice-cream maker, and freeze according to manufacturer's directions.

Yield: 4 servings

Exchange, 1 serving: ½ skim milk
Each serving contains: Calories: 53, Carbohydrates: 6 g

Cuba Ice

12 oz. can	diet cola	348 g
2 c.	skim milk	500 mL
2 T.	lime juice	30 mL
1 T.	rum flavoring	15 mL

Combine all ingredients in a bowl. Stir to mix. Pour into ice-cream maker. Freeze to desired consistency, following manufacturer's directions.

Yield: 6 servings

Exchange, 1 serving: ⅓ skim milk
Each serving contains: Calories: 31, Carbohydrates: 4 g

Wild-Irish Freeze

1 qt.	skim milk	1 L
2 T.	nondairy whipped topping mix	30 mL
3 T.	low-calorie instant chocolate-drink mix	45 mL
1 T.	almond extract	15 mL

Combine all ingredients in a bowl. Stir to completely dissolve chocolate-drink mix. Pour into ice-cream maker, and freeze according to manufacturer's directions.

Yield: 8 servings

Exchange, 1 serving: ½ low-fat milk
Each serving contains: Calories: 63, Carbohydrates: 7 g

Ice Cream Cones

2 T.	margarine, melted	30 mL
2 T.	granulated brown sugar replacement	30 mL
1 T.	granulated sugar replacement	15 mL
1	egg	1
1 t.	vanilla extract	5 mL
1¼ c.	flour	310 mL
1¼ c.	water	310 mL

Combine all ingredients in blender, food processor or mixing bowl. Beat until smooth.

For crepe pan: Pour batter into 9 in. (23 cm) pie tin. Heat crepe pan until hot, and dip crepe pan into batter. Fry batter until edges are lightly browned. With spatula, turn crepe over. Press lightly to help conform to pan. Fry until completely dry. Using spatula and cone, quickly roll batter into shape. Dry and cool on rack.

For Krumcake iron: Heat iron and place 1 T. (15 mL) mixture in center. Fry on both sides. Using spatula and cone, quickly roll batter into shape. Dry and cool on rack.

Yield: 36 cones

Exchange, 1 cone: ¼ fruit
Each serving contains: Calories: 20, Carbohydrates: 4 g

French Vanilla Ice Cream

5	egg yolks	5
¼ c.	granulated sugar replacement	60 mL
dash	salt	dash
2 c.	evaporated skimmed milk	500 mL
1 in.	vanilla bean	2.5 cm
2 c.	low-calorie whipped topping (prepared)	500 mL

Combine egg yolks, sugar replacement and salt in top of double boiler. Beat until frothy. Beat in milk and add vanilla bean. Cook and stir over simmering water until mixture is thick and vanilla bean is dissolved. Cool completely. With electric beater, beat well, and then fold in topping. Pour into freezer trays, cover with waxed paper, and freeze for 1 hour. Scrape into large bowl and beat until smooth and fluffy. Return to freezer trays. Cover. Freeze firm.

Yield: 1½ qt. (1½ L)

Exchange, ½ c. (125 mL): ½ high-fat meat
Each serving contains: Calories: 61, Carbohydrates: 14 g

Strawberry Ice Cream

1 qt.	evaporated skimmed milk	1 L
2	eggs	2
3 T.	granulated sugar replacement	45 mL
¼ t.	salt	1 mL
¼ c.	lemon juice	60 mL
2 c.	strawberries, sliced	500 mL
2 drops	red food color	2 drops

Chill milk. Beat eggs until frothy. Add sugar replacement, salt and lemon juice to the eggs, and beat well. Gradually beat in the cold milk.

For ice cream freezer: Pour mixture into 1 gal. (4 L) freezer can. Freeze as directed by manufacturer. Add strawberries and food color when cream begins to thicken.

For tray freezing: Pour into 3 freezer trays, and freeze until crystals form on edge of trays. Pour into large bowl; beat well. Add strawberries and food color, and return to trays. Repeat for lighter ice cream. Repack in ice cream or plastic cartons; freeze until firm.

Yield: 8 servings

Exchange, 1 serving: 1 nonfat milk, ⅓ fat
Each serving contains: Calories: 104, Carbohydrates: 22 g

Quick Orange Ice Cream

½ c.	orange juice concentrate, thawed	125 mL
1 env.	low-calorie whipped topping mix	1 env.
½ t.	lemon juice	2 mL

Combine all ingredients in a small narrow bowl. Whip at high speed until thick and fluffy. Pour into freezer tray and freeze until firm.

Yield: 6 servings

Exchange, 1 serving: 1 fruit, 1 fat
Each serving contains: Calories: 83, Carbohydrates: 10 g

Pineapple-Orange Ice Cream

2	eggs	2
3 T.	granulated sugar replacement	45 mL
¼ t.	salt	1 mL
1 qt.	cold evaporated skimmed milk	1 L
2 c.	unsweetened crushed pineapple, with juice	500 mL
1 c.	orange juice	250 mL
2 T.	orange rind, grated	30 mL

Beat eggs until frothy. Add sugar replacement and salt; beat well. Gradually beat in milk. Stir in pineapple, orange juice and rind.

For ice cream freezer: Pour into 1 gal. (4 L) freezer can. Freeze as directed by manufacturer.

For tray freezing: Pour into 3 freezer trays. Freeze until mushy. Pour into large bowl; beat well. Return to freezer trays. Repeat. Repack in ice cream or plastic cartons. Freeze firm.

Yield: 1 gal. (4 L)

Exchange, ½ c. (125 mL): ¼ bread
Each serving contains: Calories: 22, Carbohydrates: 8 g

Date Parfait

½ c.	dates, chopped	125 mL
1½ c.	water	375 mL
4	egg yolks, well beaten	4
½ c.	orange juice	125 mL
1 c.	low-calorie whipped topping (prepared)	250 mL

Combine dates and water in saucepan. Cook and stir occasionally over medium heat for 25 minutes; let cool. Add beaten egg yolks and orange juice; cook and stir constantly over low heat until thickened. Chill. Fold topping into date mixture, spread evenly into freezer tray, and freeze until firm.

Yield: 8 servings

Exchange, 1 serving: 1 fruit, ½ fat
Each serving contains: Calories: 55, Carbohydrates: 10 g

Mint-Chip Ice Cream

1½ t.	unflavored gelatin	7 mL
2 T.	boiling water	30 mL
2 t.	green peppermint flavoring	10 mL
¼ t.	salt	1 mL
1 env.	low-calorie whipped topping mix	1 env.
½ c.	cold water	125 mL
1 t.	vanilla extract	5 mL
¼ c.	small semisweet chocolate chips	60 mL

Sprinkle gelatin over boiling water, stirring to dissolve. Add peppermint flavoring and salt; stir well. Let mixture cool. Combine topping mix, cold water, and vanilla in bowl, and whip mixture until stiff. Fold in peppermint mixture and chocolate chips. Pour into freezer tray and freeze until firm.

Yield: 6 servings

Exchange, 1 serving: ½ fruit, 2 fat
Each serving contains: Calories: 78, Carbohydrates: 5 g

Heavenly Hash

⅓ c.	Marshmallow Crème	90 mL
1 c.	skim milk	250 mL
1 c.	almonds, chopped	250 mL
½ c.	walnuts, chopped	125 mL
1 c.	Bing cherries, pitted	250 mL
1 c.	low-calorie whipped topping (prepared)	250 mL

Dissolve Marshmallow Crème in milk over hot water; cool. Add nuts and cherries and fold in topping. Pour mixture into freezer tray; freeze until mushy. Scrape into a bowl and stir vigorously. Return to freezer tray and freeze firm.

Yield: 8 servings

Exchange, 1 serving: ⅔ full-fat milk, 1 fat
Each serving contains: Calories: 179, Carbohydrates: 21 g

Raisin Ice Cream Sandwich

½ c.	raisins	125 mL
½ c.	water	125 mL
1½ c.	flour	375 mL
1 t.	baking soda	5 mL
¼ t.	salt	1 mL
¼ c.	solid shortening, soft	60 mL
3 T.	granulated sugar replacement	45 mL
1	egg	1
⅔ c.	buttermilk	160 mL
2 c.	ice milk, softened	500 mL

Combine raisins and water in saucepan. Bring to a boil, reduce heat and simmer 5 minutes. Remove from heat; allow to cool slightly. Drain. Combine flour, baking soda, and salt in sifter, and sift twice. Return flour mixture to sifter. Cream together shortening and sugar replacement in medium mixing bowl. Add egg and beat well. Add sifted flour mixture alternately with buttermilk, beating well after each addition. Stir in drained raisins. Pour mixture into a well greased and floured 9 in. (23 cm) square pan. Bake at 350°F (175°C) for 30 to 40 minutes, or until done. Cut into 9 squares. Cut horizontally through center of each square and fill evenly with softened ice milk. Freeze until firm.

Yield: 9 servings

Exchange, 1 serving: 2 bread, 1½ fat
Each serving contains: Calories: 205, Carbohydrates: 36 g

Apricot Ice

¼ c.	granulated sugar replacement	60 mL
1 c.	water	250 mL
1 t.	cornstarch	5 mL
1 c.	unsweetened apricot purée	250 mL
2 T.	lemon juice	30 mL

Combine sugar replacement, water and cornstarch in saucepan; bring to a boil. Reduce heat and simmer 5 minutes. Add apricot purée and lemon juice. Pour into freezer tray and cover with waxed paper. Freeze until firm.

For fluffy ice: Freeze until mushy. Scrape into mixing bowl or blender and beat just until loosened. Return to freezer tray.

Yield: 6 servings

Exchange, 1 serving: 1 fruit
Each serving contains: Calories: 40, Carbohydrates: 15 g

Citrus Ice

¼ c.	granulated sugar replacement	60 mL
1 c.	water	250 mL
1 env.	unflavored gelatin	1 env.
1 c.	unsweetened grapefruit juice	250 mL
1 c.	unsweetened orange juice	250 mL
¼ c.	lemon juice	60 mL

Combine sugar replacement, water and gelatin in saucepan; bring to a boil. Reduce heat and simmer 5 minutes. Cool slightly. Stir in juices and freeze.

For fluffy ice: Freeze until mushy. Scrape into mixing bowl or blender and beat just until loosened. Return to freezer tray.

Yield: 5 servings

Exchange, 1 serving: 1 fruit
Each serving contains: Calories: 41, Carbohydrates: 23 g

Cola Sherbet

1 c.	Marshmallow Crème	250 mL
2 c.	diet cola	500 mL
dash	salt	dash
2 T.	lemon juice	30 mL

Combine all ingredients. Beat until smooth and fluffy. Pour into freezer tray and freeze until firm. Stir 2 or 3 times while freezing.

Yield: 6 servings

Exchange, 1 serving: negligible
Each serving contains: Calories: negligible, Carbohydrates: 34 g

Orange Freeze

3 c.	crushed ice	750 mL
1 pkg.	low-calorie orange drink mix	1 pkg.
½ c.	granulated sugar replacement	125 mL

Combine all ingredients in blender. Whip on high speed.

Yield: 4 servings

Exchange: negligible
Each serving contains: Calories: negligible, Carbohydrates: 32 g

Chocolate Banana Mousse

1 oz. sq.	unsweetened chocolate	28 g sq.
1 c.	evaporated skimmed milk	250 mL
3 T.	granulated sugar replacement	45 mL
2	egg yolks	2
¼ t.	salt	1 mL
1 t.	vanilla extract	5 mL
2	bananas, sliced	2

Combine chocolate, ¼ c. (60 mL) of the milk and the sugar replacement in top of double boiler. (Chill remaining milk in freezer.) Cook and stir over simmering water until chocolate melts. Pour small amount of hot chocolate mixture over egg yolks and beat well. Pour egg mixture into chocolate mixture in top of double boiler. Stir in salt. Cook and stir over hot water until mixture thickens. Cool completely. Scrape cold or slightly frozen milk into mixing bowl and beat until very stiff. Fold chocolate mixture into stiffly beaten milk. Fold in vanilla and banana slices. Spoon into mold, freezer tray, or individual cups and freeze until firm.

Yield: 8 servings

Exchange, 1 serving: 1 bread, ½ fat
Each serving contains: Calories: 69, Carbohydrates: 17 g

Pecan Mousse

½ c.	pecan, chopped	125 mL
1 t.	unflavored gelatin	5 mL
2 T.	cold water	30 mL
1½ c.	evaporated skimmed milk	375 mL
1 T.	liquid sugar replacement	15 mL
or		
2 T.	granulated fructose	30 mL
1 T.	vanilla extract	15 mL

Brown pecans in cake pan in 350°F (175°C) oven (about 10 minutes). Shake occasionally. Sprinkle gelatin over cold water and allow to rest 5 minutes to soften. Combine milk and soften gelatin in saucepan; cook and stir over medium heat until gelatin is dissolved. Remove from heat. Add browned pecans, liquid sugar replacement, and vanilla. Stir to blend well. Pour into mold, freezer tray or individual dishes and freeze until firm.

Yield: 8 servings

Exchange, 1 serving with sugar replacement: ½ full-fat milk
Each serving contains: Calories: 72, Carbohydrates: 10 g

Exchange, 1 serving with fructose: ½ full-fat milk
Each serving contains: Calories: 85, Carbohydrates: 10 g

Watermelon Granita

2 c.	watermelon (without seeds)	500 mL
1 T.	lemon juice	15 mL
2 T.	granulated sugar replacement	30 mL

Combine all ingredients in blender or food processor and beat to puree. Pour into freezer tray and freeze until firm but not hard. Scrape back into blender or food processor, beating to sherbet consistency. Cantaloupe or honeydew melon may be substituted for the watermelon.

Yield: 1 c. (250 mL)

Exchange: negligible
Each serving contains: Calories: negligible, Carbohydrates: 59 g

Pistachio Frozen Dessert

¼	Sponge Cake	¼
1 c.	low-calorie whipped topping (prepared)	250 mL
2 T.	granulated sugar replacement or granulated fructose	30 mL
¼ c.	pistachio nuts, chopped	60 mL
1 t.	almond extract	5 mL
	green food color	
1	egg white	1
dash	salt	dash

Thinly slice the sponge cake. Line bottom and sides of mold or freezer tray with two- thirds of the slices. Reserve remaining slices for top. Combine topping, sugar replacement, nuts, almond extract and a few drops of food color in mixing bowl. Beat or stir to blend. Refrigerate. Combine egg white and salt in narrow mixing bowl and beat until very stiff. Fold egg white into whipped-topping mixture. Spread evenly over sponge cake in mold. Cover with remaining slices of sponge cake, and freeze until firm. Unmold.

Yield: 6 servings

Exchange, 1 serving with sugar replacement: ½ full-fat milk
Each serving contains: Calories: 93

Exchange, 1 serving with fructose: ½ full-fat milk, ⅓ fruit
Each serving contains: Calories: 105, Carbohydrates: 18 g

Frozen Watermelon Pops

I love this recipe. Even though loads of people are at my house for summer weekends, some watermelon is always left over.

I prepare these early in the morning with leftover melon. When the crowd comes back from the beach these pops are ready. To serve on Popsicle sticks, insert sticks after the pops have been in the freezer half an hour or so.

3 c.	puréed watermelon	750 mL
1 T.	lemon juice	15 mL
1 env.	unflavored gelatin	1 env.
1 pkg.	strawberry gelatin powder, sugar-free	1 pkg.
2 c.	frozen low-fat nondairy whipped topping, softened	500 mL

In a saucepan, combine the watermelon puree, lemon juice, and unflavored gelatin. Set aside for five minutes. Heat over a low flame, stirring until the gelatin dissolves. Remove from the heat and stir in the strawberry gelatin. Mix until smooth and the gelatin is dissolved. Refrigerate for 15 minutes, to bring to room temperature. In a large mixing bowl, fold together the gelatin mixture and whipped topping. Distribute into eight 4 oz. (100 g) paper cups. Freeze. To serve, peel back the paper.

Yield: 8 servings

Exchange, 1 serving: ½ fruit; ½ fat
Each serving contains: Calories: 66, Total fat: 2 g, Carbohydrates: 9 g, Protein: 1 g, Sodium: 11 mg, Cholesterol: 0 mg

Tropical Banana Pops

These are easy to make. Keep some in the freezer for hot summer afternoons.

4	small bananas, crushed	4
1 t.	lemon juice	5 mL
1¼ c.	tropical sugar-free drink, from powder	310 mL
1 t.	coconut extract or flavoring	5 mL

Put the crushed bananas into a medium bowl. Sprinkle with lemon juice and toss. Mix in the other ingredients. Spoon into six 4 oz (100 g) paper cups. Freeze until firm. To serve, peel back the paper.

Yield: 6 servings

Exchange, 1 serving: 1 fruit
Each serving contains: Calories: 72, Total fat: 0.4 g, Carbohydrates: 18 g, Protein: 0.8 g, Sodium: 1 mg, Cholesterol: 0 mg

Honeydew Sherbet

If you don't have an ice cream machine, this won't be as creamy, but it will still taste fabulous.

½	medium honeydew melon	½
1¾ c.	frozen low-fat nondairy whipped topping, thawed	435 mL
1 T.	Triple Sec (optional)	15 mL
1 dash	aspartame sweetener to taste (optional)	1 dash

Cut the melon in half and remove the seeds. Peel the melon. Scoop the soft pulp into chunks. Purée in a food processor. Measure 1¾ cups (435 mL) of melon purée. Discard any extra, or reserve it for another use. Put the melon into a mixing bowl. Add the whipped topping. Mix to blend. Add the Triple Sec or aspartame, if desired. Process in an ice cream machine according to the manufacturer's directions.

Yield: 8 servings

Exchange, 1 serving: ⅔ fruit; ½ fat
Each serving contains: Calories: 63, Total fat: 2 g, Carbohydrates: 1 g, Protein: 0.4 g, Sodium: 8 mg, Cholesterol: 0 mg

Orange Frost

1 c.	orange juice	250 mL
2 T.	lemon juice	30 mL
1 t.	orange flavoring	5 mL
1 c.	frozen low-fat nondairy whipped topping, softened	250 mL

Combine the orange juice and lemon juice in a mixing bowl. Stir in the orange flavoring. Pour the mixture into four freezer-safe dessert dishes (i.e., paper, Pyrex, metal). Freeze. Serve with whipped topping.

Yield: 4 servings

Exchange, 1 serving: ⅔ fruit; ½ fat
Each serving contains: Calories: 70, Total fat: 2 g, Carbohydrates: 1 g, Protein: 1 g, Sodium: 1 mg, Cholesterol: 0 mg

Mixed Fruit Sherbet

This is really different. If you like fruity desserts you'll love this one.

2 c.	strawberries, fresh or whole frozen, thawed	500 mL
1	ripe banana	1
½ c.	orange	125 mL
6 pkts.	aspartame sweetener	90 mL
2 c.	frozen low-fat nondairy whipped topping, thawed	500 mL
1½ c.	skim milk	375 mL

Wash, hull, and slice the strawberries. Put them in a mixing bowl. Peel and slice the banana. Mash the two fruits together with a fork. Stir in the remaining ingredients and mix until everything is evenly combined. Process in an ice cream machine according to manufacturer's directions.

Yield: 8 servings

Exchange, 1 serving: 1 starch/bread
Each serving contains: Calories: 92, Total fat: 2 g, Carbohydrates: 15 g, Protein: 2 g, Sodium: 24 mg, Cholesterol: 1 mg

Frozen Strawberry Mousse

Lovely! You'll be proud to serve this.

2 c.	fresh strawberries, hulled	500 mL
1 T.	sugar	15 mL
½ T.	gelatin	7.5 mL
3 T.	cold water	45 mL
5 pkgs.	aspartame sweetener	5 pkgs.
2 c.	frozen low-fat nondairy whipped topping	500 mL

Cut the strawberries into a medium bowl. Sprinkle with sugar and set aside. Sprinkle the gelatin over the cold water in the top of a double boiler. Bring the water to a boil in the bottom of the double boiler. Put on the top part of the double boiler and heat the gelatin mixture until it dissolves. Remove from heat. Mash the strawberries. Fold in the gelatin and the whipped topping. Freeze.

Yield: 8 servings

Exchange, 1 serving: ½ fruit; ½ fat
Each serving contains: Calories: 60, Total fat: 2 g, Carbohydrates: 9 g, Protein: 0.3 g, Sodium: 1 mg, Cholesterol: 0 mg

Pineapple Sherbet

3¼ c.	unsweetened pineapple juice	875 mL
¼ c.	crushed pineapple in juice	60 mL
1 env.	unflavored gelatin	1 env.
5 env.	aspartame sweetener	5 env.
1 c.	low-fat milk	250 mL

In a saucepan, mix pineapple juice, crushed pineapple with juice, unflavored gelatin, and aspartame sweetener. Cook and stir until gelatin and aspartame sweetener are dissolved and mixture is slightly warmed. Remove from heat. Stir in milk. (Mixture will appear to have curdled slightly.) Mix all ingredients. Freeze in an ice-cream freezer, according to manufacturer's directions, or pour mixture into a 9 in. (23 cm) baking pan and place pan in freezer for 2 to 3 hours or until mixture is almost firm. Remove pan from freezer and break pineapple mixture into pieces. Place pieces in a chilled bowl. Beat with an electric mixer until smooth but not melted. Transfer back to pan. Cover and freeze until firm.

Yield: 8 servings

Exchange, 1 serving: 1 fruit
Each serving contains: Calories: 76, Carbohydrates: 15 g

Grape Sherbet

½ c.	grape juice	125 mL
½ c.	low-fat milk	125 mL
½ t.	vanilla extract	2 mL
⅓ c.	prepared nondairy whipped topping	90 mL

Combine grape juice, milk, and vanilla in a bowl. (Mixture will appear to have curdled slightly.) Stir to combine ingredients. Place bowl in freezer and chill until mixture is almost firm. Remove bowl from freezer and break mixture into pieces. Beat with an electric mixer until smooth but not melted. Beat in nondairy whipped topping. Cover and freeze to desired consistency.

Yield: 2 servings

Exchange, 1 serving: ½ fruit, ½ low-fat milk
Each serving contains: Calories: 108, Carbohydrates: 13 g

Strawberry Sorbet

1 env.	unflavored gelatin	1 env.
1½ c.	cool water	375 mL
1 lb. pkg.	frozen strawberries, slightly thawed	454 g pkg.
½ c.	reduced-calorie cranberry-juice cocktail	125 mL
½ c.	granulated sugar replacement	125 mL
2 T.	lemon juice	30 mL

In a medium-sized saucepan, sprinkle gelatin over cool water. Allow to soften for 1 minute. Cook and stir over low heat until gelatin has dissolved. Cool to room temperature. Meanwhile, combine strawberries and cranberry juice cocktail in a blender or food processor. Process to a puree. Blend in sweetener of your choice and lemon juice. When gelatin has cooled, blend into strawberry mixture. Pour into a 9 in (23 cm) baking pan; freeze until firm (about 3 hours). Break into pieces. Place in a large mixing bowl or food processor. With an electric mixer or food processor, beat mixture until smooth. Return to pan and refreeze. Before serving, allow sorbet to stand at room temperature for about 15 minutes or until slightly softened.

Yield: 8 servings

Exchange, 1 serving: ⅓ fruit
Each serving contains: Calories: 24, Carbohydrates: 4 g

Blackberry Buttermilk Sherbet

1-lb. bag	frozen, unsweetened blackberries	454 g bag
1	egg	1
dash	salt	dash
5 env.	aspartame sweetener	5 env.
2 c.	buttermilk	500 mL

Slightly thaw blackberries. Transfer to a food processor or blender and process to purée. Set aside. Separate egg, setting the white aside. Combine egg yolk, salt, and aspartame sweetener in a bowl. Beat until thick and lemon-colored. Gradually beat in blackberry purée. Blend in buttermilk. Beat egg white until it holds a firm peak. Fold buttermilk-blackberry mixture into beaten egg white just enough to blend. Transfer mixture to an ice-cream freezer and freeze according to manufacturer's directions, or pour mixture into a 9 in. (23 cm) baking pan and place pan in freezer for 2 to 3 hours or until mixture is almost firm. Remove pan from freezer and break mixture into pieces. Place pieces in a chilled bowl. Beat with an electric mixer until smooth but not melted. Transfer back to pan. Cover and freeze until firm.

Yield: 10 servings

Exchange, 1 serving: 1 fruit
Each serving contains: Calories: 52, Carbohydrates: 13 g

Real Lemon Sherbet

3 c.	water	750 mL
1 env.	unflavored gelatin	1 env.
5 env.	aspartame sweetener	5 env.
¾ c.	fresh lemon juice	190 mL
1 c.	low-fat milk	250 mL
1 t.	grated lemon peel	5 mL

In a saucepan, mix water, unflavored gelatin, and aspartame sweetener. Cook and stir until gelatin and aspartame sweetener are dissolved and mixture is slightly warmed. Remove from heat. Stir in lemon juice, milk, and lemon peel. (Mixture will appear to have curdled slightly.) Mix all ingredients. Freeze in an ice-cream freezer, according to manufacturer's directions, or pour mixture into a 9 in. (23 cm) baking pan and place pan in freezer for 2 to 3 hours or until mixture is almost firm. Remove pan from freezer and break mixture into pieces. Place pieces in a chilled bowl, and beat with an electric mixer until smooth but not melted. Or process pieces in a food processor in small batches using the pulse or on/off switch. Transfer back to pan. Cover and freeze until firm.

Yield: 8 servings

Exchange, 1 serving: negligible
Each serving contains: Calories: 15, Carbohydrates: negligible

Quick Orange-Yogurt Pops

6 oz. can	orange juice concentrate	210 g can
¼ c.	water	190 mL
1 c.	plain low-fat yogurt	250 mL

Combine ingredients in a blender. Process until well blended. Divide mixture evenly among eight paper drinking cups. Place in freezer and freeze until frozen. If desired, when pops are partially frozen, place a wooden stick in middle of each pop. Freeze completely.

Yield: 8 servings

Exchange, 1 serving: 1 fruit
Each serving contains: Calories: 68, Carbohydrates: 9 g

Blueberry Tofu Cream

1½ c.	fresh or unsweetened frozen blueberries	375 mL
2 t.	lemon juice	10 mL
1 env.	unflavored gelatin	1 env.
⅓ c.	water	90 mL
⅔ c.	granulated sugar replacement	180 mL
or		
⅓ c.	granulated fructose	90 mL
½ pkg. (10.5 oz.)	tofu, firm	½ pkg. (297 g)
1½ c.	low-fat milk	375 mL
1 T.	vanilla extract	15 mL
½ c.	prepared nondairy whipped topping	125 mL

Purée blueberries in a blender. Transfer to a heavy saucepan, and bring to a boil. Reduce heat and simmer, uncovered, until blueberries are reduced to about ½ c. (125 mL). Stir in lemon juice and cool to room temperature, In a small saucepan, sprinkle gelatin over water. Allow to soften for 1 minute. Cook and stir over low heat until gelatin dissolves. Set aside to cool. When the gelatin is cooled, combine gelatin, water, sweetener of your choice, and tofu in a blender. Blend until smooth. Pour in milk and vanilla. Blend until completely mixed. Add nondairy whipped topping and puréed blueberries. Blend just until mixed. Transfer to an ice-cream freezer or a 9 in. (23 cm) baking pan. Freeze according to freezer manufacturer's instructions or place pan in the freezer and freeze until firm. Break into pieces. Place in a large mixing bowl or food processor. With an electric mixer or food processor, beat mixture until smooth. Return to the pan and refreeze. To serve: Score into eight equal servings, and place on chilled serving plates. Serve immediately (Tofu Cream softens quickly).

Yield: 8 servings, with granulated sugar replacement

Exchange, 1 serving: ½ fruit, ⅓ low-fat milk
Each serving contains: Calories: 50, Carbohydrates: 7 g

Yield: 8 servings, with granulated fructose

Exchange, 1 serving: ⅔ fruit, ½ low-fat milk
Each serving contains: Calories: 92, Carbohydrates: 17 g

Tart Cherry Ice Cream

2 qts.	vanilla ice cream	2 L	
1-lb. bag	frozen, unsweetened, pitted tart red cherries	456 g bag	

Soften the ice cream in the refrigerator until it can be whipped with an electric beater. Meanwhile, thaw, drain, and pat the cherries dry with paper towels. Transfer the ice cream to a large mixing bowl. Whip the ice cream on low until smooth. Fold in the cherries. Transfer the ice cream to a covered freezer container. Freeze for several hours before serving. If the ice cream becomes solid, soften it slightly in the refrigerator before serving.

Yield: 16 servings

Exchange, 1 serving: 1 bread
Each serving contains: Calories: 98, Carbohydrates: 15 g

Grand Marnier Ice Cream

2 qts.	vanilla ice cream	2 L	
⅓ c.	Grand Marnier	90 mL	
1 recipe	candied orange peel*	1 recipe	

Soften the ice cream in the refrigerator until it can be whipped with an electric beater. Transfer the ice cream to a large mixing bowl. Whip the ice cream on low until smooth. Beat in the Grand Marnier. Transfer the ice cream to a covered freezer container. Freeze for several hours before serving. If the ice cream becomes solid, soften it slightly in the refrigerator before serving. Garnish with candied orange peel.

Yield: 16 servings

Exchange, 1 serving: 1½ bread
Each serving contains: Calories: 135, Carbohydrates: 22 g

*The actual name of the recipe is Sweetened Citrus Peel.

Maple Ice Cream Tart

1 qt.	reduced-calorie vanilla ice cream	1 L	
½ c.	chopped toasted pecans	125 mL	
2 t.	caramel flavoring	10 mL	
⅔ c.	sugar-free maple syrup	190 mL	

Soften the ice cream just enough to stir. Stir in toasted pecans and caramel flavoring. Pack into a 9 in. (23 cm) removable-bottomed tart pan, lined with plastic wrap. Refreeze until firm. To serve: Carefully remove ice cream tart from pan by turning it upside down on a decorative plate. Remove plastic wrap. Pour maple syrup over top of ice cream tart. Serve immediately.

Yield: 12 servings

Exchange, 1 serving: ⅔ bread, ⅔ fat
Each serving contains: Calories: 92, Carbohydrates: 10 g

Blueberry Mountain Dessert

1 lb. pkg.	frozen, unsweetened blueberries	456 g pkg.
5 env.	aspartame sweetener	5 env.
½ t.	lemon juice	2 mL
2⅔ c.	reduced-calorie vanilla ice cream	680 mL
8 T.	prepared nondairy whipped topping	120 mL

Remove ½ c. (125 mL) of the blueberries from the package. Set aside. Puree remaining blueberries, aspartame sweetener, and lemon juice in a food processor or blender. Pour the puréed blueberries into a heavy saucepan. Cook and stir over medium heat until mixture is very thick. Transfer to a bowl and chill for at least 30 minutes. Meanwhile, soften the ice cream. Line eight muffin or custard cups with plastic wrap. Pack each cup with ⅓ c. (90 mL) of ice cream. Freeze until firm. To serve: Turn cup upside down on a decorative plate. Remove cup and plastic wrap. Top with one-eighth of the blueberry purée. Top that with 1 T. (15 mL) of the nondairy whipped topping. Garnish with a few of the reserved blueberries. Repeat this procedure with each ice cream cup.

Yield: 8 servings

Exchange, 1 serving: ⅔ bread, ⅔ fruit
Each serving contains: Calories: 90, Carbohydrates: 21 g

Blackberry Lemon Parfait

1 lb. pkg.	frozen, unsweetened blackberries	456 g pkg.
5 env.	aspartame sweetener	5 env.
½ t.	lemon juice	2 mL
1 qt.	reduced-calorie lemon sherbet	1 L

Purée blackberries, aspartame sweetener, and lemon juice in a food processor or blender. Measure 1¼ c. (310 mL) of the blackberry purée and place in a heavy saucepan.

Reserve remaining blackberry puree for the sauce. Cook and stir over medium heat until mixture is reduced to a scant 1 c. (250 mL). Transfer to a bowl and chill for at least 30 minutes. Line a 9 × 5 in. (23 × 12.5 cm) loaf pan with plastic wrap. Transfer 1½ c. (375 mL) of the lemon sherbet to a large bowl. Fold in the reduced blackberry purée. Spread one-third of the remaining lemon sherbet in the bottom of the prepared loaf pan. Cover with the blackberry-lemon mixture. Top with the remaining lemon sherbet. Smooth the top and freeze overnight. When ready to serve, unmold parfait onto a decorative plate, allow to soften slightly, and pour reserved blackberry puree over the top. Slice into eight servings.

Yield: 8 servings

Exchange, 1 serving: ½ fruit
Each serving contains: Calories: 27, Carbohydrates: 7 g

Frozen Raspberry Mousse with Black Raspberry Sauce

2 pkgs.	sugar-free raspberry gelatin	2 pkgs.
2 c.	frozen black raspberries, slightly thawed	500 mL
¼ c.	water	60 mL
1 T.	cider vinegar	15 mL
1 stick	cinnamon	1 stick
1	egg white, beaten stiff	1
1 c.	prepared nondairy whipped topping	250 mL

Prepare both packages of raspberry gelatin together, as directed on package. Allow to completely set. Meanwhile, combine 1¼ c. (310 mL) of the black raspberries, water, cider vinegar, and cinnamon stick in a saucepan. Bring to a boil, reduce heat, and simmer for 5 to 6 minutes. If desired, strain mixture to remove seeds. Cool completely. Remove cinnamon stick. Beat the set raspberry gelatin with a wire whisk or electric mixer. Then beat ¼ c. (60 mL) of the black-raspberry sauce into the gelatin. Stir in the stiffly beaten egg white and the nondairy whipped topping. Spoon gelatin mixture into eight decorative glasses or bowls. Freeze until firm. To serve: Top frozen gelatin mixture with the remaining black-raspberry sauce. Garnish with the reserved ¼ c. (190 mL) of black raspberries.

Yield: 8 servings

Exchange, 1 serving: ⅓ fruit
Each serving contains: Calories: 22, Carbohydrates: 4 g

Triple Sherbet Dessert

2 c.	reduced-calorie raspberry sherbet	500 mL
2 c.	reduced-calorie lemon sherbet	500 mL
2 c.	reduced-calorie lime sherbet	500 mL

Slightly soften raspberry sherbet. Spread into an 8 in. (20 cm) pie pan. Refreeze until firm. Slightly soften lemon sherbet. Spread over the surface of the raspberry sherbet. Refreeze. Slightly soften lime sherbet. Spread over the surface of the lemon sherbet. Refreeze until firm. Cut into 12 wedges to serve.

Yield: 12 servings

Exchange, 1 serving: ⅔ bread
Each serving contains: Calories: 52, Carbohydrates: 9 g

Banana Sherbet

This frozen dessert is ideal for everyday eating. It's low in calories and exchanges.

1 c.	nonfat, sugar-free banana cream pie-flavored yogurt	250 mL
1 c.	mashed bananas	250 mL
1 t.	concentrated aspartame	5 mL
1 t.	vanilla extract	5 mL
½ t.	banana extract	2 mL

Combine all the ingredients in a food processor. Pour into two small yogurt containers; freeze for a few hours or overnight.

Yield: 4 servings

Exchange, 1 serving: 1 fruit + ½ milk
Each serving contains: Calories: 104, Fiber: 2 g, Sodium: 38 mg, Cholesterol: 1 mg

Frosty Frozen Dessert

Any fruit can be used in this recipe. We like nectarines for their gentle, natural sweetness.

1	egg white	1
⅓ c.	water	90 mL
⅓ c.	nonfat dry milk	90 mL
⅓ c.	egg substitute	90 mL
⅓ c.	measures-like-sugar aspartame	90 mL
¾ c.	fruit purée such as nectarines	180 mL

Use an electric mixer to beat together the first three ingredients until a stiff mixture forms. Set aside. Take a separate mixing bowl and beat together all the other ingredients until smooth. Put the bowl of beaten egg whites back under the beaters, then gently beat the fruit and egg substitute mixture into the beaten egg whites. Pour into small yogurt containers and freeze for several hours or overnight.

Yield: 11 servings, ½ c. (125 mL) each

Exchange, 1 serving: ½ milk
Each serving contains: Calories: 36, Carbohydrates: 31 g, Fiber: 1 g, Sodium: 36 mg, Cholesterol: trace

Frozen Strawberry Yogurt

This recipe works equally well with any frozen or fresh fruit.

8 oz. pkg.	frozen strawberries, no sugar added	226 g pkg.
1½ t.	lemon juice	7 mL
2 t.	aspartame	10 mL
1 T.	vanilla extract	15 mL
1½ c.	nonfat yogurt, no sugar added (plain or vanilla)	375 mL

Put fruit in food processor with flavorings. Purée; add yogurt. Freeze in small yogurt containers for easy serving.

Yield: 6 servings

Exchange, 1 serving: 1 milk
Each serving contains: Calories: 76, Carbohydrates: 7 g, Fiber: 1.6 g, Sodium: 74 mg, Cholesterol: 0 mg

Very Low Calorie Frozen Yogurt

The type of fruit you pick determines the flavor. Our taste testers preferred blueberries, raspberries, and fresh peaches. Using gelatin and lots of crushed ice makes them very, very low in calories and exchanges.

1 env.	plain gelatin	1 env.
2 T.	cold water	30 mL
⅓ c.	boiling water	90 mL
1 c.	nonfat yogurt no sugar added (any flavor)	250 mL
2 t.	aspartame	10 mL
1 t.	vanilla or almond extract	5 mL
1 c.	fresh or frozen berries or cut-up fruit (with no sugar added)	250 mL
2½ c.	crushed ice	625 mL

Sprinkle the gelatin over the cold water; let it sit for a few minutes to soften. Pour in the boiling water and stir until the gelatin is completely dissolved. Combine the yogurt, gelatin, aspartame, extracts, and fruit in a food processor or blender. Mix until well combined. Refrigerate. Just before serving, combine the crushed ice and the chilled mixture in a food processor or blender. Blend together until creamy.

Yield: 10 servings

Exchange: free
Each serving contains: Each serving contains: Calories: 21, Fiber: trace, Sodium: 16 mg, Cholesterol: 0 mg

Couldn't-Be-Easier Frozen Yogurt

This recipe is almost not a recipe.

Just place a container of yogurt in the freezer and leave until frozen. Coffee-flavored yogurt is wonderful frozen. Carefully read labels at the grocery store; be sure to buy nonfat yogurt sweetened only with aspartame. Coffee frozen yogurt is even better with a tablespoon of dietetic pancake syrup.

Yield: 2 servings

Exchange, 1 serving: ½ milk
Each serving contains: Calories: 53, Carbohydrates: 9 g, Fiber: 0, Sodium: 73 mg, Cholesterol: 0 mg

Almost Ice Cream

Using cottage cheese and dry milk powder together adds a creamy texture to this. It is very important to process the cottage cheese for the full two minutes. If you cheat on the time, cottage cheese curds may spoil the effect.

1 env.	plain gelatin	1 env.
2 T.	cold water	30 mL
1 c.	boiling water	250 mL
1⅓ c.	cottage cheese	340 mL
3 T.	nonfat dry milk	45 mL
1 T.	concentrated aspartame	15 mL
2 t.	vanilla extract	10 mL
2 t.	lemon juice	10 mL
⅓ c.	ice water	90 mL
1 c.	fruit (fresh or frozen without sugar)	250 mL

Sprinkle the gelatin on the cold water; set aside for a few minutes. Pour boiling water over the gelatin and stir until completely dissolved. Put the gelatin, cottage cheese, dry milk, aspartame, vanilla extract, and lemon juice into a food processor. Process for a full two minutes. Then put the mixture into a bowl and chill until the gelatin has set. Keep it refrigerated until shortly before serving time. Then put it into a food processor or blender with the ice water and fruit. Process for a few seconds until blended but not frothy. Serve immediately.

Yield: 8 servings per 4 c. (1 L)

Exchange, 1 serving: ½ milk
Each serving contains: Calories: 53, Fiber: trace, Sodium: 17 mg, Cholesterol: 4 mg

Hazelnut Delight

2	eggs	2
½ c.	granulated sugar replacement	125 mL
2 T.	all-purpose flour	30 mL
½ t.	baking powder	2 mL
dash	salt	dash
½ c.	finely chopped apples	125 mL
⅓ c.	finely chopped hazelnuts	90 mL

Beat eggs and sugar replacement together until foamy. Beat in flour, baking powder, and salt. Next, stir in apples and hazelnuts. Transfer to greased 8 in. (20 cm) pie pan. Bake at 325°F (165°C) for 25 to 30 minutes or until set. Chill and then cut into wedges.

Yield: 8 servings

Exchange, 1 serving: 1 fruit
Each serving contains: Calories: 72, Carbohydrates: 13

Tiramisu

This popular Italian dessert is both rich and beautiful. Try this easy yet impressive version.

1 c.	skim milk	250 mL
1 T.	butter or margarine	15 mL
1½ T.	cornstarch	23 mL
1 T.	sugar	15 mL
3 large	egg yolks, mixed lightly	3 large
2 t.	vanilla extract	10 mL
1½ c.	fat-free ricotta cheese or fat-free cottage cheese	375 mL
2 c.	frozen low-fat nondairy whipped topping, thawed	500 mL
¼ c.	strong espresso, cooled	60 mL
¼ c.	coffee liqueur	60 mL
1	angel food cake	1
2 c.	fresh raspberries, or frozen, thawed	500 mL

Warm the milk and butter in a heavy-bottom medium saucepan or the top of a double boiler, stirring constantly. In a small bowl, mix together the cornstarch, sugar, and egg yolks. Blend well. Add the vanilla and blend. Transfer the egg mixture to the warm milk. Continue to heat and mix with a wire whisk until the mixture is thick. Look for whisk patterns, which indicate that it's done. Cool. Put the cheese into a mixing bowl. Beat at high speed with an electric mixer for 3–4 minutes. Add the cooled mixture and beat the two together at a low speed until well mixed. Fold in the whipped topping until thoroughly blended. In a small bowl, stir together the espresso and liqueur.

Using a sharp knife, cut the angel food cake crosswise into three layers. Put one layer into the bottom of a serving bowl. Brush with the espresso liqueur mixture. Turn the layer over and brush the other side. Spoon one third of the milk-cheese mixture over the cake. Arrange one-third of the raspberries around edges. Brush one side of another angel food cake layer and put it (brushed-side-down) in the bowl. Brush the top and spoon on one- third of the milk-cheese mixture and raspberries. Repeat the process for the last layer. Pour any remaining espresso liqueur on top of the third layer. Smooth the top and cover tightly. Refrigerate for at least 6 hours or up to 2 days before serving.

Yield: 12 servings

Exchange, 1 serving: 3 starch/bread
Each serving contains: Calories: 242, Total fat: 3 g, Carbohydrates: 43 g, Protein: 8 g, Sodium: 295 mg, Cholesterol: 59 mg

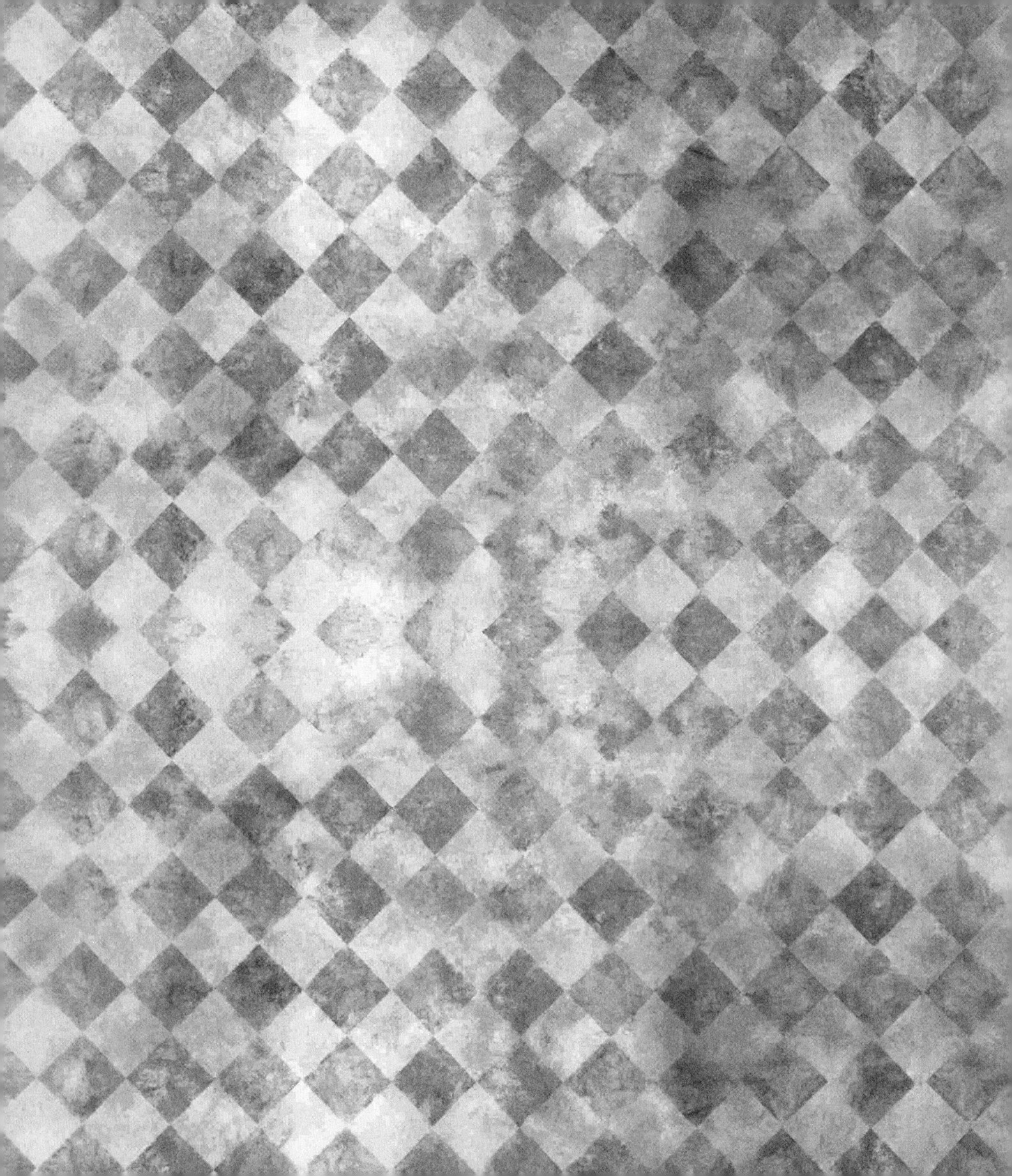

Meringues

These recipes are all based on meringue-beaten egg whites slowly baked. They are low in fat and very elegant. You might think meringues are beyond your capabilities—they are not! It's hard to go wrong if you follow a few simple rules.

- Don't use plastic when you beat the egg whites. Glass or metal bowls give the most fluff from egg whites.
- Be sure your utensils are spotless. For egg whites to beat up, the bowls, blades, and scrapers should be grease-free.
- Be sure no bits of yolk are mixed in with the whites. Separate whites and yolks into small cups or bowls, and put only pure egg whites into the mixing bowl. Should the yolk break during the separation process, put that egg aside and use another one.

- Don't bake meringues on wax paper or plain cookie sheets. Use parchment paper or the inside of clean brown paper grocery bags.
- Recognize that humidity changes meringues. On high-humidity days, meringues are chewy. On low-humidity days, meringues are dry and crispy.
- Never open the oven, even to peek, until the stated time has elapsed.
- Use reconstituted "Just Whites" powdered egg whites if you have no use for leftover yolks. They may be found in your supermarket, health food store, or gourmet shop.
- Even though egg substitutes are mostly egg whites, they don't work for meringues.
- Freeze meringues after you've made them or store them at room temperature. Always keep meringues in airtight containers.

Basic Meringue

Follow the meringue advice for best results.

3 large	egg whites	3 large	
¼ t.	cream of tartar	2 mL	
¼ c.	sugar	60 mL	

Preheat the oven to 250°F (120°C) or the temperature specified in the specific recipe. Cut a brown paper grocery bag or parchment paper to the same size as your cookie sheet. Place the paper on top of the cookie sheet. Using plates, cups, or saucers and a pencil, trace the shape specified in the recipe onto the paper. In a large glass or metal bowl, beat the egg whites with the cream of tartar using an electric mixer. When soft peaks begin to form, keep beating, but slowly add the sugar. Increase the mixer speed until stiff peaks form and the meringue is glossy. Don't beat past this point or the meringue will become too dry!

With a clean spoon or rubber scraper transfer the beaten egg white to the circles drawn on the paper. Bake in a 250°F (120°C) preheated oven for the amount of time specified in the recipe. When the time is up, turn off the oven but don't open the oven door. Leave the meringues in the turned off oven for two more hours. Then carefully remove the cookie sheets from the oven. Use a spatula to loosen the meringue from the paper.

Yield: 1 Basic Meringue recipe (4 servings)

Exchange, 1 serving: 1 starch/bread
Each serving contains: Calories: 61, Total fat: 0 g, Carbohydrates: 13 g, Protein: 3 g, Sodium: 41 mg, Cholesterol: 0 mg

Lime Kisses

1 recipe	Basic Meringue	1 recipe	
1 pkg.	sugar-free lime gelatin powder	1 pkg.	

Prepare the Basic Meringue, but add the lime gelatin along with the sugar. Use a brown paper bag or parchment paper to cover an ungreased cookie sheet. Drop the meringue by teaspoonfuls (5 mL) onto the cookie sheet. Put the kisses into a preheated 275°F (135°C) oven for 30 minutes. Turn off the oven. Keep the kisses in the oven for another 10 minutes without opening the door. Use a spatula to remove the kisses from the paper.

Yield: 5 dozen Lime Kisses

Exchange: free
Each serving contains: Calories: 4, Total fat: 0 g, Carbohydrates: 1 g, Protein: 0.2 g, Sodium: 6 mg, Cholesterol: 0 mg

Tart Orange Meringue Tarts

Thin slices of orange make a festive garnish.

1 recipe	Basic Meringue	1 recipe	
2 T.	sugar	30 mL	
4 t.	cornstarch	20 mL	
1 c.	unsweetened orange juice	250 mL	
1 T.	lemon juice (fresh is best)	15 mL	
1 t.	aspartame sweetener	5 mL	
½ c.	white topping (optional)	125 mL	

Prepare the Basic Meringue with the following variation: Draw six 4 in. (10 cm) circles on the brown paper. Spoon the meringue into the circles, building up the edges by an inch (2.5 cm), and form a depression in the middle to make a tart shell. Bake in a preheated 250°F (120°C) oven for 1 hour. Cool in the oven for two hours longer without opening the door.

After the meringues are in the oven, prepare the filling by combining the sugar and cornstarch in a saucepan. Use a whisk to blend in the orange juice. Stirring constantly, cook over a medium heat until mixture thickens. Remove from heat and stir in the orange juice, lemon juice, and aspartame. Cool and store in the refrigerator until just before serving. Then, spoon the filling into the cooked meringue shells. Top with a dollop of your favorite white topping, if desired.

Yield: 6 Orange Meringue Tarts

Exchange, 1 serving: 1 starch/bread
Each serving contains: Calories: 84, Total fat: 0.1 g, Carbohydrates: 19 g, Protein: 2 g, Sodium: 28 mg, Cholesterol: 0 mg

Valentine Tarts

1 recipe	Basic Meringue	1 recipe	
1 lb.	sweet cherries, pitted	450 g	
1 T.	sugar	15 mL	
1 T.	brandy or water	15 mL	

Prepare the meringue according to the directions for Basic Meringue. Trace eight circles or hearts about 2½ in. (12 cm) in diameter onto parchment or onto the inside of clean brown paper grocery bags cut to the size of your cookie sheets. Spoon the meringue inside the patterns and smooth to the shapes traced. Place in a preheated 250°F (120°C) oven for 30 minutes. Leave the oven door closed, turn off the heat, and let the meringue remain in the oven for two more hours. Cool on a wire rack.

Using a spatula, carefully remove the meringues from the paper. Place one meringue on each of four dessert plates. Prepare the cherry topping by putting the cherries, sugar, and brandy or water in a microwave-safe bowl. Stir. Microwave for a minute or two on high until the cherries become juicy and steamy. Alternatively, put the cherries, sugar, and brandy or water into a medium saucepan. Stir constantly and heat until the berries are soft and juicy. Put a spoonful of the sauce on top of each of the four meringues. Top each with a second meringue and then distribute the remaining cherries. Top with a dollop of your favorite white topping, if desired.

Yield: 4 Valentine Tarts

Exchange, 1 serving: 1 starch/bread, 1½ fruit
Each serving contains: Calories: 164, Total fat: 1 g, Carbohydrates: 35 g, Protein: 4 g, Sodium: 41 mg, Cholesterol: 0 mg

Tangerine Meringue Tarts

Great in the winter when tangerines are sweet.

1 recipe	Basic Meringue	1 recipe
8 oz.	fat-free cream cheese	225 g
3 T.	Triple Sec	45 mL
4 t.	cornstarch	20 mL
1⅓ c.	orange or tangerine juice, unsweetened (okay from frozen concentrate)	330 mL
3	tangerines, peeled and separated into segments, pitted	3

Prepare the Basic Meringue. To prepare the filling, put the cream cheese in a mixing bowl. Add the liqueur and beat until well mixed. Put the cornstarch into a small saucepan. Stir in the orange juice very gradually. Bring to a boil, stirring constantly. Boil for one minute. Remove from heat. Snip the center of each tangerine segment and remove the seeds. Put the seedless tangerine segments into the saucepan with the thickened juice. Put one-sixth of the cheese filling into the bottom of each meringue shell. Top with one-sixth of the tangerine mixture. Chill 1–2 hours before serving.

Yield: 6 Tangerine Cream Tarts

Exchange, 1 serving: 2 starch/bread
Each serving contains: Calories: 151, Total fat: 0.2 g, Carbohydrates: 26 g, Protein: 5 g, Sodium: 209 mg, Cholesterol: 7 mg

Traditional Pavlova

This lovely dessert was created for the graceful Anna Pavlova, the Russian ballerina who visited New Zealand and Australia in the early 1900s.

1 recipe	Basic Meringue	1 recipe
2 c.	frozen low-fat nondairy whipped topping, thawed	500 mL
2 c.	fresh strawberries, hulled	500 mL
4	ripe kiwi fruit, peeled	4

Prepare the Basic Meringue. Trace a 12 in. (30 cm) circle on the inside of a clean brown paper grocery bag or a piece of parchment paper. Put the paper on an ungreased cookie sheet. Spoon the meringue into the circle. Spread so it is evenly distributed. Bake in a preheated 250°F (120°C) oven for 1 hour. Turn off the oven. Leave the meringue in the oven for an additional 30 minutes without opening the door. Then cool on a wire rack. Carefully remove the brown paper and place the meringue on a serving plate. Just before serving, spread the whipped topping carefully over the top of the meringue. Slice the strawberries lengthwise. Place them, cut-side-down, so the points extend out past the edge of the meringue. Slice the kiwis in thin "coins" and overlap them in a ring. Arrange the remaining strawberries in the center.

Yield: 10 servings

Exchange, 1 serving: 1 starch/bread
Each serving contains: Calories: 84, Total fat: 2 g, Carbohydrates: 15 g, Protein: 2 g, Sodium: 18 mg, Cholesterol: 0 mg

Pavlova Wedges with Kiwis and Raspberry Sauce

Individual servings of a variation of the traditional Pavlova.

1 recipe	Basic Meringue	1 recipe
4	ripe kiwis	4
1 recipe	Raspberry Sauce	1 recipe

Prepare the Basic Meringue. Trace a 12 in. (30 cm) circle on the inside of a clean brown paper grocery bag or a piece of parchment paper. Put the paper on an ungreased cookie sheet. Spoon the meringue into the circle. Spread the meringue so it is evenly distributed. Bake in a preheated 250°F (120°C) oven for 1 hour. Turn off the oven. Leave the meringue in the oven for an additional 30 minutes without opening the door. Carefully cut the meringue into eight wedges. Put each wedge on a dessert plate. Peel the kiwis. Slice thinly. Arrange one-half sliced kiwi on each slice of meringue. Spoon raspberry sauce over the fruit and meringue.

Yield: 8 servings

Exchange, 1 serving: 1 starch/bread; ½ fruit
Each serving contains: Calories: 98, Total fat: 0.2 g, Carbohydrates: 21 g, Protein: 2 g, Sodium: 31 mg, Cholesterol: 0 mg

Raspberry Sauce

Seedless raspberry preserves are the best and are worth hunting down.

½ c.	no-sugar-added seedless raspberry preserves	125 mL
2 T.	Chambord liqueur or raspberry brandy	30 mL
2 T.	water	30 mL

Put the preserves into a small saucepan. Add the raspberry liqueur and water. Mix well with a wire whisk. Heat gently, stirring constantly.

Yield: ¾ cup (185 mL) or 8 servings

Exchange, full recipe: ½ fruit
Full recipe contains: Calories: 44, Total fat: 0 g, Carbohydrates: 9 g, Protein: 0 g, Sodium: 7 mg, Cholesterol: 0 mg

French Raspberry Pavlova

You will be a hit with everyone when you serve this. Don't expect leftovers!

1 recipe	Basic Meringue	1 recipe	
1 recipe	Vanilla Tart Filling	1 recipe	
2 c.	fresh raspberries	500 mL	

Prepare the Basic Meringue. Trace a 12 in. (30 cm) circle on the inside of a clean brown paper grocery bag or a piece of parchment paper cut to fit your cookie sheet. Put the paper on an ungreased cookie sheet. Spoon the meringue into the circle. Spread so it is evenly distributed. Bake in a preheated 250°F (120°C) oven for 1 hour. Turn off the oven. Don't open the door. Leave the meringue in the oven for an additional 30 minutes. Remove to a wire rack to cool.

Carefully separate the meringue from the paper using a spatula. Place the meringue on a serving plate. Prepare the Vanilla Tart Filling. Spoon on the filling. Smooth it evenly to the edges. Arrange the raspberries in concentric circles, beginning at the outside edge. Serve immediately. Meringue gets soggy in damp weather and as the filling sits on top of it. Nevertheless, my family loves the refrigerated leftovers for breakfast!

Yield: 10 servings

Exchange, 1 serving: 1 starch/bread; ½ fat
Each serving contains: Calories: 100, Total fat: 3 g, Carbohydrates: 15 g, Protein: 3 g, Sodium: 69 mg, Cholesterol: 28 mg

Peach Pavlova

This Pavlova uses ice cream or frozen yogurt along with the meringue. The combination of chewy meringue and ice cream is delightful.

1 recipe	**Basic Meringue**	1 recipe
2 c.	**fat-free vanilla ice cream or frozen yogurt, softened**	500 mL
15 oz.	**peach slices in juice, drained**	420 g

Prepare the Basic Meringue. Trace a 12 in. (30 cm) circle on the inside of a clean brown paper grocery bag or a piece of parchment paper cut to fit your cookie sheet. Put the paper on an ungreased cookie sheet. Spoon the meringue into the circle. Spread so it is evenly distributed. Bake in a preheated 250°F (120°C) oven for 1 hour. Turn off the oven. Don't open the door. Leave the meringue in the oven for an additional 30 minutes. Remove to a wire rack to cool.

Carefully separate the meringue from the paper using a spatula. Put the meringue on a serving plate. Just before serving, spread the ice cream on the baked meringue and arrange peach slices in a circle at the edge. Put any remaining peach slices in the center in a pretty pattern.

Yield: 10 servings

Exchange, 1 serving: 1 starch/bread
Each serving contains: Calories: 83, Total fat: 0 g, Carbohydrates: 18 g, Protein: 3 g, Sodium: 38 mg, Cholesterol: 2 mg

Lemon Meringue Kisses

Use a pastry bag with a ½ in. (13 mm) star tip for an even, professional look for kisses.

1 recipe	**Basic Meringue**	1 recipe
2 t.	**lemon zest, finely grated**	10 mL
½ t.	**lemon extract**	3 mL

Prepare the Basic Meringue with the following change: After peaks have formed, quickly beat in the lemon zest and extract. Cut parchment paper or brown paper grocery bags to cover the ungreased cookie sheets. Drop the meringue by teaspoonfuls (5 mL) onto the paper. Bake in a preheated 250°F (120°C) oven for 40 minutes. Turn the oven off and leave the meringues inside the closed oven for an additional 5 minutes. Remove from the oven and cool for a minute or two. Use a spatula to remove the meringues from the paper.

Yield: 5 dozen Lemon Meringue Kisses

Exchange: free
Each serving includes: Calories: 4, Total fat: 0 g, Carbohydrates: 0.9 g, Protein: 0 g, Sodium: 3 mg, Cholesterol: 0 mg

Lemon Meringue Torte

This torte has the meringue on the bottom and the top.

1 recipe	Basic Meringue	1 recipe
1 pkg.	sugar-free lemon pudding mix	1 pkg.
1¼ c.	water or skim milk	1¼ c.
2 t.	lemon juice	10 mL

Prepare the Basic Meringue. Trace two dinner plates on parchment or the inside of a brown paper bag that has been cut the same size as your cookie sheets. Put the paper on ungreased cookie sheets. Distribute the meringue between the two circles and smooth it evenly. Bake in a preheated 250°F (120°C) oven for 1 hour. Turn off the oven but do not open the door. Leave in the oven for an additional 30 minutes. Remove to wire racks to cool.

Use a spatula to remove the torte shells from the paper. Prepare the lemon pudding according to package directions, using water or skim milk. Mix in the lemon juice. Put one of the meringues on a serving plate just before you are ready to serve. Scoop half the lemon mixture on top of the meringue. Top with the second meringue. Decorate the top with dollops of the remaining pudding mix.

Yield: 8 servings

Exchange, 1 serving: 1½ starch/bread
Each serving contains: Calories: 33, Total fat: 0 g, Carbohydrates: 7 g, Protein: 2 g, Sodium: 50 mg, Cholesterol: 0 mg

Chocolate Dream Torte

1 recipe	Basic Meringue	1 recipe
1 pkg.	sugar-free chocolate pudding mix	1 pkg.
1¼ c.	water or skim milk	310 mL
1 c.	frozen low-fat nondairy whipped topping, thawed	250 mL

Prepare the Basic Meringue. Trace an 8 in. (20 cm) pie pan three times on parchment paper or the inside of a brown paper bag that has been cut the same size as your cookie sheets. Put the paper on ungreased cookie sheets. Distribute the meringue between the three circles and smooth it evenly. Bake in a preheated 250°F (120°C) oven for 40 minutes. Turn off the oven but do not open the door. Leave in the oven for an additional 30 minutes. Remove to wire racks to cool.

When you are ready to assemble the torte, remove one of the meringues carefully from the paper and place it on a serving plate. Prepare the pudding according to package directions, using the water or skim milk. (Cool, if it is a cooking recipe.) Put half the pudding on the first meringue. Smooth to the edges. Put the second meringue (with paper removed) on top and repeat with the last of the pudding and the third meringue. Cut carefully. Top each serving with a dollop of whipped topping.

Yield: 8 servings

Exchange, 1 serving: 1 starch/bread
Each serving contains: Calories: 74, Total fat: 1 g, Carbohydrates: 12 g, Protein: 4 g, Sodium: 80 mg, Cholesterol: 1 mg

Lemon Meringue Nests

2	egg whites	2
1 t.	sorbitol	5 mL
1 t.	white vinegar	5 mL
1 t.	clear vanilla flavoring	5 mL
1 pkg.*	sugar-free lemon instant pudding and pie filling	1 pkg.*
1½ c.	cold skim milk	375 mL

Beat egg whites until stiff. Gradually beat in sorbitol, vinegar, and vanilla. Continue beating until very stiff. Shape egg-white mixture into four nest-like forms on a lightly greased cookie sheet. Bake at 250°F (125°C) for 35 to 40 minutes or until surface becomes crusty. Allow to cool in oven or move to cooling rack. Combine pudding mix and skim milk in a bowl. Whip to blend. Refrigerate until completely set. Then spoon into meringue nests. Store in refrigerator.

Yield: 4 servings

Exchange, 1 serving: 1 starch/bread
Each serving contains: Calories: 77, Carbohydrates: 16 g

*four-servings size

Double Meringue Butterscotch Pie

There is meringue on the bottom (chunky), butterscotch in the middle (creamy and smooth), and meringue on top (chewy).

1 recipe	Basic Meringue, but use 4 egg whites	1 recipe
1 pkg.	sugar-free butterscotch pudding mix (use the cooked variety, not the instant)	1 pkg.
2 c.	skim milk	500 mL

Prepare the Basic Meringue with four egg whites and smooth two-thirds of the amount onto the inside of a 10 in. (25 cm) pie pan that has been coated with non-stick cooking spray. Shape the meringue into the shape of the pie pan. Save the remaining meringue in the refrigerator. Bake the pie crust in a preheated 250°F (120°C) oven for 1 hour. Turn off the oven but don't open the door; leave the pie crust in the oven to cool. Meanwhile, prepare the pudding according to package directions, using the skim milk. Just before serving, spoon the pudding into the shell. Cover with remaining uncooked meringue. Make sure the meringue topping covers the crust all the way around. Use a spoon to form peaks. Bake in a preheated 350°F (180°C) oven for 10–15 minutes. The topping will be light brown.

Yield: 8 servings

Exchange, 1 serving: ⅔ starch/bread
Each serving contains: Calories: 54, Total fat: 0.1 g, Carbohydrates: 10 g, Protein: 4 g, Sodium: 80 mg, Cholesterol: 1 mg

Meringue Chantilly

1 recipe	Basic Meringue	1 recipe
2 c.	frozen low-fat nondairy whipped topping, thawed	500 mL

Prepare the Basic Meringue. Line two ungreased cookie sheets with parchment paper or cut-up brown paper bags. Spoon the meringue onto the paper to make 12 mounds. Place the two cookie sheets into a preheated 275°F (135°C) oven. Bake for 30 minutes. Open the oven and reverse the positions of the cookie sheets. Bake for another 30 minutes. Remove the cookie sheets from the oven. Loosen and turn each meringue over. Gently depress the center of each one with the back of a spoon. Return to the oven and bake 30 more minutes. Remove from oven and cool meringues completely. Just before serving, make sandwiches with two meringues, placing the whipped topping in between.

Yield: 6 servings

Exchange, 1 serving: 1 starch/bread, ½ fat
Each serving contains: Calories: 94, Total fat: 3 g, Carbohydrates: 14 g, Protein: 2 g, Sodium: 28 mg, Cholesterol: 0 mg

Hawaiian Alaska

There is no ice cream in this pineapple baked Alaska. An advantage is that you make individual servings.

Base

⅓ c. + 1 T.	cold water	95 mL
¼ c. + 2 T.	fat-free butter and oil replacement product	90 mL
2 c.	flour	500 mL

Filling

3 oz.	fat-free cream cheese	80 g
1 large	egg	1 large
1 t.	vanilla extract	5 mL
10 slices	pineapple rings in juice, drained	10 slices

Topping

1 recipe	Basic Meringue	1 recipe

To prepare the base, put all the base ingredients in a mixing bowl. Mix with an electric mixer at low speed until well blended. Shape into a ball and transfer to a floured board. Roll out to ⅛ in. (32 mm) thickness. Cut ten 4 in. (10 cm) circles. Place the circles on cookie sheets that have been coated with non-stick vegetable cooking spray. Prick them all over with a fork. Bake in a preheated 450°F (230°C) oven for 8–10 minutes. Cool on a wire rack. Do not remove from cookie sheets.

Prepare the filling by blending all the filling ingredients except the pineapple rings. Place a pineapple ring on each of the bases. Spoon the filling evenly into the center of each ring. Return the cookie sheets to a preheated 400°F (200°C) oven for just 3 minutes. Quickly cover each cookie with the meringue. Return to the 400°F (200°C) oven and bake 8–10 minutes more. The meringue will be golden brown.

Yield: 10 servings

Exchange, 1 serving: 2 starch/bread
Each serving contains: Calories: 175, Total fat: 1 g, Carbohydrates: 36 g, Protein: 5 g, Sodium: 67 mg, Cholesterol: 23 mg

APPENDICES

Appendix A

USING THE RECIPES

All of the recipes have been developed using granulated fructose and/ or a granulated sugar replacement; diet products for syrups, toppings puddings, and gelatins; and imitation or low-calorie dairy and nondairy) products.

Most of the recipes in this book use a sweetener or sugar replacement that has the same amount of sweetness as regular sugar—be sure to check the packaging of any sweetener you intend to use, to be sure of its measurement properties. If you use a stronger product, use it in proportion to the equivalencies of that product. Remember, don't bake with an aspartame sweetener.

Read the recipes carefully; then assemble all the equipment and ingredients. Use standard measuring equipment (whether metric or customary), and be sure to measure accurately.

Customary Terms

t.	teaspoon	qt.	quart
T.	tablespoon	oz.	ounce
c.	cup	lb.	pound
pkg.	package	°F	degrees Fahrenheit
pt.	pint	in.	inch

Metric Symbols

mL	milliliter	°C	degrees Celsius
L	liter	mm	millimeter
g	gram	cm	centimeter
kg	kilogram		

Appendix B

CONVERSION & MEASUREMENT GUIDES

CUSTOMARY				METRIC	
OUNCES/POUNDS	CUPS	TABLESPOONS	TEASPOONS	GRAMS/KILOGRAMS	MILLILITERS
			¼ t.	1 g	1 mL
			½ t.		2 mL
			1 t.		5 mL
			2 t.		10 mL
½ oz.		1 T.	3 t.	14 g	15 mL
1 oz.		2 T.	6 t.	28 g	30 mL
2 oz.	¼ c.	4 T.	12 t.		60 mL
4 oz.	½ c.	8 T.	24 t.		125 mL
8 oz.	1 c.	16 T.	48 t.		250 mL
2.2 lb.				1 kg	

Keep in mind that this guide doesn't show exact conversions, but it can be used in a general way for food measurement.

CONVERSION GUIDE FOR COOKING PANS AND CASSEROLES

CUSTOMARY	METRIC
1 qt.	1 L
2 qt.	2 L
3 qt.	3 L

CANDY THERMOMETER GUIDE

Use this guide to test for doneness.

FAHRENHEIT °F	TEST		CELSIUS °C
230–234°	Syrup:	Thread	100–112°
234–240°	Fondant/Fudge:	Soft ball	112–115°
244–248°	Caramels:	Firm ball	118–120°
250–266°	Marshmallows:	Hard ball	121–130°
270–290°	Taffy:	Soft crack	132–143°
300–310°	Brittle:	Hard crack	149–154°

OVEN COOKING GUIDES

FAHRENHEIT °F	OVEN HEAT	CELSIUS °C
250–275°	very slow	120–135°
300–325°	slow	150–165°
350–375°	moderate	175–190°
400–425°	hot	200–220°
450–475°	very hot	230–245°
475–500°	hottest	250–290°

GUIDE TO BAKING PAN SIZES

Customary	Metric	Holds	Holds (Metric)
8 in. pie	20 cm pie	2 c.	600 mL
9 in. pie	23 cm pie	1 qt.	1 L
10 in. pie	25 cm pie	1¼ qt.	1.3 L
8 in. round	20 cm round	1 qt.	1 L
9 in. round	23 cm round	1½ qt.	1.5 L
8 in. square	20 cm square	2 qt.	2 L
9 in. square	23 cm square	2½ qt.	2.5 L
9 × 5 × 2 in. loaf	23 × 13 × 5 cm loaf	2 qt.	2 L
9 in. tube	23 cm tube	3 qt.	3 L
10 in. tube	25 cm tube	3 qt.	3 L
10 in. Bundt	25 cm Bundt	3 qt.	3 L
9 × 5 in.	23 × 13 cm	1½ qt.	1.5 L
10 × 6 in.	25 × 16 cm	2 qt.	3.5 L
11 × 7 in.	27 × 17 cm	3½ qt.	3.5 L
13 × 9 X 2 in.	33 × 23 × 5 cm	3½ qt.	3.5 L
14 × 10 in.	36 × 25 cm	cookie tin	
15½ × 10½ x 1 in.	39 × 25 × 3 cm	jelly roll	

Appendix C

EXCHANGE LISTS FOR MEAL PLANNING

You can make a difference in your blood glucose control through your food choices. You do not need special foods. In fact, the foods that are good for you are good for everyone.

If you have diabetes, it is important to eat about the same amount of food at the same time each day. Regardless of what your blood glucose level is, try not to skip meals or snacks. Skipping meals and snacks may lead to large swings in blood glucose levels.

To keep your blood glucose levels near normal, you need to balance the food you eat with the insulin your body makes or gets by injection and with your physical activities. Blood glucose monitoring gives you information to help you with this balancing act. Near-normal blood glucose levels help you feel better. And they may reduce or prevent the complications of diabetes.

The number of calories you need depends on your size, age, and activity level. If you are an adult, eating the right number of calories can help you reach and stay at a reasonable weight. Children and adolescents must eat enough calories so they grow and develop normally. Don't limit their calories to try to control blood glucose levels. Instead, adjust their insulin to cover the calories they need.

Of course, everyone needs to eat nutritious foods. Our good health depends on eating a variety of foods that contain the right amounts of carbohydrate, protein, fat, vitamins, minerals, fiber, and water.

The Exchange Lists are the basis of a meal planning system designed by a committee of the American Diabetes Association and the American Dietetic Association. While designed primarily for people with diabetes and others who must follow special diets, the Exchange Lists are based on principles of good nutrition that apply to everyone. Copyright © 1995 by American Diabetes Association Inc., and the American Diabetic Association.

WHAT ARE CARBOHYDRATE, PROTEIN, AND FAT?

Carbohydrate, protein, and fat are found in the food you eat. They supply you body with energy, or calories. Your body needs insulin to use this energy. Insulin is made in the pancreas. If you have diabetes, either your pancreas is no longer making insulin or your body can't use the insulin it is making. In either case, your blood glucose levels are not normal.

Carbohydrate. Starch and sugar in foods are carbohydrates. Starch is in bread: pasta, cereals, potatoes, peas, beans, and lentils. Naturally present sugars are in fruits, milk, and vegetables. Added sugars are in desserts, candy, jams, and syrups. All of these carbohydrates provide 4 calories per gram and can affect your blood glucose levels.

When you eat carbohydrates, they turn into glucose and travel in your blood stream. Insulin helps the glucose enter the cells, where it can be used for energy or stored. Eating the same amount of carbohydrate daily at meals and snacks help you control your blood glucose levels.

Protein. Protein is in meats, poultry, fish, milk and other dairy products, egg and beans, peas, and lentils. Starches and vegetables also have small amounts of protein.

The body uses protein for growth, maintenance, and energy. Protein has 4 calories of energy per gram. Again, your body needs insulin to use the protein you eat.

Fat. Fat is in margarine, butter, oils, salad dressings, nuts, seeds, milk, cheese, meat, fish, poultry, snack foods, ice cream, and desserts.

There are different types of fat: monounsaturated, polyunsaturated, and saturated. Everyone should eat less of the saturated fats found in meats, dairy products, coconut, palm or palm kernel oil, and hardened shortenings. Saturated fats can raise your blood levels of cholesterol. The fats that are best are the monounsaturated fats found in canola oil, olive oil, nuts, and avocado. The polyunsaturated fats found in corn oil, soybean oil, or sunflower oil are also good choices.

After you eat fat, it travels in your bloodstream. You need insulin to store fat in the cells of your body. Fats are used for energy. In fact, fats have 9 calories per gram, more than two times the calories you get from carbohydrate and protein.

WHAT ELSE DO I NEED TO KNOW?

Vitamins and Minerals. Most foods in the exchange lists are good sources of vitamins and minerals. If you eat a variety of these foods you probably do not need a vitamin or mineral supplement.

Salt or Sodium. High blood pressure may be made worse by eating too much sodium (salt and salty foods). Try to use less salt in cooking and at the table.

Alcohol. You may have an alcoholic drink occasionally. If you take insulin or a diabetes pill, be sure to eat food with your drink. Ask your dietitian about a safe amount of alcohol for you and how to work it into your meal plan.

HOW DO I KNOW WHAT TO EAT AND WHEN?

You and your dietitian will work out a meal plan to get the right balance between your food, medication, and exercise.

The lists of food choices (exchange lists) can help you make interesting and healthy food choices. Exchange lists and a meal plan help you know what to eat, how much to eat, and when to eat.

There are three main groups—the Carbohydrate group, the Meat and Meat Substitute group (protein), and the Fat group. Starch, fruit, milk, other carbohydrates, and vegetables are in the Carbohydrate group. The Meat and Meat Substitute group is divided into very lean, lean, medium-fat, and high-fat foods. You can see at a glance which are the lower-fat choices. Foods in the Fat group—monounsaturated, polyunsaturated, and saturated—have very small serving sizes.

WHAT ARE EXCHANGE LISTS?

Exchange lists are foods listed together because they are alike. Each serving of a food has about the same amount of carbohydrate, protein, fat, and calories as the other foods on that list. That is why any food on a list can be "exchanged," or traded, for any other food on the same list. For example, you can trade the slice of bread you might eat for breakfast for one-half cup of cooked cereal. Each of these foods equals one starch choice.

EXCHANGE LISTS

Foods are listed with their serving sizes, which are usually measured after cooking When you begin, you should measure the size of each serving. This may help you learn to "eyeball" correct serving sizes.

The following chart shows the amount of nutrients in one serving from each list.

GROUPS/LISTS	CARBOHYDRATE (GRAMS)	PROTEIN (GRAMS)	FAT (GRAMS)	CALORIES
Carbohydrate Group				
Starch	15	3	1 or less	80
Fruit	15	—	—	60
Milk				
Skim	12	8	0–3	90
Low-fat	12	8	5	120
Whole	12	8	8	150
Other carbohydrates	15	varies	varies	varies
Vegetables	5	2	—	25
Meat and Meat Substitute Group				
Very lean	—	7	0–1	35
Lean—	7	3	55	
Medium-fat	—	7	5	75
High-fat	—	7	8	100
Fat Group	—	—	5	45

The exchange lists provide you with a lot of food choices (foods from the base food groups, foods with added sugars, free foods, combination foods, and fat foods). This gives you variety in your meals. Several foods, such as beans, peas, an lentils, bacon, and peanut butter, are on two lists. This gives you flexibility in putting your meals together. Whenever you choose new foods or vary your meal plan, monitor your blood glucose to see how these different foods affect your blood glucose level.

Most foods in the Carbohydrate group have about the same amount of carbohydrate per serving. You can exchange starch, fruit, or milk choices in your meal plan. Vegetables are in this group but contain only about 5 grams of carbohydrate.

A WORD ABOUT FOOD LABELS

Exchange information is based on foods found in grocery stores. However, food companies often change the ingredients in their products. That is why you need to check the Nutrition Facts panel of the food label.

The Nutrition Facts tell you the number of calories and grams of carbohydrate protein, and fat in one serving. Compare these numbers with the exchange information to see how many exchanges you will be eating. In this way, food labels can help you add foods to your meal plans.

Ask your dietitian to help you use food label information to plan your meals.

GETTING STARTED!

See your dietitian regularly when you are first learning how to use your meat plan and the exchange lists. Your meal plan can be adjusted to fit changes in your lifestyle, such as work, school, vacation, or travel. Regular nutrition counseling can help you make positive changes in your eating habits.

Careful eating habits will help you feel better and be healthier, too. Best wishes and good eating with *Exchange Lists for Meal Planning*.

STARCH LIST

Cereals, grains, pasta, breads, crackers, snacks, starchy vegetables, and cooked beans, peas, and lentils are starches. In general, one starch is:

½ cup of cereal, grain, pasta, or starchy vegetable,
1 ounce of a bread product, such as 1 slice of bread,

¾ to 1 ounce of most snack foods. (Some snack foods may also have added fat.)

Nutrition Tips

1. Most starch choices are good sources of B vitamins.
2. Foods made from whole grains are good sources of fiber.
3. Beans, peas, and lentils are a good source of protein and fiber.

Selection Tips

1. Choose starches made with little fat as often as you can.
2. Starchy vegetables prepared with fat count as one starch and one fat.
3. Bagels or muffins can be 2, 3, or 4 ounces in size, and can, therefore, count as 2, 3, or 4 starch choices. Check the size you eat.
4. Most of the serving sizes are measured after cooking.
5. Always check Nutrition Facts on the food label.

One starch exchange equals 15 grams carbohydrate, 3 grams protein, 0–1 grams fat, and 80 calories.

Bread

Bagel	½ (1 oz.)
Bread, reduced-calorie	2 slices (1½ oz.)
Bread, white, whole wheat, pumpernickel, rye	1 slice (1 oz.)
Bread sticks, crisp, 4 in. long × ½ in.	2 (⅔ oz.)
English muffin	½
Hot dog or hamburger bun	½ (1 oz.)
Pita, 6 in. across	½
Raisin bread, unfrosted	1 slice (1 oz.)
Roll, plain, small	1 (1 oz.)
Tortilla, corn, 6 in. across	1
Tortilla, flour, 7–8 in. across	1
Waffle, 4½ in. square, reduced fat	1

Cereals and Grains

Bran cereals	½ cup
Bulgur	½ cup
Cereals	½ cup
Cereals, unsweetened, ready-to-eat	¾ cup
Cornmeal (dry)	3 Tbsp.
Couscous	⅓ cup
Flour (dry)	3 Tbsp.
Granola, lowfat	¼ cup
Grape-Nuts®	¼ cup
Grits	½ cup
Kasha	½ cup
Millet	¼ cup
Muesli	¼ cup
Oats	½ cup
Pasta	½ cup
Puffed cereal	1½ cups
Rice milk	½ cup
Rice, white or brown	⅓ cup
Shredded Wheat®	½ cup
Sugar-frosted cereal	½ cup
Wheat germ	3 Tbsp.

Starchy Vegetables

Baked beans	⅓ cup
Corn	½ cup
Corn on cob, medium	1 (5 oz.)
Mixed vegetables with corn, peas, or pasta	1 cup
Peas, green	½ cup
Plantain	½ cup
Potato, baked or boiled	1 small
Potato, mashed	½ cup
Squash, winter (acorn, butternut)	1 cup
Yam, sweet potato, plain	½ cup

Crackers and Snacks

Animal crackers	8
Graham crackers, 2½ in. square	3
Matzoh	¾ oz.
Melba toast	4 slices
Oyster crackers	24
Popcorn (popped, no fat added or lowfat microwave)	3 cups
Pretzels	¾ oz.
Rice cakes, 4 in. across	2
Saltine-type crackers	6
Snack chips, fat-free (tortilla, potato)	15–20 (¾ oz.)
Whole wheat crackers, no fat added	2–5 (¾ oz.)

Beans, Peas, and Lentils

(Count as 1 starch exchange, plus 1 very lean meat exchange.)

Beans and peas (garbanzo, pinto, kidney, white, split, black-eyed)	½ cup
Lima beans	⅔ cup
Lentils	½ cup
Miso	3 Tbsp.

Starchy Foods Prepared with Fat

(Count as 1 starch exchange, plus 1 fat exchange.)

Biscuit, 2½ in. across	1
Chow mein noodles	½ cup
Corn bread, 2 in. cube	1 (2 oz.)
Crackers, round butter type	6
Croutons	1 cup
French-fried potatoes	16–25 (3 oz.)
Granola	¼ cup
Muffin, small	(1½ oz.)
Pancake, 4 in. across	2
Popcorn, microwave	3 cups
Sandwich crackers, cheese or peanut butter filling	3
Stuffing, bread (prepared)	⅓ cup
Taco shell,	6 in. across
Waffle, 4½ in. square	1
Whole wheat fat added	4–6 (1 oz.)

Starches often swell in cooking, so a small amount of uncooked starch will become a much larger amount of cooked food. The following table shows some of the changes.

Food (Starch Group)

	Uncooked	Cooked
Oatmeal	3 Tbsp.	½ cup
Cream of wheat	2 Tbsp.	½ cup
Grits	3 Tbsp.	½ cup
Rice	2 Tbsp.	⅓ cup
Spaghetti	¼ cup	½ cup
Noodles	⅓ cup	½ cup
Macaroni	¼ cup	½ cup
Dried beans	¼ cup	½ cup
Dried peas	¼ cup	½ cup
Lentils	3 Tbsp.	½ cup

FRUIT LIST

Fresh, frozen, canned, and dried fruits and fruit juices are on this list. In general, one fruit exchange is:

1 small to medium fresh fruit,
½ cup of canned or fresh fruit or fruit juice
¼ cup of dried fruit

Nutrition Tips

1. Fresh, frozen, and dried fruits have about 2 grams of fiber per choice. Fruit juices contain very little fiber.
2. Citrus fruits, berries, and melons are good sources of vitamin C.

Selection Tips

1. Count ½ cup cranberries or rhubarb sweetened with sugar substitutes as free foods.
2. Read the Nutrition Facts on the food label. If one serving has more than 15 grams of carbohydrate, you will need to adjust the size of the serving you eat or drink.
3. Portion sizes for canned fruits are for the fruit and a small amount of juice.
4. Whole fruit is more filling than fruit juice and may be a better choice.
5. Food labels for fruits may contain the words "no sugar added" or "unsweetened." This means that no sucrose (table sugar) has been added.
6. Generally, fruit canned in extra light syrup has the same amount of carbohydrate per serving as the "no sugar added" or the juice pack. All canned fruits on the fruit list are based on one of these three types of pack.

One fruit exchange equals 15 grams carbohydrate and 60 calories. The weight includes skin, core, seeds, and rind.

Fruit

Apple, unpeeled, small fruit	1 (4 oz.)
Applesauce, unsweetened	1 (4 oz.) cup
Apples, dried	4 rings
Apricots, fresh	4 whole (5½ oz.)
Apricots, canned	½ cup
Banana, small	1 (4 oz.)
Blackberries	¾ cup
Blueberries	¾ cup
Cantaloupe, small (11 oz.) or 1 cup cubes	⅓ melon
Cherries, sweet, fresh	12 (3 oz.)
Cherries, sweet, canned	½ cup
Dates	3
Figs, fresh or 2 medium (3½ oz.)	1½ large
Figs, dried	1½
Fruit Cocktail	½ cup
Grapefruit, large	½ (11 oz.)
Grapefruit sections, canned	¾ cup
Grapes, small	17 (3 oz.)
Honeydew melon (10 oz.) or 1 cup cubes	1 slice
Kiwi	1 (3½ oz.)
Mandarin oranges, canned	¾ cup
Mango, small (5 ½ oz.) or ½ cup	½ fruit
Nectarine, small	1 (5 oz.)
Orange, small	1 (6½ oz.)
Papaya (8 oz.) or 1 cup cubes	½
Peach, medium, fresh	1 (6 oz.)
Peaches, canned	½ cup
Pear, large, fresh	½ (4 oz.)
Pineapple, fresh	¾ cup
Pineapple, canned	½ cup
Plums, small	2 (5 oz.)
Plums, canned	½ cup
Prunes, dried	3
Raisins	2 Tbsp.
Raspberries	1 cup
Strawberries	1¼ cup whole berries
Tangerines, small	2 (8 oz.)
Watermelon (13½ oz.) or 1¼ cup cubes	1 slice

Fruit Juice

Apple juice/cider	½ cup
Cranberry juice cocktail	⅓ cup
Cranberry juice cocktail, reduced-calorie	1 cup
Fruit juice blends, 100% juice	⅓ cup

Grape juice	⅓ cup
Grapefruit juice	½ cup
Orange juice	½ cup
Pineapple juice	½ cup
Prune juice	⅓ cup

MILK LIST

Different types of milk and milk products are on this list. Cheeses are on the Meat list and cream and other dairy fats are on the Fat list. Based on the amount of fat they contain, milks are divided into skim/very lowfat milk, lowfat milk, and whole milk. One choice of these includes:

	CARBOHYDRATE (GRAMS)	PROTEIN (GRAMS)	FAT (GRAMS)	CALORIES
Skim/very low-fat	12	8	0–3	90
Low-fat	12	8	5	120
Whole	12	8	8	150

Nutrition Tips

1. Milk and yogurt are good sources of calcium and protein. Check the food label.
2. The higher the fat content of milk and yogurt, the greater the amount of saturated fat and cholesterol. Choose lower-fat varieties.
3. For those who are lactose intolerant, look for lactose-reduced or lactose-free varieties of milk.

Selection Tips

1. One cup equals 8 fluid ounces or ½ pint.
2. Look for chocolate milk, frozen yogurt, and ice cream on the Other Carbohydrates list.
3. Nondairy creamers are on the Free Foods list.
4. Look for rice milk on the Starch list.

One milk exchange equals 12 grams carbohydrate and 8 grams protein.

Skim and Very Low-fat Milk

(0–3 grams fat per serving)

Skim milk	1 cup
½% milk	1 cup
1% milk	1 cup
Nonfat or low-fat buttermilk	1 cup
Evaporated skim milk	½ cup
Nonfat dry milk	⅓ cup dry
Plain nonfat yogurt	¾ cup
Nonfat or low-fat fruit-flavored yogurt sweetened with aspartame or with a non-nutritive sweetener	1 cup

Low-fat

(5 grams fat per serving)

2% milk	1 cup
Plain low-fat yogurt	¾ cup
Sweet acidophilus milk	1 cup

Whole Milk

(8 grams fat per serving)

Whole milk	1 cup
Evaporated whole milk	½ cup
Goat's milk	1 cup
Kefir	1 cup

VEGETABLE LIST

Vegetables that contain small amounts of carbohydrates and calories are on this list. Vegetables contain important nutrients. Try to eat at least 2 or 3 vegetable choices each day. In general, one vegetable exchange is:

½ cup of cooked vegetables or vegetable juice,
1 cup of raw vegetables

If you eat 1 to 2 vegetable choices at a meal or snack, you do not have to count the calories or carbohydrates because they contain small amounts of these nutrients.

Nutrition Tips

1. Fresh and frozen vegetables have less added salt than canned vegetables. Drain and rinse canned vegetables if you want to remove some salt.
2. Choose more dark green and dark yellow vegetables, such as spinach, broccoli, romaine, carrots, chilies, and peppers.
3. Broccoli, brussels sprouts, cauliflower, greens, peppers, spinach, and tomato, are good sources of vitamin C.
4. Vegetables contain 1 to 4 grams of fiber per serving.

Selection Tips

1. A one cup portion of broccoli is a portion about the size of a light bulb.
2. Canned vegetables and juices are available without added salt.
3. If you eat more than 3 cups of raw vegetables or 1½ cups of cooked vegetables, at one meal, count them as 1 carbohydrate choice.
4. Starchy vegetables such as corn, peas, winter squash, and potatoes that contain larger amounts of calories and carbohydrates are on the Starch list.

One vegetable exchange equals 5 grams carbohydrate, 2 grams protein, 0 grams fat, and 25 calories.

Artichoke
Artichoke hearts
Asparagus
Beans (green, wax, Italian)
Bean sprouts
Beets
Broccoli
Brussels sprouts
Cabbage
Carrots
Cauliflower
Celery
Cucumber
Eggplant
Green onions or scallions
Greens (collard, kale, mustard, turnip)
Kohlrabi
Leeks
Mixed vegetables (without corn, peas, or pasta)
Mushrooms
Okra
Onions
Pea pods
Peppers (all varieties)
Radishes
Salad greens (endive, escarole, lettuce, romaine, spinach)
Sauerkraut
Spinach
Summer squash
Tomato
Tomatoes, canned
Tomato sauce
Tomato/vegetable juice
Turnips
Water chestnuts
Watercress
Zucchini

MEAT AND MEAT SUBSTITUTES LIST

Meat and meat substitutes that contain both protein and fat are on this list. In general, one meat exchange is:

1 ounce meat, fish, poultry, or cheese,
½ cup beans, peas, and lentils

Based on the amount of fat they contain, meats are divided into very lean, lean, medium-fat, and high-fat lists. This is done so you can see which ones contain the least amount of fat. One ounce (one exchange) of each of these includes:

	CARBOHYDRATE (GRAMS)	PROTEIN (GRAMS)	FAT (GRAMS)	CALORIES
Very lean	0	7	0–1	35
Lean	0	7	3	55
Medium-fat	0	7	5	75
High-fat	0	7	8	100

Nutrition Tips

1. Choose very lean and lean meat choices whenever possible. Items from the high-fat group are high in saturated fat, cholesterol, and calories and can raise blood cholesterol levels.
2. Meats do not have any fiber.
3. Some processed meats, seafood, and soy products may contain carbohydrate when consumed in large amounts. Check the Nutrition Facts on the label to see if the amount is close to 15 grams. If so, count it as a carbohydrate choice as well as a meat choice.

Selection Tips

1. Weigh meat after cooking and removing bones and fat. Four ounces of raw meat is equal to 3 ounces of cooked meat. Some examples of meat portions are:
   1 ounce cheese = 1 meat choice and is about the size of a one-inch cube
   2 ounces meat = 2 meat choices, such as 1 small chicken leg or thigh or ½ cup cottage cheese or tuna
   3 ounces meat = 3 meat choices and is about the size of a deck of cards, such as 1 medium pork chop, 1 small hamburger, ½ of a whole chicken breast, or 1 unbreaded fish fillet.
2. Limit your choices from the high-fat group to three times per week or less.
3. Most grocery stores stock Select and Choice grades of meat. Select grades of meat are the leanest meats. Choice grades contain a moderate amount of fat, and Prime cuts of meat have the highest amount of fat. Restaurants usually serve Prime cuts of meat.
4. "Hamburger" may contain added seasoning and fat, but ground beef does not.
5. Read labels to find products that are low in fat and cholesterol (5 grams or less of fat per serving).
6. Peanut butter, in smaller amounts, is also found on the Fats list.
7. Bacon, in smaller amounts, is also found on the Fats list.

Meal Planning Tips

1. Bake, roast, broil, grill, poach, steam, or boil these foods rather than frying.
2. Place meat on a rack so the fat will drain off during cooking.
3. Use a nonstick spray and a nonstick pan to brown or fry foods.

4. Trim off visible fat before or after cooking.

5. If you add flour, bread crumbs, coating mixes, fat, or marinades when cooking, ask your dietitian how to count it in your meat plan.

Lean Meat and Substitutes List

One exchange equals 0 grams carbohydrate, 7 grams protein, 3 grams fat, and 55 calories.

One lean meat exchange is equal to any one of the following items.

Beef

USDA Select or Choice grades of lean beef trimmed of fat, such as round, sirloin, and flank steak; tenderloin; roast (rib, chuck, rump); steak (T-bone, porterhouse, cubed); ground round — 1 oz.

Pork

Lean pork, such as fresh ham; canned, cured, or boiled ham; Canadian bacon tenderloin, center loin chop — 1 oz.

Lamb

Roast, chop, leg 1 oz.

Veal

Lean chop, roast 1 oz.

Poultry

Chicken, turkey (dark meat, no skin), chicken (white meat, with skin), domestic duck or goose (well-drained of fat, no skin) — 1 oz.

Game: Goose (no skin), rabbit — 1 oz.

Fish

Herring (uncreamed or smoked)	1 oz.
Oysters	6 med
Salmon (fresh or canned), catfish	1 oz.
Sardines (canned) 2 medium	
Tuna (canned in oil, drained)	1 oz.

Cheese

4.5% fat cottage cheese	¼ cup
Grated Parmesan	2 Tbsp.
Cheeses with 3 grams or less fat per ounce	1 oz.

Other

Hot dogs with 3 grams or less fat per ounce	1½ oz.
Processed sandwich meat with 3 grams or less fat per ounce, such as turkey, pastrami, or kielbasa	1 oz.
Liver, heart (high in cholesterol)	1 oz.

High-Fat Meat and Substitutes List

One exchange equals 0 grams carbohydrate, 7 grams protein, 8 grams fat, and 100 calories.

Remember that these items are high in saturated fat, cholesterol, and calories and may raise blood cholesterol levels if eaten on a regular basis. One high-fat meat exchange is equal to any one of the following items.

Beef

Most USDA Prime cuts of beef such as ribs, corned beef — 1 oz.

Pork

Spareribs, gound pork, pork sausage (patty or link) — 1oz.

Lamb

Patties (ground lamb)	1 oz.

Fish

Any fried fish product	1 oz.

Cheese

All regular cheeses such as American, Blue, Cheddar Monterey Jack, Swiss	1 oz.

Other

Luncheon meat such as bologna salami, pimento loaf,	1 oz.
Sausage such as Polish, Italian smoked	1 oz.
Knockwurst, Bratwurst	1 oz.
Franfurter (turkey or chicken)	1 oz. (10/lb.)
Peanut butter (contains unsaturated fat).	1 Tbsp

FAT LIST

Fats are divided into three groups, based on the main type of fat they contain: monounsaturated, polyunsaturated, and saturated. Small amounts of monounsaturated and polyunsaturated fats in the foods we eat are linked with good health benefits. Saturated fats are linked with heart disease and cancer. In general, one fat exchange is:

1 teaspoon of regular margarine or vegetable oil,
1 tablespoon of regular salad dressings

Nutrition Tips

1. All fats are high in calories. Limit serving sizes for good nutrition and health.
2. Nuts and seeds contain small amounts of fiber, protein, and magnesium.
3. If blood pressure is a concern, choose fats in the unsalted form to help lower sodium intake, such as unsalted peanuts.

Selection Tips

1. Check the Nutrition Facts on food labels for serving sizes. One fat exchange is based on a serving size containing 5 grams of fat.
2. When selecting regular margarines, choose those with liquid vegetable oil as the first ingredient. Soft margarines are not as saturated as stick margarines. Soft margarines are healthier choices. Avoid those listing hydrogenated or partially hydrogenated fat as the first ingredient.
3. When selecting lowfat margarines, look for liquid vegetable oil as the second ingredient. Water is usually the first ingredient.
4. When used in smaller amounts, bacon and peanut butter are counted as fat choices. When used in larger amounts, they are counted as high-fat meat choices.
5. Fat-free salad dressings are on the Free Foods list.
6. See the Free Foods list for nondairy coffee creamers, whipped topping, and fat-free products, such as margarines, salad dressings, mayonnaise, sour cream, cream cheese, and nonstick cooking spray.

Monounsaturated Fats List

One fat exchange equals
5 grams fat and 45 calories.

Avocado, medium	⅛ (1 oz.)
Oil (canola, olive, peanut)	1 tsp
Olives: ripe (black)	8 large
green, stuffed	10 large
Nuts	
almonds, cashews	6 nuts
mixed (50% peanuts)	6 nuts
peanuts	10 nuts
pecans	4 halves
peanut butter, smooth or crunchy	2 tsp.
Sesame seeds	1 Tbsp.
Tahini paste	2 tsp.

Polyunsaturated Fats List

One fat exchange equals
5 grams fat and 45 calories.

Margarine: stick, tub, or squeeze lower-fat	1 tsp.
(30% to 50% vegetable oil)	1 Tbsp.
Mayonnaise: regular	1 tsp.
reduced-fat	1 Tbsp.
Nuts, walnuts, English	4 halves
Oil (corn, safflower, soybean)	1 tsp.
Salad dressing: regular	1 Tbsp.
reduced-fat	2 Tbsp.
Miracle Whip Salad Dressing®:	
regular	2 tsp.
reduced-fat	1 Tbsp.
Seeds: pumpkin, sunflower	1 Tbsp.

Saturated Fats List★

One fat exchange equals 5 grams fat and 45 calories.

Bacon, cooked	1 slice
Bacon, grease	1 tsp.
Butter: stick	1 tsp.
whipped	2 tsp.
reduced-fat	1 Tbsp.
Chitterlings, boiled	2 Tbsp.
Coconut, sweetened, shredded	2 Tbsp.
Cream, half and half	2 Tbsp.
Cream cheese: regular	1 Tbsp. (½ oz.)
reduced-fat	2 Tbsp. (1 oz.)
Fatback or salt pork, see below	
Shortening or lard	1 tsp
Sour cream: regular	2 Tbsp
reduced-fat	3 Tbsp

Use a piece 1 in. × 1 in. × ¼ in. if you plan to eat the fatback cooked with vegetables. Use a piece 2 in. × 1 in. × ½ in. when eating only the vegetables with the fatback removed.

*Saturated fats can raise blood cholesterol levels.

FREE FOODS LIST

A free food is any food or drink that contains less than 20 calories or less than 5 grams of carbohydrate per serving.

Foods with a serving size listed should be limited to three servings per day. Be sure to spread them out throughout the day. If you eat all three servings at one time, it could affect your blood glucose level. Foods listed without a serving size may be eaten as often as you like.

Fat-free or Reduced-fat Foods

Cream cheese, fat-free	1 Tbsp.
Creamers, nondairy, liquid	1 Tbsp.
Creamers, nondairy, powdered	2 tsp.
Mayonnaise, fat-free	1 Tbsp.
Mayonnaise, reduced-fat	1 tsp.
Margarine, fat-free	4 Tbsp.
Margarine, reduced-fat	1 tsp.
Miracle Whip®, nonfat	1 Tbsp.
Miracle Whip®, reduced-fat	1 tsp.
Nonstick cooking spray	
Salad dressing, fat-free	1 Tbsp.
Salad dressing, fat-free, Italian	2 Tbsp.
Salsa	¼ cup
Catsup	
Sour cream, fat-free, educed-fat	1 Tbsp.
Whipped topping, regular r light	2 Tbsp.

Sugar-free or Low-sugar Foods

Candy, hard, sugar-free	1 candy
Gelatin dessert, sugar-free	
Gelatin, unflavored	
Gum, sugar-free	
Jam or jelly, low-sugar or light	2 tsp.
Sugar substitutes	
Syrup, sugar-free	2 Tbsp.

Sugar substitutes, alternatives, or replacements that are approved by the Food and Drug Administration (FDA) are safe to use. Common brand names include: Equal® (aspartame), Sprinkle Sweet® (saccharin), Sweet One® (acesulfame-K), Sweet-10® (saccharin), Sugar Twin®, (saccharin), Sweet 'n Low® (saccharin)

Drinks

Bouillon, broth, consommé
Bouillon or broth, low-sodium

Carbonated or mineral water
Club soda
Cocoa powder, unsweetened   1 Tbsp.
Coffee
Diet soft drinks, sugar-free
Drink mixes, sugar-free
Tea
Tonic water, sugar-free

Condiments

Horseradish
Lemon juice
Lime juice
Mustard
Pickles, dill   ½ large
Soy sauce, regular or light

Taco sauce   1 Tbsp.
Vinegar
Seasonings

Be careful with seasonings that contain sodium or are salts, such as garlic or celery salt, and lemon pepper.

Flavoring extracts
Garlic
Herbs, fresh or dried
Pimento
Spices
Tabasco® or hot pepper sauce
Wine, used in cooking
Worcestershire sauce

APPENDIX D

SPICES AND HERBS

Allspice: Cinnamon, ginger, nutmeg flavor; used in breads, pastries, jellies, jams, pickles.

Anise: Licorice flavor; used in candies, breads, fruit, wine, liqueurs.

Basil: Sweet-strong flavor; used in meat, cheese, egg, tomato dishes.

Bay Leaf: Sweet flavor; used in meat, fish, vegetable dishes.

Celery: Unique, pleasantly bitter flavor; used in anything not sweet.

Chive: Light onion flavor; used in anything where onion should be delicate.

Chili Powder: Hot, pungent flavor; used in Mexican, Spanish dishes.

Cinnamon: Pungent, sweet flavor; used in pastries, breads, pickles, wine, beer, liqueurs.

Clove: Pungent, sweet flavor; used for ham, sauces, pastries, puddings, fruit, wine, liqueurs.

Coriander: Butter-lemon flavor; used for pork, cookies, cakes, pies, puddings, fruit, wine and liqueur punches.

Garlic: Strong, aromatic flavor; used in Italian, French, and many meat dishes.

Ginger: Strong, pungent flavor; used in anything sweet, plus with beer, brandy, liqueurs.

Marjoram: Sweet, semi-pungent flavor; used in poultry, lamb, egg, vegetable dishes.

Nutmeg: Sweet, nutty flavor; used in pastries, puddings, vegetables.

Oregano: Sweet, pungent flavor; used in meat, pasta, vegetable dishes.

Paprika: Light, sweet flavor; used in salads, vegetables, poultry, fish, egg dishes; often used to brighten bland-colored casseroles or entrees.

Rosemary: Fresh, sweet flavor; used in soups, meat and vegetable dishes.

Sage: Pungent, bitter flavor; used in stuffings, sausages, some cheese dishes.

Thyme: Pungent, semi-bitter flavor; used in salty dishes or soups.
Woodruff: Sweet vanilla flavor; used in wines, punches.

NOTE: Metric equivalents for the stronger spices and herbs vary for each recipe to allow for individual effectiveness at convenient measurements.

APPENDIX E

FLAVORINGS AND EXTRACTS

Orange, lime, and lemon peels give vegetables, pastries and puddings a fresh, clean flavor; liquor flavors, such as brandy or rum, give cakes and other desserts flair. Choose from the following to add some zip without calories:

Almond	Black Walnut	Butternut	Pecan
Anise (Licorice)	Blueberry	Butter Rum	Peppermint
Apricot	Brandy	Cherry	Pineapple
Banana Crème	Burnt Sugar	Clove	Raspberry
Blackberry	Butter	Coconut	Rum
		Grape	Sassafras
		Hazelnut	Sherry
		Lemon	Strawberry
		Lime	Vanilla
		Mint	Walnut
		Orange	

APPENDIX F

SUGAR AND SUGAR REPLACEMENTS

Your diet has been prescribed by a doctor or diet counselor who has been trained to determine your diet requirements by considering your daily lifestyle of exercise and calorie needs. Do not try to outguess them. Always stay within the guidelines of your individual diet and ask your counselor about additions or substitutions in your diet. If you have any questions about any diabetic recipes or exchanges, ask your diet counselor.

There have been reports stating that diabetics could eat table sugar, such as sugars made from cane or beets. The research found that refined sugar did not get into the blood any more quickly than does sugar from wheat flour or potatoes. These reports contend that because all these products are starches, they could be eaten at mealtime. Because diabetics MUST keep the numbers of calories constant in their diets, they are usually told to avoid products containing sugar.

Sugar has approximately 770 calories per cup with 199 grams of carbohydrates; refined wheat flour has approximately 420 calories per cup with 88 grams of carbohydrates and the remaining calories are made up from the 12 grams of protein. Therefore, you would have to eat 2.26 times the amount of wheat flour to gain the same amount of grams of carbohydrates from one cup of sugar. By using one of the sugar replacements or new natural sweeteners on the market, you cut out most of the carbohydrates and calories normally gained when using a cane or beet sugar.

Now, let's put this fact into a food product. Say we make a basic chocolate cake with sugar and the very same chocolate cake with one of the sugar replacements, and this cake takes one cup of sugar. In the total cake with the sugar replacement, we have reduced the calories by approximately 770. That is a lot of calories and adds up to a lot of exchange values. If we sweeten a single cup of coffee or tea with two teaspoons of sugar, we add 30 calories (¼ fruit exchange), but if we sweeten it with an aspartame product we gain only four calories and with a sugar substitute we gain approximately two to three calories. Now those are major differences in calorie counts.

Most sweeteners or sugar replacements can be found in your supermarket. They vary in sweetness, aftertaste, aroma and calories. The listing below is by ingredient name rather than product name. Check the side of the box or bottle to determine the contents of the product.

Aspartame and aspartame products are fairly new to the supermarket. Aspartame is a natural protein sweetener; it is not an artificial sweetener. Because of its intense sweetness, it reduces calories and carbohydrates in the diet. Aspartame has no aftertaste and a sweet aroma but loses part of its sweetness in heating. It does seem to complement some of the other sweeteners by removing their bitter aftertaste, however. Aspartame is recommended for use in cold products.

Cyclamates and products containing cyclamates are less intense as sweeteners than the saccharin products; but they also leave a bitter aftertaste. Many of our sugar replacements are a combination of saccharin and cyclamates.

Fructose or levulose is commonly known as fruit sugar. It is a naturally occurring sugar found in fruits and honey. The taste of fruit sugar (fructose) is the same as that of common table sugar (sucrose). But because of its intense sweetness, you use less fructose and thus reduce calories and carbohydrates in the diet. Fructose is not affected by heating or cooling and tends to add moisture to baked products.

Glycyrrhizin and products containing glycyrrhizin are sweeteners as intense as saccharin. They are seen less in supermarkets, because they give the food products a licorice taste and aroma.

Granular or dry sugar replacements containing sodium saccharin give less aftertaste to foods that are heated.

Liquid sugar replacements containing sodium saccharin are best used in cold foods or added to the food after it has partially cooled and no longer needs any heating.

Saccharin and products containing saccharin are the most widely known and used of the intense sweeteners. When used in baking or cooking, saccharin has a bitter, lingering aftertaste. You will normally find it in the form of sodium saccharin in products labelled low-calorie sugar replacements. These include liquid and granulated brown sugar replacements used in this book.

Sorbitol is used in many of our commercial food products. It has little or no aftertaste and has a sweet aroma. At present, it can only be bought in bulk form at health food stores.

APPENDIX G

CHOCOLATE PRODUCTS, CAROB, AND IMITATION CHOCOLATE

Baking cocoa is unsweetened chocolate with some of the cocoa butter removed and then powdered.

Baking or unsweetened chocolate is a pure chocolate which is molded into blocks. It is the most commonly used chocolate in baking and cooking.

Carob is not a chocolate product. People with chocolate allergies, however, can use carob and still get the chocolate flavor. Many people prefer the carob flavor to chocolate; others notice a distinct difference between the two flavors. Although many people think there is a wide calorie count difference between carob and chocolate products, one tablespoon of carob has the same calorie count as one tablespoon of cocoa. And in most carob candy products, the calorie count will equal that of a comparable chocolate product because of the addition of extra fat. Therefore, if you have an allergy to chocolate, you may use equal amounts of a carob product for any chocolate product in the recipes in this book.

Dietetic dipping or coating chocolate is a special chocolate or chocolate-flavored product formulated to reduce calories in a candy product. For this reason it is the only dipping chocolate used in this book.

German chocolate is semisweet chocolate with extra sugar added. I have not used German chocolate in this book but, rather, have added extra reduced calorie sweeteners to baking chocolate or semisweet chocolate to give the same flavor as German chocolate.

Milk chocolate is a sweet chocolate with milk added and is the chocolate used in most candy bars.

Semisweet chocolate is baking chocolate with extra cocoa butter and flavorings. We commonly use chips or bits of this type of chocolate. Chocolate sprinkles, jimmies, shot, or mounties are all considered chips or bits.

White chocolate, confectionery coating, dietetic white dipping or coating chocolate are imitation chocolates in which all or most of the cocoa butter has been replaced with another vegetable fat. It can be bought colored or can be colored and flavored at home with colored food oils.

SELECTED BIBLIOGRAPHY

American Diabetes Association. "American Diabetes Association Issues Statement on Aspartame in Diet Soft Drinks and Foods." News from American Diabetes Association, Inc. (Oct., 1983).

Chase, H. Peter. "Diabetes and Diet." *Food Technology* (Dec., 1979).

Crapo, Phyllis A. and Jerrold M. Olefsky. "Food Fallacies and Blood Sugar." *The New England Journal of Medicine* (July 7, 1983).

Crapo, Phyllis A. and Jerrold M. Olefsky, "Fructose—Its Characteristics, Physiology, and Metabolism." *Nutrition Today* (July–Aug., 1980).

Crapo, Phyllis A. and Margaret A. Powers. "Alias: Sugar." *Diabetes Forecast* (1981).

Diabetes Dateline. "FDA Approves Aspartame as Low-Calorie Sweetener." Department of Health and Human Services (July–Aug., 1981).

Dwivedi, Basant K. ed. Low-Calorie and Special Dietary Foods. The Chemical Rubber Co. (1978): 61–73.

Franz, Marion. "Is Aspartame Safe?" *Diabetes Forecast* (May–June, 1984).

Kimura, K.K. "Dietary Sugars in Health and Disease." Life Sciences Research Office (Oct., 1976).

Koivisto, Veikko A. "Fructose as a Dietary Sweetener in Diabetes Mellitus." *Diabetes Care,* Vol. 1, No. 4 (July–Aug., 1978).

Olefsky, Jerrold and Phyllis Crapo. "Fructose, Xylitol, and Sorbitol." *Diabetes Care,* Vol. 3, No. 2 (March–April, 1980).

Tolbot, John M. and Kenneth D. Fisher. "The Need for Special Foods and Sugar Substitutes by Individuals with Diabetes Mellitus." *Diabetes Care,* Vol. 1, No. 4 (July–Aug., 1978).

Public Health Service Food and Drug Administration. Department of Health and Human Services. "Aspartame: Commissioner's Final Decision." Part IV, *Federal Register,* Vol. 46, No. 142 (July 24, 1981): 38283–38308.

Index